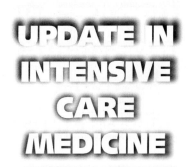

UPDATE IN INTENSIVE CARE MEDICINE

Series Editor: Jean-Louis Vincent

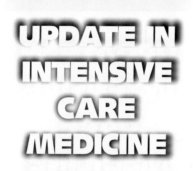

UPDATE IN INTENSIVE CARE MEDICINE

Springer
New York
Berlin
Heidelberg
Barcelona
Hong Kong
London
Milan
Paris
Tokyo

FROM NUTRITION SUPPORT TO PHARMACOLOGIC NUTRITION IN THE ICU

Volume Editors:

Claude Pichard, MD, PhD
Head of Clinical Nutrition
University Hospital
Geneva, Switzerland

Kenneth A. Kudsk, MD
Professor of Surgery
Department of Surgery
University of Wisconsin–Madison
Madison, Wisconsin, USA

Series Editor:

Jean-Louis Vincent, MD, PhD, FCCM, FCCP
Head, Department of Intensive Care
Erasme University Hospital
Brussels, Belgium

With 72 Figures and 79 Tables

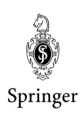

Springer

Claude Pichard, MD, PhD
Head of Clinical Nutrition
University Hospital
1211 Geneva 14
Switzerland

Kenneth A. Kudsk, MD
Professor of Surgery
Department of Surgery
University of Wisconsin–Madison
Madison, WI 53706
USA

Series Editor:
Jean-Louis Vincent, MD, PhD, FCCM, FCCP
Head, Department of Intensive Care
Erasme University Hospital
Route de Lennik 808
B-1070 Brussels
Belgium

Library of Congress Cataloging-in-Publication Data applied for

Printed on acid-free paper.

Production managed by PRO EDIT GmbH, Heidelberg, Germany.
Typeset by TBS, Sandhausen, Germany.
Printed and bound by Mercedes-Druck, Berlin, Germany.
Printed in Germany.

9 8 7 6 5 4 3 2 1

ISSN 0933-6788
ISBN 3-540-42604-3   SPIN 10851542

Springer-Verlag   New York Berlin Heidelberg
A member of BertelsmannSpringer Science+Business Media GmbH

Preface

This book has been written to help clinicians optimize their competence and understanding in managing critically ill patients with nutrition support. In each chapter, descriptions of practical applications of nutrition support are preceded by a brief yet comprehensive review of basic information, making it useful for medical students and non-medical care providers as well as clinicians on the front line of ICU medicine. While successful delivery of macronutrients, such as protein, carbohydrate, and fat, remain the key components of any nutritional strategy, this text reviews many other subtle aspects of care which are important in preserving lean body mass and the metabolic and immunologic functions of patients undergoing metabolic stress. Discussions are designed to be "state of the art," covering older issues, such as nutritional assessment, as well as new aspects of nutrition support such as modulation of the inflammatory response and host defense barriers through specific macro- and micronutrients. While clinical studies of outcome are emphasized throughout the text, authors also share new research suggesting that some molecules, such as lactate, are more than just end products of a metabolic cycle but serve as potent compounds which regulate metabolic pathways necessary for optimal nutritional management of critically ill patients. Finally, hormone therapy and receptor agonist therapy are evaluated as synergistic therapies to improve the efficacy of nutrition support.

Today, an integrated, global appreciation of the interaction between nutrition and metabolic response is essential to provide nutritional and metabolic support in an era of evidenced-based medicine and cost efficiency. This book details practical modalities useful in safe and inexpensive delivery of nutritional care which is capable of significantly improving clinical outcome. We hope you find this book both informative and useful.

Geneva, Switzerland   *Claude Pichard, MD, PhD*
Madison, Wisconsin, USA   *Kenneth A. Kudsk, MD*

Contents

List of Contributors

S.P. Allison
Department of Diabetes,
Endocrinology and Nutrition
Queen's Medical Center
Nottingham
UK

J. Alverdy
Department of Surgery
University of Chicago
Chicago, Illinois
USA

F.J. Andrews
Department of Medicine
University of Liverpool
Liverpool
UK

S. Antoun
Institut Gustave-Roussy
Villejuif
France

D. Barnoud
Département de Médecine Aiguë
Spécialisée
Unités de Réanimation
Médicale et de Nutrition Parentérale
CHU de Grenoble
Grenoble
France

M.M. Berger
Soins Intensifs de Chirurgie
CHUV
Lausanne
Switzerland

B.R. Bistrian
Department of Clinical Nutrition
Beth Israel Deaconess Medical Center
Harvard Medical School
Boston, Massachusetts
USA

M. Borhani
Department of Surgery
Washington University
St. Louis, Missouri
USA

A.P. Borzotta
Trauma Service
Bethesda North Hospital
and
Department of Surgery
University of Cincinnati
Cincinnati, Ohio
USA

N. Cano
Service d'Hépatogastroenterologie
et de Nutrition
CHP Résidence du Parc
Marseilles
France

Y.A. Carpentier
L. Deloyers Laboratory for
Experimental Surgery
Université Libre de Bruxelles
Brussels
Belgium

R. Chioléro
Surgical Intensive Care Unit
CHUV
Lausanne
Switzerland

P.S. Choban
Department of Human Nutrition
and Food Management
Ohio State University
Columbus, Ohio
USA

M. Isabel T.D. Correia
Cirurgia Geral
Nutricao Clinica
Belo Horizonte
Brazil

R. Cotter
Nutritional Sciences Worldwide
Whitehall-Robins
Madison, New Jersey
USA

D.F. Driscoll
Department of Medicine
Harvard Medical School
and
Beth Israel Deaconess Medical Center
Boston, Massachusetts
USA

I.E. Dupont
L. Deloyers Laboratory
for Experimental Surgery
Université Libre de Bruxelles
Brussels
Belgium

L.J. Flancbaum
Department of Surgery
St. Luke's-Roosevelt Hospital Center
and
Department of Clinical Surgery
Columbia University College of Physicians
and Surgeons
New York, New York
USA

P. Fürst
Institut für Biologische Chemie
und Ernährung
Universität Hohenheim
Stuttgart
Germany

C.J. Galbán Rodríguez
Sanin s/n
Los Angeles-Brion
La Coruña
Spain

L. Genton
Section Nutrition
Hôpital Cantonal Universitaire
Geneva
Switzerland

D.R. Goldhill, MD, FRCA
Department of Anaesthetics
St. Bartholomew's and
The Royal London Hospital School of
Medicine and Dentistry
London
UK

R.D. Griffiths
Department of Medicine
University of Liverpool
Liverpool
UK

J. Hasse
Transplant Services
Baylor University Medical Center
Dallas, Texas
USA

W.S. Helton
Department of Surgery
University of Illinois at Chicago
Chicago, Illinois
USA

D.N. Herndon
Department of Surgery
University of Texas Medical Branch
at Galveston
and
Shriners Hospitals for Children
Galveston, Texas
USA

D.K. Heyland
Department of Medicine and Community
Health and Epidemiology
Queen's University
and
Kingston General Hospital
Kingston, Ontario
Canada

S.B. Heymsfield
Department of Medicine
Columbia University College of Physicians
and Surgeons
and
Obesity Research Center
St. Luke's–Roosevelt Hospital Center
New York, New York
USA

K. Jeejeebhoy
Division of Gastroenterology
Department of Medicine
University of Toronto
and
St. Michael's Hospital
Toronto, Ontario
Canada

P. Jolliet
Soins Intensifs de Médecine
Hôpital Cantonal Universitaire
Geneva
Switzerland

V. Kaul
Division of Gastroenterology
and Nutrition
Albert-Einstein Medical Center
Philadelphia, Pennsylvania
USA

L. Khaodhiar
Department of Medicine
Beth Israel Deaconess Medical Center
and
Harvard Medical School
Boston, Massachusetts
USA

D.F. Kirby
Department of Medicine
Division of Gastroenterology
Section of Nutrition
Medical College of Virginia
Richmond, Virginia
USA

R.L. Koretz
Medical Center and School of Medicine
University of California, Los Angeles
and
Division of Gastroenterology
San Fernando Valley Program
Los Angeles, California
USA

K.A. Kudsk
Department of Surgery
University of Wisconsin-Madison
Madison, Wisconsin
USA

K.S. Kuhn
Institut für Biologische Chemie und
Ernährung
Universität Hohenheim
Stuttgart
Germany

X.M. Leverve
Département de Médecine Aiguë
Spécialisée
Unités de Réanimation
Médicale et de Nutrition Parentérale
Université Joseph Fourrier
Grenoble
France

G.M. Levine
Division of Gastroenterology and Nutrition
Albert-Einstein Medical Center
Philadelphia, Pennsylvania
USA

S.A. McClave
Division of Gastroenterology/Hepatology
University of Louisville School of Medicine
Louisville, Kentucky
USA

K.C. McCowen
Department of Medicine
Beth Israel Deaconess Medical Center
and
Harvard Medical School
Boston, Massachusetts
USA

M.M. McQuiggan
Food and Nutrition Services
Hermann Hospital
Houston, Texas
USA

J.M. Mirtallo
Ohio State University Medical Center
Columbus, Ohio
USA

F.A. Moore
Department of Surgery
University of Texas Houston Medical School
and
Trauma Services
Memorial Hermann Hospital
Houston, Texas
USA

G. Nitenberg
Institut Gustave-Roussy
Villejuif
France

C. Pichard
Department of Clinical Nutrition
University Hospital
Geneva
Switzerland

M.-A. Piquet
Département de Gastroentérologie
et Nutrition
CHU Côte-de-Nacre
Caen
France

J. Powell-Tuck
Department of Human Nutrition
St. Bartholomew's and
The Royal London Hospital School of
Medicine and Dentistry
London
UK

B. Raynard
Institut Gustave-Roussy
Villejuif
France

K. Robien
University of Washington
Fred Hutchinson Cancer Research Center
Seattle, Washington
USA

A.P. Sanford
Department of Surgery
University of Texas Medical Branch
at Galveston
and
Shriners Burns Hospital for Children
Galveston, Texas
USA

P.J. Schneider
College of Pharmacy
Ohio State University
Columbus, Ohio
USA

A. Shenkin
Clinical Chemistry
Royal Liverpool University Hospital
Liverpool
UK

H.L. Snider
Division of Pulmonary Medicine
University of Louisville School
of Medicine
Louisville, Kentucky
USA

W.W. Stargel
Worldwide Regulatory Affairs
Monsanto Company
Skokie, Illinois
USA

P. Stehle
Institut für Ernährungswissenschaft
Universität Bonn
Bonn
Germany

L. Tappy
Institut de Physiologie
Lausanne
Switzerland

J.A. Thomas
University of Texas Health Science Center at
San Antonio
San Antonio, Texas
USA

H.N. Tucker
Cato Research
Durham, North Carolina
USA

S.E. Wolf
Department of Surgery
University of Texas Medical Branch
at Galveston
and
Shriners Hospital for Children
Galveston, Texas
USA

Nutrition-Related Outcome in Critical Care

H.N. Tucker

Introduction

The practical limitations of conducting clinical studies in critical care patients have impacted the ability of sponsoring agencies to demonstrate convincing outcome improvements from appropriate and aggressive nutrition support. Clinical nutrition research seems to suffer from the same problems that have been identified and described by Berg [1] for the field of general nutrition; these problems include emphasis on the wrong research issues and a negligence in preparing individuals to work operationally in nutrition. Interpretation of the clinical nutrition literature is confounded by improperly designed and under-powered studies from which conclusions, which are frequently not supported by the data described, are drawn. In diligent attempts to dissect the mechanisms of energy utilization, to determine specific nutrient requirements, and to compare product formulations and routes of administration, the clinical nutrition community may have done a disservice to other healthcare providers, as well as patients. This approach may have obscured evidence suggesting that nutrient and energy balance improve outcome. Point-counter-point arguments of feeding versus no feeding and debates over the merits of one type of nutrition support versus another, while academically challenging, are not the most instructive from which to build a solid body of literature supporting the use of nutrition support. These types of arguments are not convincing to third-party payers, managed care providers, or practicing physicians who are unaccustomed to considering nutrition relevant to their medical practice.

Malnutrition in Critical Care

The past two decades have witnessed the development of overwhelming evidence that malnutrition in the hospital setting is prevalent and that it is a financial drain on the healthcare community [2–5]. Factors contributing to the continuing incidence of malnutrition in the critical care setting include the aging of the population, the higher acuity level of patients seeking care, and the treatment of chronic diseases. These factors are coupled with the continuing lack of attention to the nutrition status of patients at the time of admission. It has been demonstrated repeatedly that hospital lengths of stay and associated charges are highest for those patients who are at risk for or have evidence of protein calorie malnutrition. Figure 1 illustrates data that have been combined from two examples of the differences in average length of stay (ALOS) between low- and high-risk patients [2]. While malnutrition still exists in the critical care setting and even though there appears to be an association between malnutrition and poor outcome as measured by ALOS [5–7], the emphasis on organized nutrition support does not appear to be a high priority, as reflected by care and documentation of care [8].

Changed Financial Model

With the advent of managed care and capitated payment systems, today's financial incentives are changing from a "more-is-better" to a "less-is-better" environment. Historically, the evaluation of the clinical benefit was based, in part, on a reimbursement incentive system that gained from providing the maximum number of reimbursable services (i.e., "more-is-better"). Because of this payment system, the healthcare community has developed a methodology to evaluate and track charges, billings, and payments but frequently does not have systems to extract actual direct and indirect costs or cost savings associated with improved services. The healthcare community is struggling to catch up before bad decisions are made based on incomplete information. Without solid financial data to demonstrate costs savings, nutrition support products and services are extremely vulnerable in a "less-is-better" environment. Demonstrations of both efficacy and cost-effectiveness are required.

Financial Implication

Critics continue to review the existing evidence and state that, while nutrition support accounts for 1% of the total healthcare cost in the United States, the demonstrated clinical result does not support the expenditure [9]. The objectives to lower healthcare costs or to shorten length of stay are extremely difficult to associate with measurable, directly related clinical endpoints. Several studies have demonstrated, through single and multi-center retrospective evaluations and

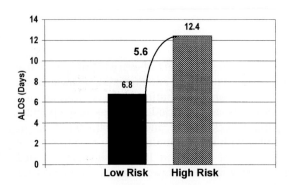

Fig. 1. The difference in ALOS in days between low- and high-risk patients. The collapsed data are from community and teaching hospitals. (Modified from [2])

chart reviews, an association between early nutrition intervention and ALOS [2–4, 10–12]. Figure 2 depicts the relationship between the day of nutritional intervention and ALOS. As days until nutrition intervention increased, so did the length of hospital stay in a ratio of 0.5. For every 2 days of earlier intervention, there was a decline by 1 day in ALOS for the average patient [2]. Retrospective reviews of economic indicators, such as ALOS and re-admission, have been used to suggest savings; however, these reviews suffer from the limited acceptability of soft data and a weak, direct association with the real cost of hospital care.

Average Length of Stay

Drawing a meaningful conclusion, even from extremely large patient trials regardless of the design, is difficult when the study objectives are broad general events, such as lowering hospital costs or changes in length of stay, that may exhibit large variances not related to nutrition support. Figure 3 is a summary of the stepwise regression model to describe the variation in ALOS in medical and surgical patients [2]. The regression model describes in percentage points the strength of influence of each of the eight factors on the number of post-intervention days. Markers for severity account for more than half of the explained variation and are similar to the findings in other studies of the effect of complications on ALOS [13]. The day of nutritional intervention, which was the only controllable factor, ranked second and accounted for 19% of the total variation for the average patient. The factors in aggregate described 15% of the total variation on ALOS observed for the group. It is clear from these data that ALOS is influenced by many uncontrollable events. Only 3% (19% of 15%) of the variation in ALOS is explainable by the day of nutritional intervention in this group of patients ($n=795$). It is important to recognize the enormous number of subjects that would be required in each group in a prospective, randomized, controlled trial (PRCT) to demonstrate an effect of nutritional intervention on these types of general outcome indicators. Based on similar considerations, Soeters commented that a change in hospital length of stay is a "questionable (and maybe suicidal) end point" for human clinical trials [14] and suggested that other endpoints would be more appropriate.

Fig. 2. The influence of early or late nutrition intervention on ALOS. The difference between groups receiving early and late nutrition intervention is 2.1 days. Late intervention was defined as being provided on day 4 or later

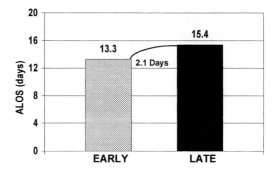

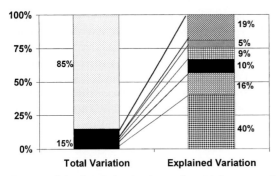

Fig. 3. Explained variation in observed ALOS for 795 medical and surgical admissions. Of the 15% explained variation, 40% was related to the number of diagnoses and 16% to the expected length of stay (indicators of severity of medical condition), 10% to gender, 9% to surgery, and 5% to height, weight, and age of patient. The day of nutrition intervention accounted for the remainder (19%)

Costs and Charges

While costs for services and products should be apparent and easily quantified, savings are often invisible and difficult to quantify. Economic reviews [9] frequently confuse charges with cost. In a true capitated managed care environment, charges are irrelevant; the costs associated with providing products and services is the only important factor. There are few sophisticated cost analyses. Figure 4 is cost-bar representation of extensive data collected by Eisenberg and colleagues to describe the cost associated with the provision of parenteral nutrition [15]. As demonstrated by these investigators, it is important to collect and understand all of the elements of cost that relate to nutrition therapy. It is also important to understand differing financial perspectives. From a hospital cash flow perspective, costs that are reimbursed must be distinguished from those that are covered in institutional general accounts in order to determine the net financial effect of the care. A good example is the reimbursable pharmacy charge for parenteral products compared with the charge for enteral products from central stores or dietary department. Reimbursed pharmacy charges represents income. Non-reimbursed dietary department charges represent loss. Also, the economic implications will be different depending on the perspective of the participant in the healthcare arena. The three participants – care receiver, care giver, and payer – have different and often conflicting financial objectives. Any discussions of costs should recognize the impact on each of the participants in the provision of healthcare. Due to the vastly different healthcare situations across the country and across institutions, published data may not relate specifically in other institutions or therapy classes. To be credible, it is usually expected that each institution will generate specific cost data based on clinical programs as practiced. The extraction of time and motion data and the exact elements of costs is demanding of both time and resource. At a time when nutrition support staff are needed to quantify the costs and net cost savings associated with nutrition and metabolic support of the critical care patient, cost pressures limit the resources. This dichotomy has made it increasingly difficult to justify nutrition support services at a time when they are most needed.

Efficacy, Effectiveness, and Cost-Effectiveness

The field of nutrition support is built on two premises. The first premise is that malnutrition is associated with increased morbidity and mortality and that the clinical result of these will increase the cost of care of the malnourished patients. The second premise is that clinical nutrition service and nutrition interventions produce net cost savings by reversing the effects of malnutrition. Increasing demands for cost control have required clinical researchers to focus on the economic benefit to the hospital business. The emphasis on cost-effectiveness has overtaken the emphasis on efficacy and effectiveness.

Efficacy is the ability of a therapeutic agent to produce a specific result when used in the treatment of specific medical conditions when administered by expert hands under ideal conditions. The most common examples of intended use are those statements published in the direction sheets or package inserts that accompany drugs and describe the approved indication for the pharmaceutical agent. Intravenous amino acids, for example, are indicated to offset negative nitrogen balance. Proof that the agent performs this function is usually demonstrated by "adequate and well-controlled" PRCTs conducted with surrogate markers of efficacy as the measured endpoints. The terms adequate and well-controlled, as well as the appropriate surrogate markers, are defined by the regulatory agency intended to grant approval.

Effectiveness, on the other hand, describes the ability of the indicated use of a product in any clinical setting to obtain a consistent clinical outcome in actual use. In the case of amino acids, offsetting negative nitrogen balance (efficacy) pro-

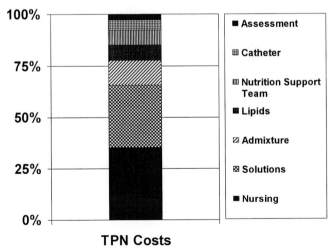

Fig. 4. Incremental cost of perioperative PN excluding the effect of ALOS. The total incremental cost was approximately $149/day. (Modified from [15])

vides a clinically measurable influence on nutrition status (effectiveness). A demonstration of efficacy may not equate to effectiveness.

In the current healthcare environment, effectiveness is not enough. Cost-effectiveness carries the effectiveness concept a large step further in that the clinical outcome desired must also be economically beneficial. The clinically significant effect must lead to a lower net cost of the care of the patient. Therapeutic approaches that have been proven both efficacious and clinically effective may not provide cost-benefit. These distinctions are important when considering a clinical trial plan for nutrition products and services. All parties need to come to a common understanding of what is to be expected by the conduct of the trial.

In some aspects, clinical nutrition suffers from the lack of regulation of safety and efficacy that is provided for drugs. When a clear distinction among efficacy, effectiveness, and cost-effectiveness becomes blurred, the resulting demands on research hold nutrition therapies to a higher standard than regulated pharmaceutical agents. In practice, this places a greater burden for proof on clinical nutrition products than on other pharmaceutical modalities that must demonstrate only safety and efficacy.

The Clinical Trial Dilemma

Providers of and payers for care have not come to a consensus regarding the tools acceptable for evaluating nutrition support outcome and agreement has not been reached regarding rational approaches for evaluating both the efficacy and cost-effectiveness of aggressive nutrition support. A comprehensive review [16] of the state of the published data illustrates conclusions (or lack thereof) that could be drawn from the existing clinical research. The consensus panel's recommendations for future studies of nutrition support during critical illness are as follows:
- Perform PRCTs to determine whether enteral nutrition support affects clinical outcome in uniform groups of critically ill patients. The control group should not receive nutrition support, but stopping rules that avoid a prolonged period of starvation (7–14 days) should be applied. Endpoints should include morbidity, mortality, organ function, length of intensive care unit and hospital stay, long-term rehabilitation, and quality of life.
- Perform additional studies to determine the optimal timing and amount of enteral nutrients needed to improve outcome.
- Perform PRCTs to determine the clinical efficacy of individual specific nutrient supplements with control groups as indicated by the effectiveness studies.

These statements are, in part, based on the belief that a PRCT with a concurrent placebo control (the gold standard) is the only credible tool for developing evidence-based support for improved clinical outcome and seem to confuse the two different issues of efficacy and effectiveness. The ability to detect evidence of broad outcome parameters, such as ALOS, morbidity, and mortality, cannot be expected from a single, reasonably sized clinical evaluation of an adjunctive or combination therapy, such as nutrition support. Nutrition support is never the primary method of treatment in the critical care setting and can only be considered supportive. The limitation of using PRCTs to study combination therapies for rheumatic diseases was discussed by Pincus [17], who concluded that new approaches, such as longitudinal databases collected over three to 5 years, would be advantageous or even required to document effectiveness of second-line therapies. The ubiquitous requirement for energy and nutrient intake and the extreme variability of both critical care patients and primary care plans confound the approaches to PRCT study designs for nutrition support. The definitive placebo-controlled, randomized, blinded clinical evaluation of the efficacy of adequate nutrition support for the critical care patient will likely be impossible to design, conduct, and finance. Changes that may be due solely to nutrient repletion are subtle and chronic in nature. The multiplicity and magnitude of other therapeutic interventions and subjectivity acute care decisions may overwhelm the detection of changes due to nutrition. Undoubtedly, the cohort sizes required to detect differences specifically related to nutrition support in any type of trial will be extremely large.

The absence of large multi-center trials in nutrition support may have a direct relation to the poor market economics of the situation [18]. The cost burden of a clinical endeavor to provide the undeniable proof of broad clinical benefit cannot be economically justified when compared with the income that might be gained from increased sales of nutrition products by pharmaceutical development sponsors. This economic disincentive has created a contradictory environment that limits the research efforts when the pharmaceutical industry is a large source of funding for trials.

Efficacy

PRCT clinical methodology is best designed to distinguish between outcomes that are related directly to defined physiologic endpoints or surrogate markers that can be isolated and result solely from the treatment studied. In addition to the standard energy, nitrogen balance, and nutrient balances, several quantitative biochemical and clinical markers have been used to indicate nutrition status, have been used to identify appropriate subjects for study, and have been used as surrogate markers to describe the efficacy of nutrition support products. Table 1 provides the usual examples derived from published studies and reviews [19–21].

Statistically significant weight changes, improved plasma albumin, or prealbumin concentrations, other nutrition biochemical, and immunologic markers may be attainable in smaller, defined subject groups. Several schemes have been proposed for the combination of multiple variables and have been correlated with both surrogate markers and physician observation [22–24]. The results based on surrogate markers are more easily correlated to the method and content of nutrition support. Even with the use of these standard surrogate markers, successful study design and protocol development are predicated on the application of several well-known concepts. Protocols must be constructed carefully with the following points in mind:
- The statistical plan must support a clearly stated study objective
- The endpoints must be directly related to and support the primary objective
- Endpoints must be measurable, clear, and simple

- The endpoints must be specifically affected by therapeutic modalities tested
- Other therapeutic effects on the endpoints must be excluded by experimental design
- Study subjects who are expected to have endpoints compromised by their clinical course or disease process should be excluded
- The clinical plan must be executable in the context of the critical care environment

While the concepts of protocol development are well known, it is apparent from a review of the clinical nutrition literature that scrupulous attention to a statistical plan and feasible study design is frequently lacking.

Studies may be designed and carried out with very different kinds of controls. Each method of control may be appropriate depending upon the objectives of the study, but none of the control methodologies are useful or adequate in every situation [25]. Selection of an appropriate control group depends largely on the hypothesis. Table 2 contains a description and examples for the types of control groups that may be considered.

The utility of such studies to defend the effectiveness of the nutrition support therapy studied depends upon convincing the clinical community that the surrogate marker correlates with improved outcome in a general clinical sense. While several investigators have demonstrated a relationship between a deterioration of nutrition status and progressively increased ALOS [4, 20, 21], the further leap of faith that the improved outcome actually reduces costs has been difficult to produce in a managed care environment.

Table 1. Indicators of nutrition status and surrogate markers for nutrition support efficacy

Indicator	Normal adult ranges	None	Mild	Nutrition depletion Moderate	Severe
Body size					
Weight	±10% ideal body weight	No loss	10% Loss	>10%	>15%
Anthropometry					
Body mass index	19.5–25	≥20	<20	<18	£17
Creatinine					
height index	100% of standard	≥95%	95%–85%	85%–70%	>70%
Plasma protein					
Albumin (g/dl)	3.5–5.0	≥3.5	3.4–3.0	2.9–2.1	<2.1
Transferrin (mg/dl)	200–400	>200	150–200	100–150	<100
Pre-albumin (mg/dl)	15.7–29.6	>15	10–15	5–10	<5
Immunologic function					
Lymphocyte (/mm^3)	2000–4000	≥1500	1200–1500	800–1200	<800
Multiple indicator					
Subjective global assessment	A	A	–	B	C
Mini-nutrition assessment	≥24	≥24	17–23.5 (at risk)	17–23.5 (at risk)	<17

Table 2. Description of possible clinical nutrition study designs

Type	Description of study design	Characteristics
A	Prospective, randomized, placebo concurrent control	Impossible for ethical and practical considerations in general feeding studies. Useful for specific single nutrient trials.
B	Prospective, randomized, no-treatment concurrent control	Difficult for ethical considerations in general feeding studies. Useful for new indications and for specific single nutrient trials. Cannot be blinded.
C	Prospective, randomized, dose-response concurrent control	Useful for differentiating between two dosages of macro- or micro-nutrients. May include a placebo (zero-dose).
D	Prospective, active (positive) concurrent control	Used to show superiority or equivalence (non-inferiority). Critical issue is the number of subjects required to appropriately power the study to distinguish differences between the groups or to determine whether either is more distinguishable than an inactive control.
E	Prospective, external control (including historical control)	Careful selection of external control group is mandatory. Includes baseline-controlled studies.
F	Prospective time series, with and without intervention	Must achieve a non-biased selection of study patients; clear definition of the method, standardization of type intervention, and careful selection of primary endpoints are critical.
G	Descriptive studies based on clinical experience	Generally considered anecdotal. May be used to propose endpoints and to support statistical plan for further study.
H	Retrospective, case-controlled analytic studies	Requires a very large number of study subjects, multi-site data collecting, and a statistical plan that will allow associative conclusions. Data supportive for planning future prospective studies.

Nutrition Intervention Trials

Various, recent reviews of the published intervention trials have provided insights into the future direction for clinical study design in critical care [26, 27], gastrointestinal surgery [28], major torso trauma [29], and severe head injury [10, 30]. Each of these trials provides accumulating evidence that nutrition intervention is beneficial. Each review article offers recommendations on patient assessment, selection of route of nutrition support, and use of specialty products. Table 3 provides examples of study designs published for the critical care patient. Most trials are conducted using active controls, and the objective of each trial is to demonstrate the benefit of providing nutrition support. The trials are characterized based on the intent to demonstrate efficacy, effectiveness, or cost-effectiveness. All of these trials were designed to demonstrate improvement or superiority of the treatment in the study group, and none were powered to demonstrate equivalency between groups. It is instructive to review the sample sizes of the studies listed and the hypothesis tested. For example, an otherwise excellent study can fail to detect an important outcome due to a sample size that is too small. Interpretations of the data from such studies only serve to confuse the issue being investigated.

Conclusion

The challenge for critical care nutrition support is a clinical trial design that will detect differences in clinical outcome and that is related to a net cost reduction. The goal for nutrition support is to prevent something that has not yet occurred or to avoid progression of malnutrition or complications due to malnutrition. With this backdrop, the goals of research must be directed to nutritional and metabolic care that guarantee that the requirements of the critical care patient are appropriately addressed at all times during the therapeutic course. A careful and creative clinical study design will be required to provide the support required for regaining the priority of nutrition support services.

Table 3. Examples of study designs in nutrition support (APCHE II Acute Physiological and Chronic Health Evaluation II; ATI Abdominal Trauma Index, EN enteral nutrition, ISS Injury Severity Score, MOF multiple organ failure, NG nasogastric, PN parenteral nutrition)

Description (type)[a]	Subjects	n	Groups	Endpoint(s)	Result	Category	Ref.
Prospective, randomized, time series (F)	Severe closed-head injury	9	Early PN at day 1 or delayed PN at day 5	Improved markers of immunologic function	Increased CD4 cells, CD4-CD8 ratios, and T-lymphocyte responsiveness to ConA	Efficacy	12
Prospective, randomized, blinded, active control (D)	Colorectal surgical patients	19	PN with structured or long-chain triglyceride emulsions	Improvement of nitrogen balance	Positive nitrogen balance in both groups, no detectable difference in the degree of nitrogen retention between the groups	Efficacy	31
Prospective, randomized, dose response control (C)	Hepatic resection	19	PN with 10 kcal/kg or 20 kcal/kg per day for 5 days	Improved nutrition markers	Retinol binding protein, pre-albumin improved, nitrogen balance normalized, urinary 3-methylhistidine decreased in the study group	Efficacy	32
Prospective, randomized, unblinded, active control (D)	Surgical patients	20	Peptide EN or amino acid EN for 1 week	Improved nutrition markers	Pre-albumin, transferrin, and cholesterol improved in Peptide EN group	Efficacy	33
Prospective, randomized, unblinded, active control (D)	Trauma, ISS 20–40	38	Early EN by NG tube or conventional fluid therapy (5% dextrose in normal saline) with oral fluid or soft diet as bowel function returned	Improved nutrition markers, fewer clinical complications, ICU days, ventilator days, and mortality	EN group had improved nitrogen balance, less body weight loss. This group had lower complication rate, shorter ICU stay, fewer ventilator days, and lower mortality	Efficacy, effectiveness	34
Multi-center, prospective, active concurrent control, unblinded (D)	Trauma, ATI 18–40, ISS 16–45	98	Immune-enhancing or standard stress EN	Improved visceral protein, acute phase reactants, lymphocyte, lymphocyte subsets, stimulated monocyte cytokine production, clinical outcome	Immune-enhancing EN increased in total lymphocytes, T-lymphocytes, and T-helper cells, this group had fewer intra-abdominal abscesses and less MOF	Efficacy, effectiveness	35

Table 3. *Continued.*

Description (type)[a]	n	Groups	Endpoint(s)	Result	Category	Ref.
Prospective, randomized, active concurrent control, unblinded (D)	300	PN to meet daily requirements or glucose alone (250–300 g/day) for 14 days or until voluntary intake resumed	Improved treatment outcome, functional and physiologic variables	No differences were detectable between groups	Effectiveness	36
Prospective, randomized, blinded (D)	80	Glutamine supplemented and standard EN	Less infectious morbidity	Incidence of pneumonia, bacteremia, and sepsis was significantly lower in the glutamine-supplemented group	Effectiveness	37
Prospective, randomized, active control and external control (D, E)	42	Immune-enhancing access EN and isocaloric EN. Non-fed comparison group	Less septic complications, antibiotic usage, hospital stay, ICU stay, ventilator days, and hospital charges	Specialty EN performed better than standard EN, fasting is inferior to both EN groups, costs did not reach statistical significance although were higher in the non-fed group	Effectiveness, cost-effectiveness	38
Prospective, block-randomized, double-blinded (D)	84	Glutamine containing PN and standard PN	Improved survival, cost per survivor	PN improves survival at 6 months and reduces costs per survivor	Cost-effectiveness	39

Subjects column values:
- Major general surgical patients regardless of nutrition status or severity (Ref. 36)
- Multiple trauma (Ref. 37)
- Severe trauma, ATI ≥25, ISS ≥21, early enteral (Ref. 38)
- Critical care, APCHE II >10, requiring PN, EN contraindicated (Ref. 39)

[a]Type of trial design defined in Table 2.

References

1. Berg A (1992) Sliding toward nutrition malpractice: time to reconsider and redeploy. American Journal of Clinical Nutrition 57:3–7
2. Tucker HN (1997) Shortened length of stay is an outcome benefit of early nutritional intervention. In: Kinney JM, Tucker HN, eds. Physiology, Stress, and Malnutrition: Functional Correlates, Nutritional Intervention. Philadelphia: Lippincott-Raven, 607–627
3. Smith PE, Smith AE (1993) Nutritional intervention influences the bottom line. Healthcare Financial Management 10:30–36
4. Shaw-Stiffel TA, Zarney LA, Pleban WE, Rosman DD, Rudolph RA, Bernstein LH (1993) Effect of nutrition status and other factors on length of hospital stay after major gastrointestinal surgery. Nutrition 9:140–145
5. Giner M, Laviano A, Mequid M, Gleason JR (1996) In 1995 a correlation between malnutrition and poor outcome in critically ill patients still exists. Nutrition 12:23–29
6. Gallagher-Allred CR, Voss AC, Finn SC, McCamish MA (1996) Malnutrition and clinical outcomes: the case for medical nutrition therapy. Journal of American Dietetic Association 96:361–366
7. McCamish MA (1993) Malnutrition and nutrition support interventions: cost, benefits, and outcomes. Nutrition 9:556–557
8. Bruun LI, Bosaeus I, Bergstad I, Nygaard K (1999) Prevalence of malnutrition in surgical patients: evaluation of nutritional support and documentation. Clinical Nutrition 18:141–147
9. Ofman J, Koretz RL (1997) Clinical economics review: nutritional support. Alimentary Pharmacology and Therapeutics 11:453–471
10. Twyman D (1997) Nutritional management of the critically ill neurologic patient. Critical Care Clinics 13:39–49
11. Wernerman J, Tucker HN (1994) Future nutritional goals in the intensive care unit. In: Kinney JM, Tucker HN, eds. Organ Metabolism and Nutrition: Ideas for Future Critical Care. New York: Raven Press Ltd, 481–495
12. Sax HC (1996) Early nutritional support in critical illness is important. Critical Care Clinics 12:661–666
13. McAleese P, Odling-Smee W (1994) The effect of complications on length of stay. Annals of Surgery 220:740–744
14. Soeters PB (1996) Glutamine: the link between depletion and diminished gut function? Journal of the American College of Nutrition 15:195–196
15. Eisenberg JM, Glick HA, Buzby GP, Kinosian B, Williford WO (1993) Does perioperative total parenteral nutrition reduce medical care costs? Journal of Parenteral and Enteral Nutrition 17:201–209
16. Klein S, Kinney J, Jeejeebhoy K, et al. (1997) Nutrition support in clinical practice: review of published data and recommendations for future research directions. American Journal of Clinical Nutrition 66:683–706
17. Pincus T (1993) Rationale for combination therapy in rheumatoid arthritis – limitation of randomized cliical trials to recognize possible advantages of combination therapies in rheumatic diseases. Seminars in Arthritis and Rheumatism 23:2–10
18. Wernerman J (1998) Documentation of clinical benefit of specific amino acid nutrients. Lancet 352:756–757
19. Jeb SA (1997) Anorexia: a neglected clinical problem. In: Kinney JM, Tucker HN, eds. Physiology, Stress, and Malnutrition: Functional Correlates, Nutritional Intervention. Philadelphia: Lippincott-Raven
20. Messner RL, Stephens N, Wheeler WE, Hawes MC (1991) Effect of admission nutritional status on length of hospital stay. Society of Gastroenterology Nurses and Associates 13:202–205
21. Smith LC, Mullen JL (1991) Nutritional assessment and indications for nutritional support. Surgical Clinics of NOrth America 71:449–457

22. Detsky AS, McLaughlin JR, Baker JP (1987) What is Subjective Global Assessment of nutritional status. Journal of Parenteral and Enteral Nutrition 11:8–13
23. Guigoz Y, Vellas B (1990) The mini-nutritional assessment (MNA) for grading the nutritional state of elderly patients: presentation of the MNA, history and validation. In: Vellas B, Garry PJ, Guigoz Y, eds. Mini Nutritional Assessment (MNA): Research and Practice in the Elderly. Vol. 1. Basel: L. Karger AG
24. Persson C, Sjoden P-O, Glimelius B (1999) The Swedish version of the patient-generated subjective global assessment of nutritional status: gastrointestinal vs urological cancers. Clinical Nutrition 18:71–77
25. ICH Steering Committee (1999) Draft Consensus Guideline: Choice of control group in clinical trials. International Conference on Harmonisation of Technical Requirements for Registration of Pharmaceuticals for Human Use
26. Jolliet P, Pichard C, Biolo G, et al. (1999) Enteral nutrition in intensive care patients: a practical approach. Clinical Nutrition 18:47–56
27. Frost P, Bihari D (1997) The route of nutritional support in the critically ill: physiological and economical considerations. Nutrition 13:58S-63 S
28. Torosian MH (1999) Perioperative nutrition support for patients undergoing gastrointestinal surgery: critical analysis and recommendations. World Journal of Surgery 23:565–569
29. McGuiggan MM, Marvin RG, McKinley BA, Moore FA (1999) Enteral feeding following major torso tauma: from theory to practice. New Horizons 7:131–146
30. Wilson RF, Tyburski JG (1998) Metabolic responses and nutritional therapy in patients with severe head injuries. Journal of Head Trauma Rehabilitation 13:11–27
31. Bellantone R, Bossola M, Carriero C, et al. (1999) Structured versus long-chain triglycerides: a safety, tolerance, and efficacy randomized study in colorectal surgical patients. Journal of Parenteral and Enteral Nutrition 23:123–127
32. Nishizaki T, Takenada K, Yanaga K, et al. (1996) Nutritional support after hepatic resection: a randomized prospective study. Hepato-Gastroenterology 43:608–613
33. Patillo D, Miller E, Schirmer B (1994) Repletion of nutritional parameters in surgical patients receiving peptide versus amino acid elemental feedings. Nutrition Research 14:3–12
34. Chuntrasakul C, Siltharm S, Chinswangwatanakul V, Pongprasobchai T, Chockvivatanavanit S, Bunnak A (1996) Early nutritional support in severe traumatic patients. Journal of the Medical Association of Thailand 79:21–26
35. Moore FA, Moore EE, Kudsk KA, et al. (1994) Clinical benefits of an immune-enhancing diet for early postinjury feeding. Journal of Trauma 37:607–615
36. Sandstrom R, Drott C, Hyltander A, et al. (1993) The effect of postoperative intravenous feeding (TPN) on outcome following major surgery evaluated in a randomized study. Annals of Surgery 217:185–195
37. Houdijk AP (1998) Glutamine reduces infection in trauma patients. Lancet 352:772–776
38. Kudsk KA, Minard G, Croche MA, et al. (1996) A randomized trial of isonitrogenous enteral diets after severe trauma. Annals of Surgery 224:531–543
39. Griffiths RD, Jones C, Palmer TEA (1997) Six-month outcome of critically ill patients given glutamine-supplemented parenteral nutrition. Nutrition 13:295–302

Host Defenses and Bacterial Assaults:
A Delicate Balance

K.A. Kudsk and J. Alverdy

In health, a symbiotic relationship exists between the human body and the bacteria which colonize its surfaces. Under normal circumstances, products of bacterial metabolism, such as short-chain fatty acids or vitamins, are critical for human well being. A single cell layer of mucosal epithelium with a complex underlying immunologic system and various innate nonspecific mechanisms allow absorption of nutrients while maintaining an effective barrier against the 1–1.5 kg of bacteria and other toxic factors. In times of illness, this balance is upset. Changes in gut permeability, inability to ingest nutrients, antibiotic pressure and many other factors alter the normal checks and balances between coexistence and absorption of toxic intraluminal products and sepsis. While two decades of research have focused on epithelial changes in permeability to toxins and bacteria, recent investigations of intestinal immunity and responses of bacteria to altered body defensives are modifying concepts of host defenses during critical illness. These new concepts in immunology and bacterial responses are the focus of this review.

Intestinal Barriers Against Bacterial Invasion

To maintain antibacterial integrity, physiologic amounts of intraluminal antigen are absorbed to educate the underlying immunologic system about the intraluminal microflora. This system, the mucosal-associated lymphoid tissue (MALT) constitutes 50% of total body immunity accounting for 70% of all antibody production [1]. By coating the mucosa with specific antibodies, particularly IgA, against those antigens, bacteria are prevented from attaching to and infecting normal mucosa [2]. By working together with various extrinsic and intrinsic barriers, this system prevents bacterial invasion.

Nonimmunologic Extrinsic and Intrinsic Barriers

There are multiple nonimmunologic barriers to bacterial invasion [3]:
- Proteolytic enzymes
- Gastrointestinal acidity
- Peristalsis

- Mucous coat
- Microvilli structure
- Enterocyte surface membrane
- Cellular junctions
- Antimicrobial proteins (e.g., defensins)
- Lactoferrin

Proteolysis and gastric acidity reduce the large number of bacteria in salivary fluid to 10^3–10^4 organisms in the duodenal fluid. Peristalsis prevents stasis and bacterial overgrowth. Mucin, a thin layer of glycoproteins of varying molecular weight, coats mucosal surfaces and contains enzymes for digestion as well as IgA for bacteria neutralization. Mucin also carries many innate microbial defenses such as lactoferrin, defensins, peroxidases, and other potent low molecular weight antimicrobial inhibitors [4–6]. Although concentration of these individual defenses vary along the GI tract, together they play important roles in antimicrobial defense.

Hemorrhage, shock, ischemia/reperfusion, lack of enteral feeding, or inadequate diets increase GI permeability to macromolecules and to bacteria [7–10]. Clinically, permeability to macromolecules increases after trauma [11], burns [12], or sepsis [13], but its relationship to subsequent complications is unclear. Translocation of bacteria, at least acutely, occurs in situations of bowel obstruction, shock, inflammatory bowel disease, burns, and sepsis but has never definitively been shown to cause extraintestinal infections such as pneumonia or intraabdominal abscess. However, this concept of a GI-driven source of subsequent multiple organ dysfunction and sepsis is supported by students of critical care medicine, but the mechanism of this process, however, is controversial.

The Immunologic Barrier

The most important antibody in gut barrier function is polymeric IgA secreted by cells residing below the mucosa. Under normal conditions, T cells secrete IL-4, IL-5, IL-6, and IL-10 which stimulate production of IgA by B cells and plasma cells in response to antigenic stimulation. These pro-IgA cytokines adequately counteract inhibitory effects of TNFβ and IFN-γ on IgA synthesis. The polymeric IgA immediately attaches to secretory component expressed on the basal membranes of epithelial cells for transport onto the mucosal cell surface. IgA can then bind to specific antigens on the microbe to prevent attachment and avoid invasion. Complement and inflammation play no role in this defense.

Surveillance and immunologic specificity occur through T cells and B cells sensitized to antigens processed within Peyer's patches of the intestine and, possibly, upper respiratory sites. Peyer's patches attract uncommitted B cells through adhesion molecules on the high endothelial venule and sensitize them to the antigens of intraluminal microbials that have been absorbed by the overlying M cells of the Peyer's patch and processed by antigen-presenting cells [18]. These cells proliferate in mesenteric lymph nodes and release daughter cells into the thoracic duct and vascular tree for distribution to submucosal lamina propria at intestinal and extraintestinal sites where IgA is produced for effective MALT barrier function (Fig. 1).

Normal oral intake stimulates maintenance of MALT cell mass and function. This effect was established in mice models of parenteral feeding where both enteric stimulation and malnutrition are avoided with parenteral feeding [19]. All compartments of the gut-associated lymphoid tissue (GALT) of the small intestine shrink by approximately 40% with a shift in the CD4/CD8 ratio of the lamina propria from a normal ratio of 2:1 to 1:1. IL-4 and IL-10 intestinal cytokine levels drop without enteric feeding presumably inducing less stimulus for IgA production by surrounding B/plasma cells [20]. This GALT "atrophy" occurs within 2 days of parenteral nutrition and recovers within 2–3 days of enteral refeeding (Fig. 2) [21].

Antimicrobial barriers are affected at both intestinal and extraintestinal sites. Within the intestine, this defect is manifested by bacterial translocation to mesenteric lymph nodes and bacterial overgrowth. Extraintestinal sites, such as the respiratory tract, are also impaired. When animals are immunized with either influenza virus or *Pseudomonas* antigen, effective barriers against these microbes are induced rapidly. Administration of H1N1 virus to mice generates a brisk IgA-mediated defense within a few weeks which eliminates virus from the upper airway [23]. Subsequent doses of virus are rapidly eliminated by these established defenses. Likewise, the administration of *Pseudomonas* antigen in liposomes also generates a brisk IgA response in mice and reduces mortality from 90% to approximately 10% to a subsequent lethal dose of intratracheal *Pseudomonas* bacteria within 10 days of immunization [24]. If parenteral nutrition is administered to animals immunized against the virus or *Pseudomonas*, mucosal immunity is impaired. Five days of parenteral nutrition results in failure to eliminate the virus in 50% of animals after viral rechallenge [25] and increases the mortality to 90%

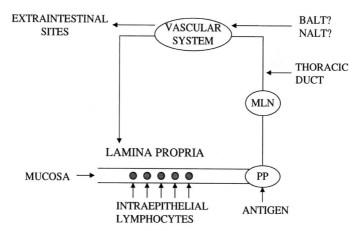

Fig. 1. Common mucosal immune system. After sensitization in the Peyer's patches (*PP*) and possibly the nasal-associated lymphoid tissue (*NALT*) and bronchus-associated lymphoid tissue (*BALT*) cells are distributed to lamina propria sites below intestinal and extraintestinal mucosal surfaces and to the intraepithelial spaces

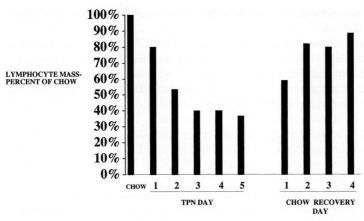

Fig. 2. Total cell atrophy and recovery with IV-TPN and chow. A generalized reduction in total cell mass of the gut-associated lymphoid tissue (*GALT*) occurs rapidly upon institution of parenteral nutrition (*TPN*) but recovers rapidly with reinstitution of an enteral diet

following intratracheal *Pseudomonas* administration [26]. Immunologic memory is not lost, however, since the reinstitution of enteral feeding returns antiviral immunity to normal within 5 days [27]. These data are consistent with the lower rates of pneumonia found in critically injured patients fed enterally [28, 29].

Support of these immunologic mechanisms may be possible, however, without direct enteral feeding. The amino acid, glutamine, is an important substrate for the unfed enterocyte, lymphocytes, and for any rapidly proliferating cell within the body [30]. Supplementation of parenteral solution with glutamine *partially* preserves GALT cell mass and antiviral [31] and antibacterial defenses [32] using the previously described models. Production of glutamine is up regulated by the body approximately six fold in times of stress and sepsis, suggesting a high biologic priority placed on this substrate. Clinically, administration of glutamine-supplemented solutions to bone marrow transplant patients normalizes microbial colonization patterns and reduces infectious complications [33], but its effectiveness in other critically injured and critically ill populations has not been determined yet.

A second potential family of clinical surrogates for enteral feeding are the neuropeptides secreted by the enteric nervous system. Nutrient delivery via the GI tract generates a brisk response with hormonal release, enzyme production, peristalsis, and stimulation of other processes of digestion. Many of these are accomplished through enteric nervous system neuropeptides such as cholecystokinin, neurotensin, and gastrin. Bombesin (BBS) is a tetradecapeptide found in frog skin analogous to gastrin-releasing peptide (GRP), a human peptide which stimulates the subsequent release of other neuropeptides. The seven amino acids important for pharmacologic function of each are identical, and bombesin is commonly used in research as a replacement for GRP. Bombesin administered three times a day prevents the reductions in GALT cell mass [34] and impairment in antibacteria [35] and antiviral mucosal immunity [36] induced by parenteral feeding.

These observations suggest many of the trophic immunologic effects of enteral nutrition are controlled through the enteric nervous system. The ability of nutrients to maintain normal mucosal immunity may be related both to their nutrient value and to their ability to stimulate neuropeptide release.

Further work on mucosal immunology should provide insights into vulnerabilities of critically ill and critically injured patients which increase susceptibilities to invasion by bacteria and viruses. But changes are not found in the defenses alone, and it appears that bacteria also respond to host and environmental changes.

The Bacterial Response in Conditions of Critical Care Medicine

The Host-Parasite Relationship

A delicate coevolutionary balance has permitted both microbes and their various hosts to live in a mutually beneficial state whereby both host and microbe share common resources. The normal intestinal flora of most mammals enjoys a warm and predictable environment and a constant food supply. From the microbes standpoint, the host will always seek shelter, maintain a predicable temperature, obtain foodstuffs, and stay mobile. These aspects of host behavior guarantee a constant supply of nutrients and if needed, the ability of the microbe to switch from one host to another.

Within the last 10,000 years a shift in the flora of humans has followed the change in foodstuffs as a result of man's transition from hunter-gatherer to sedentary food producer. The composition of the flora has also shifted as animal domestication has become a major industry. Both these transitions have occurred slowly, over millenia, allowing the immunologic apparatus of the host to adapt to the newly encountered antigens with a measured and non-phlogistic response. As with military détente, measured response is important in order to avoid unnecessary opponent aggression and ultimately self-harm. In some cases, too rapid growth in animal domestication has caused acquisition of lethal microbes resulting in plagues and crop devastation. These historical events can almost always be traced to rapid changes in either food or animal domestication [37]. In fact, the crowding of animals during domestication in order to increase production has almost invariably been associated with outbreaks of transmissible disease.

What then is the impact of the rapid advance of critical care medicine on the virulence strategy of microbes which colonize these patients? The introduction of broad spectrum antibiotics, total parenteral nutrition, vasoactive drugs, gastric acid reduction therapy, and analgesics/opiates all have independently been demonstrated to dramatically affect the quantity and composition of the intestinal flora [38, 39]. How does a luminal intestinal microbe, accustomed to a lazy life of three warm, high calorie meals a day, obtain food when all the nutrients are in the bloodstream? Furthermore, if chemically defined enteral nutrients are delivered, how do the densely populated flora in the distal intestinal tract obtain adequate nutrition when there is near complete absorption of theses foodstuffs in the proximal small bowel? To answer these questions we need to look at the world from the microbe's standpoint. There is now compelling evidence to demonstrate that microbes, like humans, obtain sensory input signals from their environment and respond appropriately. Bacteria can thus "sense" environmental changes and act in their own best interest using analogous systems such as smell, taste, and feel.

Bacterial Gene Expression

All bacteria regulate gene expression in response to different environmental signals, a property that is crucial to their ability to survive and compete with other organisms [40]. In an effort to remain metabolically economical, bacteria gene products that express survival function may predominate while virulence genes remain down regulated. Virulence genes are subject to complex regulation and cannot be in a state of constant expression. By this reasoning, during states of good health, colonizing flora are likely to have their virulence genes "turned off" in order to economize. During invasion of host tissue pathogens may need one set of genes to adhere to the host in a particular situation, such as the intestinal epithelial lining, and must immediately switch off this gene in transit through the tissues to avoid adhering to a macrophage or neutrophil. In this situation, virulence structures such as adherence appendages may be helpful one moment, and a liability the next. As one can imagine, the list of virulence phenotypes expressed in response to any number of environmental signals or cues can be infinite. The remaining discussion focuses on virulence expression on bacterial adherence to the intestinal epithelium, since adherence is the crucial initiating event for most infections. Bacteria which cannot adhere to host cells, with rare exception, cannot induce pathogenicity to the host. On the other hand bacterial adherence to the mucosal epithelium alone can result in activation of signal transduction pathways in the epithelium itself leading to multiple downstream events associated with a proinflammatory response. For example, it has been recently shown that activation of NF-κB, a global cytokine regulator in enterocytes can occur by simple adhesion of bacteria to the cell membrane without cell invasion [41]. Bacterial adherence is mediated by the expression of fimbriae or pili, which are structural adhesins on the outer surface of bacteria.

Bacteria respond to stress and dietary manipulation through the expression of the adherence phenotypes. Both stress and dietary manipulation (starvation, chemically defined enteral formulas, parenteral nutrition) result in adherence of both resident and transient intestinal bacteria to the intestinal epithelium. Adherence of bacteria, in particular *Escherichia coli* is associated with marked alterations in the permselectivity of the intestinal epithelium. In vitro studies have confirmed that bacterial adherence alone, induces a defect in epithelial barrier function at the level of the intercellular tight junction that is of sufficient magnitude to allow permeation of toxic macromolecules across this barrier [42]. Stress and starvation appear to result in adherence mediated alterations in intestinal permeability due to transformation of the intestinal flora to more adherent strains. For example, fimbrial adhesins of *Escherichia coli* (termed type I pili) increases in mice following 30% surgical hepatectomy and 48 h of starvation (Figs. 3, 4) [43]. If animals are fed normal diets following hepatectomy, or are starved but do not undergo hepatectomy, bacterial adherence to the intestinal epithelium is markedly attenuated in association with populations of *E. coli* expressing fewer pili. *E. coli* bacteria isolated from starved and stressed mice adhere to and alter the permeability of cultured mouse colon cells to a much greater extent than similar populations of *E. coli* isolated from controls, suggesting that stress and starvation increase the adherence phenotype of these particular bacterial strains [44]. These studies represent the first in vivo evidence to suggest the combination of stress and starvation result in virulence phenotype transformation of the resident intestinal flora.

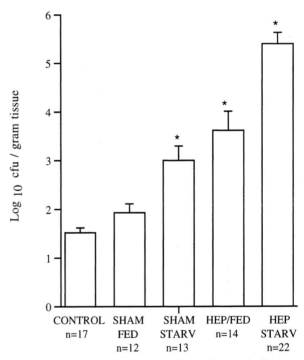

Fig. 3. The effect of starvation and hepatectomy, alone or in combination, on bacterial adherence to the cecal mucosa. Following 48 h of treatment, cecal tissues were vigorously washed, homogenized, and quantitatively cultured on media selective for gram-negative bacteria. *Cont* Untreated mice; *Sham/Fed* mice were anesthetized and underwent sham laparotomy and were fed standard chow for 48 h; *Sham/Starv* mice were treated identical to sham/fed, only were given H20 ad libitum for 48 h; *Hep/Fed* underwent a 30% hepatectomy and were fed standard chow for 48 h; *Hep/Starv* underwent 30% hepatectomy and were allowed H20 at libitum for 48 h. Results demonstrate that while starvation alone increased bacterial adherence to the cecal mucosa, the greatest increase in adherence was seen with both hepatectomy and starvation. Only in tissue containing greater than 10^5 cfu/g bacteria were alterations in mucosal electrophysiology demonstrated. This effect was completely abrogated by antibiotic decontamination, suggesting a putative role for bacteria in this response

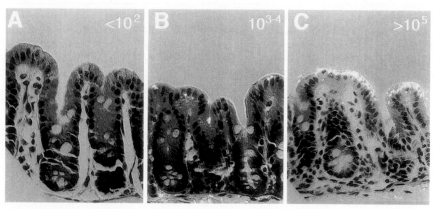

Fig. 4A–C. Bluo-Gal staining of cecal mucosa. Bluo-Gal staining measures β-galactosidase activity in gram-negative bacteria. **A** Tissues with low bacterial counts. As can be seen, gram-negative bacteria are not found to typically adhere to normal mucosal epithelia. **B** Tissues from mice who have 10^{3-4} cfu/g bacteria adherent to the cecal mucosa by culture. **C** Tissues from mice following hepatectomy and starvation in whom greater than 10^5 cfu/g tissue is typically cultured. One can see the density of bacteria is strikingly adherent to the cecal mucosa. These findings illustrate that under normal circumstance, the mucosal epithelium is sterile; however, the combination of stress and starvation results in a dramatic alteration in the host-parasite relationship

It is possible that environmental conditions within the intestinal tract during stress induce virulence genes in bacteria such that they express strategies to harm the host. A large body of in vitro evidence demonstrates that bacteria harvested from media in which the growth conditions have been manipulated can induce pathologic changes in epithelial cells which would not be observed under ideal growth conditions. For example, *Salmonella* grown under low-oxygen conditions can induce cytoskeletal changes in epithelial cells resulting in visible morphologic damage [45]. *E. coli* grown media enriched with norepinephrine express visible adherence appendages whereas in media alone, no such appendages are visible [46]. Bacteria colonized from critically ill patients are more "adherent" both structurally and functionally compared to similar strains from healthy patients [47]. These observations suggest that both the causes and treatment of critical illness may potentiate the virulence of microbes which colonize these patients inasmuch as they affect the usual and customary environment within the intestinal tract.

In the aggregate, the use of agents such as artificial nutrition, exogenous catecholamines, gastric acid reducing agents, and antibiotics, may create a unique environment whereby resistant bacteria predominate and must compete for scarce nutrients and an adequate oxygen supply. A bacterium's sense that the host is stressed and immobile, and man's unavoidable use of these therapies, may force bacteria to induce a virulence repertoire that is both life-threatening to the host and unintentional. The use of nutritional strategies which maintain mucosal immune defense at this most vulnerable time coupled with a better understanding of the induction of these virulence mechanisms, may make the intensive care unit a less hostile environment for both microbe and man.

Acknowledgements. The authors thank Doris Parsons for preparation of the manuscript. Supported by NIH grant no. 5 RO1 GM53439.

References

1. Underdown BJ, Schiff JM, Underdown JM (1986) Immunoglobulin A: strategic defense initiative at the mucosal surface. Ann Rev Immunol 4:389–395
2. Svanborg C (1994) Bacterial adherence and mucosal immunity. In: Ogra PL, Lamm ME, McGhee Jr, Mestecky J, Strober W, Bienenstock J (eds) Handbook of mucosal immunology, Academic Press, Inc., San Diego, pp 71–78
3. Pruitt KM, Rahemtulla B, Rahemtulla F, Russell MW (1999) Innate humoral factors. In: Ogra PL, Mestecky J, Lamm ME, Strober W, Bienenstock J, McGhee JR (eds) Mucosal Immunology, 2nd edn. San Diego, Academic Press, pp 65–88
4. Cone RA (1999) Mucus. In: Ogra PL, Mestecky J, Lamm ME, Strober W, Bienenstock J, McGhee JR (eds) Mucosal Immunology, 2nd edn. San Diego, Academic Press, pp 43–64
5. Lehrer RI, Bevins CL, Ganz T (1999) Defensins and other antimicrobial peptides. In: Ogra PL, Mestecky J, Lamm ME, Strober W, Bienenstock J, McGhee JR (eds) Mucosal Immunology, 2nd edn. San Diego, Academic Press, pp 89–99
6. Lehrer RI, Barton A, Daher KA, Harwig SS, Ganz T, Selsted ME (1989). Interaction of human defensins with *Escherichia coli*. Mechanism of bactericidal activity. J Clin Invest 84:553–561
7. Deitch EA, Winterton J, Ma L, Berg R (1987) The gut as a portal of entry for bacteremia: Role of protein malnutrition. Ann Surg 205:681–692
8. Deitch EA (1988) Does the gut protect or injure patients in the ICU? Perspect Crit Care 1:1–31
9. Purandare S, Offenbartl K, Westrom B, Bengmark S (1989) Increased gut permeability to fluorescein isothiocyanate-dextran after total parenteral nutrition in rat. Scand J Gastroenterol 24:678–82
10. Rothman D, Latham MC, Walker WA (1982) Transport of macromolecules in malnourished animals. I. Evidence of increased uptake of intestinal antigens. Nutr Res 2:467–474
11. Janu P, Li J, Minard G, Kudsk K (1996) Systemic interleukin-6 (IL-6) correlates with intestinal permeability. Surg. Forum 47:7–9
12. Deitch EA (1990) Intestinal permeability is increased in burn patients shortly after injury. Surgery 107:411–416
13. Ziegler TR, Smith RJ, O'Dwyer ST, Demling RH, Wilmore DW (1988) Increased intestinal permeability associated with infection in burn patients. Arch Surg 123:1313–1319
14. Lebman DA, Coffman RL (1994) Cytokines in the mucosal immune system. In: Ogra PL, Lamm ME, McGhee JR, Mestecky J, Strober W, Bienenstock J (eds) Handbook of mucosal immunology. San Diego: Academic Press pp 243–249
15. McGhee JR, Mestecky J, Elson CO, et al. (1989) Regulation of IgA synthesis and immune response by T cells and interleukins. J Clin Immunol 9:175–199
16. Marconi M. Plebani A, Avanzini MA, et al. (1998) IL-10 and IL-4 cooperate to normalize in vitro IgA production in IgA-deficient (IgAD) patients. Clin Exp Immunol 112:528–532
17. Beagley KW, Eldridge JH, Lee F, et al. (1989) Interleukins and IgA synthesis. Human and murine interleukin 6 induce high-rate IgA secretion in IgA-committed B cells. J Exp Med 169:2133–2148
18. McGhee JR, Mestecky J, Dertzbaugh MT, Eldridge JH, Hirasawa M, Kiyono H (1992) The mucosal immune system: From fundamental concepts to vaccine development. Vaccine 10:75–88
19. Li J, Kudsk KA, Gocinski B, Dent D, Glezer J, Langkamp-Henken B (1995) Effects of parenteral and enteral nutrition on gut-associated lymphoid tissue. J Trauma 39:44–52
20. Wu Y, Kudsk KA, DeWitt RC, Tolley EA, Li J (1999) Route and type of nutrition influence IgA-mediated intestinal cytokines. Ann Surg 229:662–668

21. King BK, Li J, Kudsk KA (1997) A temporal study of TPN-induced changes in gut-associated lymphoid tissue and mucosal immunity. Arch Surg 132:1303–1309
22. Alverdy JC, Aoy SE, Moss GS (1988) Total parenteral nutrition promotes bacterial translocation from the gut. Surgery 104:185–190
23. Renegar KB, Small PA Jr (1991) Immunoglobulin A mediation of murine nasal anti-influenza virus immunity. J Virol 65:2146–2148
24. Abraham E (1992) Intranasal immunization with bacterial polysaccharide containing liposomes enhances antigen-specific pulmonary secretory response. Vaccine 10:461–468
25. Kudsk KA, Li J, Renegar KB (1996) Loss of upper respiratory tract immunity with parenteral feeding. Ann Surg 223:629–635
26. King BK, Kudsk KA, Li J, Wu Y, Renegar KB (1998) Route and type of nutrition influence mucosal immunity to bacterial pneumonia.. Ann Surg 229 (2):272–278
27. Janu P, Li J, Renegar KB, Kudsk KA (1997) Recovery of gut associated lymphoid tissue (GALT) and upper respiratory tract (URT) immunity following parenteral nutrition (TPN). Ann Surg 225:707–717
28. Kudsk KA, Croce MA, Fabian TC, et al. (1992) Enteral vs. parenteral feeding: Effects on septic morbidity following blunt and penetrating abdominal trauma. Ann Surg 215:503–513
29. Moore FA, Moore EE, Jones TN, McCroskey BL, Peterson VM (1989) TEN vs. TPN following major abdominal trauma-reduced septic morbidity. J Trauma 29:916–923
30. Souba WW (1991) Glutamine: A key substrate for the splanchnic bed. Ann Rev Nutr 11:285–308
31. Li J, Kudsk KA, Janu P, Renegar KB (1997) Effect of glutamine-enriched TPN on small intestine gut-associated lymphoid tissue (GALT) and upper respiratory tract immunity. Surgery 121:542–49
32. DeWitt RC, Wu Y, Renegar KB, Kudsk KA (1999) Glutamine-enriched total parenteral nutrition preserves respiratory immunity and improves survival to a *Pseudomonas* pneumonia. J Surg Res 84:13–18
33. Ziegler TR, Young LS, Benfell K, Scheltinga M, Hortos K, Bye R, Morrow FD, Jacobs DO, Smith RJ, Antin JH, et al. (1992) Clinical and metabolic efficacy of glutamine-supplemented parenteral nutrition after bone marrow transplantation. A randomized, double-blind, controlled study. Ann Intern Med 116:821–828
34. Li J, Kudsk KA, Hamidian M, Gocinski BL (1995) Bombesin affects mucosal immunity and gut-associated lymphoid tissue in IV-fed mice. Arch Surg 130:1164–1170
35. DeWitt RC, Wu Y, Renegar KB, King BK, Li J, Kudsk KA (1999) Bombesin recovers gut-associated lymphoid tissue (GALT) and preserves immunity to bacterial pneumonia in TPN-fed mice. Ann Surg (In press)
36. Janu P, Kudsk KA, Li J, Renegar KB (1997) Effect of bombesin on impairment of upper respiratory tract immunity induced by total parenteral nutrition. Arch Surg 132:89–93
37. Diamond, Jared (1999) Gun, Germs and Steel. W.W. Norton and Co., NY, NY
38. Wells CL, Jechoredk RP, Maddaus MA, et. al. (1988) The effects of clindamycin and metronidazole on the intestinal colonization and translocation of enterococcus in mice. Aantimicrob Agents and Chemother 32:1769–1771
39. Alverdy JC, Aoys E, Moss GS (1990) Effect of commercially available chemically defined liquid diets on the intestinal microflora and bacterial translocation from the gut. JPEN 14:1–4
40. Guiney DG (1997) Regulation of bacterial virulence gene expression by the host environment. J Clin Invest 99:565–569
41. Eaves-Pyles T, Szabo C, Salzman AL (1999) Bacterial invasion is not required for activation of NF-κB in enterocytes. Infect Immun 67:800–804
42. Spitz JC, Joutsouris A, Blatt C, Alverdy JC, Hecht G (1995) Escherichia coli adherence to intestinal epithelial monolayers diminishes barrier function. Am J Physiol 31:635–639
43. Hendrickson BA, Guo J, Laughlin RJ, Alverdy JC (1998) Increased type 1 fimbrial expression among commensal Escherichia coli in the murine cecum following catabolic stress. Infect Immun 67:745–753

44. Roch F, Laughlin R, Hendrickson B, Alverdy J (1999) Virulence phenotype transformation following stress and starvation. (Submitted)

45. Francis CL, Starnbach MN, Falcow S (1999) Morphological and cytoskeletal changes in epithelial cells occur immediately upon interaction with Salmonella typhimurium grown under low-oxygen conditions. Molec Microb 21:3077–3087

46. Lyte M, Erickson AK, Arulanandam BP, Frank CD, Crawford MA, Francis DH (1997) Norepinephrine induced expression of the K99 pilus adhesin of enterotoxigenic Escherichia coli. Biochem Biophys Res Commun Mar 27;232 (3):682–6

47. Todd TR, Frnaklin A, Mankinen-Irvin P, Niederman M (1989) Augmented bacterial adherence to tracheal epithelial cells is associated with gram-negative pneumonia in an intensive care unit population. Am Rev Respir Dis 140:1586–1592

From Structure to Function: What Should Be Known About Building Blocks of Protein

P. Stehle, K.S. Kuhn, and P. Fürst

Definitions, Classifications

The name protein is derived from the greek word "proteno" – the first. Actually, the philosopher Engels defined life as the living form of protein. Proteins are associated with all forms of life, an observation that dates back to the original identification of proteins as a class by Mulder in 1838. Their importance lies in the fact that proteins are the principal nitrogenous constituents of every cell in the body (half of the dry weight, 90% as enzymes). These proteins are subject to continuous wear and replacement.

The basic structural units of proteins are the amino acids. Most naturally occurring amino acids are of the L-configuration, in turn linked together by peptide bonds. Units of two or three amino acids are called di- or tripeptides. Polymers of less than 100 amino acid residues are named polypeptides. Animal proteins can be devided into two kinds, fibrous and globular. Fibrous proteins are found in the protective and supportive tissues. Keratin is the chief protein of hair, collagen of connective tissue, fibrin of blood clot and myosin in muscle. Globular proteins are found in tissue fluids, e.g. caseinogen in milk, albumin in egg white and albumins and globulins in blood. Plant proteins are not so easily classified but, broadly speaking, most are glutelins or prolamines. Glutelins include glutenin from wheat, hordenin from barley and orzynenin from rice. Typical prolamines are gliadin from wheat and zein from maize.

Amino Acids, the Building Stones of Proteins, and Peptides

In the body, dietary proteins and peptides are broken down (catalyzed by proteolytic enzymes) to amino acids which are characterized by the presence of an amino (NH_2) component and a carboxyl group with basic and acidic properties, respectively. The rest of the molecular structure varies with the particular amino acid. There are 20 s.c. proteic amino acids found in mammalian proteins. Every species of animal has its characteristic proteins. It is the sequence of amino acids in proteins that give each species its specific immunological character and uniqueness.

Dispensable, Indispensable, and Conditionally Indispensable Amino Acids

According to the classical definition from W. Rose, amino acids are devided in *essential* and *non-essential* substrates. It could be shown that an adult human body can maintain nitrogen equilibrium on a mixture of eight pure amino acids as its sole source of nitrogen. Thus, they were called essential: isoleucine, leucine, lysine, methionine, phenylalanine, threonine, tryptophan and valine. For growth in infants, histidine is also needed. All others were thought to be exchangeable and ranked as non-essential.

This traditional classification has to be much modified [1]. On the basis of long-term clinical studies and with the availability of improved analytical technologies it became evident that some clinical conditions are associated with particular amino acid deficiencies, antagonisms or imbalances which then cause specific changes in amino acid metabolism and requirements. Accordingly, amino acids are nowadays classified as indispensable, conditionally indispensable and dispensable substrates:

– Indispensable: isoleucine, leucine, lysine, methionine, phenylalanine, threonine, tryptophan, valine
– Conditionally indispensable: arginine, cyst(e)ine, glutamine, histidine, serine, tyrosine
– Dispensable: alanine, asparagine, aspartic acid, glutamic acid, glycine, proline

This new approach of essentiality recognises functional and physiological properties of a given substrate under various pathological states [2]. Grimble proposes that, regardless of the definition used, a final judgement of the usefulness of an essential new substrate will be on the grounds of clinical and nutritional efficacy. According to a more general position, "a possible and useful direction might put more emphasis on metabolic control and its regulation of tissue and organ function and nutritional status". This definition offers suggestions as to how certain metabolic characteristics shared by some substances might be used to differentiate the various nutritionally significant substrates. This would also mean that the dietary "essentiality" of a given substrate is dependent on the ratio of supply to demand [3].

In the following, functional properties of selected pertinent amino acids will be presented.

Histidine

In the early 1970s, Fürst and Bergström could provide first evidence that histidine might be an indispensable amino acid in uremia [4]. Accordingly, supplementation of tailored intravenous as well as enteral (oral) diets given to uremic patients with histidine resulted in a considerably improved, even positive nitrogen balance [4]. At present, histidine is an integrated component for nutritional therapy in chronic uremia.

Recent studies in normal men showed that long-term histidine-deficient diet (1–8 weeks) led to a significant fall in plasma histidine levels. This observation raised the question as to whether during long term TPN supplementation with histidine might be beneficial.

Serine

In healthy adults, serine can be readily synthesized from glycine and activated formaldehyde. In all clinical situations with impaired kidney function, endogenous synthesis might not cover serine requirements resulting in low extra- and intracellular serine concentrations [5]. These findings suggest that serine may be conditionally indispensable for uremic patients on maintenance hemodialysis. It is, thus, to conclude that serine depletion may be another limiting factor for protein synthesis, thereby contributing to the increased protein requirements in these patients.

Arginine

Parenteral supplementation with arginine as an intermediate metabolite of the urea cycle significantly reduces blood ammonia, and can, thus, counteract a high ammonia load with protein hydrolysates/amino acid solutions [6].

Arginine may also be of significance in the critically ill because of its potential role in immunomodulation [7, 8]. It is hypothesized that arginine enhances the depressed immune response of individuals suffering from injury, surgical trauma, malnutrition or sepsis. In experimental animals as well as in human studies, supplementation with arginine resulted in an improved cellular response, a decrease in trauma-induced reduction in the T-cell function and a higher phagocytosis rate [7]. Innate host cellular cytotoxicity, mediated in part by natural killer (NK) and lymphokine activated killer (LAK) cells, is thought to play an important role in the inhibition of tumor growth and the reduction of metabolic spread. Arginine supplementation has been shown to enhance NK and LAK cytotoxicity (for references see [8]). Interestingly, a daily supply of 30–35 g of arginine is claimed to retard tumor growth and to diminish tumor metastasis [9, 10]. On the other hand, it has been reported that substituting ornithine for arginine in parenteral regimens will ameliorate an arginine-related increase in growth of a Ward colon tumor [11].

When dealing with the parenteral supply of arginine it is also important to note that arginine has a specific drawback in its competition with lysine for tubular reabsorption. Thus, parenteral administration of excessive amounts of arginine may result in lysine deprivation.

It is notable that 5 years ago, parenteral arginine was considered as a novel and valuable tool to improve immunity and to beneficially influence metabolism and pathophysiology in cancer and trauma. Remarkably, in the current literature the intravenous arginine approach is almost absent while great emphasis is laid on enteral arginine nutrition. Presumably, the reportedly highlighted drawbacks and disadvantages with large amounts of parenteral arginine have been slowly recognised and considered. Clinical studies administering arginine enterally have demonstrated moderate net nitrogen retention and protein synthesis compared to isonitrogenous diets in critically ill and injured patients, and following surgery for certain malignancies in elderly postoperative patients supplemental arginine (25 g/day) enhanced T-lymphocyte responses to PHA and Con-A and increased the CD_4 phenotype number. Interestingly, IGF-1 levels were about 50% higher reflecting the growth hormone secretion induced by arginine supplementation. High load of oral arginine (30 g/day) improved wound healing [9] and enhanced blastogenic response to several mitogens [12]. On the other hand, some of these studies were also associated with in vitro evidence of enhanced immunoactivity [7, 13, 14]. However, these results did not demonstrate improvements in overall patient outcome or length of hospital stay [15]. It is probable that the observed beneficial effects of this substrate were due to improved function of the immune system rather than improved gut barrier function; in the largest study clinical benefit in a subgroup of patients was claimed.

Recently, arginine was shown to be the unique substrate for the production of the biological effector molecule nitric oxide (NO). NO is formed by oxidation of one of the two identical terminal guanidino groups of L-arginine by the enzyme nitric oxide synthase (NOS). Of the three NOS isoenzymes characterized, two are constitutive, Ca^{2+} dependent [endothelial (eNOS) and neuronal (nNOS] and generate lesser levels of NO than their inducible counterpart (iNOS) [16]. iNOS is prominent in inflammatory conditions and it is also most often implicated as the producer of NO during immune response. According to recent reports, NO plays an essential role in the regulation of inflammation and immunity. Interestingly, parenteral arginine may improve myocardial ischemia in patients with obstructive coronary artery disease by producing non-stereo-specific peripheral vasodilation thereby improving endothelium-dependent vasodilation. This effect is certainly due to stimulation of insulin dependent NO release or nonenzymatic NO generation [17].

Cyst(e)ine

In healthy adults, the sulphur-containing amino acid cysteine can be synthesized from methionine via the liver-specific transsulphuration pathway. In liver tissue of fetuses and of preterm and term infants, the activity of cystathionase, key enzyme in the transsulphuration pathway, has been found to be low or undetectable [18, 19]. In liver disease, cysteine requirements of the body cannot be covered due to diminished transsulphuration capacity. In all these particular conditions, cyst(e)ine should be exogenously administered [20, 21].

Interestingly, the route of nutrient administration seems also to influence the rate of hepatic cysteine synthesis by altering the delivery of cysteine precursors to the liver. Steginck and coworkers could demonstrate in healthy men that intravenous infusion of solutions containing methionine but no cyst(e)ine resulted in depressed levels of all three forms of circulating cysteine (free cysteine, free and protein-bound cystine) [22]. This result may be interpreted as saying that parenteral solutions should not only contain sufficient methionine but additional amounts of cyst(e)ine. Presumably, such a supplementation with cyst(e)ine may be beneficial also with respect to taurine requirements during long-term TPN.

There are some highly interesting studies elucidating the potential role of sulphur-containing compounds like cyst(e)ine [23]. Macrophages act as cysteine transporters under the action of inflammatory stimuli such as endotoxin and TNF. The uptake of cysteine in macrophages is competitively inhibited by glutamate [24]. During episodes of immunosuppression or in diseases with compromised immunocompetence like AIDS and malignancy, increased extra- and intracellular glutamate concentrations are observed [25].

Cysteine also enhances a number of lymphocyte functions, such as cytotoxic T-cell activity. A high glutamate/cysteine ratio is associated with low share of T-helper cells [26]. N-acetyl-cysteine, reduced glutathione and cysteine inhibit the expression of the nuclear transcription factor in stimulated T-cell lines [27]. This observation might provide an interesting approach in the treatment of viral diseases like AIDS, since the transcription factor is necessary to express the human immunodeficiency virus (HIV) mRNA. In fact, in vitro studies demonstrate that the stimulatory effects on TNF, induced by free radicals, on HIV replication in monocytes can be inhibited by sulphydryl compounds [26]. These basic studies indicate that treatment of inflammatory diseases and AIDS with sulphydryl compounds may be beneficial, and powerful arguments have been advanced in favour of such treatment [26]. Clinical studies using this strategy are not yet available. One reason might be the lack of suitable preparations. The use of N-acetyl-cysteine in humans is not appropriate because of the lack of tissue acylases except in the kidney (vide infra) [28].

Taurine

Taurine (2-aminoethane sulphonic acid) is the most abundant free amine in the intracellular compartment [29]. The major pathway for the biosynthesis of taurine is via cysteine sulphinic acid (CSA). Taurine seems to have a functional role in stabilizing the membrane potential, in bile salt formation, in growth modulation, in osmoregulation, in antioxidation, in promoting calcium transport and calcium-binding to membranes, in vision and in exerting positive ionotropic effect on the heart as well as showing antiarrhytmic and antihypertensive effects. It is involved in many metabolic responses in the central nervous system (CNS), has an anti-convulsant action, may have an insulinogenic action and is required for eye function [30, 31]. Taurine is capable of influencing programmed cell death in a number of cell types depending upon the initiating apoptotic stimulus [32] and Fas (CD95/APO-1)-mediated neutrophil apoptosis via maintenance of calcium homeostatis [33].

There is some evidence that taurine might be indispensable during episodes of catabolic stress and in preterm infants and neonates. Trauma and infections are associated with low extra- and intracellular taurine concentrations after trauma and infection [34, 35]. Low taurine concentrations in plasma, platelets and urine have been described in infants and children and also in adult trauma patients undergoing taurine-free long-term parenteral nutrition [36–38]. Plasma taurine deficiency after intensive chemotherapy and/or radiation is more severe in those patients receiving taurine-free parenteral nutrition than in orally fed patients [39]. Low intracellular taurine concentrations in muscle are a typical feature in patients with chronic renal failure, probably due to impaired metabolic conversion of CSA to taurine [40, 41]. Intracellular taurine depletion might be associated with the well-known muscle fatigue and arrhythmic episodes in uremia.

Taurine offers protection against oxidant damage in experimental lung inflammation [42]. Experimental depletion of tissue taurine concentrations, especially in the lung, produces inflammation; administration of pro-oxidants results in severe lung oedema and interstitial fibrosis. Taurine administration ameliorates the symptoms [43]. The underlying mechanism of taurine action may be due to its interaction with H_2O_2 and Cl^- in the myeloperoxidase reaction thereby producing taurine chloramine, an oxidant with very low reactivity, partially quenching free-radical generation [23, 24].

Tyrosine

The aromatic amino acid tyrosine has been traditionally considered a non-essential amino acid for adult humans. Tyrosine is synthesized exclusively from phenylalanine by hydroxylation; inclusion of tyrosine in the diet exerts a sparing effect on the dietary phenylalanine requirement. However, under certain pathological conditions like classic phenylketonuria, liver and kidney disease, and in premature infants, tyrosine has to be considered a conditionally indispensable amino acid. The indispensability of tyrosine is attributed to severely diminshed activity of liver phenylalanine hydroxylase. In particular cases, a reduced endogenous tyrosine synthesis may also occur in full-term infants and in renal failure [44, 45].

Rudman and coworkers reported that cirrhotic patients receiving a standard TPN exhibited hypotyrosinaemia, hypocystinaemia and hypotaurinaemia [20]. They suggested that this depletion resulted from impaired liver capacity to synthesize these amino acids secondary to the pathology of the disease.

Glutamine

Glutamine is the most prevalent free proteic amino acid in the human body. In skeletal muscle, glutamine constitutes more than 60% (>19.5 mmol/l intracellular water) of the total free amino acid pool [29]. Glutamine acts not only as a precursor for protein synthesis but is also an important intermediate in a large number of metabolic pathways. It is a precursor that donates nitrogen for the synthesis of purines, pyrimidines, nucleotides and amino sugars. Glutamine is the most important substrate for renal ammoniagenesis and, thus, takes part in the regulation of the acid-base balance. As the most abundant amino acid in the blood stream, glutamine serves as nitrogen transporter between various tissues. Owing to its diverse participation in transamination reactions, glutamine can be classified as the true regulator of amino acid homeostasis.

It is well known that glutamine represents an important metabolic fuel for the cells of the gastrointestinal tract (enterocytes, colonocytes) and many rapidly proliferating cells, including those of the immune system (for references see [3]).

In addition, there is much evidence that hypercatabolic and hypermetabolic situations are accompanied by marked depressions in muscle intracellular glutamine. This has been shown to occur after elective operations, major injury,

burns, infections and pancreatitis, irrespective of nutritional attempts at repletion. Reduction of the muscle free glutamine pool (about 50% of normal) thus
appears to be a hallmark of the response to injury, and its extent and duration is
proportional to the severity of the illness [28, 46, 47].

Recent studies underlined that glutamine deprivation is mainly caused by trauma-induced alterations in the interorgan glutamine flow [48]. Muscle and, presumably, lung glutamine efflux are accelerated to provide substrate for the gut,
immune cells, and the kidneys [49, 50] explaining the profound decline in muscle
free glutamine concentration.

Two recent observations suggest that glutamine is involved in the regulation of
muscle protein balance: first, the striking direct correlation between muscle glutamine and the rate of protein synthesis, and secondly, the positive effect of maintaining intracellular glutamine content on protein anabolic processes in vitro [51,
52]. If maintenance of the intracellular glutamine pool promotes conservation of
muscle protein, there is a theoretical case for glutamine supplements in the parenteral nutrition of stressed and malnourished patients. This therapeutic potential is extensively elaborated by Fürst et al. (this volume, page 441).

Metabolism and Requirements of Amino Acids

Amino acids are subjected to series of metabolic reactions which can be catego-
rized in three major groups:
- *Endogenous protein synthesis.* Part of the free amino acid pool is incorporated
  into tissue proteins. The free amino acid pool is fed by dietary protein and
  endogenous protein breakdown.
- *Oxidative decomposition.* This process leads to loss of the carbon skeleton as
  CO_2 or its deposition as glycogen and fat, while the nitrogen is eliminated as
  urea.
- *Synthesis of N-containing metabolites.* Some free amino acids are used for synthesis of purines, pyrimidines, creatine, epinephrine and others. Amino groups
  and carbon skeletons formed during amino acid decomposition are used to
  provide endogenous indispensable amino acids.

The amount of protein synthesized daily depends on the requirements for
growth, for the manufacture of enzymes, for replacement of proteins broken
down in the cell, and for repair mechanisms. The mucosa of the small intestine is
probably renewed every one to 2 days. The red blood cells have each a life time of
about 120 days. Plasma albumin is synthesized at a rate of about 10 g/day and fibrinogen at about 2 g/day. In nutritional practice, deficient synthesis is nearly
always due to inadequacy of the amino acid supply rather than to a failure of synthetic mechanisms.

The minimum requirement for protein in the diet is estimated to yield 0.45 g
protein/kg body weight. Considering individual variations, the average safe
requirement for young adults is defined as 0.6 g/kg body weight. Daily protein
requirements are considerably higher during the first months of life; consequantly,
recommended allowances decreased progressively to the adult level (Table 1). Inter-

estingly, the proportion of total protein needs represented by essential amino acids falls from 43% for infants to 36% for older children and to 19%–20% for adults.

Effects of Stress on Protein Metabolism

The initial stimulus of trauma, injury or infection sets in motion a basic neuroendocrine response, a reflex with an efferent link composed by neural pain, pathways integration at higher central neurons system levels, and both neurologic and endocrine efferent paths. An analysis of this reflex response can be of significant importance in patient care. It has been widely accepted that the autonomic nervous system exerts CNS control over internal homeostasis.

All these alterations in neuroendocrine control mechanisms resulting from stress exert profound changes in protein metabolism. Following an acute injury without a low flow state lean body mass (LBM) is first mobilized and then lost. The major reservoir is skeletal muscle. Superimposed on that are effects of disease of the kidney, liver or intestinal tract. Loss of lean body mass, or more specifically body cell mass (BCM), can result in impaired host defense and increased morbidity and mortality with critical illness. The clinical impressions of muscle loss after injury were placed on a quantitative basis by the early work of Cuthbertson, who reported the increase in resting energy metabolism and the excretion of nitrogen, sulfur, phosphorous and creatinine following leg-bone fracture in man [53]. These observations were extended by subsequent metabolic balance studies which emphasized a negative nitrogen balance as the hallmark of the response to injury and infection [54].

Table 1. Recommended dietary allowances (RDA) of protein intake for healthy individuals (from [59])

Age (years)	Weight (kg)	RDA (g/kg BW)
Both sexes		
0–0.5	6	2.2
0.5–1.0	9	1.6
1–3	13	1.2
4–6	20	1.1
7–10	28	1.0
Males		
11–14	45	1.0
15–18	66	0.9
19–24	72	0.8
25–50	79	0.8
51+	77	0.8
Females		
11–14	46	1.0
15–18	55	0.8
19–24	58	0.8
25–50	63	0.8
51+	65	0.8

BW, body weight.

In severe traumatic conditions like acute renal failure, urinary excretion of nitrogen may reach 35–40 g N per day, the equivalent of more than 1 kg LBM [55]. Efforts made by various investigators to improve the nutrition of acute surgical patients produced conflicting results. According to one opinion, it was not conceivable to expect nitrogen utilization at the height of the catabolic response while others reported that the majority of the post-operative nitrogen loss was due to starvation, rather than being the result of obligatory neuroendocrine responses [56]. Later, it was established that an improved nitrogen balance could be approached in severe catabolic states with increasing nitrogen provision, though the augmented nitrogen loss is not reduced by the nitrogen intake [57]. The patient whose problem is primarily partial starvation can be put into positive N balance with good nutrition support, while the strongly catabolic patient cannot achieve a positive N balance by nutritional means until the peak of the catabolic drive has passed. Kinetic studies indicate that the provision of a protein intake of up to 1.5 g kg^{-1} day^{-1} can improve the N balance but that going above that level of intake merely increases the rate of protein synthesis and breakdown, without improving the nitrogen balance [58].

The extent of changes in protein synthesis and protein breakdown depend on the severity of injury. The slow wasting condition is found in mild injury, malnutrition, cancer, immobilization etc. Rapid wasting occurs after severe injury, burns, and infection. The responses are for the most part well grounded in observations in patients. It is not certain to what extent protein synthesis can rise in injury associated with inflammatory disease.

Protein Quality: Definition and Assessment

Food proteins widely differ in their amino acid composition and in the efficiency with which they are digested and the constituent amino acids are taken up. These factors determine the capacity of a given protein or protein/peptide preparation to provide nitrogen and indispensable amino acids for endogenous protein and metabolite synthesis. This protein quality influences the dietary requirement: the lower the quality, the higher the required protein intake.

There are several methods available to assess protein quality:

- *Amino acid score.* Acid or alkaline protein hydrolysis followed by a chromatographic analysis of the liberated amino acids facilitate a reliable characterization of the amino acid composition. This composition is then compared with the amino acid pattern of a high quality standard protein (generally egg white protein; protein quality=100). The chemical score (value of the limiting indispensable amino acid with the lowest percentage score) can then be used to define protein quality.
- *Biological assays in laboratory animals.* Comparative studies focusing on the effect of different protein sources on growth (e.g. protein efficiency ratio, PER) or nitrogen retention (e.g. net protein utilization, NPR) have been frequently used to predict protein quality. Since the utilization of proteins is partly species-specific, the accurate figures cannot be transferred to humans.

– *Clinical studies.* In vivo studies in healthy adults and/or patients provide the most accurate assessment of protein quality. In general, evaluation is based on nitrogen balance (nitrogen intake minus nitrogen losses in urine, faeces and surface). The main objective is to define how much protein must be fed to achieve equilibrium (zero balance).

Conclusion

Adequate delivery of amino acids in the frame of artificial nutrition is an important measure to support healing and outcome of stressed patients. Certain clinical conditions are accompanied with characteristic alterations in organ specific amino acid metabolism. Because of insufficient endogenous synthesis, some amino acids traditionally classified as non-essential must be ranked as conditionally indispensable and should be part of any nutritional efforts. Apart from their nutritive role as building blocks of proteins, amino acids possess certain "pharmacological" and/or "immunological" effects. Enteral or parenteral supply of tailored amino acid preparations can, thus, be used to modulate the immune response and to support organ function and integrity. As outlined by Fürst et al. (this volume, page 441), the transfer of this basic knowledge into routine clinical practice is an important step to improve the outcome of of seriously ill patients.

References

1. Laidlaw SA and Kopple JD (1987) Newer concepts of the indispensable amino acids. Am J Clin Nutr 46:593–605
2. Grimble GK (1994) The significance of peptides in clinical nutrition. Annu Rev Nutr 14: 419–447
3. Fürst P (1998) Old and new substrates in clinical nutrition. J Nutr 128:789–796
4. Fürst P (1972) 15N-studies in severe renal failure. II. Evidence for the essentiality of histidine. Scand J Clin Lab Invest 30:307–312
5. Bergström J, Alvestrand A and Fürst P (1990) Plasma and muscle free amino acids in maintenance hemodialysis patients without protein malnutrition. Kidney Int 38:108–114
6. Najarian N and Harper AE (1956) A clinical study of the effect of arginine on blood ammonia. Am J Med 21:832–842
7. Kirk SJ and Barbul A (1990) Role of arginine in trauma, sepsis, and immunity. JPEN 14:226S-229 S
8. Evoy D, Lieberman MD, Fahey III TJ and Daly JM (1998) Immunonutrition: The role of Arginine. Nutrition 14:611–617
9. Barbul A (1990) Arginine and immune function. Nutrition 6:53–58
10. Daly JM, Reynolds J, Sigal RK, Shou J and Liberman MD (1990) Effect of dietary protein and amino acids on immune function. Crit Care Med 18:S86-S93
11. Grossie VBJ (1996) Citrulline and arginine increase the growth of the Ward colon tumor in parenterally fed rats. Nutr Cancer 26:91–97
12. Sodeyama M, Gardiner KR, Regan MC, Kirk SJ, Efron G and Barbul A (1993) Sepsis impairs gut amino acid absorption. Am J Surg 165:150–154
13. Brittenden J, Park KG, Heys SD, Ross C, Ashby J, Ah-See A and Eremin O (1994) L-arginine stimulates host defenses in patients with breast cancer. Surgery 115:205–212

14. Beaumier L, Castillo L, Ajami AM and Young VR (1995) Urea cycle intermediate kinetics and nitrate excretion at normal and "therapeutic" intakes of arginine in humans. Am J Physiol 269:E884-E896
15. Lin E, Goncalves JA and Lowry SF (1998) Efficacy of nutritional pharmacology in surgical patients. Curr Opin Clin Nutr Met Care 1:41–50
16. Nathan C and Xie Q (1994) Nitric oxide synthases: rolls, tolls and controls. Cell 78:915–918
17. Quyyumi AA (1998) Does acute improvement of endothelial dysfunction in coronary artery disease improve myocardial ischemia? A double-blind comparison of parenteral D- and L-arginine. J Am Coll Cardiol 32:904–911
18. Gaull G, Sturman JA and Räihä NCR (1972) Development of mammalian sulfur metabolism: absence of cystathionase in human fetal tissues. Pediat Res 6:538–547
19. Zlotkin SH, Bryan MH and Anderson GH (1981) Cystine supplementation to cystine-free intravenous feeding regimens in newborn infants. Am J Clin Nutr 34:914–923
20. Rudman D, Kutner M, Ansley J, Jansen R, Chipponi JX and Bain RP (1981) Hypotyrosinemia, hypocystinemia and failure to retain nitrogen during total parenteral nutrition of cirrhotic patients. Gastroenterol 81:1025–1035
21. Chawla RK, Lewis FW, Kutner M, Bate DM, Roy RGB and Rudman D (1984) Plasma cysteine, cystine, and glutathione in cirrhosis. Gastroenterol 87:770–776
22. Stegink LD and Den Besten L (1972) Synthesis of cysteine from methionine in normal adult subjects: effect of route of alimentation. Science 178:514–516
23. Grimble RF and Grimble GK (1998) Immunonutrition: Role of sulfur amino acids, related amino acids, and polyamines. Nutrition 14:605–610
24. Grimble RF (1994) Nutritional antioxidants and the modulation of inflammation: theory and practice. New Horiz 2:175–185
25. Ollenschläger G, Jansen S, Schindler J, Rasokat H, Schrappe-Bächer M and Roth E (1988) Plasma amino acid pattern of patients with HIV infection. Clin Chem 34:1787–1789
26. Dröge W (1993) Cysteine and glutathione deficiency in AIDS patients: A rationale for the treatment with N-acetyl-cysteine. Pharmacology 46:61–65
27. Mihm S, Ennen J and Pessagra U (1991) Inhibition of HIV-1 replication and NFκB activity by cysteine and cysteine derivatives. AIDS 5:497–503
28. Fürst P (1994) New parenteral substrates in clinical nutrition. Part I. Introduction. New substrates in protein nutrition. Eur J Clin Nutr 48:607–616
29. Bergström J, Fürst P, Noree L-O and Vinnars E (1974) Intracellular free amino acid concentration in human muscle tissue. J Appl Physiol 36:693–697
30. Huxtable RJ (1992) Physiological actions of taurine. Physiol Rev 72:101–163
31. Redmond HP, Stapleton PP, Neary P and Bouchier-Hayes D (1998) Immunonutrition: the role of taurine. Nutrition 14:599–604
32. Wang JH, Redmond HP, Watson RWG, Condron C and Bouchier-Hayes D (1995) Taurine protects against stress gene induced human endothelial cell apoptosis. Br J Surg 82:
33. Neary P, Condron C, Kilbaugh T, Redmond HP and Bouchier-Hayes D (1997) Taurine inhibits fas mediated neutrophil apoptosis. Shock 7:S120
34. Askanazi J, Carpentier YA, Michelsen CB, Elwyn DH, Fürst P, Kantrowitz LR, Gump FE and Kinney JM (1980) Muscle and plasma amino acids following injury. Influence of intercurrent infection. Ann Surg 192:78–85
35. Pathirana C and Grimble RF (1992) Taurine and serine supplementation modulates the metabolic response to tumor necrosis factor α in rats fed a low protein diet. J Nutr 122:1369–1375
36. Geggel HS, Ament ME, Heckenlively JR, Martin DA, Kopple BS and Kopple JD (1985) Nutritional requirement for taurine in patients receiving long-term parenteral nutrition. N Engl J Med 312:142–146
37. Heird WC, Hay W, Helms RA, Storm MC, Kashyap S and Dell RB (1988) Pediatric parenteral amino acid mixture in low birth weight infants. Pediatrics 81:41–50

38. Kopple JD, Vinton NE, Laidlaw SA and Ament ME (1990) Effect of intravenous taurine supplementation on plasma, blood cell, and urine taurine concentrations in adults undergoing long-term parenteral nutrition. Am J Clin Nutr 52:846–853

39. Desai TK, Maliakkal J, Kinzie JL, Ehrinpreis MN, Luk GD and Ceijka J (1992) Taurine deficiency after intensive chemotherapy and/or radiation. Am J Clin Nutr 55:708–711

40. Bergström J, Alvestrand A, Fürst P and Lindholm B (1989) Sulphur amino acids in plasma and muscle in patients with chronic renal failure: evidence for taurine depletion. J Int Med 226:189–194

41. Suliman ME, Anderstam B and Bergström J (1996) Evidence of taurine depletion and accumulation of cysteinesulfinic acid in chronic dialysis patients. Kidney Int 50:1713–1717

42. Banks MA, Porter DW, Martin WG and Castranova V (1992) Taurine protects against oxidant injury to rat alveolar pneumocytes. Adv Exp Med Biol 315:341–354

43. Gordon RE, Heller RF and Heller RF (1992) Taurine protection of lungs in hamster models of oxidant injury: A morphologic time study of paraquat and bleomycin treatment. Adv Exp Med Biol 315:319–328

44. Räihä NCR (1973) Phenylalanine hydroxylase in human liver during development. Pediat Res 7:1–4

45. Alvestrand A, Fürst P and Bergström J (1982) Plasma and muscle free amino acids in uremia: influence of nutrition with amino acids. Clin Nephrol 18:297–305

46. Fürst P (1983) Intracellular muscle free amino acids - their measurement and function. Proc Nutr Soc 42:451–462

47. Fürst P, Pogan K and Stehle P (1997) Glutamine dipeptides in clinical nutrition. Nutrition 13:731–737

48. Souba WW (1991) Glutamine: a key substrate for the splanchnic bed. Annu Rev Nutr 11:285–308

49. Rennie MJ, MacLennan P, Hundal HS, Weryk B, Smith K, Taylor PM, Egan C and Watt PW (1989) Skeletal muscle glutamine transport, intramuscular glutamine concentration, and muscle-protein turnover. Metabolism 38 (suppl 1):47–51

50. Plumley DA, Souba WW and Hautamaki RD (1990) Accelerated lung amino acid release in hyperdynamic septic surgical patients. Arch Surg 125:57–61

51. Rennie MJ, Hundal HS, Babji P, MacLennan P, Taylor PM, Watt PW, Jepson MM and Millward DJ (1986) Characteristics of a glutamine carrier in skeletal muscle have important consequences for nitrogen loss in injury, infection, and chronic disease. Lancet ii:1008–1011

52. MacLennan P, Smith K, Weryk B, Watt PW and Rennie MJ (1988) Inhibition of protein breakdown by glutamine in perfused rat skeletal muscle. FEBS Lett 237:133–136

53. Cuthbertson DP (1931) The distribution of nitrogen and sulphur in the urine during conditions of increased catabolism. Biochem J 25:236–244

54. Cuthbertson DP (1932) Observations on the disturbances of metabolism produced by injury to the limbs. Q J Med 1:223–230

55. Duke JH, Jorgensen SB, Broell JR, Long CL and Kinney JM (1970) Contribution of protein to caloric expenditure following injury. Surgery 68:168–174

56. Moore FD and Brennan MR (1975) Intravenous amino acids. N Engl J Med 293:194–195

57. Shenkin A, Neuhäuser M, Bergström J, Chao L, Vinnars E, Larsson J, Liljedahl S-O, Schildt B and Fürst P (1980) Biochemical changes associated with severe trauma. Am J Clin Nutr 33:2119–2127

58. Shaw JFH and Wolfe RR (1987) Energy and protein metabolism in sepsis and trauma. Aust NZ J Surg 57:41–47

59. FAO/WHO/UNU (1985) Energy and protein requirements. WHO technical report series no 724. Geneva

Fatty Acids, Lipoproteins, and Lipid Emulsions

Y.A. Carpentier and I.E. Dupont

Introduction

In the body, fatty acids are stored essentially as triglycerides in adipose tissues and, to a more limited extent, in the liver and other organs such as skeletal muscles and the heart. While triglycerides stored in adipose tissues are hydrolysed by the hormone-sensitive lipase with a substantial release of free fatty acids into the circulation, fatty acids stored in muscles are locally oxidised.

Phospholids and (free) cholesterol represent the major constituents of cell membranes, and their relative proportion (together with the phospholipid fatty acid pattern) largely determines the physical properties of membranes. Cholesterol is also the precursor for synthesis of steroid and sexual hormones.

Transport of these different lipid components (together with lipid-soluble vitamins) in the circulation is performed by different types of lipoprotein particles, which also contain structural and exchangeable apoproteins.

Acute metabolic conditions, e.g., after an accidental or surgical trauma, markedly affect lipid and lipoprotein metabolism. Changes are characterised by an increased mobilisation of fatty acids from extrahepatic tissues and a higher rate of fat oxidation, but also an increased hepatic recycling into triglycerides and very low density lipoproteins secretion, and (often) an increased clearance of circulating triglycerides. In addition, a marked lowering of plasma low density lipoprotein and high density lipoprotein levels is observed, together with a decrease of phospholipid, cholesterol, and lipid-soluble vitamins.

Structure and Composition of Lipoproteins

Packaging of different lipid constituents into lipoproteins follows simple physical guidelines leading to the formation of discrete micellar particles. Hence the size and structure of the particles relate to the ratio between (relatively) apolar core components – triglycerides and cholesteryl esters- and surface components – phospholipids, free cholesterol and apolipoproteins (Table 1). Of interest, changes in the composition of the constituents may affect physical properties and equilibrium between surface and core components.

Table 1. Structure and composition of human plasma lipoproteins

	Chylomicrons	VLDL	IDL	LDL	HDL$_2$	HDL$_3$
Density (g/ml)	<0.950	<1.006	1.006–1.019	1.019–1.063	1.063–1.125	1.125–1.210
Size (nm)	50–500	30–80	25–30	16–25	9–12	5–9
Protein (%)	1–2	8	18	21	41	55
Phospholipids (%)	6–8	19	24	22	30	23
Free cholesterol (%)	0.8–1.6	6	6	8	5	3
Cholesteryl esters (%)	0.8–1.4	15	23	39	16	12
Triglycerides (%)	86–92	50	29	9	6	6

Triglyceride-Rich Lipoproteins

Chylomicrons

Chylomicrons are the largest lipoproteins (50–500 nm in diameter). They are formed in enterocytes after reesterification of absorbed dietary fatty acids into triglycerides (and phospholipids) and are secreted into intestinal lymphatics [1]. Chylomicrons are normally found in the plasma only after a fat-containing meal. An abnormal accumulation of chylomicrons is observed in types I and V of hyperlipoproteinemia.

About 90% of the chylomicron core mass is triglycerides, the remaining being made up of cholesteryl esters and some fat-soluble vitamins. Nascent chylomicrons contain apoproteins (apo's) B-48, A-I, and A-IV. After entering the circulation via the thoracic duct, they acquire apo E and C's (including apo C-II, which activates lipoprotein lipase), by transfer from HDL [2].

Acquisition of (more) cholesteryl esters, which are transferred from LDL and HDL following a process mediated by cholesteryl ester transfer protein (CETP) [3] together with the hydrolysis of a proportion of chylomicron triglycerides by lipoprotein lipase at the endothelium wall of extrahepatic tissues modify particle composition and lead to the formation of remnants. These particles are principally removed by the liver, mainly through apo E binding to receptors and endocytosis. Chylomicron remnants accumulate in the plasma of patients with hepatic lipase deficiency, with liver diseases, or with abnormal apo E, or else when apo E is masked or displaced.

Very Low Density Lipoproteins

Very low density lipoproteins (VLDL) are released principally from the liver and carry over 90% of plasma triglycerides in fasting conditions [1]. Still, the number of VLDL particles is increased in the postprandial state and largely exceeds that of chylomicrons. VLDL triglycerides are derived from endogenous fatty acids brought to the liver from peripheral tissues or produced in the liver itself, and from exogenous fatty acids present in the triglyceride moiety of chylomicron remnants. Major VLDL apoproteins are apo B-100, C's and E. Hepatic synthesis of triglycerides and VLDL production are stimulated by high intakes of carbohydrates (and alcohol), and by pro-inflammatory cytokines (e.g., TNF-α and interleukin-1). Impaired metabolism of VLDL triglycerides is observed in familial hyperlipoproteinemia II, IV, and V, and in conditions of insulin resistance.

As for chylomicrons, VLDL undergo CETP-mediated exchanges of neutral lipids with LDL and HDL and substantial lipolysis by lipoprotein lipase in peripheral tissues [3]. These processes convert VLDL into partially triglyceride-depleted and cholesteryl ester-enriched particles, with a density between triglyceride-rich and cholesterol-rich lipoproteins.

Intermediate Density Lipoproteins

Intermediate density lipoproteins (IDL) represent an intermediate step in VLDL catabolism [4]. They can either be removed directly by cells or undergo triglyceride lipolysis and be converted to LDL, both processes largely taking place in the liver. IDL are found only in low concentrations in normal subjects. An abnormal accumulation of IDL may be observed when the lipolytic transformation of VLDL into LDL or the uptake of IDL particles by hepatocytes (as observed in type III hyperlipoproteinemia) are impaired. Evidence for strong atherogenic properties of IDL has recently raised concern about early development of atherosclerosis caused by IDL accumulation.

Cholesterol-Rich Lipoproteins

Low Density Lipoproteins

Low-density lipoproteins (LDL) usually carry about 60%–70% of total plasma cholesterol, mainly as cholesteryl esters, which are delivered to tissues with LDL uptake. The same apo B-100 remains on the particle during conversion from VLDL to IDL to LDL. Other apo's, namely apo E, are present on particle surface. LDL particles show substantial heterogeneity with respect to their distribution into subfractions with different size and density range. A high proportion of small dense LDL (phenotype B) is found in ~25% of subjects in western countries and is associated with a markedly increased risk of developing obstructive cardiovascular disease. In addition, apo B-100 may, in some individuals, bind another apolipoprotein called apo (a), to form lipoprotein (a) which is also suggested to raise atherosclerotic risk.

LDL elimination follows different pathways. A majority of particles (~ 75% of LDL) are cleared from plasma through binding to the LDL (or apo B, E) receptor predominantly in hepatocytes [5], while the remainder follows other catabolic pathways [6]. Feedback inhibition of LDL receptors in response to intracellular cholesterol concentration avoids excessive cholesterol deposition. An insufficient number of LDL receptors or impaired recognition of LDL particles lead to plasma accumulation, as observed in type II hyperlipoproteinemia, with early and severe coronaropathy.

LDL have a fairly long half-life (3–5 days) in the circulation and, even in normal conditions, a proportion (20%–30%) of particles is sequestered in non-circulating compartments and is not taken into account by plasma determinations.

Recently, the potential for LDL to undergo peroxidative damage has been suggested to play a key role in the early steps of atherosclerotic lesion formation [6]. Small dense LDL particles are generally more sensitive to oxidative damage than normal sized LDL. Oxidation of LDL is initiated by the peroxidation of polyunsaturated fatty acids contained in phospholipids and cholesteryl esters, and is rapidly followed by alterations of apo B structure [7]. As a consequence, oxidatively modified particles are rapidly engulfed in macrophages of the arterial intima via scavenger receptors, which are not turned down by increased cell cholesterol content. Such uptake of oxidized LDL is cytotoxic for macrophages, transforms them into "foam cells", and induces the release of several mediators including pro-inflammatory cytokines, mitogenic factors and enzymes such as metalloproteinases. This process has important consequences on NO production and other endothelial functions, and on smooth muscle cell proliferation and migration in the intimal space.

Not only chronic but also several acute (e.g., post-operative or post-traumatic, septic, post-myocardial infarct) inflammatory conditions are associated with a marked lowering of plasma LDL concentration likely caused by an enhanced disposal, but the sites of removal and the consequences of this phenomenon have not been deeply evaluated.

High Density Lipoproteins

High density lipoproteins (HDL) originate from four possible sources: (a) a major part is secreted by the liver; (b) they may be formed in the plasma compartment following lipolysis of chylomicrons and release of surface remnants (phospholipids and some apolipoproteins); (c) a smaller fraction of HDL is produced as nascent particles directly released from the intestine; (d) they may originate from direct assembly of free apolipoproteins (mainly apo A-I and E) and phospholipids in interstitial fluids [4].

HDL contain the structural apoprotein A-I, alone or together with apo A-II. In addition, they serve as a reservoir of exchangeable apoproteins such as the apo C's and apo E, which are promptly transferred to triglyceride-rich lipoproteins. In acute conditions, HDL carry a major proportion of serum amyloid A (SAA), an acute phase reactant which acts as an apo.

A number of HDL subpopulations have been described which differ by particle size, composition and metabolic properties. In the circulation, nascent phospholipid-rich HDL are quickly transformed into larger, mature HDL by enrichment with free cholesterol. Subsequently, apo A-I catalyzes the enzyme lecithin:cholesterol acyltransferase (LCAT) to esterify cholesterol in the vascular compartment and cholesteryl esters are incorporated in the lipoprotein core to form HDL_3. HDL_3 largely contribute to neutral lipid exchanges with other lipoproteins, by acting as acceptors of triglycerides and donors of cholesteryl esters. These processes increase particle size (and decrease its density) to convert it in HDL_2, which can then be recycled into HDL_3 after lipolysis of triglycerides and cholesteryl ester by hepatic lipase.

Via these processes, HDL largely participate in the reverse transport of (excess) cholesterol from peripheral tissues to the liver to be excreted into the bile. This largely explains the important contribution of HDL and apo A-I against the development of atherosclerotic lesions, and the increased risk in subjects with low plasma concentration of HDL.

HDL levels are lowered in several acute conditions, particularly in prolonged episodes of severe sepsis. This may be related to other protective roles of HDL including their ability to stabilize prostacyclin, to efficiently bind (and neutralize) endotoxins, and to quench free radicals. In addition, acquisition of SAA by HDL may markedly modify their metabolism and direct them to sites of trauma and infection in order to supply healing wounds and immune cells with cholesterol and phospholipids indispensable for cell multiplication.

Lipoprotein X

In addition to the classical lipoprotein classes, another lipoprotein particle (not normally present in plasma) deserves comment. This abnormal lipoprotein is characterized by an unusually high proportion of phospholipids and free cholesterol and by a low protein content (no apo B, but some apo C and E, as well as albumin). Lipoprotein X (Lp-X) is classically found in plasma of patients with biliary obstruction [9] and familial LCAT deficiency [10] and has also been observed in neonates [11] and adults [12] receiving parenteral nutrition with some fat emulsions. During total parenteral nutrition, the particle arises from phospholipid particles present in large amounts in some 10% emulsions and co-infused with the triglyceride-rich particles (see below). These phospholipids show a high affinity for attracting free cholesterol from the surface of endogenous lipoproteins or from cell membranes to form a lipoprotein particle that is slowly cleared from plasma [12].

Lipid Emulsions

Structure and Composition

Lipid emulsions are composed of two different types of particles. One population consists of triglyceride-rich particles (TGRP), designed on the model of the endogenous chylomicron, with a core made essentially of triglycerides and stabilized by a surface layer made mainly of phospholipids. By comparison to the amount strictly required for stabilizing the triglyceride content, the phospholipid emulsifier is present in relative excess which leads to the formation of a second type of emulsion particles, the liposome-like phospholipid-rich particles (PLRP). When present in large amounts, these liposomal phospholipids can impede lipid and lipoprotein metabolism [13] and also modify the lipid composition of cell membranes [14].

Metabolic Pathways

The intravascular metabolism of emulsion TGRP involves metabolic pathways similar to those followed by chylomicrons [15–17] (Fig. 1). In fact, exogenous TGRP can be used to study particular aspects of chylomicron metabolism, both in vivo and in vitro.

Acquisition of Plasma Apoproteins

In contrast to endogenous chylomicrons, emulsion particles contain no apoprotein. Following their infusion into the circulation, TGRP rapidly acquire selected apoproteins (apo's C-I, C-II and C-III; apo E, and probably apo A-IV), mainly by transfer from the HDL pool [18]. This is the first essential step in the regulation of emulsion metabolism. The composition of both emulsion triglycerides and phospholipids can affect the physical properties of the surface layer which likely influences apoprotein acquisition [19]. On the other hand, plasma apoprotein content may substantially differ between normal subjects and is often markedly altered in patients (e.g., in intensive care, post-trauma, or in patients with severe sepsis). Apo's C-II and C-III play an important role in modulating particle binding to the receptor site of lipoprotein lipase (LPL) and the activation of triglyceride lipolysis by the enzyme. At a later stage, apo E and C-III markedly influence cellular uptake of remnant particles.

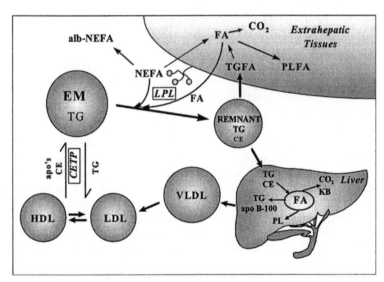

Fig. 1. Metabolism of lipid emulsion particles. The major steps shown on this fig are: acquisition of exchangeable apoproteins (*apo's*) from HDL; exchanges of triglycerides (*TG*) and cholesteryl esters (*CE*) with HDL and LDL, mediated by the cholesteryl ester transfer protein (*CETP*); hydrolysis of a proportion of core TG by lipoprotein lipase (*LPL*); uptake of remodelled remnant particles by the liver and extrahepatic tissues, with intracellular TG hydrolysis and oxidation or recycling of released fatty acids (*FA*). *PL* Phospholipids; *KB* ketone bodies

Intrasvascular Hydrolysis
of Exogenous Triglycerides and Remodeling

After binding of emulsion particles to LPL (namely at the endothelial site of adipose and muscle tissues), a substantial proportion of core triglyceride molecules are hydrolysed and the released esterified fatty acids (Nefas) are either taken by the adjacent tissues or spilled into the circulation. This process largely reduces the size of TGRP. The availability and the activity of LPL mainly depend on the type of tissue and on endogenous factors (e.g., hormonal balance, cytokine concentration, apo C content on emulsion particles). Concomitantly, emulsion particles can serve as donors of triglycerides and acceptors of cholesteryl esters in the CETP-mediated exchange process with cholesterol-rich lipoproteins [20].

These different processes reduce the size of emulsion particles and lead to the formation of remnants depleted of triglycerides and enriched with cholesteryl esters. Until recently, remnant particle uptake has been considered to take place essentially in the liver [21–22]. There is now evidence that uptake of exogenous remnants occurs at an earlier stage than for chylomicron remnants and in several extrahepatic tissues (e.g., in muscle and adipose tissues, probably in endothelial and possibly in intestinal cells).

Removal of Remnant Particles

The removal of exogenous particle remnants can proceed via cell receptors – possibly involving the low density lipoprotein receptor (LDL-R), the LDL-R-related protein (LRP) and the VLDL receptor (VLDL-R) [23–25] – or via nonreceptor-mediated pathways involving surface heparan sulfate proteoglycans (HSPG) and other ligands [26–27].

As a result of these metabolic processes, exogenous FA can be incorporated into several tissues either as Nefas released by LPL lipolysis or as whole triglycerides (or phospholipids) entering cells as components of remnant particles that undergo intracellular lipolysis in cellular lysosomes (Fig.). As mentioned, differences in the composition of lipid emulsions may substantially affect selected metabolic steps (e.g., apo acquisition, CETP-mediated lipid exchanges, LPL lipolysis, remnant clearance). For instance, LPL hydrolysis of emulsions containing a mixture of medium-chain (MCT) and long-chain triglycerides (LCT) promptly releases a major proportion of particle MCFA as Nefas [28]. In contrast, particle endocytosis is probably the dominant pathway for cell uptake of very long (>20 C atoms) polyunsaturated fatty acids (PUFAs), such as arachidonate (C20:4 n-6), eicosapentaenoate or EPA (C20:5 n-3), and docosahexaenoate or DHA (C22:6 n-3), as well as of lipid-soluble vitamins such as alpha-tocopherol [29–30].

Data from our group, obtained during controlled infusions of a physical mixture of MCT and soy LCT together with 10% fish oil, show substantial incorporation of EPA in membrane phospholipids of white blood cells (WBC) and platelets to occur within 5 h, at a time where only little amounts of EPA are present in the plasma Nefas pool and no EPA in plasma phospholipids. This clearly suggests direct uptake of fish oil-enriched remnants, followed by intracellular hydrolysis of fish oil triglycerides and EPA reprocessing into membrane phospholipids, to proceed at a rapid rate in WBC and platelets [31].

Clinical Use of Lipid Emulsions

The major purpose for developing lipid emulsions was to provide an efficient supply of energy and to reduce the load of carbohydrates, particularly in hypermetabolic patients showing variable degrees of insulin resistance. In addition, these preparations are isotonic to plasma, do not influence osmolarity, and may be administered in peripheral veins. Being made of vegetable oils, they have a high content of PUFAs or essential fatty acids (EFA), and can prevent or rapidly correct EFA deficiency which was a common complication of glucose-rich parenteral nutrition. Later, a better understanding of the roles of EFA on several key cell functions and of the balance between n-3 and n-6 EFA, as well as of the importance of a protection against free radical attacks, has led to the development of new preparations. Current views on the mechanisms of action of PUFAs and lipid-soluble antioxidants will be briefly reviewed at the end of this chapter.

The first clinically well-tolerated lipid emulsions were made of soybean or safflower oil (or of a mixture of both), and contained exclusively LCT. Since 1984, an emulsion is marketed with a 1:1 (w:w) blend of MCT and LCT in the particle core. Emulsions made of or supplemented with fish oil (containing n-3 FA), emulsions derived from olive oil and preparations made with structured triglycerides (containing both long- and medium-chain FA on the same glycerol backbone) are currently under evaluation.

Soybean Oil Based Emulsions

By comparison to recommendations for dietary FA intake in general populations (<30% saturated; 30%–40% monounsaturated and ≤30% PUFAs), soybean triglycerides contain a much higher proportion (60%–65%) of PUFAs, namely 52%–54% of linoleic acid (C18:2 n-6).

From a theoretical point of view, this may have important consequences on immune defenses, as well as on inflammatory and thrombotic reactions. However, this topic remains highly controversial when addressed to clinical practice. For instance, no difference in the incidence of bacteremia and fungemia was observed between two groups of parenteral nutrition patients undergoing bone marrow transplantation and infused with a standard dose (25%–30% energy intake) or a low dose (6%–8%) of soybean lipids [32]. In contrast, withholding the soybean derived emulsion from total parenteral nutrition components in trauma patients resulted in decreased morbidity and length of hospitalization, but these effects may be (at least partly) due to lowering caloric intake [33]. Soybean oils also contain a proportion of phytosterols which are normally poorly absorbed by the intestine. Phytosterols can accumulate in patients receiving long-term parenteral nutrition [34] and have been linked with parenteral nutrition associated cholestasis in infants.

Medium-Chain Triglyceride Containing Emulsions

Proven advantages for MCT incorporation into emulsion particles lie in their efficient hydrolysis by LPL and the rapid plasma elimination of derived small sized remnants [35]. In addition, replacing soybean LCT by MCT decreases the supply of PUFAs and the associated requirement for antioxidants. The assumption that MCFA are promptly (and completely) oxidized [36] was not confirmed in a careful study using both indirect calorimetry and isotopic methods for measuring lipid oxidation in critically ill patients receiving MCT/LCT (1:1; w:w) vs. soybean LCT [37]. Still, the possibility remains for MCFA to be preferentially oxidized, sparing higher amounts of EFA for incorporation into cell membranes.

Linseisen et al. [38] reported that the use of MCT/LCT emulsions in traumatized rats could, to some extent, better prevent the atrophy of the small bowel mucosa, submucosa and muscularis than pure soybean LCT, or a physical mixture of trinonanoin and LCT, or SCFA-containing structured triglycerides (C4-L-C4). They suggested this effect to be due to the higher ketone production induced by MCT.

With respect to immunity, the 50% reduction of n-6 FA in MCT/LCT by comparison to pure LCT emulsion was suggested to improve lymphocyte function in AIDS patients [39].

Fish Oil Containing Emulsions

Incorporation of n-3 EFA in membrane phospholipids may decrease the level of cell reactivity to various stimuli. The potential for n-3 FA to prevent cardiac arrhythmias was convincingly demonstrated in series of experiments by Leaf et al. [40] and confirmed in studies relating sudden cardiac death to dietary fish oil intake [41]. This may open new areas for investigation in patients suffering from myocardial infarct or benefiting from coronary revascularization. Of interest, n-3 EFA incorporation in cell membranes also appears to protect tissue microperfusion and to improve the function of grafted organs.

EPA does compete with arachidonic acid for the same enzymatic pathways to produce less inflammatory and non-thrombogenic prostaglandins and thromboxanes, as well as less chemoattractive leukotrienes. These properties may find applications in the treatment of chronic conditions such as inflammatory bowel disease or psoriasis, but also in more acute situations [42]. Intravenous fish oil emulsions are also suggested as a supportive measure for ARDS patients [43], as well as for patients undergoing chemo/radiation therapy [44]. Parenteral fish oil supplementation in the postoperative period reduces LTB4 production in leukocytes in favour of LTB_5 [45]. Concomitantly, n-3 incorporation in membranes was correlated with decreased circulating TNFα levels. Morlion et al. [46] have speculated that lipid emulsions with a n-3 to n-6 FA ratio of 1: 2 would induce the highest LTC_5/LTC_4 ratio and exert the most favorable modulation of lipid mediator synthesis.

Olive Oil Containing Emulsions

A lipid emulsion containing 80% olive oil and 20% soybean oil was recently developed. The rationale was to decrease (to ~ 20%) the PUFA content of soybean emulsions and to replace it with mainly (~ 63%) oleic acid (C18: 1 ω-9). From a theoretical viewpoint, this should also markedly reduce the need for antioxidants. Preliminary studies in normal subjects have shown this preparation to avoid marked changes of FA pattern in cell membrane phospholipids. Recently, Koletzko et al. [47] compared this olive oil based preparation to a soybean oil emulsion during parenteral nutrition in preterm infants and reported higher levels of C18: 3 n-6 and C20: 3 n-6 in plasma phospholipids, suggesting the lower linoleate content to enhance Δ-6 desaturation and the elongation of linoleic acid.

In addition, such new preparations are considered not to affect membrane composition and, therefore, to have little effect on eicosanoid production and immune response [48]. Clinical studies are required to confirm these points.

Mechanisms of Action of Essential Fatty Acids and α-Tocopherol

Essential Fatty Acids

EFA are important components of cell membranes and the balance between n-3 and n-6 EFA markedly affects several key metabolic pathways, namely in relation to inflammatory responses, immune defenses, and cell response to different stimuli. This involves a complex series of actions and interactions at different levels [49–52] (Fig. 2).

Action at the tissue level involves the formation of different series of eicosanoids, produced by the same enzymatic system (namely the cycloxygenase and lipoxygenase) from specific precursors such as di-homo gamma-linolenate (20:3 n-6), arachidonate (20:4 n-6), and eicosapentaenoate (20:5 n-3). Thus, different types of mediators will be produced, depending on the availability of these respective FA in membrane phospholipids. In general, prostaglandins and thromboxanes derived from n-3 EPA have much less inflammatory and thrombotic effects, and leukotrienes less chemoattractive action, than the corresponding eicosanoids derived from arachidonate.

Action at the cellular level involves the presence of respective PUFAs in cell membrane phospholipids. Indeed, PUFAs are building blocks of phospholipids and their concentration influences the physical properties (fluidity, permeability) of the membrane and the access to and function of its receptors, transporters, and enzymes.

Action at the molecular level involves intracellular signaling via the inositol triphosphate pathway and the effect of second messengers on protein kinases, as well as the regulation of gene expression via direct or indirect effects of PUFAs on nuclear transcription factors (such as nuclear factor kappa B [NFκB], peroxisome proliferator-activated receptors, sterol regulatory element binding-proteins, and a nuclear factor specifically induced by PUFAs).

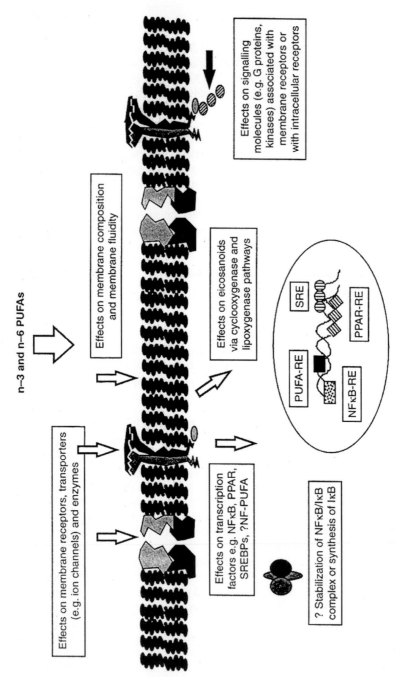

Fig. 2. The diagram shows different possible sites of action for n-3 and n-6 PUFAs, both at the site of extracellular membrane, via signaling molecules, and via effects on various nuclear transcription factors. (From [51])

This explains why PUFAs from the n-6 and n-3 series may sometimes have similar and sometimes opposing effects. Indeed, the effects of a given PUFA (e.g., EPA) may be direct or indirect (e.g., via an improvement of cell antioxidant status by expression of the gene inducing gluthatione production). Hence, the effects may markedly differ between species and cell types, but also between individuals in relation to their genotype and environmental factors.

In addition, the metabolic fate (e.g., oxidation, peroxidation, storage, elongation, incorporation into phospholipids) of administered PUFAs will depend on several factors such as tissue energy requirements, antioxidant status, efficiency of the elongase-desaturase pathway, supply of C18 EFA vs. longer chain derivatives, total calorie intake and associated lipid intake. Indeed, even if supplied primarily as metabolic modulators, a substantial proportion of EFA may "simply" get oxidized.

Antioxidants

Apart from their essential biological roles, PUFAs are highly sensitive to peroxidative stress and require an efficient protection from antioxidants, namely free radical scavengers (Fig. 3). Although antioxidant status in healthy subjects is important to counterbalance the production of free radicals at physiological levels, antioxidant intake remains below the recommended dietary allowances in a substantial proportion of elderly subjects [53]. A majority of hospitalized patients show an imbalance in oxidant/antioxidant status, either because of insufficient

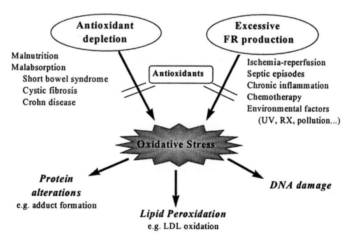

Fig. 3. Role of antioxidants in preventing oxidative stress. Oxidative stress derives from an imbalance between free radical production and antioxidant defenses. This may result from insufficient intake or absorption of antioxidants, or from an excessive production of free radicals, or both. Oxidative damage may affect proteins, lipids and DNA. These processes cause cell injury, apoptosis or death and lead to the development of illness (e.g., cancer, atherosclerosis). Supplementation with antioxidants may help preventing oxidative stress by restoring antioxidant defenses and/or scavenging free radical species

intake resulting from malnutrition or malabsorption, or because of an increased production of free radicals (as in chronic and acute inflammations, ischemia-reperfusion, septic episodes, hemodialysis), or commonly because of both. A number of recent epidemiological are currently performed to determine the beneficial clinical effects of supplementing patients with one or a combination of several antioxidants in the prevention and treatment of both chronic and acute situations.

Among antioxidants, α-tocopherol is a potent liposoluble free radical scavenger and exerts a major protection on lipid components. Due to its amphiphilic structure, α-tocopherol is inserted between phospholipids in cell membranes and in lipoprotein surfaces, where it scavenges free radical species via its phenolic function. This forms a tocopheryl radical which is restored to tocopherol by water-soluble ascorbic acid.

Besides such effect at the level of extracellular membrane, α-tocopherol may inhibit smooth muscle cell proliferation by interacting with protein kinase C [54] and modulate eicosanoid production via inhibition of phospholipase A_2 activity, leading to an inhibition of PGE_2 and a stimulation of PGI_2 production [55]. Recently, an important role was reported for α-tocopherol on nuclear transcription factors, consisting mainly in preventing NF-κB activation while stimulating activated protein-1. This would explain the anti-inflammatory effect of alpha-tocopherol, with a preservation or even an enhancement of cellular immunity [56].

Thus, in addition to radical-scavenging properties, alpha-tocopherol, and possibly other antioxidants may exert important effects on various aspects of cell function and metabolism, which may lead to novel clinical applications [57].

Conclusions

Recent progress in the understanding of factors modulating the metabolism of TG-rich lipoproteins and exogenous particles (TGRP) opens new areas in the targeting of specific compounds (e.g., nutrients, antioxidants, drugs) to specific tissues or cells. For instance, the demonstration that apo E-enriched emulsions are preferentially taken up by liver parenchymal cells rather than by Kupffer cells may represent a major breakthrough in the care of septic patients [58]. In this respect, recent observations suggest not only the composition of particle surface but also that of the triglyceride core to affect the acquisition of specific apoproteins by emulsion TGRP [59].

Major efforts have focused on developing emulsions that will not adversely affect phospholipid FA pattern in cell membranes, or will deliberately incorporate specific FA and/or lipid-soluble vitamins. In this regard, the requirements may widely vary between different types of patients and even in a given patient, throughout his or her clinical course (e.g. with respect to attempts for inhibiting or enhancing the immune response).

References

1. Gotto AM Jr, Pownall HJ, Havel RJ (1986) Introduction to the plasma lipoproteins. Methods in Enzymology 128: 3–41
2. Havel RJ, Kane JP, Kashyap MD (1973) Interchange of plasma lipoproteins between chylomicrons and high density lipoproteins during alimentary lipemia in man. J Clin Invest 52: 32–38
3. Tall AR (1986) Plasma lipid transfer protein. J Lipid Res 27: 361–368
4. Eisenberg S (1984) High density lipoprotein metabolism. J Lipid Res 25: 1017–1058
5. Brown MS, Goldstein JL (1976) Receptor-mediated control of cholesterol metabolism. Science 181: 150
6. Witztum JL, Steinberg D (1991) Role of oxidized low density lipoprotein in atherogenesis. J Clin Invest 88: 1785–1792
7. Jurgens GHF, Hoff GM, Chisolm III, Esterbauer H (1987) Modification of human serum low density lipoprotein by oxidation: characterization and pathophysiological implications. Chem Phys Lipids 45: 315–315
8. Hemhold M, Bigge J, Muche R, Mainoo J, Thiery J, Seidel D, Armstrong VW (1991) Contribution of the apo [a] phenotype to plasma Lp [a] concentrations shows considerable ethnic variations. J Lipid Res 32: 1919–1928
9. Seidel D, Alaupovic R, Furman RH, McConathy WJ (1970) A lipoprotein characterizing obstructive jaundice. II. Isolation and partial characterization of the protein moieties of low density lipoproteins. J Clin Invest 49: 2396–2407
10. Glomset JA, Norum KR, Gjone E Familial lecithin: cholesterol acyltransferase deficiency. In: Stanbury B et al. (eds) The metabolic basis of inherited disease, 5th edn. McGraw-Hill, New-York, pp 643–654
11. Griffin E, Breckenridge WC, Kuksis A, Bryan MH, Angel A (1979) Appearance and characterization of lipoprotein X during continuous Intralipid infusions in the neonate. J Clin Invest 64: 1703–1712
12. Untracht S (1982) Alterations of serum lipoproteins resulting from total parenteral nutrition with Intralipid. Biochim Biophys Acta 711: 176–192
13. Carpentier YA, Richelle M, Bury J, Bihain BE, Olivecrona T, Deckelbaum RJ (1987) Phospholipid excess of fat emulsion slows triglyceride removal and increases lipoprotein remodelling. Arteriosclerosis 7: 541a
14. Haumont D, Deckelbaum RJ, Richelle M, Dahlan W, Coussaert E, Bihain BE, Carpentier YA (1989) Plasma lipid and plasma lipoprotein concentrations in low birth weight infants given parenteral nutrition with twenty or ten percent lipid emulsion. J Pediatr 115 (5): 787
15. Olivecrona G, Olivecrona T (1998) Clearance of artificial triacylglycerol particles. Curr Opin Clin Nutr Metab Care 1: 143
16. Carpentier YA, Dubois DY, Deckelbaum RJ (1996) Plasma Lipoproteins and Intravenous Lipid Emulsions. In: Fischer JE (ed) Nutrition and Metabolism in the Surgical Patient, 2nd edn. Boston-New-York-Toronto-London, Little, Brown and Company, pp 237–265
17. Dupont IE, Carpentier YA (1999) Clinical Use of Lipid Emulsions. Curr Opin Clin Nutr Metab Care 2 (2): 139–145
18. Richelle M, Bury J, Kasry A, Deckelbaum RJ, Carpentier YA (1986) In vitro exchanges of lipids and apoproteins between HDL and exogenous fat. Clin Nutr 5: 55
19. Arimoto I, Saito H, Kawashima Y, Miyajima K, Handa T (1998) Effects of sphingomyelin and cholesterol on lipoprotein lipase-mediated lipolysis in lipid emulsions. J Lipid Res 39: 143
20. Granot E, Deckelbaum RJ, Eisenberg S, Oschry Y, Bengtsson-Olivecrona G (1985) Core modification of human low density lipoprotein by artificial triglyceride emulsion. Biochim Biophys Acta 833: 308
21. Mahley RW, Ji Z-S (1999) Remnant lipoprotein metabolism: key pathways involving cell-surface heparan sulfate proteoglycans and apolipoprotein E. J Lipid Res 40: 1
22. Cooper AD (1997) Hepatic uptake of chylomicron remnants. J Lipid Res 38: 2173

23. Beisigel U, Weber W, Bengtsson-Olivecrona G (1991) Lipoprotein lipase enhances the binding of chylomicrons to low density lipoprotein receptor-related protein. Proc Natl Acad Sci USA 88: 83
24. Niemeier A, Gafvels M, Heeren J, Meyer N, Angelin B, Beisigel U (1996) VLDL receptor mediates the uptake of human chylomicron remnants in vitro. J Lipid Res 37: 1733
25. Schneider WJ, Nimpf J, Bujo H (1997) Novel members of the low density lipoprotein receptor superfamily and their potential roles in lipid metabolism. Curr Opin Lipidol 8: 315
26. Al-Haideri M, Goldberg IJ, Galeano NF, Gleeson A, Vogel T, Gorecki M, Sturley SL, Deckelbaum RJ (1997) HSPG – mediated uptake of apo E – TG rich particles: a major pathway at physiologica particle concentrations. Biochemistry 36: 12766
27. Beisigel U, Heeren J (1997) Lipoprotein lipase (EC 3.1.1.34) targeting of lipoproteins to receptors. Proc Nutr Soc 56: 731
28. Deckelbaum RJ, Hamilton JA, Moser A, Benstsson-Olivecrona G, Butbul E, Carpentier YA, Gutman A, Olivecrona T (1990) Medium-chain versus long-chain triacylglycerol emulsion hydrolysis by lipoprotein lipase and hepatic lipase: implications for the mechanisms of lipase action. Biochemistry 29: 1136
29. Oliveira FLC, Rumsey SC, Schlotzer E, Hansen I, Carpentier YA, Deckelbaum RJ (1997) Triglyceride hydrolysis of soy oil vs fish oil emulsion. JPEN 21 (4): 224
30. Hamberger L, Carpentier YA, Hamilton J, Keyserman F, Hansen I, Schweigelsohn B, Deckelbaum RJ (1998) More efficient clearance of intravenous (I.V.) lipid emulsions containing medium-chain triglycerides (w–3 TG) as compared to traditional long-chain triglyceride (LCT) lipid emulsions in in vitro models and humans. FASEB J 12 (4): A514 (Abst)
31. Siderova VS, Dupont IE, Simoens C, Deckelbaum RJ, Carpentier YA (1998) Early enrichment of WBC and platelets with –3 fatty acids during lipid infusion results from direct FA processing in these cells. Clin Nutr 17 (1): 59 (Abst)
32. Lenssen P, Bruemmer BA, Bowden RA, Gooley T, Aker SN, Mattson D (1998) Intravenous lipid dose and incidence of bacteremia and fungemia in patients undergoing bone marrow transplantation. Am J Clin Nutr 67: 927
33. Battistella FD, Widergren JT, Anderson JT, Siepler JK, Weber JC, MacColl K (1997) A prospective, randomised trial of intravenous fat emulsion administration in trauma victims requiring total parenteral nutrition. J Trauma 43: 52
34. Clayton PT, Bowron A, Mills KA, Massoud A, Casteels M, Milla PJ (1993) Phytosterolemia in children with parenteral nutrition-associated cholestatic liver disease. Gastroenterology 105: 1808
35. Richelle M (1992) Influence of intravenous lipid emulsions on cholesterol homeostasis. Clin Nutr 11: 49
36. Bach A, Babayan VK (1982) Medium chain triglycerides. An update. Am J Clin Nutr 36: 950
37. Delafosse B, Viale J-P, Pachiaudi C, Normand S, Goudable J, Bouffard Y, Annat G, Bertrand O (1997) Long- and medium-chain triglycerides during parenteral nutrition in critically ill patients. J Am Physiol 272 (4): E550
38. Linseisen J, Wolfram G (1997) Efficacy of Different Triglycerides in Total Parenteral Nutrition for Preventing Atrophy of the Gut in Traumatized Rats. JPEN 21 (1): 21
39. Gelas P, Cotte L, Poitevin-Later F, Pichard C, Leverve X, Barnoud D, Leclercq P, Touraine-Moulin F, Trépo C, Boulétreau P (1998) Effect of Parenteral Medium- and Long-Chain Triglycerides on Lymphocyter Subpopulations and Functions in Patients With Acquired Immunodeficiency Syndrome: A Prospective Study. JPEN 22 (2): 67
40. Leaf A, Kang JX, Xiao Y-F, Billman GE (1998) Dietary n-3 fatty acids in the prevention of cardiac arrhythmias. Curr Opin Clin Nutr Metab Care 1: 225
41. Siscovick DS, Raghunathan TE, King I, Weinmann S, Wicklund KG, Albright J (1995) Dietary intake and cell membrane level of long-chain n-3 polyunsaturated fatty acids and the risk of primary cardiac arrest. JAMA 274: 1363
42. Mayer K, Seeger W, Grimminger F (1998) Clinical use of lipids to control inflammatory disease. Curr Opin Clin Nutr Metab Care 1: 179

43. Zadak Z (1997) PUFA n-3 Lipid Emulsion: A Promising Agent in ARDS Treatment. Nutrition 13 (3): 232
44. Tashiro T, Yamamori H, Hayashi N, Sugiura T, Takagi K, Furukawa K, Nakajima N, Itoh I, Wakabayashi T, Ohba S, Akahane N (1998) Effects of a Newly Developed Fat Emulsion Containing Eicosapentaemoic Acid and Docosahexaenoic Acid on Fatty Acid Profiles in Rats. Nutrition 14 (4): 372
45. Morlion BJ, Torwesten E, Lessire H, Sturm G, Peskar BM, Fürst P, Puchstein C (1996) The Effect of Parenteral Fish Oil on Leukocyte Membrane Fatty Acid Composition and Leukotriene-Synthesizing Capacity in Patients With Postoperative Trauma. Metabolism 45 (10): 1208
46. Morlion BJ, Torwesten E, Wrenger K, Puchstein C, Fürst P (1997) What is the optimum -3 to -6 fatty acid (FA) ratio of parenteral lipid emulsions in postoperative trauma ? Clin Nutr 16 (2): 49 (Abst)
47. Koletzko B, Göbel Y, Engelsberger I, Peters J, Zimmermann A, Forget D, Le Brun A, Dutot G (1998) Parenteral feeding of preterm infants with fat emulsions based on soybean and olive oils: effects on plasma phospholipid fatty acids. Clin Nutr 17 (1): 25 (Abst)
48. Yaqoob P, Knapper JA, Webb DH, Williams CM, Newsholme EA, Calder PC (1998) Effect of olive oil on immune function in middle-aged men. Am J Clin Nutr 67: 129
49. Calder P (1998) Dietary fatty acids and lymphocyte functions. Proc Nutr Soc 57: 487–502
50. Grimble RF (1998) Dietary lipids and the inflammatory response. Proc Nutr Soc 57: 535–542
51. Ross JA, Moses AGW, Fearon KCH (1999) The anti-catabolic effects of n-3 fatty acids. Curr Opin Clin Nutr Metab Care 2 (3): 219–226
52. Yaqoob P (1998) Lipids and the immune response. Curr Opin Clin Nutr Metab Care 1 (2): 153–161
53. Posner BM, Jette A, Smigelski C, Miller D, Mitchell P (1994) Nutritional risk in New England elders. J Gerontol 49 (3): M123–32
54. Boscoboinik D, Szewczyk A, Hensey C, Azzi A (1991) Inhibition of Cell Proliferation by - Tocopherol. J Biol Chem 266 (10): 6188–6194
55. Pentland AP, Morrison AR, Jacobs SC, Hruza LL, Hebert JS, Packer L (1992) Tocopherol Analogs Suppress Arachidonic Acid Metabolism via Phospholipase Inhibition. J Biol Chem 267 (22): 15578–15584
56. Traber MG, Packer L (1995) Vitamin E: beyond antioxidant function. Am J Clin Nutr 62: 1501 S – 9S
57. Grimble RF (1997) Effect of antioxidative vitamins on immune function with clinical applications. Int J Vitam Nutr Res 67 (5): 312–20
58. Rensen PCN, van Oosten M, van de Bilt E, van Eck M, Kuiper J, van Berkel TJC (1997) Human recombinant apolipoprotein E redirects lipopolysaccharide from Kupffer cells to liver parenchymal cells in rats in vivo. J Clin Invest 99 (10): 2438
59. Lontie JF, Siderova VS, Deckelbaum RJ, Carpentier YA (1998) Fish oil (FO) incorporation in mixed lipid emulsions affects the ratio between plasma apolipoprotein (APO) C and E concentrations. Clin Nutr 17 (1): 26 (Abst)

Carbohydrate and Fat as Energetic Fuels in Intensive Care Unit Patients

L. Tappy and R. Chioléro

Background

The various clinical conditions which require intensive care lead to a relatively stereotyped metabolic response called the metabolic stress response. It affects the metabolism of the three major nutrients and the whole process of energy metabolism [1, 2]. The metabolic and clinical responses to feeding are also profoundly modified.

Endogenous glucose production increases and allows the continuous release of glucose to meet the requirements of the brain and other glucose utilizing tissues, and the extra requirement of glucose for the glycolytic metabolism of inflammatory and wound tissues (Table 1). Net protein breakdown is stimulated, and the released amino acids will furnish energy and biosynthetic substrates for the immune system and for acute phase protein synthesis, as well as gluconeogenic substrate to glucose producing organs. The liver has usually been considered the sole glucose producing organ under usual conditions, but recent evidence indicates that the kidneys may also contribute substantial amounts of glucose during physiological conditions such as hypoglycemia. Its role in the metabolic stress response remains however completely unknown [3]. Adipose tissue is stimulated to release fatty acid as energy fuels. Lipolysis however exceeds fatty acid oxidation, with the consequence that considerable reesterification of fatty acid occurs in liver cells. This and the inhibition of lipoprotein lipase by stress mediators, lead to a moderate increase in plasma triglyceride concentrations [4]. The overall energy expenditure increases proportionally to the severity of the initial injury, and this thermic effect of illness is in part explained by the metabolic requirements of inflammatory tissues, and in part by other factors, including sympathetic activation, stimulation of energy requiring pathways such as gluconeogenesis and of so-called futile cycles [5–7].

An additional feature of the ICU patients is their inability to feed themselves, either as a consequence of loss of consciousness or of physical impairment, or due to the severe anorexia which occurs as part of the metabolic stress response. The metabolic response to starvation in ICU patients, however, differs from the physiological response to starvation [8] in several important aspects. Stimulation of ketogenesis failed to occur to the same extent as in starved healthy individuals, partly due to high glucose and insulin concentrations in the blood of ICU patients [9–11]. As a consequence, the sparing of endogenous protein normally elicited by ketone bodies failed to occur, and protein catabolism goes on at accelerated rates. No adaptative decreases in energy expenditure take place.

Failure to administer artificial nutrition to ICU patients would therefore lead to accelerated endogenous protein breakdown and favours early multiorgan failure and death secondary to protein wasting. The purpose of artificial nutrition is essentially to prevent such occurrence. How can this be achieved? Nutrients can be administered enterally, or parenterally if the enteral rate is not available. Current policy favours the enteral rate whenever possible for reasons which will not be reviewed here [12]. Energy supply is provided by carbohydrates and fat, in addition to protein or amino acids. The most appropriate nonprotein source of energy in critically ill patients remains yet largely unknown, due to the lack of conclusive studies showing a clear clinical advantage of either substrate. This subject is however complex and several aspects must be considered before taking any conclusion: first and most importantly, the overall clinical effect (survival, complications, infection rate, length of stay, etc.); second, the metabolic effects (protein sparing effect, thermic effect, effects on glucose and fat metabolism; third, the effects on vital organ function (particularly respiratory and liver function, immunity, inflammatory responses and antioxidant status.

In this review, we aim to specifically address the following questions concerning carbohydrate and fat as energy source in critically ill patients. Are the aforementioned aims of artificial nutrition, i.e., suppression of protein catabolism and of glucose production achieved by carbohydrate or fat supply? At which rates of nutrient administration? Do the type of nutrient and the route of administration play a role? Are lipids administered as part of parenteral or enteral nutrition as effective as carbohydrates in achieving the same goals? We will only cover the aspects directly related to energy supply, but not those concerning the effects of fat solutions on immunity, modulation of inflammatory response and antioxidant status).

Table 1. Endogenous glucose production during various metabolic conditions (from [1, 8, 13])

	Endogenous glucose production (g/h)
Healthy subjects	
Short fast	~200 g
Starvation	~100 g
Postprandial	~50 g
Trauma patients	
Fasted	300 g
Fed	>200 g
Burn patients	
Fast	300–500 g

Effects of Carbohydrates on Glucose Production and Protein Catabolism

Carbohydrates have been the sole or the main non-protein respiratory substrate in parenteral nutrition for many years. In healthy individuals, carbohydrate feeding elicits an increase in insulin secretion (Figs. 1, 2). The ensuing hyperinsulinemia, together with hyperglycemia, suppresses glucose production and stimulates splanchnic glucose uptake (essentially by promoting hepatic glycogen synthesis) [13–15]. There is ample evidence that these effects of carbohydrate feeding are markedly impaired in ICU patients. Administration of parenteral glucose solu-

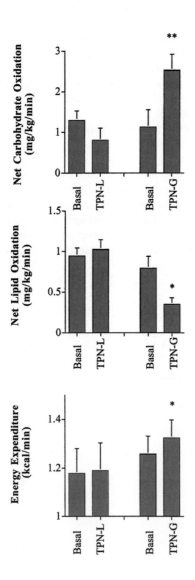

Fig. 1. Effects of isocaloric parenteral nutrition containing 15% (lipid-based total parenteral nutrition, *TPN-L*) or 70% (glucose-based total parenteral nutrition, *TPN-G*) of calories as carbohydrate on substrate oxidation. (From [26] with permission)

tions failed to suppress endogenous glucose production even at high, hyper-caloric doses [16–18]. It also fails to suppress net protein breakdown in severely injured or septic patients and to reestablish an even nitrogen balance unless very large amounts of carbohydrate and exogenous insulin are administered. This appears to be due in part to insulin resistance.

ICU patients display a marked reduction of insulin effects. Part of this insulin resistance can be reproduced by simultaneous infusions of the major hypo-glycemia counterregulatory hormones epinephrine, cortisol, glucagon, and growth hormone [19]. There is however evidence that major stress mediators, such as TNFa, IL-1, IL-2 and IL-6 also contribute to this state of insulin resistance [20]. ICU patients studied during insulin infusion show a decreased whole body glucose utilization. They also show absent or impaired suppression of glucose production, and of net protein breakdown at physiological or mildly supraphysi-ological insulin concentrations. Only pharmacological administration of insulin (resulting in plasma insulin concentrations 3–4 times above the range usually measured in ICU patients) allowed to inhibit glucose production and to restaure nitrogen balance in burn patients [21]. This was observed however during admin-istration of very large amounts of glucose to maintain euglycemia, resulting in positive energy balances. It therefore appears that parenteral carbohydrates are largely inefficient in achieving the goals of nutritional support mentioned above.

Over the past 10 years enteral nutrition has become more and more used for the nutritional support of ICU patients [12]. Enteral carbohydrate administration may have several theoretical advantages over parenteral glucose in metabolic con-trol for several reasons. First, it allows administration of complex carbohydrates, which may have a lower glycemic index [22] and hence produces lower post-pran-dial hyperglycemia. Second, it elicits the release of gastrointestinal glucoincretin GLP1 and GIP which potentialize glucose-induced insulin secretion [23]; and third, they result in portal rather than systemic delivery of glucose. As a conse-quence, portal glycemia is expected to increase, and to better inhibit glucose pro-duction at the level of liver cells [15]. Furthermore, portal glucose delivery acti-vates glucose sensors located within the portal vein which favour hepatic glucose uptake [14]. We therefore recently assessed the effects of continuous isocaloric

Fig. 2. Effects of isocaloric par-enteral nutrition containing 15% or 70% of calories as car-bohydrate on substrate oxida-tion. (From [26] with permis-sion)

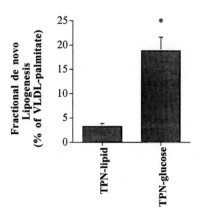

enteral nutrition containing various amounts of carbohydrate in ICU patients. Contrarily to our hypothesis we observed that enteral carbohydrate, like parenteral glucose, failed to inhibit glucose production or to suppress net protein breakdown. Furthermore, first pass splanchnic glucose uptake was measured by a dual isotope method and was observed to be nearly zero in ICU patients, suggesting that the portal signal which normally stimulates splanchnic glucose uptake was absent as a consequence of stress [24]. This study suggests that enteral carbohydrates are not more effective than parenteral glucose to limit endogenous protein losses and to inhibit glucose production.

What is the metabolic fate of glucose in ICU patients? As in normal subjects, a large part of glucose is oxidized in the glucose-dependent organs and in the wound and inflammatory tissues. In non-fed patients, endogenous glucose production largely exceeds net carbohydrate oxidation measured by indirect calorimetry [25]. This observation, however, is difficult to interprete because glucose is mainly produced from gluconeogenesis in such conditions, and therefore oxidation of this newly synthesized glucose will be computed as net protein or lipid (glycerol) oxidation. Tracer experiments nonetheless indicate that a substantial portion of glucose turnover corresponds to glucose-lactate cycling (Cori cycle) and hence to nonoxidative glucose disposal [16, 17]. Following i.v. glucose administration, the respiratory quotient increases in ICU patients, particularly in hypercaloric condition. This was also the case in a recent study performed in our ICU which compared the metabolic effects of various glucose-fat proportions during strict isocaloric conditions [26]. Similar result was however not observed in studies performed in critically ill patients after short glucose administration [27], suggesting that the metabolic adaptation to artificial feeding may be slower in ICU patients. This stimulation of glucose oxidation in ICU patients was also observed using ^{13}C-labeled glucose infusion and monitoring of $^{13}CO_2$ production. It was found to increase with increasing rates of glucose administration, but to plateau at a rate of 4–5 mg/kg/min [18]. This value is in close agreement with the one observed in healthy subjects during graded glucose – insulin infusion and indirect calorimetry [28] and therefore represents probably the maximal rate of glucose oxidation in humans.

Critically ill patients, like normal subjects, are able to efficiently utilize diets varying in their glucose-fat ratio. In ICU patients receiving isocaloric parenteral nutrition with 15% or 75% of calories as glucose, net carbohydrate oxidation assessed using indirect calorimetry was nearly identical with glucose infusion after 72 h, indicating that infused glucose was efficiently used oxidatively [26]. Respiratory quotient did not exceed 1.0, indicating no net fat synthesis. Hepatic de novo lipogenesis was measured in these experiments by means of infusion of 1-^{13}C acetate and monitoring of plasma VLDL-^{13}C palmitate enrichment (Table 2). The precursor pool ^{13}C enrichment was calculated using the mass isotopomer distribution analysis technique [29]. This technique allowed to demonstrate that overfeeding or high carbohydrate isoenergetic diet increased fractional hepatic de novo lipogenesis in healthy subjects, even though no net lipogenesis (i.e., fat synthesis in excess of fat oxidation) occurred [30–32]. In critically ill patients, it was observed that de novo lipogenesis was increased several folds during high carbohydrate parenteral nutrition, and represented about 17% of VLDL triglyc-

Table 2. Hepatic novo lipogenesis (%) in various metabolic conditions (from [26, 29–32] and unpublished data)

Healthy subjects	
Fasted	1–2
Fed	1–5
Overfeeding	15–30
Critically ill patients	
Fast	0–2
High carbohydrate	15–20
Isocaloric feeding	
Low carbohydrate	3–7

erides [26]. Although VLDL production was not monitored, this is however likely to represent only a small amount of glucose converted into fat, well below the rate of oxidation of endogenous lipids [33]. Nonetheless, increased carbohydrate oxidation and stimulation of de novo lipogenesis led to a significant 15% increase in CO_2 production in patients receiving high carbohydrate parenteral nutrition.

We recently repeated these measurements in ICU patients, receiving isocaloric continuous enteral nutrition containing various amounts of carbohydrate and made basically the same observations. Carbohydrate oxidation increased with increasing carbohydrate intake while hepatic de novo lipogenesis was stimulated. Here again, no net de novo lipogenesis was observed (JM Schwarz, data in preparation).

These studies clearly demonstrate the ability of critically ill patients to utilize diets with different glucose-fat proportions. Thus the criticall illness does not seem to abolish the metabolic acaptation required to efficiently use diets with various glucose-fat proportions.

In patients receiving total parenteral nutrition with glucose administration in excess of their energy requirements, stimulation of de novo lipogenesis becomes quantitatively very important and respiratory quotients exceed 1.0, indicating net fat deposition [34]. Recent studies performed in healthy subjects during oral/parenteral nutrition suggest that adipose tissue lipogenesis may be involved during such hypercaloric feeding regimens [35]. In ICU patients, such hypercaloric glucose administration has been shown unequivocally to have potentially serious adverse effects including respiratory failure owing to marked stimulation of CO_2 production rate, and fatty liver disease [34].

Effects of Lipids

Fat is a component of nearly all enteral formulas given to critically ill patients and is often included in TPN solutions. The addition of fat to glucose-protein solutions is claimed to offer many advantages: provision of efficiently utilized energy substrates and of essential fatty acids, high caloric content, low thermic effect, reduction of the carbohydrate supply with consequent decreased respiratory load

[36]. Besides their effect as energy source, lipids influence the phospholipid composition of cell membranes and many cell functions, while modulating prostaglandins and leukotriens synthesis.

Although lipid administration has been routinely used in total parenteral nutrition and enteral nutrition for several years, little is known of their metabolic effects in term of substrate balances! Intravenous lipid emulsions are efficiently cleared from the circulation and do not exceedingly increase plasma triglyceride concentrations [37]. However, it remains largely unknown whether they are directly oxidized as energetic fuels or whether they are temporarily stored in adipose cells. In healthy individuals, it has been shown that lipids added to a mixed meal do not promote fat oxidation [38], and have little effect on the metabolism of the carbohydrate and protein components of the meal. This indicates that exogenous lipids may merely replace endogenous fat as an energetic substrate. In stressed patients, the clearance of intravenous fat is normal or increased, particularly during sepsis [39, 40]. In such patients, fat solution alone have minimal or no significant effect on nitrogen metabolism. However, when combined with amino acids, fat induces significant protein sparing effect [40] although some of this effect can be attributed to the glycerol contained in the lipid solutions [41].

Several studies have assessed the effects of fat: glucose mixture in critically ill patients [27, 42–47]. In patients receiving full parenteral or enteral nutrition, there is no evidence that glucose-amino acids solutions have a better effect on protein metabolism (nitrogen balance and/or whole body protein breakdown and synthesis) than glucose-fat-solutions containing similar amount of energy and nitrogen. Table 3 summarizes the most relevant studies comparing glucose and fat for artificial nutrition in stressed patients in iso- and hypercaloric condition. These data demonstrate that in most citically ill patients part of the glucose can be replaced by fat as energy source without clear metabolic disadvantage. Interestingly, the addition of low to moderate insulin infusion to glucose-based TPN regimen does not seem to improve nitrogen retention [43]. It is only when adding large amount of insulin to hypercaloric glucose solution that muscle nitrogen retention is promoted in severely burned patients [21, 48]. However, it is presently not possible to recommend such hypercaloric glucose-insulin regimen for artificial nutrition in ICU patients, before the clinical beneficial effects and the lack of deleterious systemic effects, like stimulation of hepatic fatty acid synthesis and of the respiratory load, are confirmed by controlled studies. All these data suggest that there is no metabolic reason to avoid reasonable amount of fat (i.e. 20%–30% of non-protein calories) in the artificial feeding of critically ill patients. As far as energy metabolism is concerned, there is no evidence demonstrating a clear advantage for a particular source of fat solutions (i.e. triglyceride containing LCT, MCT/lCT mixture, or ω-3 fatty acids, structured lipids) in stressed patients.

Lipid administration may be associated with unwanted side effects involving mainly pulmonary function, pulmonary circulation, platelet function and immunity. Reversible worsening of gas exchange (increased intrapulmonary shunt, altered oxygenation) and transient aggravation of pulmonary hypertension have been observed in mechanically ventilated patients with ARDS during the infusion of large amount of intravenous fat solution containing LCT [49]. These alterations

Table 3. Glucose vs fat as non-protein energy supply in surgical and critically ill patients: effects on protein metabolism and pulmonary function

Reference	Clinical condition	n	Formula (fat% cal.)	Route of nutrition	Results
Isocaloric nutrition (indirect calorimetry)					
Tappy 1998	Critically ill surgical patients	16	Glucose-fat-AA (10% vs 70%)	Parenteral	Similar N balance. Increased de novo lipogenesis and CO_2 production by high glucose solution
Tappy 1999	Critically ill surgical patients	14	Glucose-fat-proteins (10% vs 57%)	Enteral	Similar N balance. Increased de novo lipogenesis by high glucose solution
Hypercaloric nutrition					
Bark 1976	Postoperative patients	9	Fat-fructose-AA vs glucose-fructose-AA (0 vs 60%)	Parenteral	Similar N balance
Baker 1984	Critically ill patients on mechanical ventilation	20	Glucose-AA vs glucose-fat-AA (0 vs 25; 0 vs 75) (crossover)	Parenteral	Similar protein turnover, synthesis, breakdown and protein balance. Increased CO_2 production by high glucose solution
Shaw 1988	Critically ill surgical patients	81	Isocaloric glucose or fat (short metabolic study)	Parenteral	Similar protein sparing effect (−15% netprotein catabolism)
Al-Saady 1989	Critically ill medical and surgical patients during weaning from mechanical ventilation	20	Glucose-fat-proteins vs Glucose-fat-proteins (30 vs 55%)	Enteral	No metabolic difference. Reduced weaning time (−42%) in the high fat group
Talpers 1992	Critically ill patients on mechanical ventilation	20	Glucose-fat-AA (5 vs 20 vs 40)	Parenteral	Similar N balance and pulmonary CO_2 excretion
de Chalain 1992	Critically ill surgical patients on mechanical ventilation	50	Glucose-AA vs glucose-fat-AA (crossover) (0 vs 50%)	Parenteral	Similar nitrogen balance and protein turnover, synthesis and breakdown
van den Berg 1994	Critically ill medical patients during weaning from mechanical ventilation	32	Glucose-fat-proteins (30 vs 55%)	Enteral	No metabolic difference. Decreased CO_2 production and RQ in the high fat group

were rapidly reversible following the end of infusion. This impairment of respiratory function is yet uncompletely understood. It has been attributed to modulation of pulmonary prostaglandin synthesis induced by fatty acids. More recent studies performed during slow or fast infusions of lipid emulsions have failed to show a direct relationship between alterations in pulmonary function and prostaglandin plasma levels [50]. MCT/lCT emulsions have been shown to exert limited effects on pulmonary gas exchange and seem to offer clinical advantage in patients with severe respiratory failure [51]. Altogether, the pulmonary effects of fat solution are limited and their clinical relevance not important. Nevertheless, it can be recommended to avoid the rapid infusion of large amounts of fat in patients with severe ARDS and compromized oxygenation. The imune function may also be altered by fat solution containg LCT. Reticuloendothelial system dysfunctions (i.e. decreased clearance rate) and depression of phagocytosis function have been described in experimental and human studies related to LCT administration [52, 53]. Increased mortality has been found in septic animals receiving intraveous fat solution containing long chain fatty acids. The clinical relevance of such finding remains yet largely unknown: there is no clear evidence that fat solutions containing long chain fatty acids exert deleterious clinical effects related to their immunodepressive effect in humans. In a prospective study 512 patients with hematological malignacies and bone marrow transplantation were randomized to receive low (6%–8% total energy) vs high dose (25%–30%) LCT solution for TPN [54]. Infection outcome (incidence of bacteremia and fungemia) was not influenced by the feeding regimen. Recent studies suggest that ω-3 fatty acid-containing Lipid emulsions improve immunity and may offer clinical advantages in patients unable to tolerate slight alterations in immunity. Such solutions may also exert beneficial effect in some critically ill patients by modulating the inflammatory response to injury. The clinical value of these new lipid solutions remain however largely unknown.

Conclusions

Both carbohydrates and carbohydrate-fat mixtures administered with proteins or amino acids have been shown to limit nitrogen losses in ICU patients. Carbohydrates and lipids administered orally or parenterally as part of an isocaloric nutrition are efficiently oxidized in ICU patients. Carbohydrate and mixtures of carbohydrate and lipids show similar sparing effects on protein breakdown. Artificial nutrition (parenteral or enteral), however, fails to completely inhibit net endogenous protein breakdown. Carbohydrate administration is also inefficient in suppressing endogenous glucose production and gluconeogenesis unless large amounts of insulin are infused concomitantly. Such insulin infusion, however, requires hypercaloric glucose administration to prevent hypoglycemia and is likely to lead to marked de novo lipogenesis and gross elevation of CO_2 production if administered for extended periods of time. In order to improve the effects of nutrition on nitrogen balance and glucose homeostasy, further studies will be required to determine the mechanisms by which stress interferes with hepatic and extrahepatic glucose metabolism.

References

1. Wilmore DW, Robinson MK (1993) Metabolism and nutritional support. In: Fischer JE and Holmes CR (eds) Surgical Basic Science. Mosby-Year Book, St-Louis, pp 125–169
2. Weissman C (1990) The metabolic response to stress: an overview and update. Anesthesiology 73:308–327
3. Stumvoll M, Meyer C, Mitrakou A, Nadkarni V, Gerich JE (1997) Renal glucose production and utilization: new aspects in humans. Diabetologia 40:749–757
4. Grunfeld C, Feingold KR (1996) Regulation of lipid metabolism by cytokines during host defense. Nutrition 12 (Suppl.):S24-S26
5. Wolfe RR, Herndon DN, Jahoor F, Miyosi H, Wolfe M (1987) Effect of severe burn injury on substrate cycling by glucose and fatty acids. N Engl J Med 317:403–408
6. Breitenstein E, Chioléro R, Jéquier E, Dayer P, Krupp S, Schutz Y (1990) Effects of beta-blockade on energy metabolism following burns. Burns 16:259–264
7. Chioléro R, Revelly JP, Tappy L (1997) Energy metabolism in sepsis and injury. Nutrition 13 (Suppl):45S-51S
8. Owen OE, Tappy L, Mozzoli MA, Smalley KJ (1990) Acute starvation. In: (eds) The Metabolic and Molecular Basis of Acquired Disease. Baillière Tindall, London, pp 550–570
9. Hartl W, Jauch K, Kimming R, Wicklmayr M, Günther B, Heberer G (1988) Minor role of ketone bodies in energy metabolism by skeletal muscle tissue during the postoperative course. Ann Surg 207:95–101
10. Monk D, Plank L, Franch-Arcas G, Finn P, Streat S, Hill G (1996) Sequential changes in the metabolic response in critically injured patients during the first 25 days after blunt trauma. Ann Surg 223:395–405
11. Schwartz MW, Seeley RJ (1997) Neuroendocrine responses to starvation and weight loss. N Engl J Med 336:1802–1811
12. Berger MM, Chioléro RL, Pannatier A, Cayeux MC, Tappy L (1997) A 10-year survey of nutritional support in a surgical ICU: 1986–1995. Nutrition 13:870–877
13. Gerich JE (1993) Control of glycaemia. Baillieres Clin Endocrinol Metab 7:551–586
14. Courtney Moore M, Connolly CC, Cherrington AD (1998) Autoregulation of hepatic glucose production. Eur J Endocrinol 138:240–248
15. Tappy L, Chioléro R, Berger M (1999) Autoregulation of glucose production in health and disease. Curr Opinion Clin Nutr Metab Care 2:161–164
16. Wolfe R, Durkot MJ, Allsop JR, Burke JF (1979) Glucose metabolism in severely burned patients. Metabolism 28:1031–1039
17. Wolfe RR (1979) Burn injury and increased glucose production. J Trauma 19:898–899
18. Wolfe RR (1996) Herman Award Lecture, 1996: relation of metabolic studies to clinical nutrition – the example of burn injufry. Am J Clin Nutr 64:800–808
19. Shamoon H, Hendler R, Sherwin RS (1981) Synergistic interactions among anti-insulin hormones in the pathogenesis of stress hyperglycemia in humans. J Clin Endocrinol Metab 52:1235–1241
20. Beisel WR (1995) Herman Award Lecture, 1995: infection-induced malnutrition – from cholera to cytokines. Am J Clin Nutr 62:813–819
21. Sakurai Y, Aarsland A, Herndon D, et al. (1995) Stimulation of muscle protein synthesis by long-term insulin infusion in severely burned patients. Ann Surg 222:283–294
22. Jenkins DJA, Thomas DM, Wolever TMS, et al. (1981) Glycemic index of foods: a physiological basis for carbohydrate exchange. Am J Clin Nutr 34:362–366
23. Thorens B (1995) Glucagon-like peptide-1 and control of insulin secretion. Diabete Metab 21:311–318
24. Tappy L, Berger M, Schwarz J-M, et al. (1999) Hepatic and peripheral glucose metabolism in intensive care patients receiving continuous high- or low-carbohydrate enteral nutrition. J Parenter Enter Nutr, in press:
25. Tappy L (1995) Regulation of hepatic glucose production in healthy subjects and in NIDDM. Diabete Metab 21:233–240

26. Tappy L, Schwarz JM, Schneiter P. et al. (1998) Effects of isoenergetic glucose-based or lipid-based parenteral nutrition on glucose metabolism, de novo lipogenesis, and respiratory gas exchanges in critically ill patients. Crit Care Med 26:860–867

27. Talpers S, Romberger D, Bunce S, Pingleton S (1992) Nutritionally associated increased carbon dioxide production. Excess total calories vs high proportion of carbohydrate calories. Chest 102:551–555

28. Thiébaud D, Jacot E, DeFronzo RA, Maeder E, Jéquier E, Felber JP (1982) The effect of graded doses of insulin on total glucose uptake, glucose oxidation, and glucose storage in man. Diabetes 31:957–963

29. Hellerstein MK, Christiansen M, Kaempfer S (1991) Measurement of de novo hepatic lipogenesis in humans using stable isotopes. J Clin Invest 87:1841–1852

30. Hudgins LC (1995) Decreased fatty acid synthesis after substitution of dietary starch for sugar. Circulation 92 (Suppl.):1–157

31. Hudgins LC, Hellerstein M, Seidman C, Neese R, Diakun J, Hirsch J (1996) Human fatty acid synthesis is stimulated by a eucaloric low fat, high carbohydrate diet. J Clin Invest 97:2081–2091

32. Schwarz J-M, Neese RA, Turner S, Dare D, Hellerstein MK (1995) Short-term alterations in carbohydrate energy intake in humans. Striking effects on hepatic glucose production, de novo lipogenesis, lipolysis, and whole-body fuel selection. J Clin Invest 96:2735–2743

33. Hellerstein M, Schwarz J, Nees R (1996) Regulation of hepatic de novo lipogenesis in humans. Annu Rev Nutr 16:523–557

34. Elwyn DH, Bursztein S (1993) Carbohydrate metabolism and requirements for nutritional support: Part I. Nutrition 9:50–66

35. Aarsland A, Chinkes D, Wolfe RR (1997) Hepatic and whole-body fat synthesis in humans during carbohydrate overfeeding. Am J Clin Nutr 65:1774–1782

36. Carpentier Y (1993) Are present fat emulsions appropriate? In: Wilmore D and Carpentier Y (eds) Update in intensive care and emergency medicine. Metabolic support of the critically ill patient. Springer-Verlag, Berlin-Heidelberg, pp 157–174

37. Carpentier YA, Simoens C, Siderova V, et al. (1997) Recent developments in lipid emulsions: relevance to intensive care. Nutrition 13) Suppl.):73S-78 S

38. Flatt J, Ravussin E, Acheson K, Jéquier E (1985) Effects of dietary fat on post-prandial substrate oxidation and carbohydrate and fat balance. J Clin Invest 76:1019–1024

39. Druml W, Fischer M, Ratheiser K (1998) Use of intravenous lipids in critically ill patients with sepsis without and with hepatic failure. J Parenter Enter Nutr 22:217–223

40. Wilmore D, Moylan J, Helmkamp G, Pruitt B (1973) Clinical evaluation of a 10% intravenous fat emulsion for parenteral nutrition in thermally injurec patients. Ann Surg 178:503–513

41. Brennan M, Fitzpatrick G, Cohen K, Moore F (1975) Glycerol: Major contributor to the short term protein sparing effect of fat emulsions in normal man. Ann Surg 182:386–394

42. Bark S, Holm I, Hakansson I, Wretlind A (1976) Nitrogen-sparing effect of fat emulsion compared with glucose in the postoperative period. Acta Chir Scand 142:423–427

43. Baker J, Detsky A, Stewart S, Whitwell J, Marliss E, Jeejeebhoy K (1984) Randomized trial of total parenteral nutrition in critically ill patients: metabolic effects of varying glucose-lipid ratios as the energy source. Gastroenterology 87:53–59

44. Shaw J, Holdaway C (1988) Protein-sparing effect of substrate infusion in surgical patients is governed by the clinical state, and not by the individual substrate infused. J Parenter Enter Nutr 12:433–440

45. Al-Saady NM, Blackmore CM, Bennett ED (1989) High fat, low carbohydrate, enteral feeding lowers PaCO2 and reduces the period of ventilation in artificially ventilated patients. Intensive Care Medicine 15:290–295

46. de Chalain T, Michell W, O'Keefe S, Odgen J (1992) The effect of fuel source on aminoacid metabolism in critically ill patients. J Surg Res 52:167–176

47. Van den Berg B, Bogaard J, Hop W (1994) High fat, low carbohydrate, enteral feeding in patients weaning from the ventilator. Intensive Care Med 20:470–475

48. Ferrando A, Chinkes D, Wolf S, Matin S, Herndon D, Wolfe R (1999) A submaximal dose of insulin promotes net skeletal muscle protein synthesis in patients with severe burns. Ann Surg 229:11–18
49. Venus B, Smith R, Patel C, Sandoval E (1989) Hemodynamic and gas exchange alterations during intralipid infusion in patients with adult respiratory distress syndrome. Chest 95:1278–1281
50. Mathru M, Dries D, Zecca A, Faareed J, Rooney M, Rao T (1991) Effect of fast vs slow Intralipid infusion on gas exchange, pulmonary hemodynamics and prostaglandin metabolism. Chest 99:426–429
51. Smirniotis V, Kostopanagiotou G, Vissiliou J, et al. (1998) Long chain versus medium chain lipids in patients on pulmonary haemodynamics and gas exchange. Intensive Care Med 24:1029–1033
52. Sobrado J, Moldaver L, Pomposelli J, et al. (1985) Lipid emulsions and reticuloendothelial system function in healthy and nurned guinea pigs. Am J Clin Nutr 42:855–863
53. Seidner D, Mascioli E, Istfan N, et al. (1989) Effects of long-chain triglycerid emlusion on reticuloendothelial system function in humans. J Parenter Enter Nutr 13:614–619
54. Lensen P, Bruemmer B, Bowden R, Gooley T, Aker S, Mattson D (1998) Intravenous lipid dose and incidence of bacteremia and fungemia in patients undergoing bone marrow transplantation. Am J Clin Nutr 67:927–933

Trace Elements and Vitamins

M.M. Berger and A. Shenkin

Introduction

In recent years there has been a growing interest in trace elements and vitamins. When facing critically ill patients with life-threatening pathologies or multiorgan dysfunction syndrome, spending time considering the requirements for minute substances like trace elements may appear futile. However research in areas such as free radical production and endogenous antioxidants has cast new light on these nutrients. Trace elements are metals and inorganic substances present in nearly undetectable concentrations in biological fluids, whereas vitamins are organic compounds. Both classes of substances together will be referred to as "micronutrients" hereafter. They have no energetic value: if deprived of them, the human body is unable to compensate for their absence, and biochemical and functional alterations develop, which end with severe deficiency states and even with death. The essentiality of these substances has been progressively established. Historically, the importance of vitamins was first demonstrated with the discovery in 1747 of the preventive and therapeutic effects of citrus fruits (vitamin C) on scurvy, and subsequently in 1911 with the property of thiamin in preventing beriberi. It is only in the past 40–50 years, that trace elements like chromium, selenium and zinc have emerged as a new category of essential nutrients. Nowadays, 10 trace elements and 13 vitamins are considered "essential" in human metabolism (Table 1).

Why Consider Trace Elements and Vitamins Together?

Trying to answer this question, a first guess might be "the editors did not have more available space, and asked the reviewer to combine them", which we believe is the wrong answer. The next guess is that "there must be a connection between trace elements and vitamins", which is the right answer. Actually, there are many physiological and biochemical reasons why they should be considered together.

The interactions are already numerous at the intestinal absorption stage and these may interfere with supplementation: vitamin C facilitates iron absorption, zinc interacts with both vitamin A [1] and iron [2], whereas copper, iron and zinc

Table 1. Essential trace elements and vitamins with main functions

Trace elements	Physiologic function	Vitamins	Physiologic function
Copper	Electron transfer, antioxidant: ceruloplasmin, CuZn superoxide dismutase, Synthesis: collagen (component of lysyl oxidase), elastin, catecholamines, melanin, Immunity	A: retinol "anti-infectious"	Immunity, growth, vision, cellular differentiation
Selenium	Antioxidant: glutathione peroxidases, thyroid hormone metabolism: deiodinases, Immunity: neutrophil function	D: Cholecalciferol "anti-rickets"	Calcium and phosphorus homeostasis and metabolism
Zinc	Antioxidant: CuZn superoxide dismutase, Immunity: cellular and humoral, endocrine: insulin, thyroid hormone, etc, Substrate metabolism: most pathways, especially nucleic acid and protein synthesis, neurologic: vision, taste	E: α-tocopherol	Antioxidant, membrane stability
Iron	Oxygen transport: hemoglobin, electron transfer, Immunity: immunoglobulins, muscle metabolism	K: phyloquinone	Coagulation, bone metabolism
Manganese	Cofactor of hydrolases, kinases, carboxylases, transferases, antioxidant: Mn superoxide dismutase	B_1: thiamin "anti-beri-beri"	Carbohydrate metabolism
Molybdenum	Sulfur metabolism: sulfite oxidases, uric acid metabolism: xanthine oxidases	B_2: riboflavin	Krebs cycle, respiratory chain
Chromium	Glucose tolerance factor, Lipid metabolism	B_3: (PP) niacin "anti-pellagra"	Carbohydrate+lipid catabolism, Krebs cycle
Fluoride	Bone and tooth (enamel) metabolism	B_5: pantothenic acid	Carbohydrate, lipid, and amino acid metabolism, Fatty acid synthesis
Iodide	Thyroid function	B_6: pyridoxine	Amino acid metabolism
Cobalt	Structure of vitamin B_{12}	B_8: (H) biotin	Carboxylation: carbohydrate+fatty acid catabolism
		B_9: folic acid	Nucleic acid synthesis, Monocarbon metabolism, homocysteine metabolism
		B_{12}: cobalamin "anti pernicious anemia"	Methyl transfer+isomerisation (eg methionin synthesis)
		C: ascorbic acid "antiscurvy"	Antioxidant, hydroxylation: collagen+carnitine+neurotransmitter synthesis. xenobiotic catabolism

compete for a common transporter (metallothionein), and free iron may affect chromium availability [3].

There are also interactions regarding availability occurring in the total parenteral nutrition (TPN) solutions: vitamin C can reduce copper from the cupric to the cuprous form which may affect utilization, whilst at the same time vitamin C is oxidized [4]. Precipitation of copper in TPN mixtures has frequently been described: this precipitation is enhanced by the addition of multi-vitamin solutions [3]. Many other complex stability problems regarding micronutrients have been reported.

During the free radical scavenging process, endogenous antioxidants depend on each other for regeneration, forming an antioxidant spiral. Indeed vitamin C, vitamin E, glutathione, and NADP are oxidized and regain activity after reduction. This has been well demonstrated in the interaction of vitamins C and E, selenium, zinc and copper to provide protection against ill-placed iron, which otherwise would cause free radical production and damage [5]. Similarly, selenium and tocopherol have long been reported to be linked, without the nature of this interaction being understood. The role of selenium in the prevention of the vitamin E dependent liver necrosis was established 40 years ago [6]. It has been discovered that animal thioredoxin reductase recycles both dehydroascorbate and ascorbyl free radical to ascorbate. Because ascorbate can recycle tocopheryl radical to tocopherol in vitro, this establishes a plausible, but still hypothetical, biochemical link between selenium and vitamin E through ascorbate [7].

For all those reasons it becomes obvious that, except in cases of proven isolated deficiency, micronutrients must be provided in combination. When added to TPN, these combinations require thorough testing. Delivering one single isolated micronutrient, or increasing strongly the amount of one of them, may introduce further disturbances into the whole system.

Micronutrient Status Assessment and the Acute-Phase Response

How should the status of a specific patient be determined? Blood level determination is the most common approach for physicians, and is usually the most accessible. In the critically ill patient, trace element and vitamin plasma levels, when available, are very difficult to interpret due to the strong impact of the systemic inflammatory response syndrome (SIRS), and of the accompanying acute phase response (APR).

SIRS with fever, tachycardia, tachypnea and leukocytosis, is indeed invariably present in the critically ill as a non-specific response to stress, injury or infection [8]. The acute phase response, in a narrow sense, refers to changes in plasma protein concentrations, that are associated with this response, and which result in part from the alterations in protein synthesis at the hepatic level [9]. C-reactive protein (CRP) is always increased during the APR, and is a good indicator of the intensity of the response. Similarly, certain metal binding proteins are also affected (Table 2), ferritin and ceruloplasmin tending to increase. On the other hand the cytokine-mediated redistribution of various proteins from the intravascular space into interstitial space, causes a lowering of protein-bound micronutrients in

Table 2. Typical changes in plasma micronutrient and carrier protein concentrations during the acute phase response (from [10])

Trace elements	Change	Vitamins	Change
Fe, Se, Zn	↓	Vitamin C	↓↓
Cu,	↑	Vitamin B1 (transketolase activity)	↓
Metal-binding proteins		Vitamin B6	↓
Albumin (Zn)	↓↓	Vitamin A	↓
Prealbumin (thyroxine: I)	↓	Vitamin E	↓
Ceruloplasmin (Cu)	↑	Vitamin D	↓
Ferritin (Fe)	↑		
Haptoglobin	↑	Vitamin-binding proteins	
Hemopexin	↓	Retinol binding protein (vit A)	↓
Transferrin	↓	LDL (vit E)	↓
Mn superoxide dismutase	↓		

plasma, independently of dietary nutrient supply. Albumin circulating levels are always depressed, with a concomitant fall in serum zinc. The reasons for these changes may be related to the property of some metal binding proteins to function as free radical scavengers. Copper and iron are trace elements which may be strongly pro-oxidant: limiting the free-fraction is hence a critical issue for the body. Accordingly, the APR induces changes in dynamics of many trace elements, particularly iron, copper, selenium and zinc [10], and causes redistribution of zinc and iron into the liver, where they are bound to metallothionein and ferritin respectively (Table 2). The APR also causes changes in dynamics of certain vitamins. A decrease in leukocyte and plasma vitamin C, and in plasma vitamin A, E and pyridoxine-5-phosphate levels is a systematic finding, causing difficulty in assessing status of those vitamins, and their requirements during APR [11].

Factors Affecting Micronutrient Status

Micronutrient status is affected by intakes (prior to or during illness), losses of biological fluids, metabolic rate, and increased oxidative stress: all these factors are modified by acute illness. The 10th edition of the US recommended daily allowances (RDA) provides recommendations for 26 nutrients including the micronutrients [12]. The RDAs are designed to cover the requirements of the general population considering broad categories like adults, children, adolescents, or pregnant women, but not individuals. Recently new concepts have emerged regarding the micronutrient requirements. The new paradigm expands the basis of RDAs beyond the simple prevention of deficiency states to include the prevention of chronic diseases like cardiovascular diseases and cancer [13], or even preventing biochemical alterations [14]. Moreover a large body of evidence is accumulating, indicating that the provision of certain micronutrients to the general population in the typical diet is probably insufficient to maintain optimal functions [15]. The changes are due to decreased micronutrient content of modern foods [15] and to changes in the eating habits, resulting in frequent borderline status in the healthy population [16]. The status may evolve into subclinical deficiency, which can be defined as a condition with depleted reserves or localized tissue deficiencies without the classical clinical signs of deficiency.

These changes in micronutrient status are of concern, since many acute and chronic diseases are either caused by an absolute or relative excess of free radical production, or at least are aggravated by it [17]. Micronutrients contribute heavily to antioxidant defense, which is strongly challenged during critical illness. During the acute phase response, the production of cytokines and oxidant molecules is part of a highly effective defense mechanism against pathogens [18]. Reactive oxygen species (ROS) enhance pro-inflammatory cytokine production. The nuclear transcription factor kappa B (NF-kB), which is now identified as a key mediator of the inflammatory response [19], is activated by cytokines, bacterial or viral products and ROS. Its activation is influenced by the redox status of the cells, and can be inhibited by a variety of antioxidants, and especially by metal chelators or –SH chelating molecules. The endogenous antioxidants involved in this modulation are glutathione, vitamins C and E, and antioxidant enzymes, like catalase, superoxide dismutases, and glutathione peroxidases, all of which are trace elements dependent.

Some categories of acute diseases, like sepsis [20], acute respiratory distress syndrome (ARDS) [21, 22], asthma, renal failure [23], major burns [24], major trauma, and brain injury [25] involve excessive production of free radicals like O_2^-, H_2O_2 and HOCl [17], at the same time as endogenous antioxidants have been observed to be depressed. Reoxygenation injury (ischemia/reperfusion injuries, post-ischemic reperfusion brain damage [26]) hypoxia, hyperoxia, and shock syndromes involve abnormal oxidation of substrates or changes in oxygen concentrations favoring lipid peroxidation. An increased free radical production contributes to the imbalance in endogenous antioxidant capacity, and to extension of primary lesions.

In addition to increased requirements related to hypermetabolism, tissue repair and to increased oxidative stress, micronutrient availability is frequently modified in the critically ill patient by (a) low intestinal absorption (altered gastrointestinal motility, short gut, ischemia, damage to the mucosa), and (b) elevated digestive losses (nasogastric aspiration, fistula, diarrhea). Further losses from "abnormal" sites are frequent due to renal replacement therapies, exudates in burns, and drains. Among patients with increased losses, burns patients have been shown to suffer significant trace element deficiencies involving predominantly copper, iron, selenium and zinc. The deficiencies are mainly explained by acute negative balances, due to extensive cutaneous exudative losses [27, 28], and to a lesser extent by urinary losses. Trauma patients also have negative selenium and zinc balances [29]. Patients on renal replacement therapy have large losses, status of vitamins A, E, C, iron, selenium and zinc being altered during chronic hemodialysis, and in critically ill patients on continuous renal replacement therapy [23, 30, 31]. Moreover many critically ill patients are dependent on artificial nutritional support, and hence on the adequacy of micronutrient prescription.

Micronutrients at Risk in the ICU

Some patients start with deficiency states, or borderline status prior to their acute illness affecting one or several micronutrients [16]. Many critically ill are hypermetabolic, and have increased nutritional requirements. Such patients will need higher levels of micronutrients, as cofactors for the metabolism of macronutrients. Further, as noted above, some categories of critically ill are at particularly high risk of developing deficiency, due to large losses of biological fluids.

Copper

Copper deficiency appears to be a particular problem of burn patients [27], where the role of copper in wound healing and antioxidant defense appears especially important. The main functions of copper are summarized in Table 1. In other categories of critically ill patients, copper deficiency is generally not a problem.

Iron

The iron requirements in the critically ill are debated. Critically ill patients often exhibit anemia and iron depletion due to frequent hemorrhagic episodes, but also due to the inflammatory response and to insufficient nutritional intakes during prolonged ICU stays [32]. More concern however comes from elevated circulating iron levels due to the infectious and oxidative risks associated with free-iron. Such changes have been documented in patients with ARDS, who compared with non-ARDS patients, exhibit complex changes in iron-oxidizing, iron-binding and free radical scavenging proteins, which reduce their phospholipid membrane protection capacity [33].

The observed reduction in iron availability, by diversion of labile plasma iron and other labile intracellular iron into a storage form, might be of particular benefit during the acute phase response, as iron is required for the growth of microorganisms [9]. Moreover the reduction of iron availability may reduce the conversion of superoxide radical to free hydroxyl radicals, thus reducing the oxidative damage to membranes. Healthy subjects have no free iron in plasma: it is all bound to iron binding proteins. When transferrin iron levels decrease below normal, pathogens have increasing difficulty surviving in hosts [34]. A study of 15 critically ill patients in septic shock showed no iron overload (no detectable free iron, with low transferrin levels and close to normal iron saturation of transferrin) [35]. Host responses occur to withhold iron more securely from potential pathogens. A few studies have shown that iron supplementation may worsen outcome of infection. It is therefore important not to alter these defense mechanisms by inappropriate iron administration. This questions the form of iron provision. Free-iron admixture to parenteral nutrition increases the likelihood of free radical formation: the dextran formulation appears safe and is devoid of lipid peroxide formation [36].

Selenium

Critically ill patients rapidly develop strongly depressed plasma selenium levels [37], which are associated with increased urinary losses, and low glutathione peroxidase activity. Some categories of patients have proven deficiencies: burns [28], trauma [29], patients on hemodialysis [23], and septic patients [38]. Considering the central role of selenium in antioxidant defense, the issue of subclinical deficiency in the critically ill should probably be addressed more systematically.

Zinc

Depletion is frequent in cases of inflammatory bowel disease, especially in presence of fistulae. In addition hypermetabolism causes increased urinary losses. Burn patients also suffer deficiency from cutaneous losses [27] and trauma patients from various drains and urine [29]. In brain injured patients early provision of zinc in amounts 2–3 times the RDA improves the neurological outcome [39].

Vitamin B Group

These are cofactors of intermediary metabolism, and as such are required for the utilization of carbohydrates and amino acids. Consequently during the hypermetabolic response their requirements increase. Thiamin (vitamin B1) status is markedly altered in the critically ill [40]: low plasma activity is associated with poor outcome, and in rare cases, to the poorly recognized Shoshin beriberi with cardiac failure and severe lactic acidosis. Deficiencies in thiamin, riboflavin, nicotinic acid and vitamin C have long been described in burn patients [41].

Vitamin C

Recent evidence based on data from a depletion-repletion study in healthy subjects suggests that the RDA for vitamin C should possibly be increased to 200 mg per day [42]. In critically ill, the requirement is greater, plasma ascorbic levels in ICU patients being markedly below reference ranges despite provision of more than 200 mg vitamin C per day [43]. In burned animals, early large ascorbic acid supplements reduce the amounts of fluid required for resuscitation [44]. As vitamin C is involved in collagen synthesis, requirements are further increased when there is a need for wound healing.

Vitamin E

This chain-breaking lipid-soluble antioxidant protects membranes from lipid peroxidation. Patients with ARDS exhibit very low alpha-tocopherol levels [21].

Lipid peroxidation mediated by ROS has been proposed to be one of the major mechanisms of secondary damage in traumatic brain injury. Animal models show that micronutrients have a protective effect on the extension of brain injury: early alpha-tocopherol supplements or alpha-tocopherol combined with ascorbic acid reduces the level of lipid peroxides in the brain [45, 46].

During TPN, unsaturated fatty acids are prone to peroxidation. This reaction occurs also during storage of the lipid emulsions. The emulsions with the highest ω-3 polyunsaturated fatty acids have the highest lipid peroxide contents. Alpha-tocopherol supplements can prevent this reaction, the inhibition of peroxidation being concentration dependent [47]. The vitamin E content of the different commercial lipid emulsions is variable, and many authors propose to increase their tocopherol content.

Micronutrients and Immunity

Alterations of copper, selenium and zinc status, will affect the entire immune system, reducing the lymphocyte and neutrophil activity, as well as antibody production. Subclinical deficiency is consequently of particular importance to immunity. There is accumulating evidence both in healthy elderly subjects and in institutionalized elderly patients of the beneficial effects of long-term micronutrient supplements on immunity. Such supplements result in a significant reduction in the number of infectious episodes per year [48, 49]. The quantities used in these studies were slightly above RDAs.

Among the critically ill, major burns are characterized by strongly depressed neutrophil activity. Early intravenous supplements of copper, selenium and zinc are associated with increases in total neutrophil counts and a significant reduction of pulmonary infectious complications [50].

Some of the positive effects observed with commercial immuno-modulatory diets like Impact (Novartis), Immun-Aid (McGaw), or Perative (Abbott) might be partly ascribed to major increases in micronutrient content of these solutions (especially selenium, zinc, vitamin, E, and vitamin C), and not only to the changes in glutamine, arginine or ω3-fatty acids. This hypothesis has not yet been investigated, but clearly deserves some attention.

What Are the Requirements in the Critically Ill?

In the absence of a clinically obvious deficiency state in a critically ill patient, blood levels only provide a limited guidance to the diagnosis of deficiency due to SIRS, and are little help in deciding how much should be provided. Moreover the analyzes are expensive, may take excessive time, and require a high quality specialized clinical chemistry laboratory. The estimation of the quantities to provide will therefore be clinical in most cases. Nonetheless, it might be suggested from our research based on balance studies [27–29], that in presence of elevated CRP levels, plasma selenium below 0.6 µmol/l (or any value associated with low glutathione peroxidase activity), plasma zinc below 8 µmol/l, and any low plasma copper level, reflects depletion. Such conditions justify provision of supplements larger than standard recommendations. In burns intravenous supplementation with quantities of trace elements, matched to compensate the exudative losses, restores serum concentrations to some extent, as well as related enzymatic activities [32, 50]: the quantities of copper, selenium and zinc used in this study were 4–7 times the usually recommended parenteral intakes. There is rarely a case to provide increased inorganic iron to the critically ill, and blood transfusion should not be used for nutritional purposes considering the associated risks [51]. Table 3 provides a summary of parenteral recommendations for the general patient [10] and of proposed micronutrient supplements in the critically ill.

When patients require TPN, all micronutrients have to be provided: multi-trace element and multi-vitamin preparations are commercially available for that purpose. Surveys show that the standard supplements are forgotten in close to a third of TPN cases [52]. Moreover, individual requirements vary greatly as a result of acute or chronic depletion of their intakes and because of acute losses during their hospital stay. As the micronutrient content of commercially available supplements are based upon expert committee recommendations, being designed to meet the requirements of most patients, while avoiding toxicity, it is not surprising that there have been numerous reports of deficiencies [3].

When patients are on enteral nutrition, the intravenous micronutrient supplements are generally reduced or stopped. This practice is highly debatable in the critically ill. Indeed the micronutrient contents of most enteral preparations are calculated to cover the "normal" requirements with the delivery of 2000 kcal per day. The worry is that, delivery of an adequate amount of enteral nutrients is difficult in the critically ill. Generally about 75% of the prescription is really provided to the patient [53]. This means that there is a real danger of delivering insufficient levels not only of energy but also of micronutrients. Further these patients may not be able to absorb the nutrients provided (see above). There is growing evidence of deficiency states occurring under enteral nutrition [54, 55].

Timing of the Supplementation

Micronutrients, and trace elements in particular, remain the Cinderella of nutrition. Although considered an essential part of parenteral nutrition [56], micronutrients are frequently not mentioned in nutrition guidelines [57]. It is therefore not surprising the timing of their introduction is generally not specified. When provided as part of artificial nutrition, the amounts delivered to the patient may not even reach the current recommendations (especially with enteral feeding), which themselves may be considered as too low for most critically ill.

There are three main ways to consider micronutrient supplements:
- To wait for a deficiency state to develop and to provide isolated elements to compensate this deficiency. This is a "negative approach", since before an obvious micronutrient deficiency occurs, biochemical alterations have long taken place. Moreover, micronutrient deficiencies are rarely recognized in the ICU.
- The "conservative attitude" is to consider provision of micronutrients as part of complete nutrition, whether enteral or parenteral, and to prescribe them at

Table 3. Recommended parenteral requirements for micronutrients "at risk" during acute illness and proposed supplements for any ICU patients and for special critically ill categories (*RE* retinol equivalent, *TE* α-tocopherol equivalent)

Micronutrient	IV requirement Weight	Molar (μmol)	Proposed supplements IV for any ICU patient	Proposed supplements for special categories
Copper	0.3–1.3 mg	5–20	1.3 mg	3.75 mg burns 2 mg biliary fistulae
Selenium	30–60 μg	0.4–0.8	100 μg also for renal replacement	375 μg burns 500 μg pancreatitis, brain injury
Zinc	3.2–6.5 mg	50–100	10 mg	40 mg burns 15 mg brain injury, hepatic failure, renal replacement therapy, organ transplant 15–30 mg enteric fistulae, diarrhea
Iron	1.2 mg	20	1.2 mg Best provided as dextran form	
Chromium	10–20 μg	0.2–0.4	20–30 μg	30–40 μg diabetes mellitus, glucose intolerance, enteric fistulae
Vitamin C	100 mg		250–500 mg	≥1000 mg burns, organ transplant
Vitamin B1	3 mg		250 mg during the first 2–3 days, then 100 mg during the acute stress	300 mg chronic alcoholism
Vitamin A	1000 μgRE			2000 μgRE wound healing
Vitamin E	10 mgTE		50 mgTE	100–200 mgTE: burns, ARDS, organ transplant, brain injury (?)

the same time as the macronutrients. But, as there is no proven benefit of early nutrition in most categories of critically ill patients, with the exception of trauma and burn patients, micronutrient provision is delayed until initiation of complete nutritional support. Although malnutrition reduces the ability to produce cytokines, high levels of nutrient intakes are associated with increased mortality in both animals and humans, whereas hypocaloric feeding for a limited period of time appears to avoid such complications [58]. Indeed, anorexia is a major feature of the response to sepsis and inflammation, and is probably best respected for a few days in most categories of patients. An adequate micronutrient intake is therefore unlikely during hypocaloric feeding.

- The "positive approach" is to attempt to prevent the occurrence of micronutrient depletion [14]. Supplementation trials have shown that early provision of large amounts of trace elements improve recovery after major burns and brain injury [39, 50]. In major burns trace elements and vitamins provided during the first hours after admission, and continued for 1–2 weeks appears effective in improving immunity and reducing oxidative damage [50]. In animals, large vitamin C supplements reduce the fluid resuscitation requirements in burns [44]. Recently an animal study on mild and severe brain injury showed that lipid peroxidation is increased by the severity of trauma, and that early α-tocopherol supplements have a protective effect against oxygen free radical-mediated lipid peroxidation [46].

In summary, animal and human evidence shows that very early provision (i.e. within the first 24 h) of micronutrients independently of nutrition is probably beneficial in highly stressed patients. Initiating the provision of micronutrients during the next 48 h in categories of patients with intermediate stress to avoid the development of the deficiencies observed after 2–3 days for vitamin B, vitamin C and selenium appears logical. The duration of the supplementation should probably extend to the entire period of acute illness. Considering the uncertainty regarding nutrient absorption in the critically ill, the intravenous route is the most effective way to ensure adequate micronutrient intake during the early phase of acute disease.

Conclusion

Considering the available evidence, we can conclude that critically ill patients generally have increased micronutrient requirements. Some micronutrients such as selenium, zinc, vitamin C and vitamin E, have a particularly strong role in antioxidant defense. Thiamin should also be specially considered, due to the elevated risk of deficiency. All micronutrients should be provided along with those mentioned above in amounts greater than generally recommended, to ensure metabolic requirements are met and to maintain essential functions, such as the immune system. The early provision of supplements to critically ill patients, before the introduction of artificial nutrition, appears reasonable as antioxidant support, and requires further investigation.

References

1. Christian P, West Jr KP. Interactions between zinc and vitamin A – An update. Am J Clin Nutr 1998; 68 (2 Suppl):435S-441 S
2. Whittaker P. Iron and zinc interactions in humans. Am J Clin Nutr 1998; 68 (2 Suppl):442S-446 S
3. Hardy G, Reilly C. Technical aspects of trace element supplementation. Curr Opin Clin Nutr Metab Care 1999; 2:277–285
4. Allwood MC. Factors affecting the stability of ascorbic acid in total parenteral nutrition infusions. J Clin Hosp Pharm 1984; 9:75–85
5. Willson RL. Vitamin, selenium, zinc and copper interactions in free radical protection against ill-placed iron. Proc Nutr Soc 1987; 46:27–34
6. Schwarz K, Foltz CM. Selenium as an integral part of factor 3 against dietary necrotic liver degeneration. J Am Chem Soc, 1957, 79: 3292–3
7. Burk RF, Hill KE. Orphan selenoproteins. BioEssays 1999; 21:231–237
8. American College of Chest Physicians/Society of Critical Care Medicine Consensus Conference: Definitions for sepsis and organ failure and guidelines for the use of innovative therapies in sepsis. Crit Care Med 1992; 20:864–874
9. Pannen BHJ, Robothan JL. The acute-phase response. New Horizons 1995; 3:183–197
10. Shenkin A. Trace elements and inflammatory response: implications for nutritional support. Nutrition 1995; 11:100–105
11. Louw JA, Werbeck A, Louw ME, Kotze TJ, Cooper R, Labadarios D. Blood vitamin concentrations during the acute-phase response. Crit Care Med 1992; 20:934–941
12. Subcommittee on the 10th edition on RDAs. Recommended Dietary Allowances, 10th ed. Washington DC: National Academy Press, 1989
13. Mertz W. Essential trace metals – New definitions based on new paradigms. Nutr Rev 1993; 51:287–295
14. King J. The need to consider functional endpoints in defining nutrient requirements. Am J Clin Nutr 1996; 63:S 983-S 984
15. Rayman MP. Dietary selenium: time to act. Br Med J 1997; 314:387–388
16. Hercberg S, Preziosi P, Galan P, Deheeger M, Papoz L, Dupin H. Apports nutritionnels d'un échantillon représentatif de la population du Val-de-Marne: III. les apports en minéraux et vitamines. Rev Epidém Santé Publ 1991; 39:245–261
17. Gutteridge JMC. Free radicals in disease processes – A compilation of cause and consequence – Invited review. Free Radical Res Commun 1993; 19:141–158
18. Grimble RF. Nutritional modulation of cytokine biology. Nutrition 1998; 14:634–640
19. Christman JW, Lancaster LH, Blackwell TS. Nuclear factor kB: a pivotal role in the systemic inflammatory response syndrome and new target for therapy. Intensive Care Med 1998; 24:1131–1138
20. Leff JA, Parsons PE, Day CE, et al. Serum antioxidants as predictors of adult respiratory distress syndrome in patients with sepsis. Lancet 1993; 341:777–780
21. Richard C, Lemonnier F, Thibault M, Couturier M, Auzepy P. Vitamin E deficiency and lipoperoxidation during adult respiratory distress syndrome. Crit Care Med 1990; 18:4–9
22. Taylor CG, McCutchon TL, Boermans HJ, DiSilvestro RA, Bray TM. Comparison of Zn and vitamin E for protection against hyperoxia-induced lung damage. Free Radical Biology and Medicine 1997; 22:543–550
23. Richard MJ, Ducros V, Foret M, et al. Reversal of selenium and zinc deficiencies in chronic hemodialysis patients by intravenous sodium selenite and zinc gluconate supplementation – Time-course of glutathione peroxidase repletion and lipid peroxidation decrease. Biol Tr Elem Res 1993; 39:149–159
24. Demling RH, Picard L, Campbell C, Lalonde C. Relationship of burn-induced lung lipid peroxidation on the degree of injury after smoke inhalation and body burn. Crit Care Med 1993; 21:1935–1943

25. Hall ED, Braughler JM. Central nervous system trauma and stroke, II: physiological and pharmacological evidence for involvement of oxygen radicals and lipid peroxidation. Free Rad Biol Med 1989; 6:303–313

26. Vanella A, DiGiacomo C, Sorrenti V, et al. Free radical scavenger depletion in post-ischemic reperfusion brain damage. Neurochem Res 1993; 18:1337–1340

27. Berger MM, Cavadini C, Bart A, et al. Cutaneous zinc and copper losses in burns. Burns 1992; 18:373–380

28. Berger MM, Cavadini C, Bart A, et al. Selenium losses in 10 burned patients. Clinical Nutrition 1992; 11:75–82

29. Berger MM, Cavadini C, Chioléro R, Dirren H. Copper, selenium, and zinc status and balances after major trauma. J Trauma 1996; 40:103–109

30. Story DA, Ronco C, Bellomo R. Trace element and vitamin concentrations and losses in critically ill patients treated with continuous venovenous hemofiltration. Crit Care Med 1999; 27:220–223

31. Peuchant E, Carbonneau MA, Dubourg L, et al. Lipoperoxidation in plasma and red blood cells of patients undergoing haemodialysis – Vitamins A, E, and iron status. Free Radical Biol Med 1994; 16:339–346

32. Berger MM, Cavadini C, Chioléro R, Guinchard S, Krupp S, Dirren H. Influence of large intakes of trace elements on recovery after major burns. Nutrition 1994; 10:327–334

33. Gutteridge JMC, Quinlan GJ, Mumby S, Heth A, Evans TW. Primary plasma antioxidant in adult respiratoy distress syndrome patients: changes in iron-oxidising, iron-binding, and free radical-scavengin proteins. J Lab Clin Invest 1994; 124:263–273

34. Weinberg ED. Editorial: Is bleomycin-detectable iron present in the plasma of patients with septic shock? Intensive Care Med 1997; 23:613–614

35. Mumby S, Maragrson M, Quinlan GJ, Evans TW, Gutteridge JMC. Is bleomycin-detectable iron present in the plasma of patients with septic shock? Intensive Care Med 1997; 23:635–639

36. Lavoie JC, Chessex P. Bound iron admixture prevents the spontaneous generation of peroxides in total parenteral nutrition solutions. J Pediatr Gastroenterol Nutri 1997; 25:307–311

37. Hawker FH, Stewart PM, Snitch PJ. Effects of acute illness on selenium homeostasis. Crit Care Med 1990; 18:442–446

38. Forceville X, Vitoux D, Gauzit R, Combes A, Lahilaire P, Chappuis P. Selenium, systemic immune response syndrome, sepsis, and outcome in critically ill patients. Crit Care Med 1998; 26:1536–1544

39. Young B, Ott L, Kasarskis E, et al. Zinc supplementation is associated with improved neurologic recovery rate and visceral protein levels of patients with severe closed head injury. J Neurotrauma 1996; 13:25–34

40. Cruickshank AM, Telfer ABM, Shenkin A. Thiamine deficiency in the critically ill. Intensive Care Med 1988; 14:384–387

41. Lund CC, Levenson SM, Green RW, et al. Ascorbic acid, thiamine, riboflavin and nicotinic acid in relation to acute burns in man. Arch Surg 1946; 55:557–583

42. Levine M, Conry-Cantilena C, Wang Y, al. et. Vitamin C pharmacokinetics in healthy volunteers: evidence for a recommended daily allowance. Proc Natl Acad Sci 1996; 93:3704–3709

43. Schorah CJ, Downing C, Piripitsi A, et al. Total vitamin C, ascorbic acid, and dehydroascorbic acid concentrations in plasma of critically ill patients. Am J Clin Nutr 1996; 63:760–765

44. Tanaka H, Matsuda H, Shimazaki S, Hanumadass M, Matsuda T. Reduced resuscitation fluid volume for second-degree burns with delayed initiation of ascorbic acid therapy. Arch Surg 1997; 132:158–161

45. Bano S, Parihar MS. Reduction of lipid peroxidation in different brain regions by a combination of alpha-tocopherol and ascorbic acid. J Neural Transm 1997; 104:1277–1286

46. Inci S, Ozcan OE, Kilinc K. Time-level relationship for lipid peroxidation and the protective effect of alpha-tocopherol in experimental mild and severe brain injury. Neurosurgery 1998; 43:330–335

47. Wu GH, Jarstrand C, Nordenström J. Phagocyte-induced lipid peroxidation of different intravenous fat emulsions and counteractive effect of vitamin E. Nutrition 1999; 15:359–364
48. Chandra RK. Effect of vitamin and trace-element supplementation on immune responses and infection in elderly subjects. Lancet 1992; 340:1124–1127
49. Girodon F, Galan P, Monget AL, et al. Impact of trace elements and vitamin supplementation on immunity and infections in institutionalized elderly patients – A randomized controlled trial. Arch Intern Med 1999; 159:748–754
50. Berger MM, Spertini F, Shenkin A, et al. Trace element supplementation modulates pulmonary infection rates after major burns: a double blind, placebo controlled trial. Am J Clin Nutr 1998; 68:365–371
51. Hébert PC, Blajchman MA, Marshall J, et al. A multicenter, randomized, controlled clinical trial of transfusion requirements in critical care. New Engl J Med 1999; 340:409–417
52. Kyle U, Jetzer G, Schwarz G, Pichard C. Utilization of total parenteral nutrition (TPN) in a university hospital: a prospective quality control study in 180 patients. Clinical Nutrition 1997; 17 (suppl 1):48
53. Berger MM, Chioléro RL, Pannatier A, Cayeux C, Tappy L. A ten year survey of nutritional support in a surgical ICU: 1986–1995. Nutrition 1997; 13:870–877
54. Camblor M, DeLaCuerda C, Breton I, Perezrus G, Alvarez S, Garcia P. Copper deficiency with pancytopenia due to enteral nutrition through jejunostomy. Clin Nutr 1997; 16:129–131
55. Yagi M, Tani T, Hashimoto T, et al. Four cases of selenium deficiency in post-operative long-term enteral nutrition. Nutrition 1996; 12:40–44
56. Shils ME, Burke AW, Greene HL, Jeejeebhoy KN, Prasad AS, Sandstead HH. Guidelines for essential trace element preparations for parenteral use. JAMA 1979; 241:2051–2054
57. ASPEN, Directors Board of. Guidelines for the use of parenteral and enteral nutrition in adult and pediatric patients. JPEN 1993; 17:1SA-51SA
58. Zaloga GP, Roberts P. Permissive underfeeding. New Horizons 1994; 2:257–263

Antioxidants in Critical Illness

M. Borhani and W.S. Helton

Introduction

Oxygen free radicals (OFR) are unstable oxygen derivatives capable of causing oxidative damage. They are produced primarily in physiologic and pathophysiologic pathways and secondarily by a variety of insults. Their actions are tightly controlled and limited by antioxidant defense mechanisms. Disturbances in oxidative balance resulting from increased OFR production or deficiencies in antioxidant defenses produce a disease state of oxidative stress in which OFR damage cellular constituents. This initiates a cascade of events that stimulates an inflammatory response by direct and indirect means. Conversely, inflammation promotes oxidation. Each process amplifies the other resulting in progressive local and systemic injury. These pathways may play a causative role in critical illnesses in which a systemic inflammatory response is a central feature. Such conditions include sepsis, adult respiratory distress syndrome (ARDS), burns and trauma. Preventing the initiation or controlling the progression of the harmful oxidative state may ameliorate or reverse the progression of disease in critically ill patients. Therapeutic approaches include inhibition of OFR production and enhancement of antioxidant defenses. Numerous strategies have been described. These approaches are in their infancy and results to date are mixed due to numerous limitations. However, several approaches show promise.

In this chapter we will review the physiology of OFR, mechanisms by which the oxidative state contributes to critical illness, potential therapeutic interventions and their limitations, and promising approaches. While not exhaustive, this review will provide the reader with an overview of the current state of oxidative stress in critical illness and recommendations for therapy based on available data.

Background

Chemistry

Oxygen free radicals (OFR) are highly reactive compounds derived from molecular oxygen and include superoxide anions (O_2^-·, hydrogen peroxide (H_2O_2), hydroxyl radicals (OH·) and singlet molecular oxygen ($^1O_2$). Like all free radicals, OFR are molecules with one or more unpaired electrons in their outer orbital shells. As a result, they are unstable and react with other molecules that serve as electron donors to pair the unpaired electrons, thus creating more stable, reduced molecules. However, this removal of electrons (oxidation) renders the donor molecules free radicals, as they now have unpaired electrons that can subsequently react with other molecules. In this way, a single free radical can initiate a chain of reactions.

Physiology

OFR Generation

OFR are produced during both physiologic and pathophysiologic conditions. OFR are formed during normal physiologic processes such as cellular respiration, arachidonic acid metabolism and inflammatory defense mechanisms [1]. Leakage of electrons from the electron transport chain or incomplete reduction of oxygen during oxidative phosphorylation generates superoxide anions. OFR are also produced during oxidative arachidonic acid metabolism driven by cyclo-oxygenase enzymes such as COX-1 and COX-2. Macrophages and neutrophils use the enzyme complex NADPH-oxidase to generate superoxide, peroxide and hypochlorous acid as antibacterial agents. Neutrophils also produce nitric oxide, another free radical that reacts with superoxide to form peroxynitrite which decomposes to the hydroxyl anion [2]. Transitional metal ions such as iron and copper contain unpaired electrons and readily participate of OFR formation. They also catalyze the conversion of OFR to the more unstable hydroxyl anion.

OFR are generated as part of the ischemia-reperfusion phenomenon. Ischemia stimulates endothelial cells to produce xanthine oxidase which catalyzes superoxide formation following reperfusion [3]. Xanthine oxidase is also produced in endothelial cells in response to endotoxin, cytokines, neutrophil adherence and acidosis [4].

Numerous exogenous agents secondarily generate OFR through their metabolism or tissue toxic effects. Such agents include medications, drugs, toxins, ethanol, tobacco and radiation. Acetaminophen is metabolized in the liver to a free radical intermediate. The pulmonary toxicity of bleomycin and cardiac toxicity of adriamycin are due to redox cycling of their metabolites [5]. Ethanol increases oxidation and decreases antioxidant defenses [6]. Tobacco contains potent nicotine-derived carcinogens that are bioactivated to form OFR metabolites by lipoxygenases and other endogenous enzymes. These oxidative effects of alcohol and tobacco not only contribute to their acute toxicities but may represent their mechanism of carcinogenesis. Tissue oxidation is thought to be the predominant toxicity associated with gamma-radiation.

OFR Defenses

In health, OFR production and consumption are balanced (Fig. 1). OFR are produced in small quantities and their activity is limited by host defense mechanisms. These defenses include enzymes that catalyze OFR metabolism, compounds with direct and indirect antioxidant properties and the sequestration of transitional metal ions.

Antioxidant enzymes include glutathione peroxidase, superoxide dismutase (SOD) and catalase. Glutathione peroxidase catalyzes the reduction of peroxide to water by oxidizing glutathione (GSH). Oxidized glutathione (GSSG) is re-reduced to GSH by glutathione reductase. Superoxide dismutase catalyzes the conversion of superoxide to peroxide. Peroxide is converted to water by catalase. These enzymes require trace metal cofactors selenium, zinc, manganese and iron.

Compounds with antioxidant properties include OFR scavengers. These are electron donors that are preferentially oxidized to neutralize OFR. The resultant oxidized forms of these scavengers are relatively unreactive and do not propagate a chain of redox reactions. Such compounds, termed "chain breaking" antioxidants, include vitamins C, E, A and β carotene [7]. Vitamin C (ascorbic acid) is a water-soluble antioxidant capable of scavenging neutrophil-generated oxidants. Vitamin E is a generic term that encompasses a collection of tocopherols and tocotrienols that originate in plant oils. Vitamin E has been described as the major chain breaking antioxidant in humans [8]. Its most active form is alpha-tocopherol. Vitamin E is lipid soluble and concentrates within cell membranes where it scavenges OFR. Additional antioxidant activities include inhibition of free radical-mediated signal transduction [9]. Vitamin A is a fat-soluble collection of retinols found in dairy products, eggs, liver and cereals. β Carotene, or provitamin A, is found in fruits and vegetables and converted to retinol in the intestinal mucosa.

GSH is central to overall antioxidant defense (Fig. 2). GSH is a tripeptide capable of either direct antioxidant activity or enzymatic activity via glutathione reductase. GSH maintains the antioxidant network in a reduced state by regenerating vitamin E by recycling ascorbate from vitamin C [10]. GSH also maintains protein sulfhydryl groups in their reduced state which is essential for proper pro-

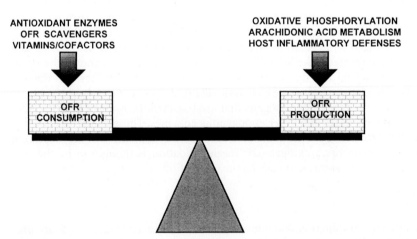

Fig. 1. Normal oxidative balance. In health, physiologic production of oxygen free radicals (*OFR*) is balanced by endogenous defense mechanisms

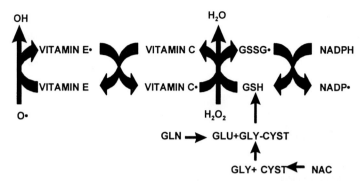

Fig. 2. Glutathione (*GSH*) is central to antioxidant defenses. GSH is a component of the enzyme, glutathione peroxidase, which catalyzes the conversion of peroxide to water. GSH also maintains vitamins C and E in their reduced states. GSH synthesis is limited by cysteine. N-acetylcysteine (*NAC*), a cysteine precursor, may be supplemented to replete GSH. *The symbol* · indicates the free radical, or oxidized form of each compound

tein function. It also has been found to modulate OFR mediated signal transduction pathways and protects endothelial cells from oxidant injury [11]. GSH is synthesized in the liver and secreted in the bile where it protects intestinal mucosa against bacterial xenobiotics and mucosal lipid peroxidation [12]. GSH depletion can lead to vitamin C and E depletion.

Transitional metal ions which can contribute to OFR formation are sequestered by binding proteins such as transferrin, lactoferrin and ceruloplasmin.

Pathophysiology

In disease, OFR may overcome host defense mechanisms, a condition known as oxidative stress. This may result from increases in OFR production, decreases in antioxidant defenses or a combination of both (Fig. 3). Once OFR load exceeds the capacity of antioxidant systems, free radical-mediated tissue damage and a corresponding immunoinflammatory response is initiated (Fig. 4). OFR directly damage cells by interacting with proteins, lipids and DNA [13]. OFR interact with membrane proteins and lipids causing lipid peroxidation and subsequent membrane disruption. Damage to DNA may be lethal or mutagenic. Damaged tissues release stores of transitional metal ions that propagate OFR production.

OFR stimulate an inflammatory response by a variety of direct and indirect mechanisms. They stimulate transcriptional factors such as NFκB which upregulate expression of cytokines and cell adhesion molecules [14]. OFR act on endothelial cells to upregulate expression of cell adhesion molecules and increase vascular permeability. Lipid peroxidation is chemotactic for neutrophils and macrophages. These changes result in neutrophil and macrophage activation and migration into local tissues where they produce OFR via oxidative bursts. Neutrophils, together with their products, also stimulate production of xanthine oxidase in endothelial cells further increasing OFR production. Secreted enzymes

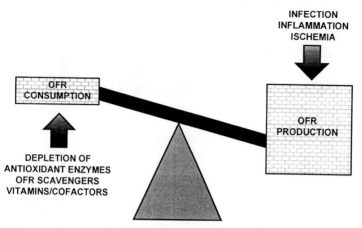

Fig. 3. Oxidative stress. Critical illness may be associated with increased OFR production, depleted OFR defenses or both. When OFR production overcomes OFR consumption, balance shifts to an oxidative state known as oxidative stress

damage surrounding tissues which propagates the local inflammatory response. Increasing levels of cytokines and OFR circulate, causing systemic effects that dominate the clinical course of many patients with sepsis, ARDS, burns and trauma. Conversely, a primary inflammatory state, such as infection, can produce oxidative stress.

OFR have been implicated in the pathogenesis of a wide variety of diseases. Mounting evidence demonstrates that oxidative stress plays a pivotal role in critical illness. Numerous investigators have reported evidence of increases in OFR formation and decreases in antioxidant defenses in critically ill patients. The most widely studied conditions are sepsis and ARDS. Evidence of increased OFR formation in these conditions includes increases in neutrophil activation, xanthine oxidase activity, hydrogen peroxide excretion and lipid peroxidation [15–22]. Deficiencies in antioxidant defenses include depletion of GSH, vitamins A, C and E and selenium [21, 23–25].

Therapy

Interventions

Critical illness is associated with increased OFR production and diminished OFR defenses. Excess OFR play an integral role in the immunoinflammatory response that is central to the pathophysiology of many critical illnesses. It follows that preventing the initiation or controlling the progression of a harmful oxidative state may ameliorate or reverse the progression of local or systemic disease processes that complicate the course of critically ill patients. General strategies for therapy are inhibition of OFR production and augmentation of antioxidant defenses. Specific therapies are listed in Table 1.

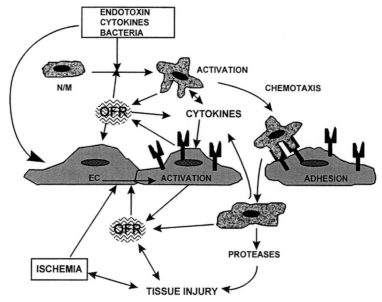

Fig. 4. Integration of OFR generation and inflammatory response. Oxidative stress generates an inflammatory response by activating macrophages (*M*) and neutrophils (*N*), stimulating cytokine production, up-regulating endothelial cell (*EC*) adhesion molecule expression and enhancing chemotaxis. This inflammatory response leads to tissue injury and further promotes OFR production and inflammation. Conversely, ischemia or inflammation can stimulate production of OFR

There are several potential approaches for antioxidant therapy to benefit critically ill patients. Augmenting antioxidant defenses is a logical approach because the generation of OFR is complex and inhibiting the process is counter-physiologic and may inhibit important steps in the response to injury and sepsis.

Supplementation of endogenous host defenses is a favored strategy. Single agent therapies with vitamin C and E have been reported in the treatment of severe burns [26–28]. A prospective randomized study reported decreased mortality in patients with sepsis and multiple organ failure who received selenium supplementation [29].

N-acetylcysteine (NAC) is attractive as a single agent because it both scavenges OFR directly and fortifies endogenous defenses as a GSH precursor [30]. In addition, NAC is a small molecule with excellent tissue penetration. Multiple prospective randomized studies have evaluated treatment with NAC in patients with lung injury and ARDS. Suter et al. reported improvements in pulmonary status as evidenced by decreased requirements for oxygen supplementation and ventilatory support in patients with lung injury who were predisposed to develop ARDS [31]. However treatment did not decrease mortality or the development of ARDS. Bernard et al. reported effective GSH repletion and decreased duration of acute lung injury with no survival benefit in ARDS patients treated with NAC [32]. Similarly, Jepsen et al. found no survival benefit from NAC in ARDS [33].

Table 1. Therapeutic approaches in the treatment of oxidative stress (*NADPH* nicotinamide adenine dinucleotide phosphate, *NSAID* non-steroidal anti-inflammatory drug, *Ab* antibody, *PAF* platelet-activating factor)

Inhibtion of OFR production	Augmentation of antioxidant defenses	
I Enzyme inhibitors	**I Enzyme supplements**	
xanthine oxidase	Superoxide dismutase	
Allopurinol	Native	
Oxypurinol	Recombinant	
Folic acid	Superoxide dismutase mimics	EUK-8
Pterin aldehyde	Modified	IgA linked
Tungsten		Polyethylene glycol
NADPH oxidase		Lysosome encapsulated
Adenosine	Catalase	
Calcium channel blockers	Native	
NSAIDs	Modified	IgA linked
Monoclonal Ab		Lysosome encapsulated
II Anti-neutrophil agents	Glutathione peroxidase	
Anti-adhesion agents	Native	
Monoclonal AB to CD11/18	Mimic	Ebselen
GMP 140	Precursors	Glutathione
PAF antagonists		*N*-acetylcysteine
BN 52021	**II OFR scavengers**	
WEB 2086	*natural*	*pharmacologic*
	Vitamin C	21 aminosteroids/lazaroids
	Vitamin E	Probucol
	Vitamin A	Salicylates
	Thiols	Mannitol
	Ubiquinol	Dimethylsulfoxide
	Flavanoids	Dimethylthiourea
	Estrogens	
	III Transitional metal sequestration/chelation	
	Transferrin	
	ceruloplasmin	
	Deferoxamine	
	Albumin	
	IV Trace element supplementation	
	Selenium	
	Zinc	
	Manganese	
	Iron	

Combination therapy by simultaneous administration of multiple antioxidants may be more beneficial due to synergy in antioxidant defenses. Galley et al. reported that the combined delivery of NAC, ascorbic acid and alpha tocopherol to patients in septic shock improved hemodynamic parameters as compared to controls [34]. Porter et al. randomized trauma patients to receive either control or a combination of NAC, vitamin C, vitamin E and selenium. They found antioxidant therapy decreased the incidence of infectious complications and multiorgan dysfunction [35].

Several synthetic compounds with antioxidant properties have been generated. Lazaroids are derivatives of methylprednisone with enhanced antioxidant properties and absent glucocorticoid and mineralocorticoid activity. As antioxidants, lazaroids inhibit lipid peroxidation, scavenge OFR, chelate iron and enhance the effects of vitamin E. Subsequent generations of lazaroids additionally inhibit NADPH oxidase. As steroid derivatives, lazaroids possess anti-inflammatory effects; they inhibit cytokine production, down-regulate cell adhesion molecule expression and inhibit neutrophil activation and migration. Therapeutic benefit has been demonstrated in numerous studies using experimental models of ischemia-reperfusion, sepsis, shock and trauma. These studies have been reviewed by Spapen et al. [36] Lazaroids are so named because of their ability to attenuate neurologic damage following cerebral ischemia. Their lipophilic moieties promote cell membrane concentration and ideally suit them for CNS delivery. Neuroprotection has been observed in animal models of stroke, trauma and cerebral ischemia. Lazaroids have been reported to improve recovery and decrease mortality following subarachnoid hemorrhage [37]. Clinical trials are currently ongoing to evaluate the effects of lazaroid treatment in ischemic stroke and head and spinal cord injury.

Antioxidant enzyme supplementation is a theoretically attractive concept. A single enzyme molecule may be able to neutralized large quantities of OFR where scavengers are consumed in a stoichiometric fashion. Marzi et al. reported recombinant SOD decreased inflammatory response, multiple organ failure, and length of ICU stay in trauma patients in a prospective randomized trial [38]. SOD supplementation is limited by its short half-life and suboptimal intracellular delivery. Linking SOD to IgA or polyethylene glycol increases its half-life. Encapsulation with liposomes confers the added benefit of improved intracellular delivery. SOD mimics are a class of compounds that exhibit SOD activity. One such compound, EUK-8, a synthetic low molecular weight complex with both SOD and catalase activity, has been shown to be effective in several models of oxidative stress. EUK-8 provided protection against LPS-mediated lung injury and prevented anoxia induced lipid peroxidation in hippocampal cultures [39, 40].

Patients at risk for OFR-mediated illness may benefit from prophylactic therapy. Patients most likely to benefit are those with impaired antioxidant defenses who are at risk for illnesses or subjected to therapies that are associated with the development of oxidative stress. Patients with chronically depleted antioxidant defenses include alcoholics, smokers, diabetics and those with chronic inflammatory disease, malnutrition, cirrhosis, and jaundice. Predisposed patients who are scheduled for elective operations which involve ischemia and reperfusion and those undergoing chemotherapy or radiation therapy may benefit from prophylactic antioxidant repletion. Preoperative or intraoperative antioxidant administration has been shown to benefit patients undergoing coronary revascularization, vascular reconstructions and solid organ transplantation [41–43].

Limitations

Therapeutic trials to date have shown mixed results due in part to numerous limitations. There is uncertainty about what targets and modes of therapy are best. Once an approach is chosen, timing of therapy, dosage, adverse effects and toxicities must be determined. The concept of simple unified enhancement of antioxidant defenses to provide blanket protection is intuitively attractive. However, the pathophysiology is far too complex and not completely understood. A wide variety of disease processes share common pathways yet there seems to be enough specificity among particular diseases to suggest that targets must be disease specific. One example is Allopurinol, which blocks OFR production by inhibiting xanthine oxidase. Its administration was effective in limiting reperfusion injury [44]. But similar benefit was not seen in experimental models of sepsis [45]. This suggests differences in the predominant mechanisms of OFR production in sepsis and ischemia reperfusion.

Antioxidant defenses GSH and vitamins E and C function synergistically to regenerate both water- and fat-soluble antioxidants [10]. Measured deficiencies of any one component may represent deficiencies of multiple antioxidants, thus necessitating multimodal therapy. To be effective, treatment must reach appropriate tissue compartments. For example, SOD catalyzes intracellular OFR metabolism and must concentrate there to be effective. Strategies to overcome this limitation include designing compounds that are maximally soluble, such as SOD mimics, or complexing them with other compounds to facilitate delivery, such as lysosome encapsulation of SOD [46]. Timing of therapy is also critical. SOD supplementation was effective when given before onset of sepsis but less so or not at all when administered after [47, 48]. Optimal doses of antioxidant therapies are unknown. Recommended doses of dietary supplements such as vitamins are based on requirements and metabolism in healthy subjects. Critical illness alters requirements and pharmacokinetics rendering standard doses meaningless. Determining optimal doses for treating oxidative stress is particularly difficult because measurements of markers of oxidation and endpoints of therapy are neither direct nor standardized. Harmful effects of these interventions are largely unknown in part because they are used primarily in critically ill patients in whom all adverse outcomes are likely attributed to illness. Certainly, OFR play a role in a variety of vital physiologic processes. Theoretically, overtreatment of oxidative stress may shift the balance toward inadequate oxidation and interfere with host defense mechanisms. Koch et al. reported the reduction of bacterial clearance in animals treated with N-acetylcysteine [49]. The clinical significance of this is not yet known. Numerous investigators have reported a paradoxical pro-oxidative effect of antioxidant therapy [50–52]. This further emphasizes the importance of appropriate dosing.

Conclusions and Recommendations

The identification of oxidative stress as a central feature of common critical illnesses has generated intense interest in this field. In vitro and animal studies provide convincing data that antioxidant therapy is a potent defense against oxidative stress. These data, considered with the facts that critical illness is associated with oxidative stress and depleted antioxidant defenses, strongly suggests that patients should benefit from antioxidant therapy. The elucidation of OFR pathways and their links to inflammatory systems has led to the identification of potential therapeutic interventions. Several strategies show promise yet none warrant widespread use at this time. Multimodal therapy designed against specific targets and disease processes is an evolving concept that appears to hold some promise for antioxidant therapy. At present, data to support routine use of antioxidants in critical illness is soft. Particular therapies, their details of administration and appropriate target populations must be better defined. Parameters for measuring oxidative states and endpoints of therapy need to be developed. The use of agents with poorly defined dosages and toxicity profiles and the administration of investigational compounds should be strictly limited to patients enrolled in clinical trials. At this time, the body of evidence suggests that supplementation of natural antioxidants and cofactors in safe, physiologic doses is reasonable in the treatment of critically ill patients or prophylaxis of high risk patients. There is no convincing data that antioxidant supplementation is beneficial when given after the insult but therapy may be considered in specific patients. We recommend replacement therapy with one gram per day of vitamin C and 1000 units per day of vitamin E in critically ill patients who were depleted prior to hospitalization, such as alcoholics, smokers and those with malnutrition and chronic jaundice. We treat all patients who are mechanically ventilated with high oxygen tension with at least 1 g/day of vitamin C as long as renal function is normal. Antioxidant therapy is probably beneficial in septic patients and those with ARDS, malabsorption, and pancreatic and biliary disease. Antioxidant therapy may be beneficial in patients who have sustained trauma and burns. More well-conceived and tightly controlled trials are needed to better focus this immense field and maximally benefit future efforts.

References

1. Maxwell SR (1995) Prospects for the use of antioxidant therapies. Drugs 49:345–361
2. Beckman JS, Beckman TW, Chen J, et al. (1990) Apparent hydroxyl radical production by peroxynitrite. Implications for endothelial injury from nitric oxide and superoxide. Proc Natl Acad Sci USA 87:1620–1624
3. Schiller HJ, Reilly PM, Bulkley GB (1993) Antioxidant therapy. Crit Care Med 21:S92–S102
4. Friedl H, Till G, Ryan U, Ward P (1989) Mediator induced activation of xanthine oxidase in endothelial cells. FASEB J 3:2512–2528
5. Cohen GM, Doherty M (1992) Free radical mediated cell toxicity by redox cycling chemicals. Br J Cancer 55 Suppl 8:46–52
6. Gerli G, Locatelli GF, Mongiat R, et al. (1992) Erythrocyte antioxidant activity, serum caeruloplasmin, and trace element levels in subjects with alcoholic liver disease. Am J Clin Pathol 97:614–618
7. Bulger EM, Helton WS (1998) Nutrient antioxidants in gastrointestinal disease. Gastroenterol Clin North Am 27:403–419
8. Packer L (1992) Interactions among antioxidants in health and disease: Vitamin E and its redox cycle. Proc Soc Exp Biol Med 200:271–276

9. Kagan V, Serbinova E, Bakalova R, et al. (1990) Mechanisms of stabilization of biomembranes by alpha-tocopherol. The role of the hydrocarbon chain in the inhibition of lipid peroxidation. Biochem Pharmacol 40:2403–2413
10. Kelly F (1994) Vitamin E supplementation in the critically ill patient: too narrow a view? NCP 9:19–25
11. Staal FJT, Anderson MT, Staal GE, et al. (1994) Redox regulation of signal transduction: Tyrosine phosphorylation and calcium influx. Proc Natl Acad Sci 91:3619–3622
12. Aw TY (1994) Biliary glutathione promotes the mucosal metabolism of luminal peroxidized lipids by rat small intestine in vivo. J Clin Invest 94:1218–1225
13. Youn YK, LaLonde C, Demling R (1991) Use of antioxidant therapy in shock and trauma. Circ Shock 35:245–249
14. Christman JW, Lancaster LH, Blackwell TS (1998) Nuclear factor κB: a pivotal role in the systemic inflammatory response syndrome and new target for therapy. Intensive Care Med 24:1131–1138
15. Bast A, Haenen GRMM, Doelman CJA (1991) Oxidants and antioxidants: State of the art. Am J Med 91 (Suppl 3 C):2S–13 S
16. Kunimoto F, Morita T, Ogawa R, et al. (1987) Inhibition of lipid peroxidation improves survival rate of endotoxemic rats. Circ Shock 21:15–22
17. Phan SH, Gannon DE, Varani J, et al. (1989) Xanthine oxidase activation in rat pulmonary artery endothelial cells and its modulation by activated neutrophils. Am J Pathol 134:1201–1211
18. Richard C, Lemonnier F, Thibault M, et al. (1990) Vitamin E deficiency and lipoperoxidation during adult respiratory distress syndrome. Crit Care Med 18:4–9
19. Bertrand Y, Pincemail J, Hanique G, et al. (1989) Differences in tocopherol-lipid ratios in ARDS and non-ARDS patients. Intensive Care Med 15:87–93
20. Takeda K, Shimada Y, Amano M (1984) Plasma lipid peroxides and alpha-tocopherol in critically ill patients. Crit Care Med 12:959–959
21. Metnitz PGH, Bartens C, Fischer M, Fridrich P, Steltzer H, Druml W (1990) Antioxidant status in patients with acute respiratory distress syndrome. Intensive Care Med 25:180–185
22. Keitzmann D, Kahl R, Muller M Burchardi H, Kettler D (1993) Hydrogen peroxide in expired breath condensate of patients with acute respiratory failure and with ARDS. Intensive Care Med 19:78–81
23. Gadek JE, Pacht ER (1996) The interdependence of lung antioxidants and antiprotease defense in ARDS. Chest 110:273S–277 S
24. Keller G, Burke R, Harty J, et al. (1985) Decreased hepatic glutathione levels in septic shock. Arch Surg 120:941–945
25. Cross CE, Forte T, Stocker R, et al. (1990) Oxidative stress and abnormal cholesterol metabolism in patients with adult respiratory distress syndrome. J Lab Clin Med 115:396–404
26. Matsuda T, Tanaka H, Williams S, Hanumadass M, Abcarian H, Reyes H (1991) Reduced fluid volume requirement for resuscitation of third-degree burns with high-dose vitamin C. J Burn Care Rehabil 12:525–532
27. Matsuda T, Tanaka H, Hanumadass M, et al. (1992) Effects of high-dose vitamin C administration on postburn microvascular fluid and protein flux. J Burn Care Rehabil 13:560–566
28. Chai J, Guo Z, Sheng Z (1995) Protective effects of vitamin E on impaired neutrophil phagocyte function in patients with severe burn. Chung Hua Cheng Hsing Shao Shang Wai Ko Tsa Chih 1:32–35
29. Zimmermann T, Albrecht S, Kuhne H, Vogelsang U, Grutzmann R, Kopprasch S (1997) Selenium administration in patients with sepsis syndrome. A prospective randomized study. Med Klin 92 (Suppl 3):3–4
30. Henderson A, Hayes P (1994) Acetylcysteine as a cytoprotective antioxidant in patients with severe sepsis: potential new use for an old drug. Ann Pharmacother 28:1086–1088

31. Suter PM, Domenighetti G, Schaller MD, Laverriere MC, Ritz R, Perret C (1994) N-acetylcysteine enhances recovery from acute lung injury in man. A randomized, double-blind, placebo-controlled clinical study. Chest 105:190–194

32. Bernard GR, Wheeler AP, Arons MM et al. (1997) A trial of antioxidants N-acetylcysteine and procysteine in ARDS. The Antioxidant in ARDS Study Group. Chest 112:164–172

33. Jepsen S, Herlevsen P, Knudsen P, Bud MI, Klausen NO (1992) Antioxidant treatment with N-acetylcysteine during adult respiratory distress syndrome: a prospective, randomized, placebo-controlled study, Crit Care Med 20:918–923

34. Galley HF, Howdle PD, Walker BE, Webster NR (1997) The effects of intravenous antioxidants in patients with septic shock. Free Radic Biol Med 23:768–774

35. Porter JM, Ivatury RR, Azimuddin K, Swami R (1999) Antioxidant therapy in the prevention of organ dysfunction syndrome and infectious complications after trauma: early results of a prospective randomized study. Am Surg 65:478–483

36. Spapen H, Zhang H, Vincent JL (1997) Potential therapeutic value of lazaroids in endotoxemia and other forms of sepsis. Shock 8:321–327

37. Hall ED (1995) Inhibition of lipid peroxidation in central nervous system trauma and ischemia. J Neurol Sci 134 (Suppl):79–83

38. Marzi I, Buhren V, Schuttler A, Trentz O (1993) Value of superoxide dismutase for prevention of multiple organ failure after multiple trauma. J Trauma 35:110–119

39. Gonzalez PK, Zhuang J, Doctorow SR (1995) EUK-8, a synthetic superoxide dismutase and catalase mimetic, ameliorates acute lung injury in endotoxemic swine. J Pharmacol Exp Ther 275:798–806

40. Musleh W, Bruce A, Malfroy B, Baudry M (1994) Effects of EUK-8, a synthetic catalytic superoxide scavenger, of hypoxia- and acidosis-induced damage in hippocampal slices. Neuropharmacology 33:929–934

41. Novelli GP, Adembri C, Gandini E, et al. (1997) Vitamin E protects human skeleton muscle from damage during surgical ischemia-reperfusion. Am J Surg 173:206–209

42. Schiller HJ, Andreoni KA, Bulkley GB (1991) Free radical ablation for the prevention of post-ischemic renal failure following renal transplantation. Klin Wochenschr 69:1083–1094

43. Yau TM, Weisel RD, Mickle DA, et al. (1994) Vitamin E for coronary bypass operations: A prospective, double-blinded, randomized trial. J Thorac Cardiovasc Surg 108:302–10

44. Allan G, Cambridge D, Lee-Tsang-Tan L, et al. (1986) The protective action of allopurinol in an experimental model of hemorrhagic shock and reperfusion. Br J Pharmacol 89:148–155

45. Shatney CH, Toledo-Pereyra LH, et al. (1980) Experiences with allopurinol in canine endotoxic shock. Adv Shock 4:119–121

46. Turrens JF, Crapo JD, Freeman BA (1984) Protection against oxygen toxicity by intravenous injection of lisosome-entrapped catalase and superoxide dismutase. J Clin Invest 73:87–95

47. Broner CW, Shenep JL, Stidham GL, et al. (1988) Effect of scavengers of oxygen derived free radicals on mortality in endotoxin challenged mice. Crit Care Med 16:848–851

48. Broner CW, Shenep JL, Stidham GL, et al. (1989) Effect of antioxidants in experimental Escherichia coli septicemia. Circ Shock 29:77–92

49. Koch T, Heller S, Heibler S, et al. (1996) Effects of N-acetylcysteine on bacterial clearance. Eur J Clin Invest 26:884–892

50. Koch T, Heller S, Heibler S, et al. (1996) Effects of N-acetylcysteine on bacterial clearance. Eur J Clin Invest 26:884–892

51. Aruima OI, Evans PJ, Kauer H, et al. (1990) An evaluation of the antioxidant and potential pro-oxidant properties of food additives and of Trolox-C, vitamin E and probucol. Free Rad Res Commun 10:143–157

52. Yim MB, Chock PB, Stadtman ER (1990) Copper-zinc superoxide dismutase catalyses hydroxyl radical production form hydrogen peroxide. Proc Natl Acad Sci USA 87:5006–5010

Strategies for Motility and Dysmotility in Nutrition Support

V. Kaul and G.M. Levine

Introduction

Among the many variables which affect enteral nutrient delivery, gastrointestinal motility is of paramount importance. The overall integrity of this 'organ' determines the success of enteral nutritional support. We shall review the management of motility and dysmotility states and suggest strategies which may help to optimize this aspect of critical care management.

Regulation of Gastrointestinal Motility

The regulation of gastrointestinal motility is governed by a complex interaction of neuromuscular, hormonal, humoral, mechanical, luminal and metabolic factors. Research advances in the fields of smooth muscle physiology, electrophysiology, neurohormonal regulation, flow dynamics as well as molecular biology have led to a better understanding of gastrointestinal motility.

The autonomic nervous system (ANS) initiates, maintains and coordinates gastrointestinal peristaltic activity. Parasympathetic nerves predominantly innervate the upper gastrointestinal tract and colorectum, providing pathways for central nervous system afferent and efferent interactions. Sympathetic fibers may act directly on secretory-absorptive enterocytes and on blood vessels, or indirectly via the intestinal plexus of nerves. Partial control of the exocrine and endocrine functions of the gastrointestinal tract also depends on the ANS [1].

Numerous neuropeptides and hormones are involved in the regulation of intestinal transit. The cyclic occurrence of the propulsive migrating motor complex (MMC) is linked to peripheral hormonal factors and is influenced by luminal contents [2]. Motilin is the major hormone triggering the gastric MMC whereas somatostatin and enkephalins are implicated in the propagation of contractions along the small intestine. Gastrointestinal transit may be altered in some patho-physiologic situations where CRF, TRH and some cytokines (IL 1 β, TNF α) play an important role [1].

Feeding suppresses intestinal MMC's and propulsive transit, increasing the contact time for nutrient absorption. Intraduodenal feeding maintains a fed motility pattern while intragastric feeding stimulates the normal variation between fed and fasting patterns [3]. Post-prandial inhibition of motility is a function of the caloric content of the meal rather than the infusion rate. After several hours of continuous infusion of a formula into the duodenum, MMC activity returns [4]. A lipid containing meal has a stronger inhibitory effect than a carbohydrate meal, that in turn, is more potent than a protein meal [5]. Parenteral nutrition also may effect motility, but the interaction of lipid, amino acids and glucose are complex. Lipid emulsion and hypertonic glucose slow gastric emptying and peristaltic activity. Amino acids stimulate gastric and pancreatic secretion and peristaltic activity [6]. However, high dose intravenous amino acids also modulate antro-duodenal motility, decreasing antral contractions and gastric emptying, with a concomitant slowing in small bowel transit [7].

Management Strategies for Dysmotility States in the Critically Ill

Gastro-Esophageal Reflux Disease and Aspiration Syndromes

The risk of reflux related aspiration is extremely high in patients with oropharyngeal dysphagia or cricopharyngeal dysfunction from acute neurological events. In patients with pre-existing reflux disease who are critically ill, enteral feeding frequently worsens gastroesophageal reflux [8]. Recurrent aspiration commonly is seen, leading to nosocomial pneumonia and interruption in nutritional support. Patients are often nursed for prolonged periods in the supine position, exacerbating reflux [9]. A recent prospective study demonstrated that after 5 days of mechanical ventilation, about half of the patients had erosive esophagitis. This finding was related to bile rather than acid reflux since all patients were on acid suppressive therapy [8]. Stress induced gastroparesis leads to high gastric volumes that worsen gastroesophageal reflux [10]. Other complications of reflux include dysphagia, regurgitation, chest pain, intractable nausea, abdominal bloating and bleeding.

Placement of naso-enteric feeding tubes may reduce the risk of aspiration especially if the feedings are delivered beyond the ligament of Treitz [11]. However, duodenal or jejunal feeding may stimulate gastric secretion through neurohumoral mechanisms [12]. The diameter of feeding tubes is not an important factor in producing reflux [13].

Considerable controversy exists as to whether intermittent or continuous nasogastric feedings are preferable in order to limit the risk of aspiration [14, 15]. Several simple measures such as raising the head of the bed to 30°–45° elevation and frequent checking of gastric residuals has been recommended to reduce the risk of reflux aspiration [11]. Enterally administered cisapride, a serotonin (5-HT_4) agonist or metoclopramide, a dopamine antagonist with serotonergic agonist effects, may benefit patients in the ICU setting. These drugs increase lower esophageal sphincter tone, increases esophageal acid clearance and gastric emptying [16].

Proton pump inhibitors are indicated for severe esophagitis, and soon shall be available in parenteral form in the USA. The best results are obtained by combining cisapride with a high dosage of an H_2 receptor blocker or a proton pump inhibitor [17]. Physicians must be aware of the arrhythmogenic effects of cisapride. This compound can lengthen the cardiac QT interval and induce torsades de pointes tachycardia that can eventuate in ventricular fibrillation [18]. This drug should not be given to patients receiving systemic azole antifungals (i.e., fluconazole, ketoconazole) or macrolide antibiotics (i.e. erythromycin, clarithromycin etc). Metoclopramide, can be administered parenterally when the oral/enteral routes are not feasible. It may have disturbing extrapyramidal side effects, especially tardive dyskinesia [16], that may limit its utility.

Gastroparesis

Delayed gastric emptying has a variety of mechanical and non-mechanical causes [19]:
- Mechanical obstruction
  - Status post gastric surgery
  - Duodenal, pyloric, gastric ulcer
  - Gastric malignancy
  - Pancreatic pseudocyst
- Non-mechanical obstruction (gastroparesis)
  - ICU "stress" (pain, sepsis, hypoxia, supine position)
  - Medications (narcotics, anticholinergics, calcium channel antagonists)
  - Electrolyte disorders (potassium, calcium, magnesium, phosphate)
  - Metabolic (hyperglycemia, hypothyroidism, hyperthyroidism)
  - Neurologic (neurosurgery, cranial trauma)
  - Neuromuscular (diabetic enteropathy, connective tissue disease)
  - Infiltrative (malignancy, amyloidosis)
  - Infectious (viral)
  - Post-vagotomy

ICU patients have one or more etiologic factors causing gastroparesis including sepsis, pain, hypoxia and administration of opioids. Mechanical ventilation has been reported to impair gastric emptying [10]. Neurosurgical patients and those patients suffering from cranial trauma are likely to develop gastroparesis [20].

Uncontrolled or long-standing diabetes and gastric surgery also slow gastric emptying. Anticholinergics, opiates, tricyclic anti-depressants, phenothiazines, and α and β adrenergic agents are commonly used in the ICU setting and may exacerbate gastroparesis [19].

Management of gastroparesis encompasses a multi-modality approach. Efforts at reversing the underlying etiology should be combined with drug therapy and modification of feeding routes. Jejunal feeding is helpful in many patients [21], enabling post-pyloric delivery of nutrients. Jejunal feeding in head injury patients enables enteral delivery of nutrients in a safe and efficient way enabling a higher caloric input and a better nitrogen balance [20]. The development of prokinetic agents has improved the treatment of gastroparesis. Studies have documented that cisapride is beneficial, both acutely and chronically [22, 23]. Although available only for enteral administration, cisapride, in doses of 10–20 mg is usually effective in increasing the rate of gastric emptying as well as increasing peristalsis. Patients may experience diarrhea as a side effect. Metoclopramide has similar pharmacologic effects to cisapride. It has the advantage, being availability in a parenteral form. Erythromycin also promotes gastric emptying via a stimulatory effect on the motilin receptor as well as direct cholinergic actions. Enteral (250–500 mg doses) or parenteral administration of 3 mg/kg q.8 h. is effective [24]. Unfortunately, the utility of this drug is limited because it frequently induces nausea. Erythromycin also has been used to facilitate placement of nasoduodenal tubes [25]. Several other therapeutic agents have prokinetic properties with potential clinical use in gastroparesis. These include misoprostol, a prostaglandin analogue and the narcotic antagonists, naloxone and naltrexone [26]. These agents have shown some promise, but additional studies in humans need to confirm their role in the treatment algorithm of gastroparesis. Strict control of diabetes has shown some benefit in reversing the severity of gastroparesis [27]. In a study of 26 patients with diabetic gastroparesis, jejunostomy tube placement improved overall health, decreased hospitalizations and improved symptoms of nausea and vomiting [21].

Intestinal Motility Disorders

These motility problems are broadly classified into ileus, predominantly small bowel, or pseudo-obstruction if predominantly colonic. (Obviously, mechanical obstruction must be considered first and treated appropriately if present.) The various causes are:

- Acute Ileus
  - Intraabdominal inflammation (appendicitis, cholecystitis, pancreatitis, diverticulitis)
  - Postoperative
  - Mesenteric ischemia
  - Electrolyte disorders (potassium, calcium, magnesium, phosphate)
  - Medications (narcotics, anticholinergics, calcium channel antagonists)
  - Toxic megacolon
- Pseudoobstruction
  - Diabetes mellitus
  - Neuromuscular diseases
  - Metabolic disorders
  - Paraneoplastic syndromes
- Mechanical obstruction
  - Adhesions/bands
  - Hernias
  - Volvulus
  - Fecal impaction
  - Tumors
  - Ischemia
  - Intussuception

It is important to differentiate between these causes as the management and prognosis differ in each case. Fluid and electrolyte resuscitation and correction of acid-base imbalance take precedence. Due to the risk of aspiration from increased luminal secretions, nasogastric suction is appropriate. The use of long nasoenteral decompression tubes (Cantor, Miller-Abbott) is controversial [28]. Rectal tube decompression may be helpful in some cases. There is no consensus regarding the role of urgent (therapeutic) colonoscopic decompression for acute colonic pseudo-obstruction [29, 30]. Withholding drugs causing hypomotility (opiates, anticholinergics, calcium channel blockers, etc.) is prudent. Recently Ponec et al. reported on the use of neostigmine in acute colonic pseudo-obstruction [31]. An intravenous dose of 2 mg of the drug produced decompression in 10 of 11 subjects compared to no improvement in placebo treated controls. This dramatic response makes neostigmine the treatment of choice as long as the patient does not have a resting bradycardia or hypotension. Both these cardiovascular responses transiently occur with neostigmine making monitoring mandatory.

Cisapride may be beneficial in acute hypomotility states, as it significantly accelerates transit of solids and liquids, increasing stool frequency through its effect on smooth muscle. There is no evidence that cisapride is effective in chronic intestinal pseudo-obstruction associated with extrinsic neuropathy or a myopathic disorder [32]. Mechanical obstruction must be ruled out prior to any trial with prokinetics. Parenteral erythromycin in low doses (3 mg/kg q.8 h) appears to increase duodenal contractions and has been tried as an adjunctive treatment in ileus [24]. There are also anecdotal reports of its efficacy in acute colonic pseudo-obstruction or spinal ileus [33].

Bacterial Overgrowth

Total bacterial counts in excess of 100,000 colony forming units per ml of small bowel contents, invariably in the setting of altered motility, is often used to define bacterial overgrowth [34]. The following conditions are associated with bacterial overgrowth:
- Pernicious anemia
- Atrophic gastritis
- Proton pump inhibitor therapy
- Billroth II gastrectomy
- Truncal vagotomy
- Intestinal obstruction
- Intestinal diverticula
- Collagen vascular diseases
- Intestinal pseudo-obstruction
- Diabetes mellitus
- Crohn's disease
- Immunodeficiency syndromes

Attenuation of MMC activity plays a causal role in the pathogenesis of bacterial overgrowth [35]. In patients with or predisposed to bacterial overgrowth, care should be taken to avoid drugs that interfere with gut motility (anticholinergics, neuroleptics, sedatives etc.). Inhibitors of acid secretion should be prescribed with caution since hypochlorhydria predisposes to bacterial overgrowth [36]. Awareness of the long term nutritional and metabolic consequences of overgrowth like anemia, vitamin deficiencies and osteomalacia is crucial, since these are all preventable and treatable. Management includes efforts to reverse the primary underlying pathology. Often, an empiric trial of antibiotics for 7–10 days is warranted [37]. Patients with chronic recurrent overgrowth will need various antibiotics on a rotating basis. Common first line choices include amoxicillin/clavulanate, tetracycline and/or metronidazole, but clindamycin, the quinolones and chloramphenicol are also effective. The role of prokinetic drugs is not clear but cisapride has been tried with varying success [34].

Diarrhea

Diarrhea is a frequently encountered complication in the ICU, affecting a large number of patients [38]. The etiology of acute diarrhea can be determined in the vast majority of patients. Although tube feedings are often blamed, and the initial management often involves changing the type of formula, this strategy rarely is the correct one. Investigation into the cause of diarrhea should begin with an attempt to describe the quantity and content of the stool. Guenther et al. have devised a novel, easy to use system for this purpose, using estimates of the stool consistency and frequency [39]. Patients with small amounts of diarrhea, who are otherwise stable may not need an extensive evaluation. The patient with frequent loose stools, with abdominal distention or pain merits evaluation. Diarrhea while fasting should suggest a secretory process. Several approaches can be used based on pathophysiologic principles such as the distinction between osmotic versus secretory diarrhea, or, the presence or absence of signs and symptoms of inflammation or mechanical obstruction. Oftentimes measurement of stool electrolytes can point to the cause of diarrhea.

However, in our experience, a knowledge based assessment of the common causes of ICU diarrhea can be performed. Figure 1 The medication Kardex is a good place to start the evaluation. In some studies, over half the diarrheal illnesses are caused by medications [38]. Is the patient receiving elixirs or solutions compounded with poorly absorbed carbohydrates such as mannitol or sorbitol [40]? Are osmotically active salts (magnesium, phosphate etc.) being administered to correct an electrolyte disturbance? Have any medications known to cause diarrhea been ordered such as metoclopramide, cisapride, quinidine, colchicine or antibiotics?

If the patient is receiving antibiotics, *Clostridium difficile* diarrhea or colitis may be present. Stool samples should be obtained for analysis, most commonly by toxin assay. However, the sensitivity of the assay may be no better than 70% because some strains of *C difficile* do not produce the toxin assayed. Up to 3 samples may need to be checked to maximize the possibility of identifying the toxin [41]. Patients with large volume diarrhea should have antibiotics stopped if possible, and treated with enteral metronidazole, 250 mg q.i.d. Enteral vancomycin,

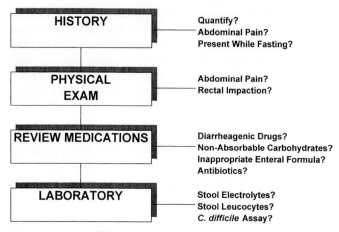

Fig. 1. Evaluation of diarrhea

125 mg, q.i.d, and/or cholestyramine, 4 g, q.i.d. are alternatives if metronidazole cannot be used [42]. In severely ill patients with an ileus, intravenous metronidazole 250–500 mg q.8 h. may be effective. Many physicians empirically treat patients with metronidazole when diarrhea occurs in the ICU patient receiving antibiotics. Patients with *C. difficile* diarrhea can be treated with antidiarrheal drugs if fever, abdominal distention and pain are absent.

Medications and antibiotics probably account for 80% of ICU diarrhea [38]. If these causes of diarrhea are not apparent, other problems should be considered. Fecal impaction with "overflow" diarrhea is often overlooked because a recent rectal exam has not been done. A plain abdominal X-ray will often suggest the diagnosis. Intolerance to the content and composition of enteral diets is rarely responsible for diarrhea, unless the patient is receiving a formula containing lactose or high fat content. Although, fiber containing formulas are promoted widely, there are few, if any, well documented reports that these preparations ameliorate or prevent diarrhea in ICU patients [43]. Heimburger et al. recently reported that small peptide containing formulas caused diarrhea more than twice as frequently as a whole protein formula [44].

Diarrhea may occur if inappropriate volumes and rates of administration are used. Intermittent administration of large volumes of hypertonic formula into the small bowel often causes diarrhea. Has a previously placed nasogastric tube migrated into the small bowel? Is the formula being bolused rather than infused slowly? Have feedings begun at too high a rate in a patient who has fasting induced gut atrophy?

Other common causes of diarrhea in the ICU patient include ischemic colitis, inflammatory bowel disease and malabsorptive disorders. Fever, abdominal pain and blood in the stool usually accompany mesenteric ischemia and ischemic colitis. These findings should be evaluated with an obstruction series and/or a CT scan. A patient with a prior history of inflammatory bowel disease may develop a flare when hospitalized for other reasons. The new onset of malabsorption is very uncommon and should prompt consideration of bacterial overgrowth, pancreatic insufficiency or small bowel disease.

Empiric treatment of diarrhea with anti-motility agents is safe if impaction and inflammatory processes are ruled out. We prefer to start therapy with loperamide 4 mg initially and if needed, 2–4 mg three or four times daily. Alternate therapies include paregoric in 5 ml doses or tincture of opium in 1 ml doses. We avoid using anticholinergic agents such as atropine or tincture of belladonna because these drugs affect several other body systems causing tachycardia, urinary retention and inspissated secretions.

Constipation

Few ICU patients are fortunate to have a normal, formed stool each day. For those patients not suffering from diarrhea, the opposite extreme often occurs. (Fig. 2). Once hospitalized for a serious illness requiring ICU care, there are multiple factors causing constipation such as narcotics administered for pain relief, or drugs with antimotility side effects (calcium channel blockers, anticholinergics, etc.). Other inciting causes include prolonged immobility in a supine position, depressed state of consciousness and electrolyte disturbances such as hypokalemia, hypomagnesemia, hypophosphatemia and hypercalcemia.

Evaluation of constipation begins with a review of medications, and a careful abdominal and rectal exam. Fecal impaction requires manual disimpaction before use of enemas or laxatives. An abdominal X-ray may be needed if there is concern over obstruction or ileus. If possible, decrease or modify the dosing of drugs with antimotility effects. In the patient with a normal abdominal exam (active bowel sounds and no abdominal tenderness), constipation can be treated initially with tap water or phosphate containing enemas. Oral or tube administered laxatives play an important role in treating and preventing recurrent constipation. Lactulose syrup, 30–60 ml once or twice a day is effective in most

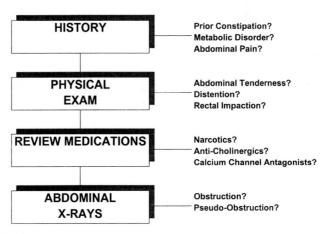

Fig. 2. Evaluation of constipation

patients. Titrate the daily dose in order to maintain normal fecal frequency. Other osmotic laxatives such as magnesium citrate 8–16 ounces or a sorbitol solution, 30–60 ml, also are effective. Recalcitrant constipation may respond better to administration of a saline-PEG solution. Although widely used, the sulfosuccinates are ineffective [45].

Biliary Motility Disorders

ICU patients are prone to biliary stasis for several reasons. First, prolonged periods of fasting or the administration of parenteral nutrition preclude normal, frequent gallbladder emptying, eventuating in sludge and stone formation [46]. This problem may be prevented in patients receiving TPN with high doses of amino acids in the infusion [6]. Second, anticholinergic drugs and calcium channel blockers impair gallbladder contraction [47]. Octreotide, frequently used to decrease mesenteric blood flow in patients with gastrointestinal bleeding and in patients with intractable diarrhea or fistulas, inhibits gallbladder smooth muscle [48].

Enteral feeding may adequately stimulate release of endogenous cholecystokinin from the duodenum, stimulating the highest density of CCK neuroendocrine cells [48]. Ledeboer et. al. reported that continuous administration of a polymeric diet intragastrically produced a sustained rise in CCK concentrations, maintained gallbladder contractile activity and led to a reduced gallbladder volume [49].

Biliary stasis may be prevented with intermittent administration of sincalide 0.02 µg/kg [50]. An intravenous bolus of sincalide, several times a week may be sufficient to empty the static gallbladder of sludge and microlithiasis.

Conclusions

Motility disorders are frequently encountered in ICU patients. Gastroesophageal reflux is a common complication of mechanical ventilation, enteral feeding and prolonged supine positioning. Pharmacologic therapy and care in feeding can obviate reflux. Impaired GI motility often results in gastroparesis, constipation, bacterial overgrowth and pseudo-obstruction. Identification of underlying causes such as motor inhibitory medications, poorly controlled diabetes and will help guide therapy. Diarrhea is commonly caused by medications given to ICU patients, rarely caused by enteral feeding. A systematic approach to diagnosis leads to rational therapy

References

1. Goyal RK, Hirano I (1996) The enteric nervous system. N Engl J Med 334:1106–1115
2. Bueno L, Fioramonti J (1994) Neurohormonal control of intestinal transit. Reprod Nutr Dev. 34 (6): 513–25

3. Ledeboer M, Masclee AA, Coenraad M, Vecht J, Biemond I, Lamers CB (1999) Antroduodenal motility and small bowel transit during continuous intraduodenal or intragastric administration of enteral nutrition. Eur J Clin Invest 29:615–623

4. Riachi G, Ducrotte P, Guedon C, et al. (1996) Duodenojejunal motility after oral and enteral nutrition in humans: a comparative study. JPEN 20:150–155

5. Hammer J, Hammer K, Kletter K (1998) Lipids infused into the jejunum accelerate small intestinal transit, delay ileocolonic transit of solids and liquids. Gut 43:111–116

6. Masclee AA, Gielkens HA, Lam WF, De Boer SY, Lamers, CB (1996) Effects of parenteral nutrients on gastrointestinal motility and secretion. Scand J Gastroenterol 218:50–55 (suppl)

7. Gielkens HA, van den Biggelaar A, Vecht J, Onkenhout W, Lamers CB, Masclee AA (1999). Effect of intravenous amino acids on interdigestive antroduodenal motility and small bowel transit time. Gut 44:240–5

8. Wilmer A, Tack J, Frans E, et al. (1999) Duodenogastroesophageal reflux and esophageal mucosal injury in mechanically ventilated patients. Gastroenterology 116:1293–1299

9. Torres A, Serra-Batlles J, Ros E, et al. (1992) Pulmonary aspiration of gastric contents in patients receiving mechanical ventilation: the effect of body position. Ann Intern Med 116:540–543

10. Heyland DK, Douglas G, King D, Cook DJ (1996) Impaired gastric emptying in mechanically ventilated patients. Intensive Care Med 22:1339–1344

11. Kirby DF, De Legge MH, Fleming CR (1995). American Gastroenterological Association medical position statement: guidelines for the use of enteral nutrition. AGA technical review on tube feeding for enteral nutrition. Gastroenterology 108: 1282–1286

12. Chendrasekhar A (1996) Jejunal feeding in the absence of reflux increases nasogastric output in critically ill trauma patients. Am Surg 62:887–888

13. Ferrer M, Bauer TT, Torres A, Hernandez C, Pierra C (1991) Effect of nasogastric tube size on gastroesophageal reflux and microaspiration in intubated patients. Ann Intern Med 130:991–994

14. Ciocon JO, Galindo-Ciocon DJ, Tiessen C, Galindo D (1992) Continuous compared with intermittent tube feeding in the elderly. JPEN 16:525–528

15. Jacobs S, Chang RWS, Lee B, Bartlett FW (1990) Continuous enteral feeding: a major cause of pneumonia among ventilated intensive care unit patients. JPEN 14:353–356

16. Wiseman LR, Fauld D (1994). Cisapride: An updated review of its pharmacology and therapeutic efficacy as a prokinetic agent in gastrointestinal motility disorders. Drugs 47: 116–152

17. Vigneri S, Termini R, Leandro G, et al. (1995) A comparison of five maintenance therapies for reflux esophagitis. N Engl J Med 333:1106–1110

18. Vitola J, Vukanovic J, Roden DM (1998) Cisapride-induced torsades de pointes. J Cardiovasc Electrophysiol 9:1109–1113

19. Horowitz M, Dent J, Fraser R, Sun W, Hebbard G (1994) Role and integration of mechanisms controlling gastric emptying. Dig Dis Sci 39:7S-13 S (suppl)

20. Altmayer T, O'Dell MW, Jones M, Hawkins HH (1996) Cisapride as a treatment for gastroparesis in traumatic brain injury. Arch Phys Med Rehabil 77:1093–1094

21. Fontana RJ, Barnett JL (1996) Jejunostomy tube placement in refractory diabetic gastroparesis: a retrospective review. Am J Gastroenterol 91:2174–2178

22. Kendall BJ, McCallum RW (1993). Gastroparesis and the current use of prokinetic drugs. Gastroenterologist: 1:107–14

23. Richards RD, Valenzuela GA, Davenport KG, Fisher KLK, McCallum RW (1993) Objective and subjective results of a randomized, double-blind, placebo-controlled trial using cisapride to treat gastroparesis. Dig Dis Sci: 38: 811–16

24. Camilleri M (1993) The current role of erythromycin in the clinical management of gastric emptying disorders. Am J Gastrenterol 88:69–171

25. Stern MA, Wolf DC (1994) Erythromycin as a prokinetic agent: a prospective, randomized, controlled study of efficacy in nasoenteric tube placement. Am J Gastroenterol 89:2011–2013

26. Mittal RK, Frank EB, Lange RC, McCallum RW (1986). Effects of morphine and naloxone on esophageal motility and gastric emptying in man. Dig Dis Sci: 31: 936–42
27. Koch KL (1999) Diabetic gastropathy: gastric neuromuscular dysfunction in diabetes mellitus: a review of symptoms, pathophysiology and treatment. Dig Dis Sci 44:1061–1075
28. Fleshner PR, Siegman MG, Slater GI, Brolin RE, Chandler JC, Aufses AH Jr (1995) A prospective, randomized trial of short versus long tubes in adhesive small-bowel obstruction. Am J Surg 170:366–370
29. Sloyer AF, Panella VS, Demas BE et al. (1988) Ogilvie's syndrome: successful management without colonoscopy. Dig Dis Sci 33:1391–1396
30. Jetmore AB, Timmcke AB, Gathright JB Jr, Hicks TC, Ray JE, Baker JW (1992) Ogilvie's syndrome: colonoscopic decompression and analysis of predisposing factors. Dis Colon Rectum 35:1135–1142
31. Ponec RJ, Saunders MD, Kimmey, MB (1999) Neostigmine for the treatment of acute colonic pseudo-obstruction. N Engl J Med 341:137–141
32. Coulie B, Camilleri M (1999) Intestinal pseudo-obstruction. Annu Rev Med 50:37–55
33. Bonacini M, Smith OJ, Pritchard T (1991) Erythromycin as therapy for acute colonic pseudo-obstruction. J Clin Gastroenterol 13:475–476
34. Husebye E (1995) Gastrointestinal motility disorders and bacterial overgrowth. J Int Med 237:419–427
35. Soudah HC, Hasler WL, Owyang C (1991) Effect of octreotide on intestinal motility and bacterial overgrowth in scleroderma. N Engl J Med 325:1461–1467
36. Fried M, Siegrist H, Frei R et al. (1994) Duodenal bacterial overgrowth during treatment in outpatients with omeprazole. Gut 35:23–26
37. Farrugia G, Camilleri M and Whitehead WE (1996). Therapeutic strategies for motility disorders. Gastroenterol Clin N America 25:225–246
38. Edes TE, Walk BE, Austin JL (1990) Diarrhea in tube-fed patients: feeding formula not necessarily the cause. Amer J Med 88:91–93
39. Guenther PA, Settle RG, Perlmutter S, Marino PL, DeSimone G, Rolandelli RH (1991) Tube feeding-related diarrhea in acutely ill patients. JPEN 15:277–280
40. Hill DB, Henderson LM, McClain CJ (1991) Osmotic diarrhea induced by sugar-free theophylline solution in critically ill patients. JPEN 15:332–336
41. Bliss DZ, Johnson S, Savik K, Clabots CR, Willard K, Gerding DN (1998) Acquisition of *Clostridium difficile* and *Clostridium difficile*-associated diarrhea in hospitalized patients receiving tube feeding. Ann Intern Med 129:1012–1019
42. Bartlett JG (1985) Treatment of *Clostridium difficile* colitis. Gastroenterology 89:1192–1195
43. Dobb GJ, Towler SC (1990) Diarrhoea during enteral feeding in the critically ill: a comparison of feeds with and without fibre. Intensive Care Med 16:252–255
44. Heimburger DC, Geels WJ, Bilbrey J, Redden DT, Keeney C (1997) Effects of small-peptide and whole-protein enteral feedings on serum proteins and diarrhea in critically ill patients: a randomized trial. JPEN 21:162–167
45. Chapman RW, Sillery J, Fontana DD, Matthys C, Saunders DR (1985) Effect of oral dioctyl sodium sulfosuccinate on intake-output studies of human small and large intestine. Gastroenterology 89:489–493
46. Roslyn JJ, Pitt HA, Mann LL, Ament ME, Denbesten L (1983) Gallbladder disease in patients on long-term parenteral nutrition. Gastroenterology 84:148–154
47. Kapicioglu S, Senturek O, Ilgun K, Ovali, E (1998) Effect of long-acting somatostatin analogue (octreotide, SMS 201–995) plus calcium channel blocker (verapamil) on gallbladder contraction. Hepatogastroenterology 45:420–423
48. Stolk MF, Van Ercpecum KJ, Hiemstra G, Jansen JB, Van Berge-Henegouwen GP (1994) Gallbladder motility and cholecystokinin release during long-term enteral nutrition in patients with Crohn's disease. Scand J Gastroenterol 29:934–939
49. Ledeboer M, Masclee AA, Biemond I, Lamers CB (1998) Effect of intragastric or intraduodenal administration of a polymeric diet on gall bladder motility, small bowel transit time and hormone release. Amer J Gastroenterol 93:2089–2096

50. Sitzman JV, Pitt HA, Steinhorn PA et al. (1990) Cholecystokinin prevents total parenteral nutrition induced biliary sludge in humans. Surg Gynecol Obstet 170:25–31

The Value of Organized Nutritional Support Service in Intensive Care Unit Care

P.J. Schneider and J.M. Mirtallo

The development of the technique of intravenous feeding in 1968 was a breakthrough in medical care (Wilmore and Dudrick 1968). Since then, the use of specialized nutrition support has become a standard tool in the care of patients. Much has been learned about the appropriate and safe indications, use and administration of enteral and intravenous nutrition. This chapter addresses the safe preparation and administration of intravenous nutrition in critical care medicine so that treatment decisions optimize patient outcome, but do not compromise patient safety.

Risks Associated with Intravenous Nutrition

It was recognized early in the evolution of intravenous feeding that it was of great, often life saving benefit to patients, but also potentially risky because of problems with infection, glucose balance, fluid and electrolyte balance and acid-base balance. These problems were found to be common unless the preparation and administration of the formula prescribed was not done properly. In 1973, Goldmann and Maki reported rates of sepsis between 6 and 27% in hospitals who used intravenous nutrition. In hospitals with higher infection rates, it was found that formalized procedures for preparing and the formulations or caring for the access site were not in place. The authors stated in their conclusion "A survey by the Centers for Disease Control and a review of the literature indicate that the risk of infection can be substantially reduced if stringent infection control measures are practiced. Accordingly, the Center's Hospital Infections Section has developed infection control guidelines for total parenteral nutrition programs" (Goldmann and Maki 1973).

Kaminski and Stolar surveyed hospitals using intravenous feedings and discovered significant deviations from standards of care. Areas in which practice was found unacceptable included skin preparation, catheter care, evaluation of fever, sterility of the infusion system, electrolyte and fluid balance and glucose concentration. As a result of these deviations from standards of care, it was found that 12.1% of patients experienced complications related to catheter placement (e.g. pneumothorax, hydrothorax), 42% had glucosuria, 5% became dehydrated, 28% had fluid and electrolyte abnormalities (usually hypokalemia) and 42% had fevers that could not be traced to non-hyperalimentation causes (Kaminski and Stolar 1974). These authors recommended:

- That each hospital develop or adopt a set of parenteral nutrition procedures based on published and generally accepted guidelines.
- That this protocol be developed by a joint effort of the medical, nursing and pharmacy staffs.
- That the protocol be rigidly followed.
- That all personnel involved in any aspect of parenteral nutrition therapy receive proper training and instruction.

Evidence Supporting Standardization and a Team Approach

It is possible to improve the safety of intravenous nutrition by standardizing procedures and using professionals who are knowledgeable about this complex form of therapy. Several studies have demonstrated this to be true. Skoutakis et al. reported an incidence of complications that was lower that those reported by Kaminski and Stolar following the implementation of a detailed protocol in conjunction with a total parenteral nutrition team. The incidence of sepsis was less than 1%, electrolyte abnormalities was 2.7% and glucosuria was 5%. Because of the these favorable complication rates compared to previous reports, these authors recommended implementing rigid protocols and the use of a team approach to administering intravenous nutrition (Skoutakis et al. 1975). Brown and Grenkoski reported a reduction in the incidence of sepsis from 12.5%–5.1% in a community hospital after the institution of rigid protocols concerning catheter insertion and care, a nursing care plan and a metabolic flow sheet (Brown and Grenkoski 1977). Nehme studied clinical outcomes in patients receiving intravenous nutrition in two hospitals; one with and one without a nutrition support team. Two groups of patients receiving intravenous nutrition were compared in a prospective study over 24 months. A nutrition support team consisting of a properly trained physician, dietitian, nurse and pharmacist managed nutrition in one group of 211 patients. A variety of physicians managed the nutritional therapy of another group of 164 patients. In the group being managed by the team, 3% of the patients developed sepsis, there were no patients with glucose imbalance and 3% of patients had electrolyte imbalance. In contrast, ten patients in the group managed by a variety of physicians died from complications resulting from glucose imbalance and 36% of patients had electrolyte abnormalities. The authors concluded that a protocol strictly adhered to by knowledgeable persons is necessary for the proper administration of intravenous nutrition in hospitalized patients (Nehme 1980). Further, Trujillo et al. found the metabolic and monetary costs associated with parenteral nutrition use were improved when provided by a nutrition support service as compared with individual clinicians prescribing the therapy (Trujillo et al. 1999). Specifically, better compliance to appropriate parenteral nutrition use [based on national guidelines (A.S.P.E.N. Board of Directors 1993)] was observed (82% vs. 56%) as well as fewer complications (34% vs. 66%) and therapies with duration <5 days (16% vs. 35%).

Nutrition Care of the Critically Ill

Critical illness is associated with marked hypermetabolism and hypercatabolism that leads to dramatic nutrient alterations, including increased gluconeogenesis, glycogenolysis and lipolysis. These metabolic effects have a significant impact on the nutritional condition of the patient and tolerance and efficacy to the provision of exogenous nutrients. Early enteral feedings have been shown to reduce septic mortality post laparotomy (Moore and Jones 1986) and have improved outcomes in children with burns (Alexander et al. 1980) and following head injury (Young et al. 1987). In the critically ill, enteral feeding is the preferred route of nutrient administration. Advances in endoscopic and laparoscopic techniques of tube placement as well as the composition of enteral nutrition formulations have improved the ability to use the gastrointestinal tract for nourishment during periods of critical illness. Applications of nutrition to the critically ill is accomplished by the appropriate assessment of nutrition status, use of the enteral route and reserved application of the parenteral route to those circumstances when the enteral route fails or is contraindicated. Despite this information, parenteral nutrition continues to be overused. In a recent audit of our intensive care unit, the appropriate use of parenteral nutrition for a specific group of surgeons ranged from 16.7%–50%. Use of parenteral nutrition was not in compliance with the hospital's evidence based guidelines because the patients either expired, had an inadequate or no trial of enteral tube feeding or were not severely malnourished and transitioned to an enteral diet within 5 days of therapy. Frequently, the critically ill patient has an impaired tolerance to nutrition support where the risks of therapy are increased disproportionate to the benefit that can be achieved. For example, Chang et al. found a 53.3% mortality among ICU patients treated with parenteral nutrition (Chang et al. 1986). This suggests the patients had a poor prognosis at the start of therapy. Further, a meta-analysis of the literature found that parenteral nutrition in the critically ill had no effect on mortality (10%–12%) and was associated with a higher complication rate as compared with no nutrition (Hegland et al. 1998).

Nutrition Care Process

Nutrition support in the critically ill patients is fraught with complications with clear benefits of therapy difficult to discern. Proper use of nutrition in the critically ill requires specific skills to determine the appropriate time and route of nutrient delivery. As such, it is important to consider a system (Fig. 1) of nutrition support that supports the safe and efficacious use of nutrition in these patients. An important component of the nutrition care process is the nutrition screen that identifies the patient at high nutrition risk – the patient most likely to benefit from nutrition support. Specific indicators of severe malnutrition are useful and may include prealbumin <10 mg/dl (normal 17–42 mg/dl), weight loss >10% of body weight over 1 month, body weight <75% of ideal or 80% of usual and/or a prolonged period of inadequate oral intake that is expected to continue >7 days. It has already been introduced that an interdisciplinary team provides nutrition

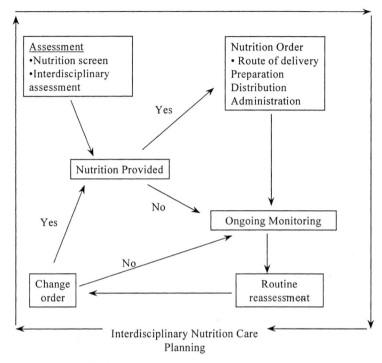

Fig. 1. Nutrition care process critical illness

care more effectively than individuals acting independently. Nutrition support is a collaborative responsibility between the nutrition support service and the multiple disciplines involved with the patient's care. Specific functions need to be performed in order to assure quality nutrition outcomes (Table 1). A nutrition support service provides all of these functions. If a NSS does not exist, specially trained individuals from other disciplines may provide certain functions but not in the comprehensive manner of a NSS. The NSS serves a gatekeeping function, assuring that the appropriate nutrition support is provided (Fig. 2). Since parenteral nutrition tends to be overused, a summary of its indications is provided (Table 2).

Measuring the Performance
of the Nutrition Support Process

An important principle of assuring the quality and improving the performance of any process, including the nutrition support process, includes establishing performance goals or aims (Schneider et al. 1999). The emphasis of these goals is the expectation of patients and on the clinical outcome of the patient, not on the structure and process of how specialized nutrition support is provided. These

Table 1. Interdisciplinary nutrition care[*NSS* nutrition support service consisting of a nurse (*RN*), dietitian (*RD*), pharmacist (*RPh*), and physician (*MD*), + personnel are capable of performing specific nutrition care functions if trained adequately]

Nutrition care functions	Personnel responsible				
	NSS	RD	RPh	RN	MD
Nutrition assessment	+	+			
Determine energy and protein needs	+	+	+		+
Determine the severity of malnutrition	+	+			
Enteral/parenteral nutrition indicated appropriately	+	+			+
Assess the adequacy of access for nutrition therapy	+			+	+
Initiate and manage enteral and parenteral nutrition Complete orders	+		+		+
Document in patient record	+	+	+	+	+
Daily patient assessment	+	+	+	+	+
Recommend changes to therapy	+	+	+	+	+
Transition feedings: parenteral to enteral to oral	+	+	+	+	+

If an NSS does not exist, the nutrition care functions must be performed by the individual disciplines that may or may not be aware of the assignment or have the necessary skills to perform the functions adequately.

Table 2. Parenteral nutrition indications: critical illness

Malnourished and unable to eat adequately (including tube feeding) for more than 7 days	Objective indicators of malnutrition are present
The benefits of parenteral nutrition outweigh the risk	Patient is in a clinical condition to respond favorably to parenteral nutrition
Patient is normally nourished and expected to be NPO including tube feeding for >14 days	
Use parenteral nutrition only when:	The enteral route is contraindicated as with paralytic ileus, mesenteric ischemia, short bowel syndrome, gastrointestinal fistula The intestinal tract has severely diminished function due to underlying disease or treatment

goals should be stated in a way that performance can be measured. Examples of performance aims framed as measurable goals include:

1. Nutrition support should be indicated. No patient should receive expensive, potentially risky treatment unless it is clearly needed.
   Goal: We will improve the ordering system so that 100% of patient records demonstrate clinical indication before treatment begins.
2. The route of administration should be appropriate. The improper method for providing specialized nutrition support can result in unnecessary costs and risk.

Goal: We will improve the selection of access route so that 100% of patients who can be fed enterally are fed via this route.

3. The patient should benefit from therapy. No patient should receive expensive, potentially risky treatment unless there is meaningful clinical improvement.
   Goal: We will improve the monitoring of nutrition therapy so that 100% of patients who receive nutrition support are shown to improve clinically.

4. The incidence of complications should be low. Complications are inevitable, but using proper techniques can minimize their rate.
   Goal: We will standardize ordering, preparing and administering nutrition support so that the infection rate, glucose imbalance, fluid and electrolyte imbalances and acid-base disturbances are reduced.

5. The patient should understand the risks and benefits of therapy. The choice to use expensive or risky treatment should involve the patient.
   Goal: We will improve patient education so that 100% of patients understand the risks and benefits of nutrition support before treatment is initiated.

6. The proper quantity of nutrition substrate should be ordered. Too much or too little substrate can predispose patients to harm.
   Goal: We will improve the ordering process so that the appropriate quantities of nutrition support substrates are ordered for 100% of patients.

7. The proper quantity of nutrition support should be administered. If nutrition support is administered incorrectly, the wrong quantities of nutrition support substrates will be given even if the order is correct.
   Goal: We will improve the method of administering nutrition support so that 100% of patients receive the appropriate quantity of nutrition support substrate.

8. The patient should not experience a detrimental drug-nutrient interaction. Nutrition can interact negatively with other prescribed drug treatment if not properly monitored.
   Goal: We will improve the process of screening orders in the pharmacy and monitoring patients who receive nutrition support so that no patients have predictable and preventable drug-nutrient interactions.

9. The patient should receive nutrition support in a timely manner. Nutrition therapy should be provided promptly after treatment decisions are made.
   Goal: We will reduce the cycle time from order to start of treatment to 2 h.

Measurement is critical to assuring and improving the performance of the nutrition support process so that it can be determined if a change in practice results in an improvement.

Improving the quality of nutrition support requires regular measurement after performance goals have been established. When a goal has not been met, practices can be changed and tested to determine whether performance improvement results. Goals can continually be evaluated to determine whether further changes better meet patient needs. Based on the goals listed above, the following measurement tools could be used.

1. Measure and track the percentage of patients for whom nutrition support is indicated based on predefined standards.

2. Measure and track the percentage of patients for whom the proper route of administration is used to administer nutrition support.

3. Measure and track the percentage of nutrition support patients with improved nitrogen balance.
4. Measure and track the incidence of hyper/hypoglycemia, fluid and electrolyte imbalance, and acid-base imbalance in nutrition support patients.
5. Measure and track the number of nutrition support patients who understand the risks and benefits of therapy.
6. Measure and track the percentage of nutrition support patients with improved nitrogen balance.
7. Measure and track the number of patients who are given nutrition support that deviates from the prescribed treatment.
8. Measure and track the number of patients who experience a detrimental drug-nutrient interaction.
9. Measure and track the number of patients who receive nutrition support more than 2 h after a treatment decision is made.

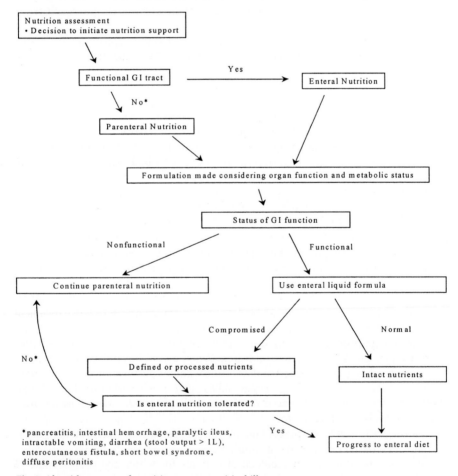

Fig. 2. Algorithm-route of nutrition support critical illness

Plotting performance using a "run"chart (measurement of performance over time) helps nutrition support providers determine how closely they are achieving their aim. It also enables the measurement of the impact of procedural changes on the quality of care. For example, if it is decided that a nutrition support team is no longer needed to provide specialized nutrition support, the impact of such a change can be measured with a good monitoring system.

Changes in practice that can be used to improve performance can be adopted from known process improvement principles. For example, it is well recognized that standardization improves quality. This could be applied to nutrition support through the concept of a standard order form. A standard order form might be postulated to improve the safety of nutrition support because orders are easier to write and interpret. A standardized order form might affect the percentage of patients who receive therapy that deviates from prescribed treatment. A standard order form might affect the number of patients who are overfed if the standard order incorporates guidelines for selecting the proper quantity of substrate. Other change concepts that could be tested to determine if they improve nutrition support include: developing treatment guidelines or critical pathways, academic detailing or education, implementing a total nutrient admixture program, implementing a nutrition support team, the use of multilumen catheters, or the use of semipermeable dressings.

Nutrition Support Clinical Guidelines

Clinical practice guidelines serve to educate clinicians on consistent methods in carrying out patient care activities. Evidence-based guidelines are derived from literature which is graded according to quality; with prospective, randomized, double-blinded trials being the highest quality followed by consensus statements derived from literature review and expert opinion and finally, expert opinion in which there is no literature support. Guidelines are used to assist organizations in developing a consensus on the methods of patient care for areas where controversy exists or where large deviations in the use of treatments and procedures as well as costs occur. Parenteral and enteral nutrition is an example of a high cost therapy, used in patients in which benefit separate from the treatment of the primary disease is difficult to discern and opinions differ on if, when, and by what route nutrition should be provided. Development of an evidence-based clinical guideline should be useful in educating staff on the appropriate use and safe delivery of enteral and parenteral nutrition as well as assisting in identifying problems that need to be addressed. Appropriate use of parenteral nutrition at our institution was monitored before and following the development of clinical practice guidelines. Parenteral nutrition was considered appropriate if the patient was severely malnourished and met one of the following criteria: (a) failed enteral nutrition with an appropriate tube placement; (b) enteral nutrition was contraindicated as in paralytic ileus, mesenteric ischemia, small bowel obstruction, and gastrointestinal fistula and; (c) there was an expected transition to an enteral diet >7 days. Inappropriate parenteral nutrition use occurred in the following circumstances: (a) transition to an oral diet in 5–7 days, (b) inadequate documentation of failed enteral trial or contraindication to appropriate enteral tube placement, (c) cancer unresponsive to chemotherapy, (d) clinical illness precluded an appropriate response to therapy or, (e) there was an inadequate trial of medical management to treat hyperemesis gravidarum. Using these criteria, the frequency of appropriate parenteral nutrition use was 67%. This frequency fell to 41% when medical staff support was removed from the nutrition support service. This resulted in a 53% increase in patient days of therapy and a 36% increase in cost for parenteral nutrition despite the presence of clinical practice guidelines. The following actions were taken to improve appropriate parenteral nutrition use: (a) create an executive summary of clinical practice guideline making it user friendly that includes an algorithm (Fig. 2); (b) establish a process to continually monitor compliance to guidelines that identifies areas where education is needed; (c) improve documentation in the medical chart of the outcome of an enteral nutrition trial, the contraindication to enteral nutrition and objective evidence of gastrointestinal dysfunction. With these efforts, appropriate use of parenteral nutrition was increased to 80% resulting in a 50% decrease in the cost of parenteral nutrition. The next phase of the guideline implementation will include whether patients were initiated appropriately on enteral nutrition when indicated.

The Team Approach to Providing Nutrition Support

A nutrition support service (team) consists of a director, usually a physician, a dietitian, nurse and a pharmacist as core members. A formal service, when present, is consulted to provide either parenteral or enteral nutrition and serves the primary responsibility of assuring that if indicated the patient receives nutrition support via the appropriate route. The service obtains access and is responsible for the access device for nutrition support and initiates and manages nutrition therapy until which time the patient tolerates an enteral diet or is stabilized on tube feedings and care can be transferred back to the primary care team. As healthcare environments evolved, the concept of nutrition support services has changed. Many services have had staff reallocated or reduced and organizations have had various disciplines cross-trained to perform the functions (Table 2) that formal services once provided. The focus on reducing length of stay in intensive care units has created challenges in continuity of nutrition care as patients move back and forth between various areas of the hospital. Staff familiar with providing enteral tube feedings to complicated patients may be lacking in some areas that patients are transferred. Staffing may not allow for performing nutrition care functions to the extent or quality of that provided by a formalized service. The current emphasis is on teamwork rather than teams and the recognition that quality nutrition outcomes result from collaboration. This collaboration (and documentation) may be accomplished by having a specific nutrition support service responsible for providing specialized nutrition support or by multiple discipline involvement integrated with the patient care team not necessarily existing as a distinct team. It is evident that having no team or collaborative responsibility by individuals trained in providing specialized (enteral and parenteral) nutrition support results in poor patient outcomes. Therapy is used when not indicated and results in significant septic and metabolic complications. If a nutrition support service is not present, it is important to assure that staff are competent to perform nutrition support functions and a system is in place to monitor process and outcome indicators that reflect the quality of patient care being provided.

Summary

Nutrition support is a potentially life saving treatment. It is also expensive and risky, particularly in the hands of untrained health care providers. This is particularly true in the critically ill. The evidence-based standard for optimizing treatment outcomes for administering nutrition support effectively and safely is the interdisciplinary team approach. Fewer complications result when this method is in place. It has yet to be demonstrated that clinicians using standardized clinical guidelines can achieve the same clinical performance as a nutrition support team. It is likely that this approach is superior to leaving the use of nutrition support to individual clinicians with no special training in the use of this treatment. In any case, the measurement of clinical performance and use of the principles of continuous quality improvement are essential to assuring that patients receive the optimal benefit from this important, but risky form of treatment.

References

1. Alexander JW. MacMilan BG, Stinner JD, et al. (1980) Beneficial effects of aggressive protein feeding in severely burned children. Ann Surg 192: 505–517
2. A.S.P.E.N. Board of Directors. Guidelines for the use of parenteral and enteral nutrition in adult and pediatric patients (1993) J Parenter Enter Nutr 17 (Suppl): 1SA-52SA
3. Brown RS and J Grenkoski (1977) Total parenteral nutrition: a safe procedure in the small hospital? Crit Care Med 5:241-4
4. Chang RWS, Hatton I, Henley J, et al. (1986) Total parenteral nutrition: a four-year audit. Br J Surg 73: 656–658
5. Goldmann, DA and DG Maki (1973) Infection control in total parenteral nutrition. JAMA 223:1360-4
6. Hegland DK, MacDonald S, Keefe L and Drover JW (1998) Total parenteral nutrition in the critically ill patient. A meta-analysis. JAMA 280: 2013–2019
7. Kaminski MV and MH Stolar (1974) Parenteral hyperalimentation – A quality of care survey and review. Am J Hosp Pharm 31:228-35
8. Moore EE, Jones TN (1986) Benefits of immediate jejunostomy feeding after major abdominal trauma-a prospective, randomized study. J Trauma 26: 874–881
9. Nehme AE Nutritional support of the hospitalized patient (1980) JAMA 1906–8
10. Schneider PJ, A Bothe and M Bisognano (1999) Improving the nutrition support process: Assuring that more patients receive optimal nutrition support. Nutr Clin Pract. 14: 221–6
11. Skoutakis, VA, DR Martinez, WA Miller, et al. (1975) Team approach to total parenteral nutrition. Am J Hosp Pharm 32:693-7
12. Trujillo EB, Young LE, Chertow GM, et al. (1999) Metabolic and monetary costs of avoidable parenteral nutrition use. J Parenter Enter Nutr 23: 109–113

13. Wilmore DW and SJ Dudrick (1968) Growth and development of an infant receiving all nutrients exclusively by vein. JAMA 203:860–4
14. Young B, Ott L, Twyman D, et al. (1987) The effect of nutritional support on outcome from severe head injury. J Neurosurgery 67: 668–676

Enteral Versus Parenteral Feeding in Critical Illness

K.A. Kudsk

Hypermetabolic, critically ill patients rapidly mobilize lean tissue, releasing large quantities of amino acids into the circulating amino acid pool for distribution to the liver, intestine, bone marrow, and injured or healing tissues. Within these sites, gluconeogenesis, immune cell proliferation, and fibroblast proliferation support the body's attempts to seal and heal its injuries while maintaining defenses against bacterial challenges. Glutamine and alanine synthesis up-regulated through the metabolism of branched-chain amino acids by skeletal muscle provide specific fuels for enterocytes and rapidly proliferating immunocytes as well as sources of carbon skeletons for gluconeogenesis [1]. In addition, amino acids from the general amino acid pool are synthesized by the liver into acute-phase production to upregulate effectiveness of the reticuloendothelial system in clearing foreign material from the bloodstream [2]. While current opinion suggests that well-nourished patients can maintain a vigorous metabolic response for a week or perhaps longer, certain mechanisms of mucosal defenses may be influenced by nutrition support even in well-nourished patients. These defenses are described by Kudsk and Alverdy (this volume), and this chapter addresses the clinical implications of those mechanisms. Malnourished patients, however, may not be able to generate a prolonged, vigorous metabolic response because of pre-existing defects in protein-calorie deficiencies, rendering them vulnerable to bacterial assaults and wound healing problems.

In both well-nourished and malnourished patients, the timing, route, and generalized use of nutrition support has generated a significant body of both clinical and experimental data, attempting to define the role of nutrition support in these diverse patient populations. While there is little doubt that parenteral nutrition is lifesaving in patients with total loss of the gastrointestinal tract secondary to embolism, repeated resections for inflammatory bowel disease, prolonged obstruction, etc., its use in the critical care unit has recently been debated due to several studies. In 1991, 395 malnourished patients in Veterans Administration Hospitals of North America requiring laparotomy or noncardiac thoracotomy were randomized to one to 2 weeks of preoperative nutrition or no perioperative nutrition support [3]. Significantly more infectious complications developed in the patients receiving parenteral nutrition with no corresponding significant decrease in noninfectious complications. Only in severely malnourished patients did parenteral nutrition provide obvious benefits by significantly reducing noninfectious complications, such as wound or anastomotic dehiscence, without increasing infectious complications. Subsequently, in a randomized, prospective trial of 117 well-nourished to moderately malnourished patients randomized to postoperative parenteral nutrition or IV fluids alone, intra-abdominal abscess and major complications were significantly greater in parenterally fed patients [4]. Some support for parenteral nutrition was noted, however, in a study by Fann et al. who demonstrated benefit of parenteral nutrition in patients undergoing resection of hepatocellular carcinoma [5]. Postoperative morbidity was significantly reduced with the perioperative parenteral nutrition due to fewer septic complications compared to patients fed an oral diet alone. Notwithstanding this final study, and with experimental data suggesting that enteral delivery of nutrients provides benefits not gained when nutrients are delivered intravenously [6–8], comparisons of enteral and parenteral feeding in patients sustaining severe injuries or undergoing major surgical procedures have been carried out. While the preponderance of studies were performed in patients with blunt and penetrating trauma of the torso, other categories of patients, such as those with head injuries, transplantation, pancreatitis, etc., have also been studied. This chapter evaluates those studies.

Blunt and Penetrating Trauma of the Torso

Moore et al. [9] randomized trauma patients requiring celiotomy at moderate risk of infectious complications by the calculated Abdominal Trauma Index (see Enteral Access chapter for table of ATI) to early enteral feeding or delayed (after 5 days) parenteral nutrition. Over the first 5 days of hospitalization, patients received no nutrition other than the intravenous glucose. The intra-abdominal abscess rate was significantly increased in patients receiving delayed parenteral nutrition, providing support to early experimental studies comparing enteral versus parenteral nutrition. Subsequently, patients with similar risks of infectious complications by the ATI were randomized to early enteral feeding or early parenteral nutrition [10]. Pneumonia was significantly reduced in patients receiving early enteral feeding with nonsignificant intra-abdominal abscesses. Our group randomized 98 patients with a moderate to severe risk of infectious complications by the ATI or Injury Severity Score (ISS) to either early enteral feeding with a defined formula diet or to parenteral solution with similar concentrations of fat, carbohydrate, and protein [11]. Both pneumonia and intra-abdominal abscess was significantly reduced in patients receiving early enteral feeding (Table 1), but it was clear that the benefit was noted only in the most severely injured patients (Table 2). There was no benefit (and a low risk of infectious complications) in patients with lesser degrees of injury, but patients with an abdominal trauma index (ATI) >25 or an injury severity >20 had a significant reduction in infections.

Two studies have demonstrated no benefit with early enteral feeding but warrant close inspection to explain the discrepancy with the three articles mentioned above. Adams et al. [12] randomized 46 patients to early enteral or parenteral feeding after trauma laparotomy. There were no differences in infectious complications, but there appeared to be a significant breakdown in the random-

Table 1. Septic morbidity (*ENT* enteral, *TPN* total parenteral nutrition)

	ENT		TPN		
	n	%	n	%	P
Pneumonia	6/51	11.8	14/45	31	<0.02
Intra-abdominal abscess	1/51	1.9	6/45	13.3	<0.04
Empyema	1/51	1.9	4/45	9	NS
Line sepsis	1/51	1.9	6/45	13.3	<0.05
Fasciitis/dehiscence	3/51	5.9	4/45	8.9	NS
Abscess (intra-abdominal and/or empyema)	2/51	3.9	8/45	17.8	<0.03
Pneumonia and/or abscess	8/51	13.7	17/45	37.8	<0.02
Pneumonia, abscesses, and/or line sepsis	9/51	15.7	18/45	40	<0.02

Table 2. Frequency of infections (pneumonia, intra-abdominal abscess, or empyema) after stratification of patients by mechanism and severity of injury (*ENT* enteral, *TPN* total parenteral nutrition, *ISS* Index Severity Score, *ATI* Abdominal Trauma Index)

Variable	ENT		TPN		Odds ratio	P
	n	%	n	%		
ISS ≤20	3/17	17.7	4/20	20.0		0.9
ISS >20	5/34	14.7	13/25	52.0	6.3 ×	<0.002
ATI ≤24	5/24	20.8	7/24	29.2		0.6
ATI >24	3/27	11.1	10/21	47.6	7.3 ×	<0.005
ATI >24 and ISS >20	3/20	15.0	8/12	66.7	11.3 ×	<0.003
Blunt	4/16	25.0	6/10	60	3.0 ×	0.08
Penetrating	4/35	11.4	11/35	31.4	3.6 ×	<0.05

ization process. Although ISS scores were similar, the early enteral feeding group had twice the number of head injuries, three times as many *severe* thoracic injuries, and three times the number of pelvic fractures (Table 3). Since fever, leukocytosis, and infiltrate on chest X-ray were used as diagnostic criteria for pneumonia, the incidence of severe chest injury may have biased the outcome toward a higher diagnosis rate of pneumonia in the early enteral group. Eyer et al. [13] randomized 52 patients with blunt trauma with an ISS greater than 13 to early feeding or delayed feeding. Total infectious complications were significantly greater in the group randomized to early enteral feeding primarily due to increased pneumonia and urinary tract infections, but it is not stated whether there was a difference in the number of patients developing infections. The types of injuries were not provided; however, there appeared to be more severe chest injuries in the blunt trauma patients randomized to early enteral feeding as measured by depressed PaO_2/FiO_2 ratio (Table 4). Almost 60% of the patients in the early fed group had a PaO_2/FiO_2 ratio less than 150, indicating a shunt factor of

Table 3. Patient injuries (from [12])

	Jejunostomy (*n*=23)	TPN (*n*=23)
Age (years)	29±10	29±10
Injury Severity Score	39±12	36±12
Prognostic Nutrition Index	63±15	57±18
Blunt injury	20 (87%)	13 (56%)
Head injury	9 (39%)	5 (22%)
Severe chest injury	12 (52%)	4 (17%)
Pelvic fracture	9 (39%)	3 (13%)
Soft tissue	6 (26%)	1 (4%)

Table 4. Demographics and outcome data (from [13])

	Early feeding (*n*=19)	Late feeding (*n*=19)
Age (years)	44±22	41±18
Injury Severity Score	34±11	32±9
Admission PaO_2/FiO_2	11 (58%)	4 (21%)
Pneumonia	8	4
Urinary tract	4	2
Abdominal abscess	1	0
Wound infection	3	1
Catheter sepsis	1	1
Bacteremia	2	0
Sinusitis	9	6
Eye infection	1	0

approximately 25%; whereas, approximately 20% of the patient receiving delayed feeding had this severe ventilation-perfusion mismatch. Since pneumonia was diagnosed by fever, leukocytosis, or infiltrates as well as "significant growth on sputum cultures," an over diagnosis of pneumonia has been postulated as the primary reason for lack of benefit or infectious complications in the group randomized to early feeding. Additional infections of the urinary tract, sinuses, and eye, noted in the early enteral group are unlikely to be affected by route of nutrition (Table 4).

In summary, early enteral delivery of nutrients in patients sustaining severe blunt and penetrating trauma of the torso appears to benefit the patient by reducing infectious complications compared to parenteral nutrition, delayed enteral feeding, or IV fluids alone.

Head Injury

Several studies compare enteral and parenteral feeding in head injured patients, but only one [14] of the five published studies randomizing patients have noted any benefit with early enteral feeding compared to TPN or IV fluids alone. Typical of these studies, gastroparesis complicating the head injury often delayed advancement of enteral feeding over the first 5–10 days.

Rapp et al. [15] studied patients within 8 h of severe head injury, randomizing them to parenteral nutrition or intragastric feedings after gastric residuals had dropped below 300 cc. Mortality rate was significantly higher in the enteral group although almost all of the deaths were attributed to the head injury itself. One-third of the patients in the enteral group developed septic complications, but the septic rate in the parenterally fed group was not reported. Typical of this patient population, gastroparesis limited gastric emptying, resulting in a mean calorie intake of only 500 kcal/day in the enteral group over the first 7 days compared with 2000 calories in the TPN group. None of the enteral patients received more than 600 kcal/day during the first week or more than 1000 kcal/day over the first 10 days. Unfortunately, the reduced mortality with early parenteral nutrition following head injury was not confirmed in a second study by the same group [16]. Neurologic outcome was similar in this study, and a 30% incidence of sepsis was found in both enteral and parenteral groups. Although an early improvement in Glasgow Coma Scale score (GCS) was noted at 3 months with parenteral feeding, there were no differences between the groups at late follow-up.

Hadley et al. [17] randomized 45 head injured patients with a GCS ≤10 to intragastric feeding or parenteral nutrition but noted no differences in complication rate or infectious complications over the course of the study. Similar results were found by Borzotta [18] who randomized 48 head injured patient with a GCS ≤8 to parenteral nutrition or surgically placed jejunostomies. There appeared to be no differences in significant clinical outcome between the two patient populations.

Grahm et al. [14] published the only positive study randomizing 22 patients with a GCS <10 to either nasojejunal feeding within 36 h of injury or intragastric feedings when GI tract function returned. Infectious complications, notably fewer bacterial infections within the pulmonary tract, were noted in patients receiving early intrajejunal feeding.

In summary, although either enteral or parenteral nutrition can meet nutrient goals, there is little convincing evidence that positively influences infectious morbidity or neurologic outcome following severe head injury. This discrepancy with results of blunt and penetrating trauma studies may reflect the character of the patients and their neurosurgical management. Head injured patients undergo prolonged intubation, immobilization, and paralysis to minimize increases in intracranial pressure. This intensive neurosurgical management may lasts seven to 10 days or longer and precludes ventilator weaning and even effective pulmonary toilet in some situations. Given the inherent pulmonary assault of this management, pneumonia may be inevitable despite any nutrition support.

General Surgical Patients

Benefits of nutrition and effect of route of nutrition on outcome of general surgical patients appears limited to patients with more advanced degrees of malnutrition prior to surgical procedure. The studies by The VA Cooperative Group [3] and Brennan et al. [4] noted can confirm this. This concept is also consistent with observations that complication rates after upper gastrointestinal surgical procedures are very low in well-nourished patients, and it is unlikely that nutrition support is likely to positively influence clinical outcome [19]. Further support is provided in Heslin et al.'s [20] study in which 195 well-nourished patients undergoing esophageal, gastric, or pancreatic surgery were randomized to early enteral feeding or IV fluids alone. Feeding did not influence the number of major, minor, or infectious complications resulting in difference in hospital mortality or length of stay. Similarly, Dogietto [21] noted no benefit of protein-sparing therapy in 678 patients with normal nutritional status or mild malnutrition undergoing major elective abdominal surgery.

When stratified by degree of malnutrition, some studies do demonstrate a benefit of early enteral feeding in general surgical patients. Shirabe et al. [22] studied 26 patients undergoing major hepatic resection randomized to either early feeding or parenteral nutrition and noted significantly higher immunologic parameters, such as lymphocyte number and PHA response, in patients receiving early enteral nutrition. Infectious complications were also higher in the parenteral group (31%) versus the enteral group (8%), but this did not reach statistical significance. Gianotti [23] randomized patients undergoing pancreatic, duodenal, or gastric surgery to enteral diets or parenteral nutrition. Postoperative infection rate was the highest in the parenterally fed group (28%) compared with patients receiving enhanced enteral diet. Length of stay also was significantly increased in patients receiving parenteral nutrition. A group randomized to a standard enteral diet had infection rates and hospital stays midway between the parenteral group and the patients receiving the enhanced diet, suggesting that benefits of both route and type of nutrition in these patients undergoing major surgical procedures.

Sand et al. [24] randomized 29 patients undergoing total gastrectomy to either jejunal feeding or parenteral nutrition. There were fewer infective complications in the enteral group (23%) compared with the parenteral group (31%), but this failed to reach statistical significance. Bier-Holgersen randomized patients undergoing major abdominal surgery to either enteral nutrition supplements or placebo via a duodenal feeding tube. Infectious complications were significantly lower in the group receiving the nutritional supplements.

Interpretations of data from heterogeneous patient populations of general surgical patients with varying nutritional status and stress is not as clear as patients undergoing several blunt trauma. There is a tendency towards a reduction in infectious complications with early enteral feeding which reaches statistical significance in a few studies, but it appears that preexisting malnutrition may be an important factor. One can speculate that just as benefits are only gained in severely injured trauma patients, benefits of nutrition therapy on outcome in general are likely to be obvious only when preexisting malnutrition is evident at the time of surgical stress.

Inflammatory Bowel Disease

Patients with inflammatory bowel disease are often in negative nitrogen balance as a result of poor oral intake, inadequate absorptive surface, acute and chronic inflammation, and the catabolic effects of steroid therapy. In patients with ulcerative colitis, enteral and parenteral therapy are equally effective as therapeutic agents and produce similar rates of disease remission [25]. Gonzales-Huiz [26] randomized 42 patients to either a polymeric enteral nutrition or to an isocaloric, isonitrogenous parenteral solution in patients with a moderate to severe degree of malnutrition. There were fewer adverse advents, fewer postoperative infections, and an improvement in serum albumin in the group randomized to early enteral feeding.

Bowel obstruction frequently complicates the ability to deliver enteral nutrition in patients with Crohn's disease, and there are no randomized, prospective studies comparing enteral and parenteral feeding. Although several studies suggested that an elemental enteral diet is equivalent to steroid therapy in inducing disease remission, it is unclear whether enteral feeding provides any additional benefit compared to parenteral nutrition.

Organ Transplant

The results following liver transplant have been relatively inconsistent. In a study of 24 patients randomized to jejunal feeding or parenteral nutrition, Wicks and colleagues [27] demonstrated no difference in outcome between the two groups. Hasse et al. [28], however, randomized 50 transplant patients to jejunal feeding or IV fluids and noted excellent tolerance to enteral feeding. Of the 31 patients completing the study, there was a significant reduction in viral infections in patients fed via the gastrointestinal tract and a trend toward a reduction in bacterial infections as well (29.4% vs. 14.3%). These findings are consistent with improvement in mucosal immunology addressed in Chapter 2. These changes in clinical outcome, however, did not affect hospital costs, ventilator days, length of stay, or rejection.

Recently, Mehta [29] placed jejunostomy tubes at the time of liver transplantation and administered enteral feeding with a semi-elemental diet and parenteral nutrition to 21 patients. Early enteral feeding increased the incidence of diarrhea (73% vs. 25%) but stimulated resumption of oral nutrition sooner and reduced the incidence of prolonged postoperative ileus compared to parenteral nutrition. In most cases, the diarrhea induced by enteral feeding lasted three to 5 days and responded rapidly to antimotility drugs.

Pancreatitis

Relatively few studies have investigated patients with pancreatitis since upper intestinal feeding was considered a contraindication to intragastric feeding to avoid stimulation of pancreatic secretions. In cases of severe pancreatitis, gastric decompression is necessary and, unless access distal to the ligament of Treitz can be obtained at the time of surgery, intravenous nutrition is almost unavoidable. In conditions of mild pancreatitis, however, access beyond the ligament of Treitz is possible without surgery. McClave [30] randomized 30 patients admitted with mild, acute pancreatitis to either nasojejunal feeding or to isocaloric, isonitrogenous parenteral nutrition. Both cost of nutrition care and stress-induced hyperglycemia was significantly increased with parenteral nutrition, and clinical outcome parameters measured by the Ranson criteria improved significantly in the enterally fed group. Windsor et al. [31] stratified patients according to severity of acute pancreatitis and randomized them to either parenteral nutrition or enteral nutrition for 7 days. The markers of the system inflammatory response syndrome, sepsis, organ failure, and ICU stay were improved in enterally fed patients with improvements in the acute-phase response and disease severity scores. These latter two parameters remained unchanged in patients given parenteral feeding.

In summary, these studies suggest a benefit of enteral delivery of nutrients in patients in whom appropriate access can be obtained in cases of mild to acute pancreatitis. There are no studies of patients with severe pancreatitis randomized to enteral versus parenteral feeding.

Pediatric Studies

Few isolated studies of enteral and parenteral feeding have been noted in the pediatric population, suggesting some benefits with enteral delivery of nutrients. In a study of 29 consecutive pediatric patients requiring extracorporal membrane oxygenation (ECMO) [32], patients were administered either parenteral nutrition or total enteral nutrition during their hospital stay. There was no difference between the time needed to achieve caloric goals from initiation of ECMO, and there were no complications associated with enteral feeding. Survival was higher in the enteral fed group (100% vs. 79%) although this did not reach statistical significance. Cost for nutrition support was less with enteral nutrition.

Summary

Considering the body of data investigating the role of nutrition support and differences in route and type of nutrition, several basic principles became evident. The majority of patients tolerate either enteral or parenteral feeding. In patients who recover quickly and have a low risk of complications, there is no benefit gained by enteral delivery of nutrients and, in fact, complications can increase when parenteral nutrition is used. This is most obvious in well-nourished or mildly malnourished patients undergoing general surgical procedures. In patients who are severely malnourished, parenteral nutrition appears to be beneficial. In almost clinical studies of patients responsive to nutrition support, there appears to be an advantage to delivering nutrients via the gastrointestinal tract including reduced infectious complications and earlier return in GI tract function. The ability to feed enterally, however, is influenced by the ability to obtain access at an appropriate point in the gastrointestinal tract (See Kirby and Kudsk's Chapter). If appropriate access is obtained, malnutrition exists, or the degree of stress and insult is significant enough to warrant nutrition support, under almost all circumstances enteral delivery of nutrients delivers results which are comparable to or better than the use of parenteral nutrition.

References

1. Wilmore DW, et al. (1988) The gut: A central organ following surgical stress. Surgery 104: 917–923
2. Kudsk KA, Minard G, Wojtysiak SL, Croce ML, Fabian T, Brown RO (1994) Visceral protein response to enteral vs. parenteral nutrition and sepsis in trauma patients. Surgery 116 (3):516–523
3. The Veteran Affairs Total Parenteral Nutrition Cooperative Study Group: Perioperative total parenteral nutrition in surgical patients (1991) N Engl J Med 325:525–532
4. Brennan MF, Pisters PWT, Posner M, Quesada O, Shike M (1994) A prospective, randomized trial of total parenteral nutrition after major pancreatic resection for malignancy. Ann Surg 220:436–444
5. Fan St, Lo CM, Lai EC, Chu KM, Liu CL, Wong J (1994) Perioperative nutritional support in patients undergoing hepatectomy for hepatocellular carcinoma. N Engl J Med 331:1547–52
6. Kudsk KA, Carpenter G, Petersen S, Sheldon GF (1981) Effect of enteral and parenteral feeding in malnourished rats with E. coli-hemoglobin adjuvant peritonitis. J Surg Res 31:105–110
7. Kudsk KA, Stone JM, Carpenter G, Sheldon GF (1983) Enteral and Parenteral Feeding Influences Mortality After Hemoglobin-E. coli Peritonitis in Normal Rats. J Trauma 23: 605–609
8. Kudsk KA, Renegar KB, Li J (1996) Loss of upper respiratory tract immunity with parenteral feeding. Ann Surg 223:629–638
9. Moore EE, Jones TN (1986) Benefits of immediate jejunostomy feeding after major abdominal trauma– a prospective, randomized study. J Trauma 26:874–879
10. Moore FA, Moore EE, Jones TN, McCroskey BL, Peterson VM (1989) TEN versus TPN following major abdominal trauma– reduced septic morbidity. J Trauma 29:916–923
11. Kudsk KA, Croce MA, Fabian TC, et al. (1992) Enteral versus parenteral feeding: effects on septic morbidity after blunt and penetrating abdominal trauma. Annals of Surgery 215 (5):165–173
12. Adams S, Dellinger EP, Wertz MJ, Oreskovich MR, Simonowitz D, Johansen K (1986) Enteral versus parenteral nutritional support following laparotomy for trauma: a randomized prospective trial. J Trauma 26:882–891
13. Eyer SD, Micon LT, Konstantinides FN, et al. (1993) Early enteral feeding does not attenuate metabolic response after blunt trauma. J Trauma 34:639–44
14. Grahm TW, Zadrozny DB, Harrington T (1989) The benefits of early jejunal hyperalimentation in the head-injured patient. Neurosurgery 25:729–35
15. Rapp RP, Young B, Twymand D, Bivins BA, Haack D, Tibbs PA, Bean JR (1983) The favorable effect of early parenteral feeding on survival in head injured patients. J. Nuerosurg 58:906–911
16. Young B, Ott L, Haack D, et al. (1987) Effect of total parenteral nutrition upon intracranial pressure in severe head injury. J Neurosurg 67:668–676
17. Hadley MN, Grahm TW, Harrington T, et al. (1986) Nutritional support in neurotrauma: a critical review of early nutrition in 45 acute head injury patients. Neurosurgery 19:367–73
18. Borzotta AP, Penning S, Papasadero B, Paxton J, Mardesic S, Borzotta R, Parrott A, Bledsoe F (1994) Enteral vs parenteral nutrition after severe closed head injury. J Trauma 37:459–68
19. King BK, Blackwell AP, Minard G, Kudsk, KA (1997) Predicting patient outcome using preoperative nutritional markers. Surg Forum 48:592–595

20. Heslin MJ, Latkany L, Leung D, Brooks AD, Hochwald SN, Pisters PW, Shike M, Brennan MF (1997) A prospective, randomized trial of early enteral feeding after resection of upper gastrointestinal malignancy. Ann Surg 226:567–77

21. Doglietto GB, Gallitelli L, Pacelli F, Bellantone R, Malerba M, Sgadari A, Crucitti F (1996) Protein-sparing therapy after major abdominal surgery: lack of clinical effects. Ann Surg 223:357–62

22. Shirabe K, Matsumata T, Shimada M, Takenaka K, Kawahara N, Yamamoto K, Nishizaki T, Sugimachi K (1997) A comparison of parenteral hyperalimentation and early enteral feeding regarding systemic immunity after major hepatic resection– the results of a randomized prospective study. Hepatogastroenterology 44:205–9

23. Gianotti L, Braga M, Vignali A, Balzano G, Zerbi A, Bisagni P, Di Carlo V (1997) Effect of route of delivery and formulation of postoperative nutritional support in patients undergoing major operations for malignant neoplasms. Arch Surg 132:1222–9

24. Sand J, Luostarinen M, Matikainen M (1997) Enteral or parenteral feeding after total gastrectomy: prospective randomized pilot study. Eur J Surg 163:761–766

25. Dickerson RJ, Ashton MG, Axon HTR, et al. (1980) Controlled trial of intravenous hyperalimentation and total bowel rest as a adjunct to routine therapy of acute colitis. Gastroenterology 79:1199–1205

26. Gonzalez-Huix F, Fernandez-Banares F, Esteve-Comas M, Abad-Lacruz A, Cabre E, Acero D, Figa M, Guilera M, Humbert P, de Leon R, et al. (1993) Enteral versus parenteral nutrition as adjunct therapy in acute ulcerative colitis. Am J Gastroenterol 88:227–32

27. Wicks C, Somasundaram S, Bjarnason I, Menzies IS, Routley D, Potter D, Tan KC, Williams R. Comparison of enteral feeding and total parenteral nutrition after liver transplantation. Lancet 344:837–840

28. Hasse JM, Blue LS, Liepa GU, Goldstein RM, Jennings LW, Mor E, Husberg BS, Levy MF, Gonwa TA, Klintmalm GB (1995) Early enteral nutrition support in patients undergoing liver transplantation. JPEN 19:437–43

29. Mehta TL, Alaka KJ, Filo RS, Leapman SB, Milgrom ML, Pescovitz MD (1995) Nutrition support following liver transplantation: comparison of jejunal versus parenteral routes. Clin Transplant (Denmark) 9:364–369

30. McClave SA, Greene LM, Snider HL, Makk LJK, Cheadle WG, Owens NA, Dukes LG, Goldsmith LJ (1997) Comparison of the safety of early enteral vs parenteral nutrition in mild acute pancreatitis. JPEN 21 (1):14–20

31. Windsor AC, Kanwar S, Li AG, Barnes E, Guthrie JA, Spark JI, Welsh F, Guillou PJ, Reynolds JV (1998) Compared with parenteral nutrition, enteral feeding attenuates the acute phase response and improves disease severity in acute pancreatitis. Gut 42:431–435.

32. Pettignano R, Heard M, Davis R, Labuz M, Hart M (1998) Total enteral nutrition vrsus total parenteral nutrition during pediatric extracorporeal membrane oxygenation. Crit Care Med 26:358–363

Obtaining and Maintaining Access for Nutrition Support

D.F. Kirby and K.A. Kudsk

Whenever possible, enteral delivery of nutrients is the preferred route for specialized nutrition support in critically ill patients. In addition to obvious economic benefits, substantial clinical data demonstrates improved clinical outcome in certain groups of critically ill or critically injured medical and surgical patients.

The appropriate access technique for an ICU patient depends upon multiple factors including the following: (a) need for laparotomy; (b) the functional status of the gut; (c) how long access will be needed; (d) an estimate of the patient's risk of aspiration; (e) the patient's co-morbidities and others as defined in Table 1. The foremost is the functional status of the gastrointestinal tract. The only absolute contraindication to enteral feeding is complete mechanical obstruction, but protracted vomiting, intestinal dysmotility, severe malabsorption and diarrhea, or inability to obtain safe access to an adequate GI surface area for absorption (e.g., distal to a fistula) can create special challenges for the safe, effective use of the GI tract. Under some circumstances, enteral feeding may be successful if access to specific sites is available; for example, in patients with delayed gastric emptying secondary to head injury, diabetes mellitus, sepsis, or gastric outlet obstruction secondary to stress ulceration, access beyond the ligament of Treitz may allow successful enteral delivery while intragastric feeding is doomed to failure. Direct small intestinal feeding may be safe in hemodynamically stable patients capable of shunting blood to the gastrointestinal tract for digestion and absorption but may carry significant risk for intestinal ischemia and necrosis under conditions of hemodynamic instability requiring pressors. Under these circumstances, intragastric feeding may still be safe since a high gastric residual will identify the patient incapable of safe enteral feeding.

Estimated length of time for access becomes an important step in selecting the access site. For short term use (less than 30 days), a nasoenteric tube may be adequate, but for long-term use (greater than 30 days), a tube enterostomy may be more appropriate although exceptions to this guidelines do occur [1].

Risk of aspiration depends on several factors. If oropharyngeal dysphagia is present, the patient may aspirate his secretions and oral food or fail to protect the airway from gastroesophageal reflux of feedings. Videofluoroscopy may be clinically helpful in the assessment of stable ICU patients suspected of these conditions. Intubated, sedated, supine patients are at risk of tube feeding-related reflux, which could increase mortality and morbidity. Mittal et al. noted that catheters

Table 1. Questions to address while considering ICU enteral feeding (adapted and used with permission of Ross Products Division, Abbott Laboratories, Columbus, Ohio, from 17th Ross Roundtable. 1997 Ross Products Division, Abbott Laboratories)

1	Is the GI tract functional: obstructed? intact?
2	Does the patient have an underlying condition that might lead to delayed gastric emptying (e.g., head injury, diabetes mellitus, sepsis)?
3	Does the patient have a feeding tube in place, and if so, where is its tip located?
4	Is the patient on a ventilator? hemodynamically stable? on pressors?
5	Is the patient conscious and cooperative?
6	Is the patient able to be placed in a head up (30–45°) position or must the patient continuously lie flat?
7	Can the patient be transported to the Radiology Department, if necessary? or is there a bedside fluoroscopy unit available?
8	Is bedside endoscopy available?
9	Are there any contraindications to feeding tube placement?

crossing the lower esophageal sphincter aggravate reflux and aspiration by increasing transient lower esophageal sphincter relaxation [2]. Feeding beyond the stomach may seem a reasonable goal in this situation, but effectiveness has not been proven. Many studies of this problem have failed to document the position of the postpyloric feeding tube [3, 4]. Gastric reflux and subsequent gastroesophageal reflux may be common unless access is obtained distal to the ligament of Treitz. Elevation of the head of the bed reduces aspiration, but does not eliminate it in ventilated patients [5, 6], and nasogastric tube decompression of the stomach does not reduce its risk [7]. Gastric feeding is safe and the incidence of reflux is low in the critically ill patient if the head of the bed is elevated and gastric residuals remain low (<100 ml every 4 h). However, the safest site for feeding in vulnerable patients is into the distal duodenum or past the ligament of Treitz which reduces tube feeding-related aspiration complications [8, 9].

Underlying conditions also influence successful feeding. Intragastric feeding will be less successful with delayed gastric emptying due to diabetes, head injury, or severe sepsis unless these conditions are correctable. Similarly, enteral feeding is unwise in patients with diffuse peritoneal metastases, significant ascites, diffuse adhesions, or other processes causing high-grade, partial, intestinal obstructions unless access can be obtained in uninvolved bowel with residual surface area adequate for digestion and absorption. However, ICU patients without such obvious contraindications have a number of potential sites for accessing the gastrointestinal tract (Fig. 1), and the choice is determined most commonly by indications for laparotomy to manage the primary disease and the opportunity for direct enteral access at that time.

Access in Patients Undergoing Celiotomy

If surgical therapy by celiotomy is required for the management of a primary disease state, certain populations will benefit from direct enteral access. Since intra-

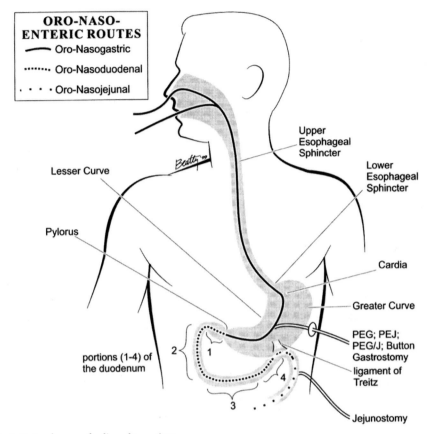

Fig. 1. Enteral access feeding alternatives

gastric feeding is unreliable due to gastroparesis early following surgical procedures, access in trauma and surgical patients should be obtained beyond the ligament of Treitz. Trauma patients requiring laparotomy should have direct access
if they have spinal cord injuries, an Abdominal Trauma Index=25 (Table 2), Injury
Severity Score (ISS)=20 [10], severe closed head injuries, multiple lower extremity fractures and/or soft tissue injuries requiring surgical/orthopedic procedures,
or a high likelihood of sepsis or delayed oral intake [11–17]. In general, patients
with major trauma to two major anatomic regions, such as the chest and
abdomen, the head and lower extremity, etc., have an ISS of 20 or greater. Surgical judgment is necessary to determine general surgical patients likely to have
delayed oral intake and require specialized nutrition support. Patients with an
albumin <32.5 g/l experience a higher risk of postoperative complications than
well-nourished patients [18–19]. Access beyond the ligament of Treitz can be
accomplished in one of three ways: advancement of a nasal and/or oral tube
through the stomach and into the small intestine, placement of a transgastric
jejunostomy [20, 21], or placement of a jejunal catheter [22, 23].

Table 2. Calculated risk of sepsis by the abdominal trauma index (from [11, 39])

Organ Injured	Risk factor	Scoring
High Risk		
Pancreas	5	1. Tangential 2. Through and through (duct intact) 3. Major débridement or distal duct injury 4. Proximal duct injury 5. Pancreaticoduodenectomy
Large intestine	5	1. Serosal 2. Single wall 3. ≤25% wall 4. >25% wall 5. Colon wall and blood supply
Major vascular	5	1. ≤25% wall 2. >25% wall 3. Complete transection 4. Interposition grafting or bypass 5. Ligation
Moderately high risk		
Duodenum	4	1. Single wall 2. ≤25% wall 3. >25% wall 4. Duodenal wall and blood supply 5. Pancreaticoduodenectomy
Liver	4	1. Nonbleeding peripheral 2. Bleeding, central, or minor débridement 3. Major débridement or hepatic artery ligation 4. Lobectomy 5. Lobectomy with caval repair or extensive bilobar débridement
Moderate risk		
Stomach	3	1. Single wall 2. Through and through 3. Minor débridement 4. Wedge resection 5. >35% resection
Spleen	3	1. Nonbleeding 2. Cautery or hemostatic agent 3. Minor débridement or suturing 4. Partial resection 5. Splenectomy
Low risk		
Kidney	2	1. Nonbleeding 2. Minor débridement or suturing 3. Major débridement 4. Pedicle or major calyceal 5. Nephrectomy
Ureter	2	1. Contusion 2. Laceration 3. Minor débridement 4. Segmental resection 5. Reconstruction

Table 2. *Continued*

Bladder	1	1. Single wall 2. Through and through 3. Debridement 4. Wedge resection 5. Reconstruction
Extrahepatic biliary	1	1. Contusion 2. Cholecystectomy 3. ≤25% wall 4. >25% wall 5. Biliary enteric reconstruction
Bone	1	1. Periosteum 2. Cortex 3. Through and through 4. Intra-articular 5. Major bone loss
Small bowel	1	1. Single Wall 2. Through and through 3. ≤25% wall 4. >25% wall 5. Wall and blood supply or >5 injuries
Minor vascular	1	1. Nonbleeding small hematoma 2. Nonbleeding large hematoma 3. Suturing 4. Ligation of isolated vessels 5. Ligation of named vessels

Nasal Placement of Enteric Tubes

At surgery, a tube is advanced through the stomach and guided thorough the duodenum into the small intestine. Because this can be technically challenging, a Kocher maneuver may be helpful, but with practice, either a small-bore feeding tube or an NG/NJ tube can be used. Unfortunately, dislodgment in the ICU is not uncommon, and nursing personnel must be well trained to avoid this problem [24]. A major advantage is that no additional violation of the gastrointestinal tract is required. Fortunately, direct enteral access does not increase the incidence of intraperitoneal sepsis even if prior GI tract violation has not occurred.

Direct Small Bowel Access (Jejunostomy Tubes)

Either of two types of jejunostomy tubes are currently used: large-bore 14-, 16-, 18-F or larger jejunostomy tubes or the needle catheter jejunostomy. A needle catheter jejunostomy should be used when required for less than 3 weeks since they cannot be replaced if clogged or dislodged [22, 23]. Larger bore tubes provide the advantage of replacement.

Jejunostomy construction must be meticulous. The site of tube insertion in the small intestine must be far enough from the ligament of Treitz to avoid tension and dislodgement from a too short afferent limb if the patient becomes distended. After advancing the tube into the small intestine at the enterotomy site through a pursestring suture, five 3-0 silk sutures placed over a distance of 5 cm should be used to create a Witzel tunnel over the tube. By leaving the needles on the first, the third, and the fifth suture, these sutures can be used to attach the jejunostomy to the anterior abdominal wall and avoid tube dislodgement into the peritoneum or volvulus at the attachment site, the two complications which can occur if a single stitch is used to attach the jejunostomy to the anterior abdominal wall. An additional stitch placed above the tube insertion site is used to isolate the tube from the peritoneal cavity. In circumstances in which the bowel is too edematous to create a Witzel tunnel around a larger bore catheter, a needle catheter jejunostomy can still be used in most circumstances. The jejunostomy should be brought out either just lateral to the rectus sheath to minimize chances of small bowel herniation above the jejunostomy attachment site.

In any direct small bowel access technique, feeding should not be started until patients are hemodynamically stable and advanced cautiously, recognizing the variability in tolerance typical of critically ill patients [25–27]. Although chemically defined diets were recommended for direct small bowel feedings, particularly through small-bore needle catheter jejunostomies, these restrictions are not necessary [28], and fiber-containing diets can be administered through a 5-F needle catheter jejunostomy [29]. However, some limitations with 5-F small-bore tubes are necessary. Protein supplement added to tube feedings will clog 5-F tubes as will some of the immune-enhancing diets. There are no contraindications to either the addition of protein supplements or the use of an immune-enhancing diet (diets supplemented with glutamine and/or arginine and/or omega-3 fatty acids, et al.) in patients with the 7-F needle catheter jejunostomy. Medications should not be administered via the needle catheter because of clogging due to feeding "coagulation" and difficulty in replacing or opening an occluded tube. Larger bore jejunostomy tubes can be replaced if clogging occurs, allowing their use for medication administration.

All jejunostomies should be irrigated every 6 h. In the occasional instance of obstruction of a needle catheter jejunostomy within the first 48 h, the cause is usually a tube "kink" at the fascial level. By simultaneously flushing and withdrawing the tube, the kink straightens and flow resumes immediately. The kink can be cut off and the needle reattached. This complication never occurs a second time.

Transgastric Jejunostomy

Transgastric jejunostomies allow simultaneous decompression of the stomach and bypass problems of gastroparesis by providing access beyond the pylorus [20, 21]. The tube design should have a postpyloric tube long enough to allow positioning of the distal port beyond the ligament of Treitz and not just into the duodenum. Proximal intraduodenal feeding stimulates pancreatic and biliary secretions which can cause fluid and electrolyte problems while direct intestinal feedings do not. In some circumstances, these losses can be 2–3 l/day with some loss of feedings as well. Transgastric jejunostomies are easily placed and the use of a stylette available in some kits eases advancement of the tube through the pylorus into the duodenum. Feedings into the small intestine should not be started unless patients are hemodynamically stable and capable of shunting blood to the gastrointestinal tract in response to enteral delivery of nutrients to minimize the chance of intestinal ischemia or necrosis.

Access in Patients with no Indications for Celiotomy

Most ICU patients requiring enteral access have no indication for celiotomy, and radiologic, laparoscopic, and endoscopic techniques can be used in these circumstances. Access is determined by the availability of resources and expertise available in an institution for placing access devices. ICU management by nursing personnel ultimately determine the longevity and success in maintaining these tubes.

Oro- and Nasoenteric Access

When no gastroparesis exists and there are no anatomic restrictions or contraindications to tube placement, simple intragastric feeding is successful in the majority of patients. Orally placed enteric tubes may be necessary in patients sustaining facial fractures and nasal deformity that prevents use of the nasal route. Alert patients do not tolerate oroenteral tubes well, and this access route is usually reserved for patients who are sedated and/or intubated. These tubes can be used to deliver nutrients into the stomach and, if necessary, into the duodenum or jejunum. They may be placed "blindly" at the bedside or using endoscopy, fluoroscopy, or even with manual manipulation during an abdominal procedure. For short-term feeding (<30 days) nasogastric (NG), nasoduodenal (ND), or nasojejunal (NJ) tubes are generally used because of their ease of placement and low cost [1]. The disadvantage of these tubes is clogging of the tubes or dislodgment. If enteric access is required beyond the ligament of Treitz with these tubes, nursing personnel must take special precautions during movement of patients, suctioning, extubation, etc., to avoid dislodgment of the tubes. In addition, medications should be avoided, if possible, because elixirs cause tube feedings to clog the tube. While this is less of a problem if intragastric positioning is satisfactory since the tube can usually be easily replaced, it becomes a significant issue if success depends upon small bowel feeding. If enteral administration of medications is absolutely necessary, the tubes must be compulsively irrigated with at least 20 cc of water both before and after administration in addition to normal flushing protocol.

Nasogastric Tubes

These tubes are easily placed and replaced and can be used for medications or for enteral feeding. Endoscopic placement is rarely required unless an anatomic deformity (stricture or diverticulum) exists or where repeated attempts to gain intragastric placement are unsuccessful. NG tubes can be used for feeding but care must be taken, particularly in the ICU patient, to monitor residuals (<100–150 cc every 4 h) to minimize the chance of gastroesophageal reflux and aspiration. Under all circumstances, the head of the bed should be elevated to 30°. The smallest tube that allows reliable gastric aspiration should be used; typically this is a 7- or 10-F size. Large-bore nasogastric tubes used for NG decompression should not be used for feedings if at all possible because of the high rate of reflux, but unfortunately this is a fairly common practice.

Nasoduodenal and Nasojejunal Tubes

Access beyond the stomach is most often necessary to reduce aspiration risk or to bypass gastroparesis. Blind bedside placement or facilitated maneuvers, such as the corkscrew technique or pharmacologic agents, can result in advancement into the small bowel in most patients [1, 30]. ICU placement teams trained in this technique are particularly successful in this regard, but if unsuccessful, fluoroscopic and endoscopic technics may be necessary. Success rates of 86%–91% have been reported using fluoroscopic guidance with a low major complication rate (0.4%) [31]. Unfortunately, transport of the critically ill patient to radiology may be necessary due to the unavailability of bedside fluoroscopy. This labor-intensive and potentially dangerous transport may be contraindicated in certain critically ill patients, and other techniques for gaining enteral access, or the use of parenteral nutrition, may be more appropriate.

Endoscopic placement provides several advantages in the ICU and account for approximately 25% of nutrition support teams' endoscopic services at one of the author's institutions (DFK). Two types of devices may be placed orally or nasally: standard small-bore, single-lumen nasoenteric tubes or combined nasogastric/nasojejunal (NG/NJ) tubes. The use of the former is technically more difficult. A 10-F tube can be guided technically into the small bowel by grasping a suture placed at its end, if one is not present on the tube. Although 105 cm, 125 cm, or 145 cm tubes can be used successfully [32], a 105 cm tube leaves very little length at the nose for proper fixation creating nursing problems. Simple small bowel tubes are best for patients who are not on ventilator support since NG tubes used in ventilated patients can dislodge small-bore feeding tubes if they require removal or replacement.

A successful option to ventilated patients is the combined NG/NJ tube (an example shown in Fig. 2) that provides gastric decompression and a second lumen for feeding into the jejunum. In a series of 54 critically ill patients using this tube [33], placement was 94% successful with an average placement time of approximately 12 min. These tubes can be placed by a radiologist or as a combined endoscopic and fluoroscopic procedure as reported by Baskin et al. [34]. To offset the expense of endoscopic placement compared to parenteral nutrition, the tube must be in use for at least 5–7 days before becoming cost effective so that nursing and physician education is critical to longevity of the tube. Medications should not be administered via either port unless absolutely necessary to minimize clogging. Crushed medications should be placed through the gastric port

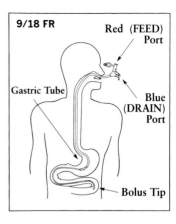

Fig. 2. Example of a combined nasogastric/nasojejunal feeding tube. Provided by Novartis Nutrition Corporation (Minneapolis, Minn., USA)

and liquid medications should be flushed through the small bowel port as long as the principles noted above-frequent and complete flushing-are followed. Medications at high risk of clogging tubes are fiber-containing laxatives, exchange resins, and coating agents in addition to elixirs. Use of medications can considerably shorten the usefulness of the tube and should be given via the tube only when absolutely necessary.

Percutaneous Endoscopic Gastrostomy, and Jejunostomy Techniques

Tube gastrostomy or enterostomy should be considered in patients requiring extended tube feedings (>30 days). They eliminate frequent dislodgment in the ICU, prevent the complications of sinusitis and mucosal and nasal erosions, and in the case of PEGs, provide long-term access for the administration of feedings as well as medications with minimal tube clogging.

PEGs

Although occasionally difficult to predict prolonged need for a feeding tube, certain populations, such as elderly stoke patients, patients with severe facial trauma, patients following major head and neck surgery with complications such as fistula, or patients with severe head injury, are usual candidates. If the patient recovers, the PEG can be removed by traction and the site heals rapidly although some PEG models require endoscopic removal. PEG placement is usually reserved for patients with low gastric residuals, no gastroesophageal reflux nor aspiration, and no evidence of gastroparesis. In supine patients, a large PEG (24 or 28 F) can be placed and, if necessary, converted to a PEG/J tube if unexpected contraindications to gastric feeding occur (Fig. 3). Most PEGs have inner bumpers that are pliable or firm. The firm bumper is most valuable in patients likely to pull out the PEG tube-intentionally or unintentionally – although any PEG tube can be dislodged with enough traction. Pressure necrosis and tube migration though the

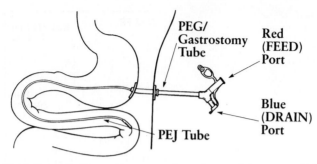

Fig. 3. Example of a percutaneous endoscopic gastrojejunostomy (*PEG/J*). Provided by Novartis Nutrition

stomach wall due to excess tightness occurs occasionally and is referred to as the "buried bumper" syndrome. To avoid this complication, the external bumper should be loosened at regular intervals and the PEG tube advanced 1 centimeter into the stomach with a 360° twist to test that the internal bumper moves easily [35]. Most complications of PEG tubes are minor and easily dealt with, and Table 3 lists potential complications.

Table 3. Endoscopic and radiologic tube enterostomy complications (*MRSA* methicillin-resistant *Staphylococcus aureus*) (From [40])

Aspiration	Bleeding	Bowel obstruction
Buried bumper syndrome	Candida cellulitis	Clogged tube
Colocutaneous fistula	Dehydration	Extrusion/migration[a]
Gastric outlet obstruction	Hematoma	Hypopharyngeal/esophageal tube impaction
Ileus		
Prolonged	Inability to transilluminate	Incisional pain
From migrated PEG		
Intraperitoneal placement	Intraperitoneal displacement	Mallory-Weiss tear of esophagus
Misplaced T-fastener	MRSA skin infection†	Multiple punctures of stomach
Necrotizing fasciitis	Peritonitis	Placement/technical failure
Pneumoperitoneum	Pneumonia	Small bowel perforation
Stomal leakage	Suture/wire breakage	Subcutaneous emphysema
Tube deterioration	Tube displacement	Volvulus
Wound infection		

[a]May also be part of the buried bumper syndrome.

Endoscopic Jejunostomy Techniques

Feeding jejunostomies are usually required in patients with a significant history of aspiration, gastroparesis, and those in whom previous surgical resection pre-empts PEG tube placement. The first PEJ tubes (today, these would be considered endoscopic duodenostomies) were reported by Ponsky and Aszodi and were small extension tubes that were hard to position and usually only reached the first or second portion of the duodenum [36]. The tubes clogged easily and frequently flipped back into the stomach. Contemporary PEJs have both gastric and small bowel feeding ports and are commonly referred to a percutaneous endoscopic gastrojejunostomies (PEG/Js) or jejunal extensions of PEGs (JET-PEGs). Prior gastric resection with either Billroth I or Billroth II procedures is not a contraindication to endoscopic tube placement and have been described but are uncommon in the ICU setting. If gastric anatomy is altered with a Billroth I anastomosis, the tube may be advanced through the abdominal and stomach wall into the duodenum [37]. Prior Billroth II procedures may not allow gastric transillumination for safe placement, but a tube may be advanced into the efferent jejunal limb [37]. Occasionally direct percutaneous placement into the jejunum is possible but is difficult due to the smaller size and mobility of the jejunal limb. Mellert et al. safely performed this procedure in 45 patients [38].

Most PEG or PEG/J tubes are placed after patients have survived the critical illness and are ready for long postinjury rehabilitation or nursing home placement. If there is need for early placement of a PEJ in an ICU patient, a 12-F small-bore tube can be placed over a guide wire through a 24- or 28-F PEG, and with experience, a 95%–98% success rate of small bowel advancement is possible. In these circumstances, the preferred tube placement is beyond the ligament of Treitz but, at a minimum, should be to the third portion of the duodenum to eliminate tube feeding-related reflux [8, 9]. More commonly in an ICU setting, the NG/NJ tube allows simultaneous decompression in patients with gastroparesis and feeding into the small intestine. It is ideal for patients sustaining severe head injury that do not require an operation or who sustain prolonged gastroparesis from a variety of causes and can be placed within the first few days after hospital admission and in patients who are supine. As gastroparesis resolves, the tube can be replaced with a nasoenteric tube or, if longer access is necessary, a PEG tube.

Summary

A large variety of techniques are available for gaining successful access into the gastrointestinal tract of critically ill and critically injured patients. Endoscopic, fluoroscopic, and surgical techniques should provide a broad armamentarium for the nutrition support specialist. The majority of ICU patients can be successfully fed via the gastrointestinal tract if a proactive approach to enteral access is assumed by the clinical team.

Acknowledgements. The authors would like to thank Mary Beatty of the McGuire Veterans Affairs Medical Center Medical Media Department in Richmond, Virginia for her illustration of Fig. 1.

References

1. Kirby DF, DeLegge MH, Fleming CR (1995) American Gastroenterological Association technical review on tube feeding for enteral nutrition. Gastroenterology 108:1282–1301
2. Mittal RK, Stewart WR, Schirmer BD (1992) Effect of a catheter in the pharynx on the frequency of transient lower esophageal sphincter relaxations. Gastroenterology 103:1236–1240
3. Lazarus BA, Murphy JB, Culpepper L (1990) Aspiration associated with long-term gastric versus jejunal feeding: a critical analysis of the literature. Arch Phys Med Rehabil 71:46–53
4. Strong RM, Condon SC, Solinger MR, et al. (1992) Equal aspiration rates from postpylorus and intragastric-placed small-bore nasoenteric feeding tubes: a randomized, prospective study. JPEN 16:59–63
5. Torres A, Serra-Battles J, Ros E, et al. (1992) Pulmonary aspiration of gastric contents in patients receiving mechanical ventilation: the effect of body position. Ann Intern Med 116:540–543
6. Ibañez J, Penafiel A, Raurich JM, et al. (1992) Gastroesophageal reflux in intubated patients receiving enteral nutrition: effect of supine and semirecumbent positions. JPEN 16:419–422
7. Ferrer M, Bauer TT, Torres A, et al. (1999) Effect of nasogastric tube size on gastroesophageal reflux and microaspiration in intubated patients. Ann Intern Med 130:991–994
8. Duckworth PF Jr, Kirby DF, McHenry L, et al. (1994) Percutaneous endoscopic gastrojejunostomy (PEG/J) made easy: a new over-the-wire technique. Gastrointest Endosc 40:350–353
9. DeLegge MH, Duckworth PF Jr, McHenry L Jr, et al. (1995) Percutaneous endoscopic gastrojejunostomy: A dual center safety and efficacy trial. JPEN19:239–243
10. Kudsk KA, Minard G. Injury severity scoring for penetrating trauma. In: Ivatury RR, Cayten CG, eds. Textbook of Penetrating Trauma. Williams & Wilkins, Philadelphia, PA, 1996, pp 142–150.
11. Moore EE, Dunn EL, Moore JB, Thompson JS (1981) Penetrating Abdominal Trauma Index. J Trauma 21:439–445
12. Moore EE, Jones TN (1986) Benefits of immediate jejunostomy feeding after major abdominal trauma– a prospective, randomized study. J Trauma 26:874–879
13. Moore FA, Feliciano DV, Andrassy RJ, McArdle, AH, et al. (1992) Early enteral feeding, compared with parenteral, reduces postoperative septic complications: the results of a meta-analysis. Ann Surg 216:172–183
14. Moore FA, Moore EE, Jones TN, McCroskey BL, Peterson VM (1989) TEN versus TPN following major abdominal trauma– reduced septic morbidity. J Trauma 29:916–923.
15. Moore FA, Moore EE, Kudsk KA, et al. (1994) Clinical benefits of an immune-enhancing diet for early postinjury enteral feeding. J Trauma 37:607–15
16. Kudsk KA, Croce MA, Fabian TC, et al. (1992) Enteral versus parenteral feeding: effects on septic morbidity after blunt and penetrating abdominal trauma. Annals of Surgery 215 (5):165–173
17. Kudsk KA, Minard G, Croce MA, et al. (1996) A randomized trial of isonitrogenous enteral diets following severe trauma: an immune-enhancing diet (IED) reduces septic complications. Ann Surg 224:531–543
18. King BK, Blackwell AP, Minard G, Kudsk KA (1997) Predicting patent outcome using preoperative nutritional markers. Surg Forum 48:592–595
19. The Veteran Affairs Total Parenteral Nutrition Cooperative Study Group: Perioperative total parenteral nutrition in surgical patients (1991) NEJM 325:525–532

20. Winkler MJ, Korunda MJ, Garmhausen L, Kudsk K (1995) Jejunal cannulation via Stamm gastrostomy: an improved technique for feeding jejunostomy at laparotomy. Surg Rounds 18:469–474
21. Minard G, Schurr MJ, Croce MA, et al. (1996) A prospective analysis of tee in the diagnosis of traumatic disruption of the aorta. J Trauma 40:225–230
22. Page CP: Edgar J. Poth lecture (1989) The surgeon and gut maintenance. Am J Surg 158:485–490
23. Delany HM, Carnevale NJ, Garvey JW (1973) Jejunostomy by needle catheter technique. Surgery 73 (5):786–790
24. McClave SA, Sexton LK, Spain DA, et al. (1999) Enteral tube feeding in the intensive care unit: Factors impeding adequate delivery. Crit Care Med 27:1252–1256
25. Chang RWS, Jacobs S, Lee B (1987) Gastrointestinal dysfunction among intensive care unit patients. Crit Care Med 15:909–914
26. Jones BJM (1986). Enteral feeding: techniques of administration. Gut 27:47–50
27. Jones TN, Moore FA, Moore EE, McCloskey BL (1989) Gastrointestinal symptoms attributed to jejunostomy feeding after major abdominal trauma – a critical analysis. Crit Care Med 17:1146–50
28. Mowatt-Larssen CA, Brown RO, Wojtysiak SL, Kudsk KA (1992) Comparison of Tolerance and Nutritional Outcome between a Peptide and a Standard Enteral Formula in Critically Ill, Hypoalbuminemic Patients. JPEN 16:20–24
29. Collier P, Kudsk KA, Glezer J, Brown RO (1994) Fiber-containing formula and needle catheter jejunostomies: a clinical evaluation. Nutr Clin Pract 9:101–103
30. Zaloga GP (1990) Bedside method for placing small bowel feeding tubes in critically ill patients – a prospective study. Chest 100:1643–6
31. Gutierrez ED, Balfe DM (1991) Fluoroscopically guided nasoenteric feeding tube placement: results of a 1-year study. Radiology 178:759–762
32. Mathus-Vliegen EMH, Tytgat GNJ, Merkus MP (1993) Feeding tubes in endoscopic and clinicla practice: The longer the better? Gastrointest Endosc 39:537–542
33. Patrick PG, Marulendra S, Kirby DF, DeLegge MH (1997) Endoscopic nasogastric/jejunal feeding tube placement in critically ill patients. Gastrointest Endosc 45:72–76
34. Baskin WN, Johanson JF (1995) An improved approach to delivery of enteral nutrition in the intensive care unit. Gastrointest Endosc 42:161–165
35. Boyd JW, DeLegge MH, Shamburek RD, Kirby DF (1995) The buried bumper syndrome: A review of the literature and a new technique for safe, endoscopic PEG removal. Gastrointest Endosc 41:508–511
36. Ponsky JL, Aszodi A (1984) Percutaneous endoscopic jejunostomy. Am J Gastroenterol 79:113–116.
37. Shike M, Schroy P, Ritchie MA, Lightdale CJ, Morse R (1987) Percutaneous endoscopic jejunostomy in cancer patients with previous gastric resection. Gastrointest Endosc 33:372–374
38. Mellert JK, Fischer H, Grund KE (1993) Direct endoscopic percutaneous jejunostomy (EPJ): An alternative for operative catheter-jejunostomy. Gastrointest Endosc 39:254 (abstract)
39. Borlase BC, Moore EE, Moore FA (1990) The abdominal trauma index: a critical reassessment and validation. J Trauma 30:1340
40. Kirby DF, DeLegge MH (1994) Enteral nutrition: the challenge of access. In: Kirby DF, Dudrick SJ (eds) Practical handbook of nutrition in clinical practice. CRC, Boca Raton, p 98

Formulation of Parenteral and Enteral Admixtures

D.F. Driscoll

Introduction

The use of parenteral and enteral nutrition admixtures in the intensive care unit (ICU) requires a high level of clinical expertise in order to safely provide efficacious nutrition support. During critical illness, numerous physiological responses are produced by the host to appropriately defend against injury, and to reestablish homeostasis in an attempt to maintain cardiopulmonary function and hemodynamic stability. Critical care clinicians often facilitate these physiological adaptations through aggressive monitoring with invasive intravascular catheters, pharmacological interventions such as through the use of vasopressors, inotropic agents and resuscitative fluid therapy, and respiratory support through mechanical ventilation. The combination of the body's metabolic response to injury and critical care interventions produces an array of changes in nutrient and metabolic homeostasis. Whether parenteral or enteral nutrition are given, or even when combined parenteral and enteral therapy are chosen, such conditions challenge the clinician who attempts to meet the nutritional and metabolic demands during this metastable state. Each mode of delivery has its attendant risks that may assume clinical significance. The purpose of this review is to examine the major pharmaceutical issues that determine the stability and compatibility of parenteral and enteral nutrition admixtures in the critical care setting, in order to avoid significant physicochemical combinations that may produce therapeutic failures and/or increase the risk of morbidity and mortality.

TPN Admixtures

The physicochemical stability and compatibility of TPN admixtures is complex given the multitude of individual chemical entities that comprise the typical formulation. A TPN admixture may contain up to 50 different compounds including 15–20 crystalline amino acids, glucose, lipids, 10–12 electrolytes, 5–7 trace minerals, 12 vitamins, and even various medications when used as a drug delivery vehicle. The final formulation can vary with the clinical condition of the patient, which in the critical care setting can widely fluctuate on a daily basis. In contrast, more stable institutionalized patients or those receiving home TPN therapy will generally receive admixtures that have little to no formulation changes on a daily basis. These regimens tend to be more standardized, whereas ICU patients with significant end-organ dysfunction, tend to be patient-specific with frequent changes in the daily formulation. The degree to which this occurs depends on the both the clinical status of the patient and the extent of use of the TPN admixture as the primary infusion to accomplish metabolic homeostasis. When the TPN admixture is used to correct severe electrolyte disturbances, manage acid-base disorders and be used as a drug delivery vehicle, the stability and compatibility of the final formulation poses significant, yet manageable physicochemical challenges. Using the TPN admixture in these ways may greatly assist in the metabolic management of ICU patients in a single 24-h infusion [1].

The application of the TPN admixture in this fashion must be closely monitored to avoid incompatibilities or unstable products that may produce harmful physiological effects. However, when such practices are undertaken by experienced personnel, they can favorably assist the metabolic management of common clinical disorders in the ICU, such as fluid overload [2, 3]. For example, consolidating the number and volumes of separate infusions that would normally be used if the following three therapies were prescribed for an ICU patient could be beneficial: (a) 100 mmol of hydrochloric acid in 1000 ml over 24 h; (b) 40 mmol of KCl in 100 ml given every 4–6 h; (c) an H2-receptor antagonist in 50 ml every 6–8 h. In the present example, all of these three components could be added to a lipid emulsion-free TPN admixture. However, if given separately, they would require 1.5–1.8 l parenteral fluid daily. In contrast, using the TPN admixture, which also serves as the drug vehicle would require total daily volumes of 190–250 ml per day to deliver the same parenteral therapies. These clinical maneuvers can reduce daily volume intakes by approximately 1/10 of usual amounts and will greatly assist in achieving fluid balance, and reduce the potential for adverse sequelae of volume overload.

Composition of the TPN Admixture

As a result of the normal metabolic response to acute injury, the typical composition of the TPN admixture in the ICU setting is, in one case is simplified, yet in another context can become more complex. This apparent paradox can be explained on the basis of the amount of nutrients that can be supplied, and the increased physicochemical issues that arise from the need to limit fluid intake because of issues related to volume overload. Thus, concentrated TPN admixtures are frequently prescribed that increases the risk of physicochemical incompatibilities and unstable formulations. In extreme situations, maximally concentrated TPN admixtures are given which are essentially comprised of fluid from stock bottles of nutrients with no additional fluid ("free water") added, such as sterile water for injection, to bring the admixture to its final volume [4]. In less concentrated TPN admixtures, pharmacists routinely q.s. ad (add a sufficient quantity to make) with sterile water for injection to fill the TPN admixture to its final, prescribed volume.

Simplification of the TPN admixture in the ICU setting occurs by virtue of the physiological limits imposed by the metabolic response to injury that restricts the total amounts of nutrients that can be safely supplied. Unfortunately however, when excess nutrients are given intravenously, they appear to be well-tolerated except for seemingly benign changes in metabolic homeostasis. For example, although hyperglycemia is acknowledged as a normal component of the injury response, resulting from endogenous increases in the serum concentrations of catecholamines, cortisol, glucagon, and other neurohumoral mediators [5], the additional and sustained effects of hyperglycemia by exogenous glucose infusion increases the risk of septic complications [6]. In diabetic patients, the infectious risks are magnified in this setting [7]. Unless meticulous attention is paid to these metabolic details and, if appropriate adjustments in the dose of carbohydrate and insulin are not made, the uninterrupted supply of intravenous nutrients continues, such as glucose, and will produce significant morbidity.

Therefore, recognizing these issues, the composition of the TPN admixture is simplified in that the total quantities of all nutrients that can be safely provided are limited, given the common clinical presentation of ICU patients. Thus, early nutrition support using TPN therapy in the ICU is frequently a hypocaloric regimen [8–10]. However, because of the increased endogenous production of anti-natriuretic hormone, insulin, and antidiuretic hormone during acute metabolic stress, critically ill patients will retain fluid. Consequently, volume restrictions are frequently imposed in ICU patients, often leaving as little as 1000 ml for nutrition support purposes [1]. Under such conditions, despite limiting the total amounts of protein, energy and electrolytes prescribed, the TPN volume allotment of 1000 ml produces a concentrated admixture that increases the risk of physicochemical instabilities and incompatibilities, and therefore, in this setting, increases the chemical complexity of the final formulation.

For example, a hypocaloric regimen for early parenteral nutrition support can be designed to provide at least 1 g/kg/day of protein, with the remaining TPN volume used to provide energy at approximately 50%–60% of needs (total kcal=15 kcal/kg/day), and leaving at least 5% of this volume for additives such as electrolytes, vitamins, minerals and drugs. With the advent of automated compounding devices, the pharmacy tasks of TPN preparation of such specialized mixtures has been greatly simplified [11]. Thus, in 1000 ml of total fluid, a variety of concentrated TPN regimens can be produced as depicted in Table 1. However, in some cases leaving 5% of the remaining TPN volume for additives is not enough, and may slightly exceed the prescribed final volume of 1000 ml, especially when large volumes of TPN additives are prescribed. Thus, in some cases, the usual infusion rate of 42 ml/h may need to be increased to deliver the daily nutrition and metabolic support within 24 h. In contrast, Table 2 depicts the full needs of adult patients in the absence of volume restrictions.

Significant Physicochemical Issues Affecting TPN Compatibility and Stability

The examples below are not inconclusive, but rather represent the most common types of incompatibilities that may influence the clinical course of hospitalized patients. Therefore, the most significant examples of incompatible and/or unstable TPN admixtures will be presented.

Table 1. Hypocaloric 1000 ml TPN regimens as a single- vs. mixed-fuel system in ICU patients

Weight (kg)	Total kcal/day[a]	Single-fuel		Mixed-fuel		
		Amino acids[b]	Glucose[c]	Amino acids	Glucose	Lipids[d]
40	600	40 g or 266 ml (4%)[e]	128 g or 183 ml (12.8%)[e]	40 g or 266 ml (4%)[e]	75 g or 107 ml (7.5%)[e]	20 g or 100 ml (2%)[e]
50	750	50 g or 333 ml (5%)[e]	160 g or 228 ml (16%)[e]	50 g or 333 ml (5%)[e]	96 g or 137 ml (9.6%)[e]	24 g or 120 ml (2.4%)[e]
60	900	60 g or 400 ml (6%)[e]	192 g or 275 ml (19.2%)[e]	60 g or 400 ml (6%)[e]	115 g or 164 ml (11.5%)[e]	29 g or 145 ml (2.9%)[e]
70	1050	70 g or 466 ml (7%)[e]	224 g or 320 ml (22.4%)[e]	70 g or 466 ml (7%)[e]	135 g or 192 ml (13.5%)[e]	34 g or 170 ml (3.4%)[e]
80	1200	80 g or 533 ml (8%)[e]	256 g or 366 ml (25.6%)[e]	80 g or 533 ml (8%)[e]	154 g or 220 ml (15.4%)[e]	39 g or 195 ml (3.9%)[e]

[a]Calories from the hypocaloric regimen consists of 1 g/kg/day protein and 15 kcal/kg/day total or approximately 50%–60% of needs. Hypocaloric regimens that are intended as permissive underfeeding are often prescribed for patients whose present weight is within 10% of ideal body weight.
[b]Assumes a stock bottle of 15% amino acids at 4.1 kcal/g.
[c]Assumes a stock bottle of 70% hydrated dextrose at 3.4 kcal/g.
[d]Assumes a stock bottle of 20% lipid emulsion at 9 kcal/g and providing approximately 20% of total calories.
[e]Final concentration of nutrient in 1000 ml TPN fluid, to illustrate the chemical complexity that results during severe fluid restrictions.

Table 2. Eucaloric, euvolemic TPN regimens as a single vs. mixed-fuel system in ICU patients

Weight (kg)	Total kcal/day[a]	Single-fuel		Mixed-fuel		
		Amino acids[b]	Glucose[c]	Amino acids	Glucose	Lipids[d]
40	1000	60 g or 400 ml	222 g or 317 ml	60 g or 400 ml	166 g or 237 ml	21 g or 105 ml
50	1250	75 g or 500 ml	277 g or 396 ml	75 g or 500 ml	208 g or 297 ml	26 g or 130 ml
60	1500	90 g or 600 ml	333 g or 476 ml	90 g or 600 ml	250 g or 357 ml	31 g or 155 ml
70	1750	105 g or 700 ml	388 g or 554 ml	105 g or 700 ml	290 g or 414 ml	37 g or 185 ml
80	2000	120 g or 800 ml	444 g or 634 ml	120 g or 800 ml	333 g or 476 ml	42 g or 210 ml

[a]Calories from the eucaloric and euvolemic regimen consists of 1.5 g/kg/day protein, 25 kcal/kg/day and 25 ml/kg/day. Eucaloric and euvolemic regimens are in conformance with the ASPEN Guidelines for safe TPN formulations and intended for patients whose present weight is within 10% of ideal body weight.
[b]Assumes a stock bottle of 15% amino acids at 4.1 kcal/g.
[c]Assumes a stock bottle of 70% hydrated dextrose at 3.4 kcal/g.
[d]Assumes a stock bottle of 20% lipid emulsion at 9 kcal/g and providing approximately 25% of total calories.

Calcium Phosphate Compatibility

One of the most common and potentially lethal physicochemical compatibility issues that arise from TPN admixtures is the formation of the insoluble product, dibasic calcium phosphate. The 1994 FDA Safety Alert in which two deaths and two near fatal injuries associated with an incompatible mixture of calcium phosphate attests to the significance of this interaction [12]. It is the product of an interaction between soluble calcium and phosphate salts, and is known as the double replacement or metathesis reaction characteristic of calcium ions [13]. In essence, when providing full and balanced nutrition support intravenously, it is necessary to supply both calcium and phosphorus supplements as part of the recommended dietary allowance (RDA). In adults, the parenteral equivalent of the oral RDA for calcium is approximately 5 mmol or 200 mg of elemental calcium per day, and for phosphorus, it approximates 30 mmol or 1000 mg of elemental phosphorus daily. For most adult central venous alimentation admixtures, these quantities can be met in the majority of TPN formulations. However, during acute illness the concentrations of these ions in TPN admixtures can increase significantly as a result of either fluid restrictions imposed or heightened requirements.

The key to understanding the complex chemical interactions of calcium and phosphate salts in multicomponent admixtures, such as in TPN formulations is related to the availability of the free, dissociated fractions of ions that are present at any given time. For it is only the free ions that are capable of forming the insoluble product. Because of the number of ionically active species in a TPN admixture, these ions can form soluble complexes, such as with certain amino acids, that reduce their interaction potential and can improve the compatibility of the final formulation. As phosphorus is a trivalent anion, there are three potential salts that may arise from this interaction, namely, mono-, di-, and tri-basic calcium phosphate. Of these, only the monobasic and dibasic calcium phosphate salt forms are important in TPN admixtures under their usual final pH conditions, that typically range from 5.0–6.5. Therefore, the pH of the TPN admixture medium is critical to the compatibility of the formulation. For example, at ambient room temperature conditions, higher pH levels foster the formation of the more dangerous dibasic calcium phosphate (aqueous solubility ~ 0.3 g/l), whereas under the same conditions, lower pH levels favor monobasic calcium phosphate formation (aqueous solubility ~ 18 g/l). Table 3 outline the conditions of calcium phosphate precipitation while Fig. 1 illustrates the general significance of pH in this regard. Thus, with a 60-fold difference in solubility, it is clear that pH and the availability of either monobasic or dibasic phosphate anions will dictate the compatibility and safety of the final admixture. In the cases reported in the FDA Safety Alert[14], the effect of pH of the admixtures on calcium phosphate precipitation was subsequently tested, and infused into laboratory animals at two different values, namely 5.86 and 6.68. The product with a pH of 5.86 had no adverse effects on the animals after receiving three days of parenteral nutrition. In contrast, in the animals receiving the product with a pH of 6.68, it resulted in the onset of respiratory distress and death within four hours of the first infusion. According to the calculations illustrated in Figure 1 for estimating the amount of the dibasic phosphate ions present, the 5.86 product would have 4.4% of the ions present, whereas the

Table 3. Calcium phosphate salts

	Monobasic	Dibasic	Tribasic
Structure	CaH2PO4	CaHPO4	Ca3 (PO4)2
Aqueous Sol.	18 g/l	0.3 g/l	insoluble
pH conditions	acid	neutral	alkaline
Factor in TPN	Yes	Yes	No

Fig. 1. The Influence of final pH on the formation of dibasic calcium phosphate on the compatibility and safety of the TPN admixture. As the dibasic phosphate ion represents the most dangerous form of the types of calcium phosphate precipitants possible in TPN admixtures, the above calculation demonstrates the significance of pH on the reaction. Clearly, as pH rises, greater amounts of the dibasic phosphate ions form that increases the risk of interaction with free, ionized calcium present in the admixture, and the subsequent formation of the insoluble dibasic calcium phosphate product

Henderson-Hasselbach Equation

For Acids: pH = pKa + log ([A-]/[HA])

⇩

rearranged to:

% ionized = 100/ [1 + antilog (pka - pH)]

CONDITIONS
Source: inorganic phosphate
pKa of dibasic phosphate: 7.2
pH range: 4.0 –9.0

pH	% ionized
4.0	0.06%
5.0	0.6%
6.0	6.0%
7.0	39%
8.0	86%
9.0	98%

Example:

pH = 6.0: % ionized = 100/[1 + antilog (7.2 - **6.0**)] = 5.9%

pH = 9.0: % ionized = 100/[1 + antilog (7.2 – **9.0**)] = 86.3%

6.68 product has 23.2% present. This case demonstrates the subtle differences between a safe and a lethal TPN formulation. Although not universally available, the use of organic phosphate salts, such as sodium glycerophosphate, reduces the risk of this physicochemical incompatibility.

Finally, there continues to exist two divergent opinions on the use of in-line filters to prevent harm from unstable or incompatible parenteral nutrition admixtures, such as an incompatible calcium phosphate infusion. In cases where in-line filters were used, yet catheter occlusion or other overt signs suggesting the post-filter presence of calcium phosphate precipitants occurred [15, 16], neither case resulted in death, whereas in the absence of such filters, fatalities occurred [12]. This would at least suggest that the filter reduced the lethal dose of precipitants, and therefore can be lifesaving. Even with the routine use of in-line filters during infusion, extemporaneous compounding practices by the Pharmacy must be regularly reviewed and optimized wherever possible [17]. In conclusion, an inline filter will reduce the exposure of potentially embolic matter, especially solid precipitates, and therefore routine use of such filters for complex parenteral admixtures such as TPN, are strongly recommended [12].

Compatibility of Acidifying Agents

In the treatment of severe metabolic alkalosis that requires rapid correction, the use of acidifying salts, such as hydrochloric acid (HCl), or HCl precursors, ammonium chloride and arginine monohydrochloride are frequently employed [18]. Of these, HCl is the most direct and safest way to treat alkalemia, without the risk associated with precursors that may exacerbate the clinical management of patients with nitrogen accumulation disorders, whether they be of renal and/or hepatic origin. Although initial estimates of acid requirements during severe metabolic alkalosis may exceed 300–400 mmol [18], prudent replacement is often accomplished gradually, administering 100 mmol of HCl daily until the alkalemia satisfactorily resolves. In lipid emulsion-free TPN admixtures, HCl has been shown to be compatible in concentrations up to 100 mmol/l [19].

Major physicochemical issues arise as a result of the changes in the pH of the admixture that affects drug compatibility, as well as interactions with certain catheter materials. For example, if a concentrated TPN admixture is prescribed (i.e., 1000 ml), and 100 mmol of HCl are provided (0.1 N), according to the Sorenson pH scale, the pH of the final admixture is 1.0. In reality, it is slightly higher (between pH 1–2) due to the presence of buffers found in the amino acid formulation or because of certain salts normally prescribed. In any event, such low admixture pH values may result in the precipitation of acid drugs with low dissociation constants or pKa values. In general, for an acid drug to be nearly completely ionized (i.e. at least 99% ionized), and therefore be water-soluble, it must reside in a pH medium that is at least two units above its pKa value. The pKa values of common medicinal compounds have been reported previously [20, 21]. Otherwise, a precipitate of the unionized fraction may occur and could produce an embolic syndrome. In addition, higher final concentrations of HCl (i.e., >0.2 N) may not only be excessive in clinical terms, but induces substantial physical deterioration of the components of intravascular catheters [22].

Compatibility of Alkalinizing Agents

In the treatment of severe metabolic acidosis that requires immediate correction, the use of alkalinizing salts such as sodium bicarbonate, tromethamine, and sodium or potassium acetate are frequently employed. Of these sodium bicarbonate is most often used [23]. However, in TPN admixtures, sodium bicarbonate produces an incompatibility in the presence of calcium ions and can form an insoluble precipitate, calcium carbonate, which if infused without an in-line filter, will almost certainly be fatal. Not only is there little to no compatibility data with tromethamine in TPN admixtures, it is also associated with serious side effects that restricts its use in the treatment of severe acidemia [23]. A safer alternative to these therapies is the use of either sodium or potassium acetate salts that does not pose the compatibility issues of sodium bicarbonate, nor the safety issues of tromethamine.

Stability of Intravenous Lipid Emulsions

Intravenous lipid emulsion (IVLE) is intended as either a source of essential fatty acids for long-term TPN therapy and/or used as an alternative energy source to glucose where a portion of the carbohydrate calories are substituted with fat on a daily basis [24]. When used as a daily caloric source, IVLEs are often added to a TPN infusion to form an all-in-one or total nutrient admixture. The addition of IVLE to TPN admixtures results in disrupting the stability of the emulsion. Specifically, the emulsifier is an anionic mixture of egg yolk phosphatides that surrounds the surface of each lipid droplet constituting a highly effective electromechanical barrier to the coalescence of neighboring droplets that could form enlarged fat globules. As cations such as sodium, potassium and especially divalent species, calcium and magnesium are added to the admixture, they lessen the negative surface charge, fostering an increase in the number of adhesive collisions among lipid droplets. Even minute amounts of trivalent cations, such as ferric oxyhydroxide or iron dextran are capable of destabilizing phospholipid-stabilized lipid emulsions [25]. As the emulsion becomes less stable, coalescence proceeds forming large numbers of fat globules in excess of 5 µm in diameter that are capable of obstructing pulmonary capillaries and may produce an embolic syndrome. When compounding any TPN admixture, the pharmacist must ensure the final formulation does not progress to such unstable conditions during the infusion period that it produces physiological harm [26]. When ICU patients require high concentrations of electrolytes, and are managed through a low final volume TPN admixture, the use of an all-in-one mixture should be reserved until such deficiencies are adequately supplemented or higher final TPN volumes (i.e., >1000 ml) can be given.

Stability and Compatibility of Ascorbic Acid

The use of ascorbic acid in pharmacological doses as an antioxidant in quantities up to 2000 mg has been suggested. Commercially available ampuls of up to 500 mg/ml make the task of extemporaneous addition to TPN admixtures a relatively easy maneuver. However, the instability of ascorbic acid in TPN admixtures is well-documented [27]. Oxalic acid is a known terminal degradation product of ascorbic acid and can readily interact with calcium ions. In fact, such a reaction has been reported in a TPN admixture with the formation of a precipitate that was subsequently identified as calcium oxalate [28]. This occurred in a "batch-prepared" (stored for several hours before they are used) TPN with conventional doses of ascorbic acid found in a commercial multivitamin dosage form that contained 1/20 (100 mg) of the advised maximum antioxidant dose. Thus, if ascorbic acid is used in doses exceeding the amounts usually provided in a standard parenteral multivitamin mixture, it should not be included in the TPN admixture.

Enteral Nutrition Admixtures

The use of enteral nutrition in the ICU has been advocated, whenever possible, versus parenteral nutrition. The major determinant of success with enteral nutrition in ICU patients is a functioning gastrointestinal tract that will assimilate nutrients delivered. In patients incapable of digesting the enteral supply of nutrients, the typical physiological response of excessive nutrients would manifest as gastrointestinal intolerance, thus limiting the amounts that can be reasonably supplied. Even then, non-patient factors within the ICU such as improper ordering, frequent interruptions and inappropriate cessation of enteral feeding, impede the delivery of adequate enteral nutrition support [29]. In essence, it is difficult to overfeed by the enteral route, principally because of GI limitations, among other factors, whereas in contrast, it is quite easy to overfeed with parenteral nutrition without such overt signs of intolerance or the need to interrupt nutritional therapy.

Frequently in the ICU, the GI tract is compromised, in large part, as a consequence of the normal metabolic response to injury wherein splanchic vasoconstriction occurs in order to preserve blood flow to critically dependent vital organs. Consequently, delivery of nutrients to the small bowel may inappropriately re-direct blood flow to the gut which, in hemodynamically unstable patients, may lead to bowel ischemia or infarction [30]. Thus, when initiating enteral nutrition during critical illness, it is important to ensure that the metabolic stresses present do not increase the risk of serious complications, particularly those related to the central circulation. Patients requiring continuous vasopressor drug infusion(s) should probably receive little to no enteral nutrition support until such pharmacological therapy is no longer needed and the patient is hemodynamically stable.

Composition of the Enteral Nutrition Admixture

There are a variety of enteral nutrition formulations that are commercially available, and they span an entire spectrum of nutritional components that not only differ in the amounts provided, but also in their chemical composition. For example, protein is available as monomeric formulas consisting of individual crystalline amino acids, oligomeric formulas consisting of di- and tri-peptides, and polymeric formulas as intact casein hydrolysates. Similarly, carbohydrate sources can be composed of mono-, oligo-, or polysaccharides. Lipid calories also varies widely with the formulation, and exist as long- or medium-chain triglycerides, or in combination as physical or even structured mixtures that may exert certain beneficial therapeutic effects through alterations in prostaglandin metabolism, as well as influence GI tolerance [31]. With respect to the physicochemical compatibility and stability of enteral feeding formulations, these compositional differences in macronutrients may pose additional chemical interactions with various extemporaneous additives, causing mechanical problems affecting the delivery of nutrition support. Moreover, if drugs are involved in these unfavorable interactions, the consequences of these effects on bioavailability may assume clinical significance.

Significant Physicochemical Issues Affecting Enteral Nutrition Compatibility and Stability

The examples presented below principally represent issues related to mechanical blockage of the enteral feeding tube. Therefore, for the most part, these issues are of lesser clinical consequence when compared to the previous physicochemical issues associated with parenteral nutrition. For example, the inadvertent infusion of dibasic calcium phosphate precipitants into the central circulation can have immediate and possibly life-threatening consequences, whereas a mechanical blockage resulting from an incompatible enteral mixture temporarily interrupts the delivery of nutrition support. Nevertheless, the interference of drug bioavailability may assume some degree of clinical significance particularly if a therapeutic failure results from the interaction. An extreme, but plausible example of this would be inadequate anti-ulcer protection resulting in a major gastrointestinal bleed.

Extemporaneous Addition of Nutritional Components

At times, certain critically ill patients may need the extemporaneous addition of other nutritional components to fully support the nutrient requirements of patients receiving enteral nutrition therapy. These additional supplements are often added as a result of patient-specific conditions that preclude the ability to meet the nutritional needs using commercial enteral feeding formulations. For example, ICU patients may be fluid-restricted, have heightened electrolyte needs or other clinical conditions necessitating modification of the conventional commercial enteral formulation.

In patients who are fluid overloaded, one option may be to use a high density formula (>1 kcal/ml) or to add modular components to a less dense commercial formulation, such as protein or carbohydrate, to extemporaneously produce a more concentrated enteral formula. These components are frequently available as dry powders to be dispersed into the commercial formulation. The latter method of feeding may be more cost effective, as calorically dense formulations tend to be significantly more expensive. When modular nutritional components are added, significant changes in the physical characteristics of the original product occur, such as an increase in viscosity. Moreover, the powders added must be sufficiently hydrated for adequate dispersion. Otherwise, if a small bore feeding tube is used, the flow of nutrients may be impeded leading to an obstruction. This may interrupt the infusion temporarily, if the blockage can be successfully cleared, or worse, require replacement of the feeding tube that substantially increases the costs of nutritional therapy. Another cause of incompatibility that can result in the blockage of feeding tubes includes the addition of certain liquid supplements, such as electrolytes, to concentrated EN formulations. For example, the addition of supplemental calcium chloride to a high density EN formula composed of protein from casein hydrolysates can produce the insoluble product calcium caseinate, that can also obstruct enteral feeding tubes. In essence, when high density EN formulations are used, whether they be of commercial or extemporaneous origin, the addition of supplemental nutrients should be carefully undertaken, being especially mindful of interactions that yield partially solubilized powders or insoluble co-precipitates.

Enteral Nutrition Admixtures as Drug Vehicles

Using the EN admixture as a drug delivery vehicle poses additional concerns beyond the formation of an insoluble product that produces a mechanical blockage of the feeding tube. For such interactions may also reduce the bioavailability of the drug and may result in therapeutic failures. Interactions affecting the compatibility [32], stability [33], and absorption [34] of drugs added to EN formulations have been described. Clearly, the occurrence of any of these interactions will affect the bioavailability of drugs added. Thus, because of the lack of sufficient data on these matters, the addition of medications to EN formulations is not recommended [34].

Instilling Medication Via the Enteral Feeding Tube

As an alternative to using the enteral nutrition formulation as a drug vehicle, the use of the enteral feeding tube to deliver oral medications provides another option for drug delivery. Of course, it is important to ensure the feeding tube is cleared of any enteral formula prior to instilling the medication (s). The following method has been suggested previously:[30]
1. Stop the enteral infusion and flush the tube with 20–30 ml of water.
2. Use liquid medications whenever possible. If not available, a slurry can be made in water from crushed tablets or capsule contents and instilled via a syringe (controlled or sustained release products are inappropriate).
3. After the medication is instilled, flush the tube again with 20–30 ml of water.
4. Re-start the enteral feeding infusion.

Although this practice should reduce the incidence of clogged feeding tubes, it does present additional problems. First, it is labor-intensive, especially if multiple medications are delivered in this manner over the course of the day. Additionally, as described previously, it will also cause numerous interruptions in the delivery of enteral nutrition that may affect the delivery of a desired level of nutrition per 24 h. Finally, although liquid medications are most desirable when administered in this manner, they are often hypertonic [35] and thus may induce gastrointestinal intolerance. Extreme caution and suitable selection of both medications and patient conditions is advised when medications are administered via the enteral feeding tube.

Conclusion

The formulation of enteral and parenteral feeding mixtures requires great care to ensure the final formulations are safe for administration to hospitalized patients. This requirement is heightened when those formulations are provided to critically ill, ICU patients. As with any medication, parenteral formulations present the greatest danger of patient harm if an incompatibility or unstable mixture gains access to the central circulation. An incompatibility usually presents as a precipitate, and if administered intravenously, will almost surely produce an embolic syndrome. Unstable mixtures also carry a risk, especially if the outcome of the reaction produces a reactive species that forms a precipitate. Unstable mixtures may also produce therapeutic failures that may assume clinical significance. Although incompatibility and instability issues can occur in enteral formulations, they tend to be less dangerous in their clinical presentation. Nevertheless, because of the complex compositions of these formulations, every effort should be made to ensure that these untoward events are minimized and patient care is not compromised. As medications are often involved in these reactions, pharmacists are best suited to monitor and direct the extemporaneous manipulation (s) of any feeding formulation. This is especially true in the critical care setting.

References

1. Driscoll DF (1989) Drug-induced metabolic disorders and parenteral nutrition in the intensive care unit: A pharmaceutical and metabolic perspective. DICP, Ann Pharmacother 23:363–371
2. Simmons RS, Berdine GG, Seindenfeld JJ et al. (1987) Fluid balance and adult respiratory distress syndrome. Am Rev Respir Dis 135:924–9
3. Lowell JA, Schifferdecker C, Driscoll DF et al. (1990) Postoperative fluid overload: Not a benign problem. Crit Care Med 18:728–733
4. Driscoll DF, Bistrian BR, Baptista RJ et al. (1987) Base solution limitations and patient-specific TPN admixtures. Nutr Clin Prac 2:160–3
5. Wolfe RR. (1987) Carbohydrate metabolism in critically ill patients. Crit Care Clin 3:11–24
6. Khaodhiar L, McCowen K, Bistrian BR. (1999) Perioperative hyperglycemia, infection or risk? Curr Opin Clin Nutr Metab Care 7:79–82
7. Pomposelli JJ, Baxter JK, Babineau TJ et al. (1998) Early postoperative glucose control predicts nosocomial infection rate in diabetic patients. JPEN 22:77–81
8. Echenique MM, Bistrian BR. (1982) Theory and techniques of nutritional support in the ICU. Crit Care Med 10:546–9
9. McMahon M, Driscoll DF, Bistrian BR. (1989) Design of nutritional therapy for the fluid-restricted patient. In: Perspectives in Clinical Nutrition. Kinney J, Borum P (eds). Baltimore-Munich, Urban and Schwarzenberg, pp 169–80
10. Zaloga GP, Roberts P. (1994) Permissive underfeeding. New Horizons 2:257–63
11. Driscoll DF. (1996) Clinical delivery of nutritional therapy: automated compounders and patient-specific feeding. [Editorial] Nutrition 12:461–2
12. Food and Drug Administration. (1994) Safety alert: hazards of precipitation associated with parenteral nutrition. Am J Hosp Pharm 51:1427–8
13. Driscoll DF, Newton DW, Bistrian BR. (1994) Precipitation of calcium phosphate from parenteral 11 nutrient fluids. Am J Health Syst Pharm 51:2834–6
14. Hill SE, Heldman LS, Goo EDH et al. (1996) Fatal microvascular pulmonary emboli from precipitation of a total nutrient admixture solution. JPEN 20:81–87
15. Robinson LA, Wright BT. (1982) Central venous catheter occulsion caused by body-heat-mediated calcium phosphate. Am J Hosp Pharm 39:120–1
16. Knowles JB, Cusson G, Smith M et al. (1989) Pulmonary deposition of calcium phosphate crystals as a complication of home parenteral nutrition. JPEN 13:209–13
17. Driscoll DF. (1996) Ensuring the safety and efficacy of extemporaneously prepared infusions. [Editorial] Nutrition 12:289–90

18. Adrogue HJ, Madias NE. (1998) Management of life-threatening acid-base disorders. Part 2 N Engl J Med 1998;338:107–111

19. Mirtallo JM, Rogers KR, Johnson JA et al. (1981) Stability of amino acids and the availability of acid in total parenteral nutrition solutions containing hydrochloric acid. Am J Hosp Pharm 38:1729–31

20. Newton DW, Kluza RB. (1978) pKa values of medicinal compounds in pharmacy practice. Drug Intell Clin Pharm 12:546–54

21. Raymond GG, Born JL. (1986) An updated pKa listing of medicinal compounds. Drug Intell Clin Pharm 20:683–6

22. Kopel RF, Durbin CG Jr. (1989) Pulmonary artery catheter deterioration during hydrochloric acid infusion. Crit Care Med 17:688–9

23. Adrogue HJ, Madias NE. (1998) Management of life-threatening acid-base disorders. Part N Engl J Med 1998;338:26–34

24. Driscoll DF, Adolph M, Bistrian BR. (1999) Lipid emulsions in parenteral nutrition. In Parenteral Nutrition. Rombeau J.L., Rolandelli R. (eds), W. B. Saunders Company, Philadelphia, PA

25. Driscoll, D.F., Bhargava, H.N., Li, L. et al. (1995) The physicochemical stability of complex intravenous lipid dispersions as total nutrient admixtures. Am J Hosp Pharm 52:623–34

26. Driscoll D.F. (1995) Total nutrient admixtures: Theory and practice. Nutr Clin Pract 10:114–9

27. Allwood MC. (1984) Factors influencing the stability of ascorbic acid in total parenteral nutrition. J Clin Hosp Pharm 9:75–85

28. Gupta VD. (1986) Stability of vitamins in total parenteral nutrient solutions. Am J Hosp Pharm 43:2132

29. McClave SA, Sexton LK, Spain DA et al. (1999) Enteral tube feeding in the intensive care unit: Factors impeding adequate delivery. Crit Care Med 27:1252–6

30. Daly BJ, Cahill S, Driscoll DF, Bistrian BR. (1993) Parenteral and enteral nutrition. In Wolfe MM (ed). Gastrointestinal Pharmacotherapy. W. B. Saunders Company, Philadelphia PA, pp. 293–316

31. Kenler AS, Swails WS, Driscoll DF et al. (1996) Early enteral feeding in postsurgical cancer patients: Fish oil structured lipid-based polymeric formula versus a standard polymeric formula. Ann Surg 1996;223:316–33

32. Cutie AJ, Altman E, Lenkel L. (1983) Compatibility of enteral products with commonly employed drug additives. JPEN 1983;7:186–91

33. Strom JG, Miller SW. (1990) Stability of drugs with enteral nutrient formulas. DICP, Ann Pharmacother 24:130–4

34. Engle KK, Hannawa TE. (1999) Techniques for administering oral medications to critical care patients receiving continuous enteral nutrition. Am J Health-Syst Pharm 1999; 56:1441–4

35. Dickerson RN, Melnik G. (1988) Osmolality of oral drug solutions and suspensions. Am J Hosp Pharm 832–4

Drug-Nutrient Interactions in the Critically Ill

J.A. Thomas, W.W. Stargel, and R. Cotter

Introduction

Drug-nutrient interactions in the critically ill patient have the potential to lead to decreased drug efficacy and/or increased drug toxicity. With the increased use of specialized nutritional support in patients requiring multiple medications, there is genuine concern about the possibility for pharmacologic-nutritional interactions, and the consequences of therapeutic outcomes [1, 2]. The frequency of drug interactions can be high in the critically ill patient because of the large number of drugs that they receive [3]. According to Sierra, et al. [3] most of these interactions are designated as being of moderate clinical importance with digoxin being the most frequently implicated drug.

Critically ill patients may receive upwards of 14 different therapeutic agents [3], and significant correlations were noted between the incidence of interactions and the age of the patient. The incidence of drug-nutrient interactions may be accentuated in the elderly [4, 5]. Geriatric patients may experience age-related changes in the pharmacokinetics of a drug. Physiological aging decreases the reserve of the geriatric patient, making them more susceptible to the stress associated with illness, drugs and surgery [6]. The ability to predict drug interactions has improved with the growing understanding of substrates, inhibitors, and inducers of CYP-450 isoenzymes [7].

Metabolic complications associated with electrolytes and drug management can be complex [8]. It is very important to monitor electrolytes very closely during parenteral and enteral nutritional support and to correct acute physiological imbalances. Also, the widespread use of enteral tubes requires that consideration be given to the location of the tube as well as problems associated in crushing and administering solid dosage forms of certain medications [9].

If nutritional support is necessary, enteral support rather than parenteral support has been advocated. However, there are many considerations depending upon the clinical circumstances [10]. Nutritional support may be indicated in a variety of medical conditions, some of which are straightforward (e.g., dyshagia, unconsciousness, etc.). Total parenteral nutrition (TPN) can be provided using peripheral veins when the need is short-term (e.g., critically ill) and the majority of the patient's energy is supplied by isotonic fat solutions. Long-term TPN requires placement of a central vein catheter. Increasing evidence supports the use of enteral nutrition over TPN whenever possible [11, 12]. Parenteral support is associated with more infectious, metabolic and fluid complications than enteral nutrition.

The purpose of this review is to describe some underlying physiologic factors that can affect therapeutic responsiveness in the critically ill patient. An examination of various therapeutic agents, and how they can be influenced by gastrointestinal activity, by fluid and electrolyte homeostasis, and by hepatic and renal function is reviewed in the critically ill patient receiving concomitant nutritional support.

Physiological and Pharmacokinetic Considerations

Absorption

Most clinically significant nutrient-drug interactions involve the absorption process [13]. Adrenergic mechanisms play a significant modulating action upon gut motility, blood flow and mucosal transport [14]. Both α and β-subtypes of adrenoceptors are involved at different levels of the gastrointestinal tract, and are involved in the regulation of motility and secretion. Thus, they may influence drug-nutrient interactions. α_1-Adrenoceptors are located post-junctionally on mostly smooth muscle cells, while α_2-adrenoceptors can be found both at pre- and post-synaptic sites. Several agents can act selectively as agonists as well as antagonists (Table 1).

Excluding ethanol, few drugs are absorbed to any significant degree in the stomach; most acidic or basic drugs are absorbed in the small intestine. Thus, gastric function has a major effect upon both the rate and degree of drug absorption, as changes in gastric motility can affect the residence time the food and/or drug in the gastrointestinal tract. The composition of the diet and the timing of meals can also influence drug absorption; for example, delays in gastric emptying time may be caused by fatty foodstuffs and thus affect a drug's absorption.

Food can sometimes facilitate the drug's absorption from the G-I tract (Table 2). A host of different mechanisms are involved in these interactions. Dicumarol and phenytoin, both of which might be indicated in the critically ill patient, can delay gastric emptying time. Table 3 reveals some of the mechanisms involved in hindering drug absorption. In critically ill patients, digoxin is frequently involved in interactions [3]. Foods high in fiber content or high in pectins can delay the G-I absorption of cardiac glycosides.

Drug-nutrient interactions involve several physiological factors whereby a drug affects processes relating to eating, sensory appreciation of food, swallowing, digestion, gastric emptying, nutrient absorption, nutrient metabolism or renal excretion of nutrients [15]. Hence, physiological interactions can also include reactions in which the absorption, metabolism or elimination of a drug is changed by food ingestion. The mechanisms of food-drug interactions are not well characterized, but involve both direct and indirect factors (Table 4). While the exact number of drugs which influence gastrointestinal absorption is not known, estimates suggest over 100 separate agents can elicit such actions.

Table 1. Gastrointestinal receptors affecting secretion and motility (from [52, 53])

	α_1	α_2	Receptor type β_1	β_2	β_3
Distribution in the gut	Smooth muscle Gastric neurons	Adrenergic neurons (autoreceptors) Myenteric neurons (heteroceptors)	Smooth muscle Enteric neurons (?)	Smooth muscle	Smooth muscle
Functional response	Smooth muscle contraction or relaxation Neuronal depolarization	Smooth muscle presynaptic-inhibition Smooth muscle contraction	Smooth muscle relaxation Smooth muscle relaxation	Peripheral noradrenergic neurons (?)	Smooth muscle relaxation
Selective agonists	Phenylephrine, methozamine, cirazoline	Clonidine, azepexole	Xamoterol, prenalterol	Facilitation of transmitter release	
Selective antagonists	Prazosin, corynanthine	Yohimbine, idazoxan, rauwolscine	Betaxolol, atenolol	Terbutaline, salbutamol, ritrodrine	

Table 2. Drug-nutrient interactions that affect absorption (from [20, 53, 54])

Drug	Mechanism
Atovaquone	High fat meal facilitates absorption
Carbamazepine	Increased bile production; enhanced dissolution and absorption
Cyclosporin	Increased bioavailability
Diazepam	Food enhances enterohepatic recycling of drug; increased dissolution secondary to gastric acid secretion
Dicumarol	Increased bile flow; delayed gastric emptying permits dissolution and absorption
Erythromycin	Unknown
Griseofulvin	Drug is lipid-soluble, enhanced absorption
Hydralazine	Food reduces first-pass extraction and metabolism, blocks enzymic transformation in gastrointestinal tract
Hydrochlorothiazide	Delayed gastric emptying enhances absorption from small bowel
Labetalol	Food may reduce first-pass extraction and metabolism
Lithium citrate	Purgative action decreases absorption
Lovastatin	Unknown
Metoprolol	Food may reduce first-pass extraction and metabolism
Misoprostol	Food decreases its side effects
Nitrofurantoin	Delayed gastric emptying permits dissolution and increased absorption
Phenytoin	Delayed gastric emptying and increased bile production improves dissolution and absorption
Propoxphene	Delayed gastric emptying improves dissolution and absorption
Propranolol	Food may reduce first-pass extraction and metabolism
Spironolactone	Delayed gastric emptying permits dissolution and absorption; bile may solubilize

Table 3. Mechanisms involved in delaying absorption of drug (from [53–55])

Drug	Mechanisms
Acetaminophen	High pectin foods act as absorbent and protectant
Ampicillin	Reduction in stomach fluid volume
Amoxicillin	Reduction in stomach fluid volume
Aspirin	Direct interference; change of gastric pH
Atenolol	Mechanism unknown, possibly physical barrier
Cephalosporins	Mechanism unknown
Cimetidine	Mechanism unknown
Digoxin	High-fiber, high-pectin foods bind drug
Furosemide	Mechanism unknown
Glipizide	Unknown
Metronidazole	Mechanism unknown
Piroxicam	Mechanism unknown
Quinidine	Possibly protein binding
Sulfonamides	Mechanism unknown; may be physical barrier
Valproic acid	Mechanism unknown

Table 4. Drug-fluid/drug-food interactions

Indirect mechanisms affecting absorption
°Drug-induced alterations in gastrointestinal motility (e.g., anticholinergics)
°Drug-induced malabsorption syndromes (e.g., neomycin)
Direct mechanisms affecting absorption
°Drug-induced pH alterations in gastrointestinal tract (e.g., antacids)
°Drug-induced changes in bioavailability (e.g., absorption to drug-kaolin/pectin)
°Drug-induced retardation of absorption (e.g., charcoal)
°Drug-binding/chelation (e.g., anionic exchange resins-cholestyramine; metal ions-iron, calcium)

Oral administration of drugs is convenient, and associating drug doses with daily routines such as mealtimes often improves patient compliance. However, this association can result in an increased incidence of nutrient-drug interactions by altering bioavailability, solubility in gastric fluid and gastric emptying time [16]. Delayed drug absorption does not necessarily imply that less total drug is actually absorbed, but that peak blood levels of the drug may be achieved over a longer period of time. Drugs that bind or complex to nutrients are often unavailable for absorption, or at least their absorption is delayed.

Metabolism and Bioavailability

Bioavailability describes that fraction of the drug's dosage that reaches the systemic circulation metabolically unchanged [17]. Several factors affect a drug's disposition including diet, genetic traits, age, sex and pregnancy [18]. Bioavailability can be modified by food, and thus result in a drug's pharmacokinetics and pharmacodynamics being altered. Food can influence drug bioavailability as a result of physicochemical or chemical interactions between a specific nutrient or other food component (s) and the drug molecule in the gastrointestinal tract.

Foodstuffs can affect the bioavailability of drugs by binding directly to the drug. They may also change luminal pH, gastric emptying, intestinal transit, mucosal absorption and splanchnic-hepatic blood flow [19, 20]. Food-induced changes in the bioavailability of some drugs may be partially dependent upon hepatic biotransformation, as evidenced by absorbed nutrients competing with drugs for first-pass metabolism in the intestine or the liver. Drugs may undergo metabolic transformation by enteric micro-organisms that may in turn be affected by nutrients, hence affecting the drug's metabolism. Parenteral nutritional regimens may affect oxidative drug metabolism.

Excretion

Drugs are excreted from the body either unchanged or as metabolites. The organs of excretion (e.g., kidney, skin, liver and lungs) eliminate polar compounds (i.e., water-soluble) more efficiently than drugs that are lipid-soluble. Lipid-soluble drugs are usually poorly excreted unless they have undergone some degree of biotransformation to render them more water-soluble.

The kidney plays a major role in the excretion of drugs and their metabolites. Renal excretion of drugs involves three processes: glomerular filtration, active tubular secretion and passive tubular reabsorption. Drugs excreted in the feces are primarily unabsorbed orally ingested drugs (or their metabolites) or are excreted into the bile and not reabsorbed from the gastrointestinal tract.

Organic acid and organic base renal transport mechanisms exert important roles in the elimination of non-filterable molecular species. Many drugs undergo such elimination processes via these organic acid and organic base systems (Table 5) [22]. The mechanism of action of some drugs may be dependent upon these transport systems, yet other drugs involve proximal tubular transport systems as a major route of elimination from the body. Drugs transported by the organic ion system may cause nephrotoxicity either directly or indirectly. Obviously, any renal impairment present in the critically ill patient could have a profound affect upon the elimination of various acidic or basic drugs.

Drugs and Nutritional Support

Gastrointestinal

The presence of food within the G-I tract can markedly affect the oral bioavailabilty of drugs [23]. The presence of food in the G-I tract impacts significantly on transit profiles, pH, and its solubilitization capacity. Ordinarily, the presence of food in the GI tract has been regarded as a barrier to absorption. Often there is a physicochemical basis to altered bioavailability when drugs are administered postprandially. Despite the physical and chemical interactions that may occur between

Table 5. Renal transport systems and drug excretion (from [51])	
	Organic acid system
	Phenylbutazone
	Salicylate
	Cephalothin
	Sulfonamides
	Chlorothiazide
	Furosemide
	Penicillin
	Methotrexate
	Probenecid
	Organic base system
	Isoproterenol
	Quinidine
	Morphine
	Procaine
	Tolazoline
	Mecamylamine
	Piperidine

drugs and specific food components, altered postprandial absorption is usually related to changes associated with conversion from the fasted to the fed state. Changes may be due to altered secretion of gastric acid, bile, or pancreatic fluids, and to modified gastric motility and fluctuations in visceral blood and lymph flow. Changes in postprandial gastric physiology are delineated by the slowing of gastric emptying time and a significant rise in pH. Such changes impact primarily upon gastric dissolution, with the magnitude of these changes being dependent upon the degree of ionization (i.e., pKa) and the solubility of the drug [23].

Nutritional support, more specifically that involving enteral feeding, often leads to diarrhea. Diarrhea can be a major clinical issue in the critically ill patient [24]. Patient intolerance to enteral formula may be improved by using fiber-containing products. Enteral nutrition may be administered by nasogastric, nasojejunal, gastrostromy, jejunostomy, or combined gastrojejunostomy tubes. Bowel sounds are commonly used as a diagnostic criteria for evaluating G-I function [25]. However, the passage of flatus or stools is a better marker of peristalsis and bowel function. If diarrhea is present in the enterally fed patient, it is necessary to determine whether the patient's medications were switched from the intravenous to the enteral route when enteral feeding was initiated. Some orally administered medications may contain sorbitol and magnesium which can cause osmotic diarrhea. Several other pharmacologic agents are associated with diarrhea in enterally fed patients (Table 6). Drugs must be ruled out as the etiology of diarrhea when G-I intolerance develops in the critically ill patient [2]. It has been reported that medications are the most frequent cause of diarrhea in patients receiving enteral tube feeding [26]. Over three-fourths of the cases with diarrhea can be caused directly by medications or pseudomembraneous colitis (PMC) secondary to antibiotic therapy. There appears to be an association between the use of antibacterial antibiotics and PMC. To determine the cause of watery stools that have developed during certain antibiotic therapy, it may be necessary to rule out *Clostridium difficle* toxin [2].

Many other pharmacologic agents have been associated with causing G-I pathologies, and these can affect the normal ingestion and processing of nutrients. Several drugs have been implicated in causing acute pancreatitis [27, 28] (Table 7). The thiazide diuretics and the tetracyclines would most likely be con-

Table 6. Agents associated with diarrhea during enteral-tube feeding (from [2])	Sorbitol Aminophylline solution Theophylline solution Acetaminophen elixir
	Magnesium Magnesium-containing antacids Magnesium citrate
	Electrolyte solutions Potassium chloride Sodium phosphate Potassium phosphate
	Antibiotics

siderations in the critically ill patient. Other agents, including doxycycline, potassium chloride, tetracyclines, minocycline and aspirin can cause esophagitis [2].

Renal and Electrolytes

Drugs that modify electrolytes can also affect the excretion of a drug (Table 8) [22]. Agents or drugs that induce renal dysfunction can cause excessive urinary loss of vital anions or cations. Thiazides may exert an opposite action. Oftentimes such losses coexist with either defects in the urinary concentrating-diluting mechanism or renal acidosis. Some of these agents act directly upon the kidneys, which others may act indirectly.

Several major clinical syndromes in nephrology caused by drugs (and by other chemicals) can ultimately affect drug-nutrient interactions [22]. The magnitude of nephrotoxicity depends upon the dose, duration of treatment/exposure, and several other factors known to affect pharmacological activity (e.g., age, sex, hepatic function, etc.). Aminoglycoside antibiotics commonly lead to proximal tubular injury in 10%–15% of therapeutic regimens. Likewise, nephrotoxicity is seen following amphotericin B and cis-platinum therapy.

Although hepatotoxicity or liver damage may vary depending on the type, severity and duration of injury, there are only a few mechanisms that alter a drug's excretion [18]. Drug elimination may be modified due to decreased enzyme activity resulting from hepatic parenchymal cell disease, altered hepatic blood flow, hypoalbuninemia or a combination of these factors or conditions. Hypoalbuninemia can affect the protein binding of a drug in the serum and change its pharmacodynamics. In cirrhosis, reduced functional hepatic cell mass may lead to diminished enzyme complement.

Sodium homeostasis can be complex because many drugs are actually marketed as sodium salts. Further, these drugs may be administered in normal saline piggybacks. There are a large number of antibiotics (e.g., carbenicillin, ticarcillin, azlocillin, ceftizoxime, etc.) that provide an added sodium load. Finally, sodium loading may be indicated in instances where the drug may cause renal toxicity (e.g., amphotericin B).

Conversely, sodium restriction can also lead to drug interactions [29]. Acute renal failure can be precipitated by sodium restriction and concomitant angiotensin–converting enzyme inhibitors, nonsteroidal anti-inflammatory drugs and immuno-suppressive drugs. Sodium restriction can enhance the renal tubular reabsorption of drugs such as lithium, leading to toxic side effects. Also, calcium antagonists exhibit greater efficacy when prescribed to salt-replete hypertensive patients [29].

Potassium homeostasis, like sodium homeostasis, can likewise be affected by both diuretic and non-diuretic agents (Table 8). Enhanced urinary elimination of potassium commonly occurs with loop diuretics, corticosteroids, amphotericin B and selected penicillins (e.g., ticarcillin). The potassium content of nutritional formulas may need to be decreased significantly should hyperkalemia develop. An enteral formula with reduced potassium may be required in patients who are unable to tolerate the potassium levels present in standard formulas [2].

Table 7. Drugs implicated as causing acute pancreatitis (from [27, 28])

	Definite	Probable	Possible
Azathioprine	Cimetidine	Bumetanide	ERCP contrast media
	Indomethacin	Anticholinesterase	Ethacrynic acid
Cisplatin	Mefenamic acid	Carbamazepine	Isoniazid
Colaspase	Estrogens	Chlorthalidone	Isotretinoin
(L-asparaginase)	Opiates	Clonidine	Mercaptopurine
Furosemide	Paracetamol	Colchicine	Methyldopa
Tetracycline	Phenformin	Coricosteroids	Metronidazole
	Valproic acid	Cotrimoxazole	Nitrofurantoin
Thiazides	Fonofos	Cyclosporin	Oxphenbutazone
Sulfonamides	Diazinon	Cytarabine	Piroxicam
		(cytosine arabinoside)	
		Diazoxide	Procainamide
		Enalapril	Rifampicin
		Ergotamine	Salicylates
			Sulindac

Table 8. Drug-induced electrolyte disturbances (from [22])

Sodium
Hyponatremia – drugs that impair water excretion
Hypernatremia – saline
Anti-inflammatory steroids
Potassium
Cardiac glycosides
Anti-inflammatory steroids
Hypokalemia
Diuretics
Antibiotics
Tocolytic agents
Licorice
Hyperkalemia
Potassium supplements
Potassium-sparing diuretics
Selected antihypertensive drugs
Calcium
Hypocalcaemia
Aminoglycoside antibiotics
Thiazide diuretics
Vitamin D supplements
Phosphorus
Hypophosphatemia
Parenteral nutrition
Hyperphosphatemia
Cytotoxic drugs

Several agents can also affect phosphorus homeostasis, and in fact, may be a major cause of severe hypophosphatemia in hospitalized patients [30]. Theophylline administration has been linked to hypophosphatemia [31]. Patients receiving enteral nutrition can have phosphate salts supplemented into their formulas.

Magnesium homeostasis is important in critical care. Urinary magnesium wasting can occur with several agents including thiazide diuretics, amphotericin B, aminoglycosides, cyclosporine and cisplatin [25, 32–34]. Hypomagnesemia can lead to reduced potassium and calcium.

Anticoagulants

There is some evidence to indicate that Warfarin resistance can be caused by the concomitant administration of enteral feedings [2, 35]. Although the amount of vitamin K content has been lowered in enteral formulas, such Warfarin resistance is still evident [36]. It is possible that this resistance develops as a result of Warfarin sequestration rather than by excessive vitamin K.

Patients undergoing Warfarin treatment with enteral formulations should be monitored for prothrombin times. Several other drugs interact with anticoagulants [38]. Warfarin may interact with antibiotics, cardiac medications and central nervous system-acting drugs. The potential for Warfarin to interact with other drugs, resulting in a change in its anticoagulant effect, is widely recognized among health professionals and informed patients. Drug-food interactions involving Warfarin can lead to potentiation, inhibition or no effect (Table 9) [38]. Agents cited represent those where there is a high probability of interaction. Other drugs may also interact, but generally are less likely to do so [38, 39]. Vitamin K content in foods and the quantity of vitamin K supplementation may affect the action (s) of oral anticoagulant therapy. Further, supplements of vitamins A, E and C may affect the efficacy of oral anticoagulant therapy. Drugs that do exhibit a high probability of affecting coagulation are not necessarily contraindicated, but may necessitate an increased awareness or more prudent therapeutic monitoring.

Respiration

Theophylline is frequently used in mechanically ventilated patients with severe chronic obstructive pulmonary disease (COPD). Theophylline may increase bronchodilation and improve diaphragmatic breathing. Continuous nasogastric feedings may interfere with the oral absorption of theophylline [40]. Theophylline treatment may be initiated using the intravenous route. Jonkman [41] has reported that diets high in fat and low in protein can facilitate the absorption of theophylline leading to toxic concentrations. Some studies, however, have failed to demonstrate any significant effects of enteral feeding upon the absorption of sustained-release theophylline tablets [42, 43].

The time to maximum drug interaction (i.e., onset and termination) is dependent upon the time required for the inhibited drug to reach a new steady state [44,

Table 9. Anticoagulants (Warfarin) and drug interactions

Potentiation	Inhibition	No effect
Alcohol[a]	Barbiturates	Alcohol
Amiodarone	Carbamazine	Antacids
Cimetidine	Chlordiazepoxide	Atenolol
Clofibrate	Cholestryramine	Bumetanide
Co-trimoxazole	Griseofulvin	Diflunisal
Erythromycin	Nafcillin	Enoxacin
Fluconazole	Rifampin	Famotidine
Isoniazid	Sucralphate	Felodipine
Metronidazole	Vitamin K (foods)	Fluoxetine
Miconazole	Dicloxacillin	Ketorolac
Omeprazole	Gisapride	Metoprolol
Phenylbutazone	Amiodarone	Moricizine
Piroxicam	Fluconazole	Naproxen
Propafenone	Itraconazole	Nitrazepam
Propranolol	Ketoconazole	Nizatidine
Sulphinpyrazone	Erthyromycin	Psyllium
	Omeprazole	Ranitidine

[a]Concomitant liver disease.

45]. When, for example, cimetidine-theophylline interact, the maximum increases in theophylline concentrations are not evident for about 2 days because this is the time required for theophylline to reach a new steady state [46]. The interactions between theophylline and enteral feeding formulas is discussed further in Section IV, 1 – Enteral Feeding.

Central Nervous System

Phenytoin if often used to control seizures in both acute and chronic conditions. It may be indicated in the critically ill patient for acute seizure control as well as during the post-traumatic period for seizure prophylaxis. Phenytoin is among one of the most frequently reported drugs to interact with enteral feeding [47]. The oral route of phenytoin administration is preferred in patients requiring chronic prophylaxis because of the risk of hypotension linked to the intravenous administration and because of the reduced availability from the intramuscular administration [2]. Enteral feeding leads to a decrease in serum phenytoin level; cessation of feeding results in a rise in drug levels. In critically ill patients, there are a number of factors that lead to decreased total phenytoin concentrations regardless of whether this drug is administered with enteral feeding. Such factors include decreased protein binding and the increased clearance of phenytoin. About 90% of phenytoin is bound to protein, primarily albumin. Accordingly, during hypoalbuminemia and kidney dysfunction, there can be an exaggerated pharmacologic effect of phenytoin. It appears that critically ill trauma patients exhibit increased phenytoin clearance. Hence, without aggressive phenytoin dosing and monitoring, subtherapeutic concentrations are more apt to occur in this patient population [48].

Nutritional Effects on Drug Therapy

Enteral Feeding

Table 10 provides a summary of interactions between oral medications and enteral feeding formulas [2]. Various mechanisms of interaction have been proposed including protein binding, altered solubility and chelation (e.g., antibiotics). Early enteral feeding, compared with parenteral feeding, reduces postoperative septic complications [11]. There is increasing support to use enteral nutrition in preference to TPN whenever possible [11, 12]. The trend toward enteral-tube feeding in critically ill patients who are receiving many therapeutic agents enhances the possibility of drug-nutrient interactions.

Parenteral Feeding

Over three-fourths of the drugs used in patients receiving parenteral nutrition caused some degree of altered nutritional support [49]. Parenteral support is linked to more infectious, metabolic, and fluid complications than enteral nutrition. Extended TPN may lead to atrophy of the G-I tract and to hepatic complications [50].

Drug disposition studies in patients receiving TPN indicate that the route of administration of nutrients may affect hepatic microsomal activity [20]. Ethanol interferes with many nutritional factors, including the type and amount of dietary fat, protein and amino acids. These interactions provide the rationale for the parenteral administration of complete amino acid mixtures to patients with severe alcoholic liver disease [51]. While dietary deficiencies (i.e., reduced food intake) may play a role in alcoholic liver injury, supplementation with S-adenosyl-L–methionine (SAM) and polyunsaturated lecithin may significantly offset some of the toxic manifestations of ethanol.

Short-chain peptides have been considered for parenteral nutrition. Such use is based on the assumption that specially concocted amino acid solutions will enhance the therapeutic benefits to patients receiving parenteral nutrition. Dipeptide-based parenteral solutions exhibit low osmolarity, thus enabling them to fulfill the nitrogen requirements of patients with severe fluid restriction. Synthetic peptides are rapidly eliminated and amounts of these solutes do not significantly accumulate in biological fluids. L-alanyl-L-glutamine has undergone clinical evaluation, and other dipeptides are certain to be tested for their potential efficacy. It is difficult to predict any clinically significant drug-dipeptide interactions.

Table 10. Summary of drug interaction–enteral feeding (*EFF* enteral feeding formulas) from [2]

Drug	Postulated mechanisms	Suggested interventions
Phenytoin	Binding proteins in EFF	Stop EFF 2 h before/after oral drug
	Binding electrolytes in EFF	IV phenytoin administration
	Altered drug solubility by EFF	Cycling EFF with drug dosing during "off" time
Theophylline	Drug inactivation by EFF	Stop EFF 1 h before/after oral dose and
	Drug precipitation by EFF	use rapid-release theophylline products
Warfarin	Binding proteins in EFF–	Increase dose of Warfarin cautiously and
	vitamin K content of EEF	monitor prothrombin time frequently
Ciprofloxacin	Chelation with cations in EFF	Change to an alternative oral antibiotic Cycling EFF with drug dosing during "off" time

TPN should be reserved for patients with conditions that result in a non-accessible or non-functional G-I tract. If TPN is indicated, there should be frequent evaluations to determine the suitability of switching to enteral support.

Conclusions

Drug efficacy and drug toxicity can be affected by pharmacotherapy-nutritional interactions. Therapeutic outcomes must be monitored very closely, particularly in the critically ill patient. A host of metabolic complications can be associated with acutely administered therapeutic agents including electrolyte balance, seizure control (or lack of), G-I homeostasis and patency of respiratory passageways. Special conditions prevail in the critically ill patients and increased vigilance is required to minimize drug-nutrient interactions.

References

1. Sacks GS, Brown RO (1994) Drug-nutrient interactions in patients receiving nutritional support. Drug Therapy, March, 35–42
2. Mowatt-Larssen C, Brown R (1994) Drug-nutrient interactions. In: Nutrition in Critical Care, Zaloga GP, ed. Mosby Co., St. Louis, MO, 487–503
3. Sierra P, Castillo J, Gomez M, Sorribes V, Monterde J, Castano J (1997) Servicio de anestesioilogia, Fundacion Puigvert, Barcelona. Rev Esp Anestesiol Reanim (Spain), Dic., 44 (10), 383–387
4. Thomas JA, Tschanz C (1994) Nutrient-drug interactions. In Nutritional Toxicology, Kotsonis FN, Mackey M, Hjelle JJ (eds.), Target Organ Toxicity Series, Raven Press, New York, pp. 139–148
5. Thomas JA, Burns RA (1998) Important drug-nutrient interactions in the elderly. Drugs and Aging, Sept., 13 (3), 199–209
6. Johnson JC (1993) General concepts of geriatric medicine. Clin Podiatr Med Surg, 10 (1) 23–33

7. Landrum-Michalets E (1998) Update: clinically significant cytochrome P-450 drug interactions. Pharmacotherapy, 18 (1), 84–112

8. Seshadri V, Meyer-Tettambel OM (1993) Electrolyte and drug management in nutritional support. Crit Care Nurs Clin North Am, March, 5 (1), 31–36

9. Varella L, Jones E, Meguid M (1997) Drug-nutrient interactions in enteral feeding: a primary care focus. The Nurse Practitioner, 22 (6):98–104

10. Parrish CR, MCCray SF, Wolf AM, Wolf AMD (1999) When is nutrition support appropriate? Hospital Medicine, 50–55

11. Moore FA, Feliciano DV, Andrassy RJ et al. (1992) Early enteral feeding, compared with parenteral, reduces postoperative septic complications. Ann Surg, 216, 172–178

12. Windsor ACJ, Kanwar S, Li AG, et al. (1998) Compared with parenteral nutrition, enteral feeding attenuates the acute phase response and improves disease severity in acute pancreatitis. Gut, 42, 431–439

13. Tschanz C, Stargel WW, Thomas JA (1996) Interactions between drugs and nutrients. Advances in Pharmacology, 35, 1–26

14. DePonti F, Giaroni C, Cosentino M, Lecchini S, Frigo G (1996) Adrenergic mechanisms in the control of gastrointestinal motility: from basic science to clinical applications. Pharmacology and Therapeutics, 69, 59–78

15. Roe DA (1993) Drug and food interactions as they affect the nutrition of older individuals. Aging: Clinical Experimental Research, 5, 51–53

16. Trovato A, Nuhlicek DN, Midtling JE (1991) Drug-nutrient interactions. American Family Physician, 44, 16541–1658

17. Winstanley PA, Orme ML'E (1989) The effects of food on drug bioavailability. British Journal of Clinical Pharmacology, 28, 621–628

18. Hoyumpa AM, Schenker S (1982) Major drug interactions: effect of liver disease, alcohol, and malnutrition. Annual Reviews of Medicine, 33, 113–149

19. Anderson KE and Kappas A (1987) How diet affects drug metabolism. Hospital Therapy, April, 93–102

20. Anderson KE (1988) Influences of diet and nutrition on clinical pharmacokinetics. Clinical Pharmacokinetics, 14, 325–346

21. Pantuck EJ, Pantuck CB, Weissman C, et al. (1984) Effects of parenteral nutritional regimens on oxidative drug metabolism. Anesthesiology, 60, 534- 536

22. Bennett WM and Porter GA (1993) Overview of clinical nephrotoxicity. In Toxicology of the Kidney, 2 edn, Hook JB and Goldstein RS (eds), Target Organ Toxicity Series, Raven Press, New York, Chapter 3, 61–97

23. Charman WN, Porter CJH, Mithani S, Dressman JB (1997) Physicochemical and physiological mechanisms for the effects of food on drug absorption: The role of lipids and pH. Journal of Pharmaceutical Sciences, 86, 3, 269–282

24. Bliss DZ, Guenter PA, Settle RG (1992) Defining and reporting diarrhea in tube- fed patients – what a mess! AM J Clin Nutr, 55, 753–759

25. Zaloga GP, Chernow B, Pock A, et al. (1984) Hypomagnesemia is a common complication of aminoglycoside therapy. Surg Gynecol Obstet, 158, 561–565

26. Edes TE, Walk BE, Austin JL (1990) Diarrhea in tube-fed patients: feeding formula not necessarily the cause. Am J Med, 88, 91–93

27. Banerjee AK, Patel KJ, and Grainger SL (1989) Drug-induced acute pancreatitis: a critical review. Med. Toxicol. Adverse Drug Exp., 4, 186–198

28. Rünzi M, Layer P (1996) Drug-associated pancreatitis: facts and fiction. Pancreas, 13 (1), 100–109

29. Bennett WM (1997) Drug interactions and consequences of sodium restriction. American Journal of Clinical Nutrition, 65, 6785–6815

30. Halevy J, Bulvik S (1988) Severe hypophosphatemia in hospitalized patients. Arch Intern Med, 148, 153–155

31. Brady HR, Ryan F, Cunningham J, et al. (1989) Hypophosphatemia complicating bronchodilator therapy for acute severe asthma. Arch Intern Med, 149, 2367- 2368

32. Sheehan J, White A (1982) Diuretic-associated hypomagnesemia. BMJ, 285, 1157–1159
33. Nozue T, Kobayashi A, Kodama T, et al. (1992) Pathogenesis of cyclosporine- induced hypomagnesemia. J Pediatr, 120, 638–640
34. Schilsky RL, Anderson T (1979) Hypomagnesemia and renal magnesium wasting in patients receiving cisplatin. Ann Intern Med, 90, 929–931
35. Parr MD, Record KE, Griffith GI, et al. (1982) Effect of enteral nutrition on Warfarin therapy. Clin Pharm, 1, 274–276
36. Martin JE, Lutomski DM (1989) Warfarin resistance and enteral feedings. JPEN, 13, 206–208.
37. Kuhn TA, Garnett WR, Wells BK, et al. (1989) Recovery of Warfarin from an enteral nutrient formula. Am J Hosp Pharm, 46, 1395–1399
38. Wells S, Holbrook AM, Crother NR, Hirsh J (1994) Interactions of Warfarin with drugs and food. Annals of Internal Medicine, 121, 676–683
39. Harris JE (1995) Interaction of dietary factors with oral anticoagulants: review and applications. Journal of the American Dietetic Association, 95, 580–584
40. Gal P, Layson R (1986) Interference with oral theophylline absorption by continuous nasogastric feedings. Ther Drug Monitor, 8, 421–423
41. Jonkman JHG (1989) Food interactions with sustained-release theophylline preparations: a review. Clin Pharmacokinet, 16, 162–179
42. Plezia PM, Thornley SM, Kramer TH, et al. (1990) The influence of enteral feedings on sustained-release theophylline absorption. Pharmacotherapy, 10, 356–361
43. Schaaf LJ, Bhargava VO, Berlinger WG, et al. (1989) Effect of an enteral formula on sustained-release theophylline absorption (abstract). Pharmacotherapy, 9, 185
44. Coutts RT (1994) Polymorphism in the metabolism of drugs, including antidepressant drugs: comments on phenotyping. J Psychiatry Neurosci, 19, 30- 44
45. Soto J, Alsar MJ, Sacristan JA (1995) Assessment of the time course of drugs with inhibitory effects of hepatic metabolic activity using successive salivary caffeine tests. Pharmacotherapy, 15, 781–784
46. Shinn AF (1992) Clinical relevance of cimetidine drug interactions. Drug Safety, 7, 245–267
47. Bauer LA (1982) Interference of oral phenytoin absorption by continuous nasogastric feedings. Neurology, 32, 570–572
48. Boucher BA, Rodman JH, Jaresko GS, et al. (1988) Phenytoin pharmacokinetics in critically ill trauma patients. Clin Pharmacol Ther, 44, 675–683
49. Schneider PJ, Mirtallo J (1983) Medication profiles in TPN patients. Nutr Supp Serv, 3, 40–46.
50. Gottschlich MM, Matarse LEA, Shronts EP. Nutrition Support Dietetics Core Curriculum, 2 ed., Silver Spring, MD: Aspen, 1992
51. Lieber CS (1994) Mechanisms of ethanol-drug-nutrition interactions. Clinical Toxicology, 32, 631–681
52. Hussar DA (1988) Drug interactions in the older patient. Geriatrics, 43, 20–30
53. Thomas JA, Stargel WW, Tschanz C (1998) Interactions between drugs and diet. Nutrition and Chemical Toxicity, ed. C Ioannides, J Wiley & Sons Ltd., p 161- 182
54. Katz NL, Dejean A (1985) Interrelationships between drugs and nutrients. Pharm Index, December, 9–15
55. Kirk JK (1995) Significant drug-nutrient interactions. Am Fam Physician, 51 (45), 1175–82
56. Mehta S, Nain CK, Sharma B, Mathur VS (1982) Disposition of four drugs in malnourished children. Drug-Nutrient Interactions, 1, 205–211

A Practical Approach
to Feeding Intensive Care Patients

P. Jolliet and C. Pichard

Introduction

The conjunction of prolonged survival of critically ill patients and increased prevalence of malnutrition prior to hospitalization [1] represents a challenge to the ICU physician, faced with the difficult task of reconciling apparently opposed goals while trying to provide the best nutritional support to his patient [2–4]. Many nutritional issues still remain the subject of ongoing controversies [5–8], many of which are discussed in detail in other chapters of this book. These controversies notwithstanding, adequate nutritional support instituted early in the course of severe critical illness is regarded as an integral part of proper patient management [2]. To that end, various practical aspects must be considered, and it is the purpose of this chapter to provide the reader with such basic information derived from the published litterature and the authors' experience [4, 9, 10]. In that perspective and with focus on practical issues, enteral and parenteral nutrition will first be considered independently, then their possible combined uses will be discussed. No attempt is made to review in depth all such issues, but emphasis will be placed on those most often referred to by ICU physicians in daily practice.

Enteral Nutrition

Route of Feeding and Choice of Tube

Various routes of enteral feeding are available. From a practical point of view, in surgical patients with extensive gut resection or impossibility to use gastric feeding, a perioperative [11] or percutaneous [12] jejunostomy should be considered, while the initial approach in all other cases should be a trial of nasogastric feeding. Indeed, the latter preserves the reservoir function of the stomach and the gastric stages of digestion, and is hence the most physiologic route and the easiest to access. In patients with persistent gastroparesis and intolerance to gastric feeding despite adequate prokinetic treatment, endoscopic placement of a naso-duodenal tube should be the next step [13], while naso-jejunal tubes should be used only as a last resort, since they are technically the most difficult to place, and do not protect from aspiration or duodenogastric reflux [14]. Percutaneous gastrostomy has become an attractive route of feeding when long term (≥4–6 weeks) enteral nutritional support is required [15].

Whatever the elected route of feeding, one caveat that should always be kept in mind is that even though the risk of aspiration of feeding solution is decreased when the latter is administered in the jejunum it is by no means abolished [16, 17], and mandates that airway protective measures such as inclination of the torso 30 degrees above the horizontal plane, endotracheal intubation or tracheostomy be considered.

Regarding the choice of naso-enteric feeding tube, the most comfortable for patients undergoing nutrition are silicone or polyurethane small diameter (6–12 F) tubes, whose length depends on the location of feeding (stomach 90 cm, duodenum 110 cm, jejunum ≥120 cm). It should be remembered though that when preparations of slightly higher viscosity such as fiber-enriched solutions are used, administration through the smaller diameter tubes might be more difficult unless a constant infusion pump is used. Furthermore, if aspiration of gastric content is necessary, a larger tube is mandatory. Consequently, since gastric aspiration is often required in ICU patients, it is preferable to use the latter in the initial period of ICU stay, and to switch to the smaller feeding tubes after that time if enteral nutrition is well tolerated and is expected to last for more than 10 days.

Finally, after placement of the nasoenteric tube, an abdominal X-ray should be performed to verify its proper placement, and avoid the risk of feeding solution administration in case of tube malpositioning (e.g. loops in the oral cavity or lower esophagus, intratracheal position, intracranial introduction in head trauma patients) [18, 19].

Type of Feeding Solution

The first feeding solutions used for enteral nutrition were prepared from nutrients mixed together and homogenized in hospital kitchens. This approach entails numerous potential complications for the patients, such as nutritionally unbalanced solutions, water and electrolyte disorders, and diarrhea due to excessive osmolality of the preparation. Furthermore, severe nosocomial infection can result from bacterial contamination of the solution [20, 21]. These problems have led to the development of standardized, industrially prepared feeding solutions, the most commonly used being iso-osmotic (approximately 300 mOsm/l) and containing 1–1.5 kcal/ml, obtained with varying proportions of carbohydrates (45%–60%), lipids (20%–35%), and proteins (15%–20%). All solutions are free of lactose and gluten.

Standard feeding preparations are known as polymeric solutions, and are made up of a homogenized mixture of substrates similar to those found in normal feeds. Thus, digestion and absoprtion of carbohydrates, lipids and proteins follow the same steps within the digestive tract as the latter [22]. Conceptually, however, these processes could be severely altered in patients with major gastrointestinal dysfunction, a concern that has led to the development of semi-elemental or elemental solutions. In these preparations, maltodextrins (semi-elemental) or oligosaccharides (elemental), hydrolyzed proteins (semi-elemental) or amino acids (elemental), and medium-chain triglycerides replace standard carbohydrates, polypeptides and long-chain triglycerides, respectively. Some studies have shown that semi-elemental enteral nutrition might be better tolerated and lead to improved nitrogen retention [23] in selected subgroups of patients with severe small-bowel disease [24], but the bulk of evidence demonstrates no advantage of such preparations [23, 25, 26], and even suggests major possible side effects such as atrophy of gut villosities [27]. Consequently, polymeric solutions should be preferred as the first line of enteral nutrition, and semi-elemental preparations should be considered in selected patients with very severe small bowel disease or extensive intestinal resection.

Adding fibers to enteral feeding solutions can prove beneficial, as the insoluble fibers (cellulose, lignin) adsorb water, which leads to improved regulation of intestinal transit and a reduced incidence of diarrhea [28], while the soluble fibers (pectin, gums, mucilages) are degraded into short-chain fatty acids, which enhance colonic water and electrolyte absorption and provide fuel for the colonic cells [29]. Since there are very little side effects or risks associated with their use, these fiber enriched solutions should be used in most ICU patients.

Finally, in patients receiving 1500 ml/day of enteral nutrition, and in the absence of prior severe micronutrient deficiency (e.g. chronic alcoholism), or of conditions known to associate increased needs and major losses (e.g. hemodialysis, burns, etc.) [30, 31], there is no need to add vitamin or trace elements to standard feeding preparations.

Conditioning and Delivery Apparatus

The optimal volume of the feeding bottle is around 500 ml, which, even though such containers entail a higher workload (most ICU patients receive around 1500 ml/of solution/day), are easier to store, manipulate and fit into bedside organization. Furthermore, there is a reduced risk of bacterial contamination associated with large volume containers (>1 l) but some wasting of solution when only partial administration of required needs is possible.

The connector set linking the patient's feeding tube to the container should undergo regular changing. Indeed, leaving the set in place for longer than 24 h can result in a markedly increased rate of bacterial contamination [32]. It is thus recommended to change the connector set every 24 h, and to bear in mind that proper hand washing or antisepsis remains a golden rule of hospital hygiene that applies to the manipulation of enteral nutrition preparations and apparatus [33].

Enteral nutrition can be delivered to the patient by gravity or with a constant delivery pump. The former has the benefit of simplicity and bears no additional cost. However, the gravity method is less precise than the pump technique, and carries the possibility of accidental bolus administration of large amounts of solution, which has been shown to increase the risk of gastroesophageal reflux and the possibility of broncho-aspiration [34]. Conversely, improved tolerance and a reduced incidence of diarrhea have been documented with continuous compared to bolus feeding [35, 36]. These points are of particular importance in ICU patients, in which a high incidence of both delayed gastric emptying [14, 37] and diarrhea [38, 39] has been demonstrated, two problems liekly to be exacerbated by bolus feeding. Avoiding these pitfalls through a better tolerance to enteral nutrition allows an improved protein and calorie intake, at least in some patients [40]. Thus, constant delivery should be the preferred method in ICU patients, as it presents many advantages that justify the added cost of using a pump.

Monitoring Enteral Nutrition

Critically ill patients very often present with delayed gastric emptying and impaired gastroduodenal motility, the etiology of which is multifactorial [14, 37, 41]. This problem represents a major interference with the proper adminstration of enteral nutrition, ans is an often cited cause of incomplete delivery of the prescribed daily feed [42, 43]. Measuring gastric residuals by aspiration is often used as a monitoring tool on which decisions to continue, forego, or change the administration rate of enteral nutrition are made [43]. One of the main drawbacks of this approach is that the cutoff value for effecting those changes is difficult to determine, as it depends on key factors such as the timing of gastric residuals determination, the duration of interruption of enteral nutrition before measurements are made, and the volume of gastric secretions. An arbitrary value above which enteral nutrition is usually given at a slower rate or discontinued is 150 ml [44]. However, this volume might considerably overestimate the risk of digestive tract intolerance, and lead to inappropriate decision-making [45], thereby leading to underfeeding of patients [42, 43]. In our view, gastric residuals should be measured once daily, at the same time each day, and volumes up to 300 ml considered normal. If residuals are >300 ml, the infusion rate should be reduced by half for approximately 6 h, and progressively returned to normal over the next 24–48 h. During that time, residuals should be measured twice daily, and prokinetic drugs (cisapride or erythromycin) administered to promote gastric emptying [46, 47].

Diarrhea During Enteral Nutrition

Diarrhea is a frequent problem in ICU patients receiving enteral nutrition, and has often been atttributed to the latter, mainly to its osmotic effect [38, 48]. However, even though the early preparations described above often had a high osmolarity (up to 1200 mOsm/kg), most standard polymeric industrial feeds have much lower values (≤380 mOsm/kg). Furthermore, various studies attempting to determine the etiology of diarrhea in enterally fed patients have identified several possible factors not related to nutrition itself, such as antibiotics and other medication, osmotically active excipients, Clostridium difficile colitis, hypoalbuminemia, sepsis, fever and previous suspension of enteral nutrition [38, 39, 48–51]. Thus, enteral nutrition should not systematically be discontinued when diarrhea appears in a tube-fed patient. If diarrhea is severe, nutrition flow rate should be recalculated (as an excessive flow rate can induce diarrhea) and slowed if necessary, and tests performed searching for other causes (e.g. stool cultures for *Clostridium difficile* toxin, review of currently prescribed drugs). The use of fiber enriched solutions should also be considered, as well as the administration of antidiarrheal agents (motility and gut secretion regulators such as loperamide) or exogenous microflora components (such as *Saccharomyces boulardii* or inactivated *Escherichia coli*) in particular patients [39].

Parenteral Nutrition

Venous Access

One of the many often cited downsides of parenteral nutrition is the need for central venous access, and the associated risks of pneumothorax, arterial puncture and catheter-related infection [52]. However, even though these risks should not be minimized, it should be remembered that central venous lines are often present in ICU patients for other reasons (e.g. hemodynamic monitoring, administration of various drugs). Hence, in severely ill ICU patients, it is very rarely that a central venous line must be placed solely for the purpose of parenteral nutrition. In any case, the placement of a central venous catheter requires experienced personnel to minimize the risk of complications, while its subsequent management should be focused on means to prevent catheter-related infection, by addressing the issues of catheter material, duration, dressing, as well as apparatus and manipulations for injection of drugs or infusions [53–55].

Parenteral nutrition is possible using a peripheral venous catheter [56]. However, due to the difficulty of durably administering adequate caloric and protein intake, plus the needed electrolytes, by this route (thrombophlebitis due to high osmolarity, fluid overload), central venous access is preferable for anything but short duration support. The choice of central venous access site should be guided by whether or not a central line is already in place, in which case it should be used to minimize the risk of a new puncture site. In the absence of a preexisting line, either subclavian or internal jugular sites are preferred, and both have advantages and disadvantages. The former has a lower risk of infection and dressing care is easier, but the risk of pneumothorax or subclavian artery puncture is higher, both complications bearing potentially devastating effects in unstable ICU patients. The risk of these two complications is much lower with internal jugular vein catheterization, but carotid artery puncture is more frequent, as is infection of the insertion site [54, 57]. Final choice should be guided by the experience of the operator with one particular site, whether or not the patient has an added source of infection close to the insertion point (e.g. tracheotomy and internal jugular vein), presence or absence of cutaneous lesions, burn, prior radiotherapy, and deep vein thrombosis, as well as an estimation of the patient's tolerance to a possible pneumothorax. Subcutaneously tunneled catheters should be reserved for long-term parenteral support (>3–4 weeks), such as in bone marrow transplantation associated with multiple intensive i.v. therapy.

Risk of Infection

Besides the risk of catheter-related infection, parenteral nutrition may cause infection due to bacterial or fungal growth if solutions are contaminated during packaging, if they are improperly stored, or if left too long connected to the patient [58]. Indeed, nutrition solutions potenitally constitute a culture medium for these micro-organisms [59, 60]. The issue of nosocomial infection due to parenteral nutrition has been addressed by various studies, which have led to the conclusion that while infection does occur in this context, it is very difficult to differentiate between catheter-borne and solution-caused infection, and that the overall risk is quite small if care is taken to avoid contaminating the solutions [58–60]. All-in-one solutions may decrease the risk of infection by reducing the need for manipulation of i.v. lines and connectors (see below).

Type of Feeding Solution, Conditioning, and Mode of Administration

Most commercially available parenteral nutrition solutions comprise glucose, triglycerides and amino acids in varying proportions, either as separate plastic pouches or glass bottles, or in 2-3- compartment all-in-one pouches [61, 62]. The latter represent an attractive alternative to the former, as they entail less workload to change the various containers, easier storage, reduced infectious risk due to decreased number of manipulations, connections and stopcocks, and are less costly to use [62]. One major drawback is the fixed proportion of their various constituants, which can sometimes prompt discontinuation of nutrition (e.g. potassium, phosphorus and magnesium in the presence of acute renal failure).

As with enteral feeding solutions, there is a wide range of available preparations on the market, containing various proportions and classes of the three basic constituents. A detailed review of the pros and cons of these possible combinations is to be found elsewhere in this book. Suffice it to say that for routine parenteral nutrition needs, the all-in-one approach is the most convenient, because most such solutions contain balanced proportions of feeds in various concentrations, and all the clinician has to do is determine the patient's energy requirement and choose the appropriate solution.

The preferred mode of administration in ICU patients is continuous as opposed to cyclic, since it avoids intermittent hyperglycemia, improves metabolic tolerance and improves the efficiency of substrate utilization [63].

Compatibility Between Parenteral Nutrition Solutions and Additives

These solutions contain up to 40 components, which are known to be compatible. However, this large number of components carries a high risk of incompatibilities when other i.v. drugs (such as electrolytes, antibiotics, etc) are infused simultaneously through the same i.v. line, which can potentially lead to clinical accidents (occult precipatation and intravenous embolization of particles, inactivation of drugs, etc.). The best preventive measure is to reserve a catheter for parenteral nutrition administration whenever possible. If this is not possible, one option is to administer drugs as far away as possible downstream from the site of nutrition solution infusion, in order to limit contact time between these agents. Another option is to transiently interrupt parenteral nutrition during the drug infusion, provided the latter does not require continuous i.v. administration.

Practical Approach in the ICU

The choice between enteral and parenteral nutrition in ICU patients has sparked a debate vaguely reminiscent of the colloid vs cristalloid controversy in fluid resuscitation [5]. However, even though solid evidence-based proof allowing definitive guidelines might still be lacking, there is from our standpoint sufficient data available to recommend a practical strategy in the nutritional approach to such patients (Fig. 1).

First, a considerable body of data suggests that using the digestive tract to provide nutrition exerts several beneficial effects, such as favoring intestinal villous trophicity, promoting gut motility, reducing the risk of bacterial translocation from the gut, decreasing the number of infectious complications associated with parenteral nutrition, and lowering costs [64–66]. Hence, it seems logical to use the gut whenever possible, and nowadays most would agree that in the presence of a functional gut, enteral nutrition should be preferred (Table 1).

Second, optimal timing of the onset of enteral nutrition is crucial. There is often unnecessary delay due to the fear of regurgitation associated with decreased gastroduodenal motility [42, 43]. This delay can prolong negative nitrogen balance and cause further weight loss or organ dysfunction [67], and, even though there is some evidence that nutritional support can be delayed by as much as 5–7 days without deleterious effects [3, 68], this period seems excessive in the presence of prior malnutrition and/or highly catabolic illness. Thus, a compromise must be made between reaching nutritional objectives as quickly as possible and avoiding the complications associated with a functional but slowed down digestive tract (Fig. 1). In our view, enteral nutrition should be started within 48 h of ICU admission, not necessarily with the goal of providing the patient's total energy requirements, but with that of stimulating gut function and trophicity, thus preventing intestinal disuse atrophy which will render enteral feeding even more difficult. Indeed, there is some evidence that this goal can be attained with only minimal amounts of enteral nutrition [69]. In such patients, parenteral nutrition should not be used from the onset.

The above should naturally be influenced by the nutritional assessment and energy requirement of the patient, taking into consideration simple parameters of patient history and evaluation of present condition (Table 2). In patients with severe catabolic illness, and/or those with a poorly functional gut, parenteral nutrition should be started concomitantly, to allow protein and energy requirements to be met and attempt to minimize excessive muscle wasting [70, 71]. Like-

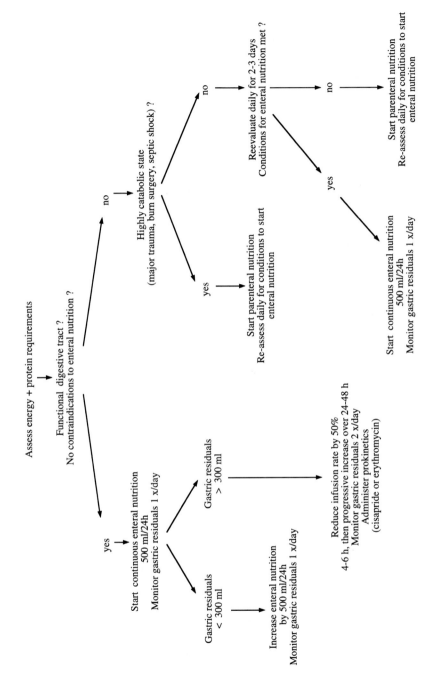

Fig. 1. Proposed practical approach to the nutrition of intensive care patients

Table 1. Indications, contraindications and timing of enteral nutrition (EN) in critically ill patients (from [9])

General statement

Whenever artificial nutrition is indicated, the enteral route is preferred to parenteral nutrition

Practical indications

Present malnutrition, whatever the etiology, in a patient unable to eat

Prolonged fasting (more than 3–4 days) in a well-nourished patient unable to resume oral nutrition

Supplementation of insufficient oral intake for >3–4 days

Severe trauma and burns: there is accumulating evidence that early EN is beneficial

Maintenance of gut mucosa, prevention of atrophy, stimulation of compensatory hypertrophy after small bowel resection

Opening of digestive tract and peparation of oral feeding

Contraindications

Absolute

Non functional gut: anatomic disruption, obstruction, gut ischemia

Generalized peritonitis

Severe shock states

Relative

Expected short period of fast, except in severely injured patients

Abdominal distension during EN

Localized peritonitis, intraabdominal abcess, severe pancreatitis

Patients with terminal disease

Comatose patients at risk of aspiration (especially gastric feeding)

Extremely short bowel (less than 30 cm)

Timing

Early EN (within 24–48 h): severe trauma, burn, highly catabolic state

Standard EN (after 2–3 days): moderate stress in a patient unable to eat

---

Table 2. Practical elements of nutritional assessment in intensive care patients (from [9])

Patient history

Disease states associated with heightened risk of malnutrition (e.g. chronic debilitating disease)

Recent severe body weight loss ($\geq$5% of usual body weight in 3 weeks or $\geq$10% in 3 months)

History of chronic low food intake, drug abuse, alcoholism, chronic psychiatric disorders)Assessment of present condition

Diseases associated with hypermetabolism and prolonged catabolic activity (polytrauma, burns, persistent fever, sepsis, multiple organ failure)

Signs of malnutrition on physical examination (e.g. cachexia, muscle atrophy, edema)

Body mass index [body weight in kg/(height in m)^2] <20 kg/m^2

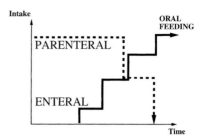

Fig. 2. Conceptual diagram of suggested progressive replacement of parenteral nutrition by early enteral nutrition, with the goal of promoting gut function and facilitating the ultimate reinstitution of normal oral feeding. (From [4], with permission)

wise, parenteral nutrition should replace enteral nutrition if patients develop major intolerance or any other contraindication to the latter during ICU stay.

In any case, regular attempts should be made to start or increase enteral feeding, with the goal of gradually replacing parenteral nutrition (Fig. 2).

Conclusion

The goal of nutritional support in ICU patients is to avoid the excessive muscle wasting and its associated morbidity and mortality in the presence of protracted critical illness. There is considerable evidence that this goal can best be achieved by the use of enteral nutrition, in the form of pre-conditioned ready-to-use 500 ml containers of a iso-osmotic fiber-containing solution, with the added benefit of improving digestive tract function. There are however situations where intolerance or absolute contraindications mandate that protein-calorie requirements be met with parenteral nutrition, to avoid the risks and complications of underfeeding patients with highly catabolic disease. In those cases, all-in-one solutions represent the most attractive option, both from a physiologic and economic standpoint. However, the ease of use of these solutions should not deter the ICU physician from regularly testing tolerance to even minimal amounts of enteral feeding, with the priority of always trying to replace parenteral feeding with the more physiologic enteral route. In some cases, a combined approach using both routes can be used during a transient period.

References

1. Giner M, Laviano A, Meguid MM, Gleason JR (1996) In 1995 a correlation still exists between malnutrition and poor outcome in critically ill patients still exists. Nutrition 12: 23–29
2. Cerra FB, Benitez MR, Blackburn GL, et al. (1997) Applied nutrition in ICU patients. A consensus statement of the American College of Chest Physicians. Chest 111: 769–778
3. Klein S., Kinney J., Jeejeebhoy K., et al. (1997) Nutrition support in clinical practice: review of published data and recommendations for future research directions. JPEN 21: 133–156
4. Jolliet P, Pichard C, Chevrolet JC (1998) Nutritional support in the ventilator-dependent patient. Eur Respir Mon 8: 84–113

5. Lipman TO (1998) Grains or veins: is enteral nutrition really better than parenteral nutrition? A look at the evidence. JPEN 22: 167–182
6. Koretz RL (1994) Feeding controversies. In: Zaloga G (ed). Nutrition in critical care. Mosby. St. Louis, pp 283–296.
7. Koretz RL (1995) Nutritional supplementation in the ICU. How critical is nutrition for the critically III? Am J Respir Crit Care Med 151: 570–573
8. Heyland D.K., Cook D.J., Guyatt G.H. (1994) Does the formulation of enteral feeding products influence infectious morbidity and mortality rates in the critically ill patient? A critical review of the evidence. Crit Care Med 22: 1192–1202
9. Jolliet P, Pichard C, Biolo G, et al. (1998) Enteral nutrition in intensive care patients: a practical approach. Intensive Care Med 24: 848–859
10. Pichard C, Kyle U, Chevrolet JC, et al. (1996) Lack of effects on muscle function of recombinant growth hormone in patients requiring prolonged mechanical ventilation: a prospective randomized controlled study. Crit Care Med 24: 403–413
11. Gorman R, Morris J, Metz C, Mullen J (1993) The button jejunostomy for long-term jejunal feeding: results of a prospective randomized trial. JPEN 17: 428–431
12. Shike M, Latkany L, Gerdes H, Bloch A (1997) Direct percutaneous endoscopic jejunostomies for enteral feeding. Nutr Clin Pract 12: S38-S42
13. Stark SP, Sharpe JN, Larson GM (1991) Endoscopically placed nasoenteral feeding tubes. Indications and technique. Ann Surg 57: 203–205
14. Dive A, Moulart M, Jonard P, Jamart J, Mahieu P (1994) Gastroduodenal motility in mechanically ventilated critically ill patients: a manometric study. Crit Care Med 22: 441–447
15. Russell T, Brotman M, Norris F (1984) Percutaneous gastrostomy. Am J Surg 148: 132–137
16. Kadakia SC, Sullivan HO, Starnes E (1992) Percutaneous endoscopic gastrostomy or jenunostomy and the incidence of aspiration in 79 patients. Am J Surg 164: 114–118
17. Cogen R, Weinryb J, Pomerantz C, Fenstemacher P (1991) Complications of jenunostomy tube feeding in nursing home facility patients. Am J gastroenterol 86: 1610–1613
18. Breach CL, Saldanha LG (1988) Tube feedings: a survey of compliance to procedures and complications. Nutr Clin Practice 3: 230–234
19. Butters M, Campos AC, Meguid MM (1992) High frequency-low morbidity mechanical complications of tube feeding: a prospective study. Clin Nutr 11: 87–92
20. Anderton A (1993) Bacterial contamination of enteral feeds and feeding systems. Clin Nutr 12: S16-S32
21. Levy J, Van Laethem Y, Verhaegen G, Perpête C, Butzler JP, Wenzel RP (1989) Contaminated enteral nutrition solutions as a cause of nosocomial bloodstream infection: a study using plasmid fingerprinting. JPEN 13: 228–234
22. Caspary WF (1992) Physiology and pathophysiology of intestinal absorption. Am J Clin Nutr 55: 299S-308 S
23. Rees RG, Hare WR, Grimble GK, Frost PG, Silk DB (1992) Do patients with moderately impaired gastrointestinal function requiring enteral nutrition need a predigested nitrogen source? A prospective crossover controlled trial. Gut 33: 877–881
24. Heimburger DC, Geels WJ, Bilbrey J, Redden DT, Keeney C (1997) Effects of small-peptide protein enteral feedings on serum proteins and diarrhea in critically ill patients: a randomized trial. JPEN 21: 162–167
25. Mowatt-Larssen CA, Brown RO, Wojtysiak SL, Kudsk KA (1992) Comparison of tolerance and nutritional outcome between a peptide and a standard enteral formula in critically ill, hypoalbuminemic patients. JPEN 16: 20–24
26. Jones BJ, Lees R, Andrews J, Frost P, Silk DB (1983) Comparison of an elemental and polymeric enteral diet in patients with normal gastrointestinal function. Gut 24: 78–84
27. Aguilar-Nascimento JE, Garcia A, De Lima SA, Pereira ACC (1997) Effect of an elemental diet on the morphology of the colon in rats. Nutrition 14: 287–290
28. Homan HH, Kemen M, Fuessenich C, Senkal M, Zumtobel V (1994) Reduction of diarrhea incidence by soluble fiber in patients receiving total or supplemental enteral nutrition. JPEN 18: 486–490

29. Scheppach W.M., Bartram H-P. (1993) Experimental evidence for and clinical implications of fiber and artificial enteral nutrition. Nutrition 9: 399–405
30. Shenkin A. (1995) Trace elements and inflammatory response: implications for nutritional support. Nutrition 11: 100–105
31. Berger MM, Cavadini C, Bart A, et al. (1992) Cutaneous zinc and copper losses in burns. Burns 18: 373–380
32. Kohn CL (1991) The relationship between enteral formula contamination and length of enteral delivery set usage. JPEN 15: 567–571
33. Pittet D, Dharan S, Touveneau S, Sauvan V, Pernegger TV (1999) Bacterial contamination of the hands of hospital staff during routine patient care. Arch Intern Med 26: 821–826
34. Coben RM, Weintraub A, DiMarino AJ, Cohen S (1994) Gastroesophageal reflux during gastrostomy feeding. Gastroenterology 106: 13–18
35. Jones BJ, Payne S, Silk DB (1980) Indications for pump-assisted enteral feeding. Lancet 17: 1057–1058
36. Ciocon JO, Galindo-Ciocon DJ, Tiessen C, Galindo D (1992) Continuous compared with intermittent tube feeding in the elderly. JPEN 16: 525–528
37. Heyland DK, Tougas G, King D, Cook DJ (1996) Impaired gastric emptying in mechanically ventilated, critically ill patients. Intensive Care Med 22: 1339–1344
38. Ringel AF, Jameson GL, Foster ES (1995) Diarrhea in the intensive care patient. Crit Care Clin 11: 465–477
39. Bleichner G, Bléhaut H, Mentec H, Moyse D (1997) *Saccharomyces boulardii* prevents diarrhea in critically ill tube-fed patients. Intensive Care Med 23: 517–523
40. Pichard C, Roulet M (1984) Constant rate enteral nutrition in bucco-pharyngeal cancer care. A highly efficient nutritional support system. Clin Otolaryngol 9: 209–214
41. Bosscha K, Nieuwenhuijs VB, Vos A, Samson M, Roelofs JMM, Akkermans LMA (1998) Gastrointestinal motility and gastric tube feeding in mechanically ventilated patients. Crit Care Med 26: 1510–1517
42. Heyland D, Cook DJ, Winder B, Brylowski L, Van de Mark H, Guyatt G (1995) Enteral nutrition in the critically ill patient: a prospective survey. Crit Care Med 23: 1055–1060
43. Adam S, Batson S (1997) A study of problems associated with the delivery of enteral feed in critically ill patients in five ICUs in the UK. Intensive Care Med 23: 261–266
44. McClave SA, Snider HL, Lowen CC, et al. (1992) Use of residual volume for enteral feeding intolerance: prospective blinded comparison with physical examination and radiographic findings. JPEN 16: 99–105
45. Lin HC, Van Citters GW (1997) Stoping enteral feeding for arbitrary gastric residual volume may not be physiologically sound: results of a computer simulation model. JPEN 21: 286–289
46. Spapen HD, Duinslaeger L, Diltoer M, Gillet R, Bossuyt A, Huyghens LP (1995) Gastric emptying in critically ill patients is accelerated by adding cisapride to a standard enteral feeding protocol: results of a prospective, randomized, controlled trial. Crit Care Med 23: 481–485
47. Frost P, Edwards N, Bihari D (1997) Gastric emptying in the critically ill – the way forward? Intensive Care Med 23: 243–245
48. Fuhrman MP (1999) Diarrhea and tube feeding. Nutr Clin Pract 14: 83–84
49. Heimburger DC (1990) Diarrhea in tube-fed patients: will the real cause please stand up. Am J Med 88: 89–90
50. Edes TE, Walk BE, Austin JL (1990) Diarrhea in tube-fed patients: feeding formula not necessarily the cause. Am J Med 88: 91–93
51. Keohane PP, Attrill H, Love M, Silk DB (1984) Relation between osmolality of diet and gastrointestinal side effects in enteral nutrition. Br Med J 288: 678–680
52. Schlichtig R, Ayres SM (1988) Modes of delivery: rationale, implementation, and mechanical complications. In: Schlichtig R, Ayres S (ed). Nutritional support of the critically ill. Year Book Medical Publishers Inc. Chicago, London, Boca Raton, pp 75–95.
53. Giuffrida DJ, Bryan-Brown CW, Lumb PD, Kwun KB, Rhoades HM (1986) Central vs. peripheral venous catheters. Crit Care Med 90: 806–809

54. Reed CR, Sesler CN, Glauser FL, Phelan BA (1995) Central venous catheter infections: concepts and controversies. Intensive Care Med 21: 177–183
55. Cook D, Randolph A, Kernerman P, et al. (1997) Central venous catheter replacement strategies: a critical review of the literature. Crit Care Med 25: 1417–1424
56. Hansell DT (1989) Intravenous nutrition: the central or peripheral route? Int Ther Clin Monit 10: 184–190
57. Kemp CL, Burge J, Chonban P, Harden J, Mirtallo J, Flancbaum L (1994) The effect of catheter type and site on infection rate in total parenteral nutrition. JPEN 18: 71–74
58. Thompson B, Robinson LA (1991) Infection control of parenteral nutrition solutions. Nutr Clin Pract 6: 49–51
59. Mehrson J, Nogami W, Williams JA, Yoder C, Eitzen HE, Lemons JA (1986) Bacterial/fungal growth in a combined parenteral nutrition solution. JPEN 10: 498–502
60. Parr MD, Bertch KE, Rapp RP (1985) Amino acid stability and microbial growth in total parenteral nutrient solutions. Am J Hosp Pharm 42: 2688–2691
61. Leutenegger A, Frutiger A (1986) All-in-one: conventional versus two different all-in-one solutions for total parenteral nutrition surgical intensive care patients. World J Surg 10: 84–94
62. Baddeley J, Thomas M, Chatterjee R, Page C, Nicholas A (1996) Pharmacoeconomic analysis of a new TPN service compared with on-site hospital manufacture. Br J Int Care Oct: 290–296
63. Forsberg E, Soop M, Lepape A, Thörne A (1994) Metabolic and thermogenic response to continuous and cyclic total parenteral nutrition in traumatised and infected patients. Clin Nutr 13: 291–301
64. Lew JL, Rombeau JL (1993) Effects of enteral nutrients on the critically ill gut. In: Wilmore D, Carpentier Y (ed). Metabolic support of the critically ill patient. Springer-Verlag. Berlin, Heidelberg, New York, pp 175–197.
65. Buchman AL, Moukarzel AA, Bhuta S, et al. (1995) Parenteral nutrition is associated with intestinal morphologic and functional changes in humans. JPEN 19: 453–460
66. Frost P, Bihari D (1997) The route of nutritional support in the critically ill: physiological and economical considerations. Nutrition 13: 58S-63 S
67. Weekes E, Elia M (1996) Observations on the patterns of 24-h energy expenditure changes in body composition and gastric emptying in head-injured patients receiving nasogastric tube feeding. JPEN 20: 31–37
68. American Society for Parenteral and Enteral Nutrition (1993) Guidelines for the use of parenteral and enteral nutrition in adult and pediatric patients. JPEN 17: 1SA-51SA
69. Zaloga GP, Black KW, Prielipp P (1992) Effect of rate of enteral nutrient supply on gut mass. JPEN 16: 39–42
70. Arnold J, Campbell IT, Samuels TA, et al. (1993) Increased whole body protein breakdown predominates over increased whole body protein synthesis in multiple organ failure. Clin Sci 84: 655–661
71. Finn PJ, Plank LD, Clark MA, Connolly AB, Hill GL (1996) Progressive cellular dehydration and proteolysis in critically ill patients. Lancet 347: 654–656

Nutritional Assessment of Intensive Care Unit Patients

M. I. T.D. Correia

Introduction

Human survival is certainly jeopardized without adequate nutrition. Almost all of the body's physiological functions rely on the external supply of nutrients for good metabolism. It's known that long periods of fasting, above 8 weeks, can lead to death due to loss of lean tissue (loss of more than 1/3 of the original weight) and its correlated complications, such as decreased immune response and higher infectious complications [1]. Malnutrition has been associated with an increase in morbidity and mortality [2–4]. Thus, the nutritional status of the patient should be routinely assessed in the hospital setting.

Centuries ago, primitive cultures searched for food that was thought to have magical and healing qualities that would purify the body [5]. At present, and despite its well documented role in the caring of the sick, nutritional therapy is still underused worldwide [6, 7], although in many centers it has gone into the arena of molecular biology. Moreover, simple routines such as nutritional screening and/or assessment are often overlooked in hospitals. One of the reasons for this oversight is concern about the relevance and the reliability of the currently available methods in predicting a patient's outcome [8]. On the other hand, providing nutrition to a patient without a previous assessment of his or her nutritional status is like blood transfusing a patient with blood based on the color of his or her mucosa without having a red cell count. Therefore, identifying those patients in poor nutritional condition or at risk of developing nutritional deficiencies is of utmost importance for the quality of caring.

Intensive care patients are a unique group, represented almost always by hypermetabolic individuals who usually suffer from acutization of previous illness, which could have compromised their nutritional status, or acute trauma. In any of the aforementioned situations, the nutritional status should be assessed, especially if nutritional therapy is foreseen. Hippocrates wrote: "Let us inquire, therefore what is admitted to be medicine... to me it appears... that nobody would have sought medicine at all, provided the same kinds of diet had suited with men in sickness as in good health" [9].

The Role of Nutritional Assessment

Nutritional assessment determines patients [1] who are either malnourished or at risk of developing malnutrition [2], the type of nutritional therapy required [3], for what period of time nutrition therapy should continue and [4] the effectiveness of the feeding regimen.

There are several ways of assessing nutritional status. Some techniques are very sophisticated and expensive, while others are less complicated and available in most hospitals. Among the options, there has yet to be a technique that is sensitive and specific enough to be considered the gold standard in diagnosing malnutrition [8]. Creating such a gold standard is difficult for several reasons, the most fundamental of which is that malnutrition has not been defined in terms of outcome.

Defining Malnutrition

Viewed as a physical state, malnutrition is a disorder of body composition characterized by macro- and/or micro-nutrient deficiencies and resulting from an insufficient intake or an increased demand for, and/or altered use of nutrients [10]. Jellife defined [11] malnutrition as a morbid state secondary to a deficiency or excess, relative or absolute, of one or more essential nutrients. Also, malnutrition can be classified as either acute (kwashiorkor type) which is usually represented by an edematous state secondary to loss of protein stores, or chronic (marasmatic), where there is a predominant loss of fat (energy) deposits. Waterlow [12] states that malnutrition can be either primary (as in community famines), where there is a protein-energy-deficient state due to lack of food, or secondary (as in the disease per se) where the type and duration of the insult is the main cause. Regardless of whether malnutrition is acute or chronic malnutrition, it leads to reduced organ function, abnormal results of blood chemistry tests, reduced body mass, poor clinical outcomes and higher mortality. However, acute malnutrition is much more severe in terms of outcome, as the body is not able to develop mechanisms of adaptation [12].

According to the literature 30%–50% of hospitalized patients have some degree of malnutrition [13–16]. Malnutrition in hospitalized patients is a consequence of several factors: previous nutrient deficiencies due to socio-economical problems and the disease per se, types of medications, length of hospitalization, psychological derangements, long periods of fasting for diagnostic tests and also, the medical teams lack of awareness of the patient's nutrient requirements and the importance of nutritional therapy [7, 16].

Unlike starvation or undernutrition, where the loss of protein is minimized by its reduced utilization as a source of energy, in hypercatabolic patients (whether postoperative, in sepsis or due to politrauma), protein catabolism occurs to provide energy and to support increased protein synthesis. Both visceral and muscle protein are broken down to provide fuel and metabolic substrate; the more severe and prolonged the hypermetabolic status, the greater the chances of malnutrition [17]. Thus, most ICU patients are at imminent risk of developing malnutrition and should have their nutritional status routinely assessed. However, at the moment, there is no available test that is both highly sensitive and specific for the assessment of malnutrition in critically ill patients. For this reason, the advantages and disadvantages of available methods used in clinical practice will be reviewed.

Nutritional Assessment

Anthropometry

Body Weight and Weight Loss

Body weight is a simple measure of total body mass. It is either compared to an ideal weight based on the weight of healthy populations or, used to calculate body mass index (BMI). BMI is obtained by dividing the weight (in kilograms) by the height squared (in meters). The normal values for BMI are 20–25 kg/m². A BMI of 14–15 kg/m² is associated with a significant mortality rate [18]. Loss of body weight has been related with poor nutritional status, morbidity, and mortality. A loss of more than 10% of the usual body weight suggests malnutrition and is associated with higher morbidity and mortality [19, 20]. A loss of more than 1/3 of the original weight is associated with imminent death [1]. However, weight loss is difficult to determine. Morgan et al. [21] have shown that the accuracy of weight loss by history was 0.67 and the predictive power was 0.75. This data suggests that 33% of those patients who had lost weight would have been overlooked and 25% of those who had been weight stable would have been diagnosed as having lost weight. Moreover, in most intensive care patients, the measured weight may not reflect the real body mass, since the patients are usually edematous as a result of resuscitation and stress.

Weight loss alone may not have any nutritional significance, since it is influenced by a wide range of confounding factors, mainly changes in hydration status.

Skinfolds and Circumferences

Anthropometry measured as skin folds and arm circumferences represent body compartment measurements of adipose tissue and muscles. In edematous states, these measurements are also altered. They suffer the influence of intra- and inter-observers errors and are compared to tables derived from healthy populations, which are very controversial. The most commonly used standard tables comparing triceps skinfold and midarm muscle circunference are those from Jellife [11] and Frisancho [22]. Both of these tables pose questions about the methodology used. Jellife based his tables on measurements of European male military personnel in service in Greece and, on low income American women. As for Frisancho tables, they were based on measurements of both white men and women participating in the 1971–1974 US Health and Nutrition Survey. According to Thuluvath and Triger [23], 20%–30% of healthy controls would be considered malnourished based on the standards of the aforementioned tables. In addition, these authors found a poor correlation between the Jellife and Frisancho standards.

Laboratory Tests

Serum Proteins

Hepatic proteins such as albumin, transferrin, retinol binding protein and prealbumin have been used as nutritional markers.

Albumin is one of the most extensively studied proteins. There have been about 19,000 citations of albumin over the last 30 years [18]. Several studies have shown the correlation between a low albumin concentration and an increased morbidity and mortality [24, 25]. Serum albumin represents an equilibrium between hepatic synthesis and albumin degradation and losses from the body. It is also influenced by intravascular and extravascular albumin compartments and water distribution. About one third of the albumin pool is in the intravascular compartment and two thirds in the extravascular. Once albumin is released into the plasma, its half life is about 21 days. In a steady state, a total of 14 g (200 mg/kg) albumin are synthesized and degraded, every day. Protein-calorie malnutrition leads to a decrease in albumin production due to lack of nutrients which are fundamental to its synthesis. However, in chronic malnutrition states, the plasma albumin concentration is often normal because of the compensatory effect (lower degradation and a shift from the extracellular compartment to the intracellular). In acute stress due to infection, surgery and politrauma, albumin levels are generally very low as a consequence of decrease synthesis, increased degradation, transcapillary losses and fluid replacement [26–29]. Albumin losses from plasma to extravascular space were increased three fold in septic shock patients [18]. Albumin might be altered due to factors other than malnutrition, such as in hepatic disorders, protein losses (in fistula, peritonitis, nephrotic syndromes, etc), and acute infection or inflammation. All of these situations are common in ICU patients and, therefore, albumin is a poor tool to assess nutritional deficiencies or to measure the effectiveness of nutritional support.

Other hepatic protein such as transferrin and prealbumin have also been used as nutritional markers and predictors of outcome [30]. However, they also suffer influence by other non-nutritional situations, such as hepatic and renal failure, hormone infusion and infection [18].

Creatinine Height Index

The creatinine height index is derived from the measurement of 24 h urinary creatinine excretion and is compared to standard values for a given height. From it, one can estimate the proportion of lean body mass. Any other factor that might interfere with creatinine excretion, such as age, renal disease, stress and diet, may also change or alter its interpretation [18].

Nitrogen Excretion

In the human body only protein is composed of nitrogen, thus measuring nitrogen excretion is a method to assess protein metabolism. Nitrogen balance can be used to estimate needs, assess nutritional therapy and follow the metabolic status. One gram of nitrogen represents 30 g lean tissue. Dietary protein averages about 16% nitrogen. Most nitrogen is lost in the urine as urea, very little in the stools and skin, and those patients with fistulas and diarrhea might have increased losses. Measuring urine urea nitrogen (UUN) and adding a factor for non-urinary losses (usually not more than 4 g/day), one can estimate the nitrogen lost in a day, with reasonable accuracy. Nitrogen balance (NB) is then calculated based on nitrogen losses and nitrogen intake, as the following formula:

$$NB=(dietary\ protein \times 0.16)-(UUN+2\ g\ stool+2\ g\ skin)$$

From this formula, the catabolic index (CI) can also be derived, which indicates the excess nitrogen created from catabolism of lean tissue:

$$CI=UUN-[0.5 \times protein\ intake \times 0.16)+3\ g]$$

A CI below five indicates a moderate stress and when above five represents severe stress [31].

A positive nitrogen balance is the goal of feeding. However, this should be followed with caution and based on clinical parameters. It is naive to think that by offering high amounts of protein (above 2 g/kg/day) to catabolic patients and achieving nitrogen balance one is accomplishing anabolism. If counterregulatory hormones are still increased, high protein intake will result in a protein futile cycle and nitrogen balance will be inaccurate, and falsely positive.

Nitrogen excretion should be obtained by serial measurements of 24 h urine collections, which depend on the good cooperation of the nursing staff. However, it is a non-expensive technique that can be used, especially, as a tool to measure catabolic stress.

Immune Response Tests

Malnutrition has been related to decrease immune response. Delayed cutaneous hypersensitivity which results from inoculation of antigens such as Candida, Trichophyton, mumps, and others, has been used to measure immunological competence and, indirectly, nutritional status. In ICU these tests are influenced by a number of other situations that cause anergy, such as different drugs (especially steroids and antirejection drugs), presence of infection, malignancy and burns, among others [32].

Nutritional Indexes

Nutritional indexes, such as the Prognostic Nutrition Index (PNI), are mathematical derived equations that combine measurements of albumin, triceps skinfold thickness, transferrin and delayed hypersensitivity skin testing. Each measurement has its own restrictions, but when put together have been shown to increase the sensitivity of predicting major morbidity in surgical patiens [33]. PNI has not been evaluated well in ICU and in medical patients.

Functional Tests

Functional tests assess nutritional status by examining the adductor pollicis muscle, handgrip dynamometry, ability to perform work in an ergometer, changes of heart rate during maximal exercise and respiratory muscle strength [34, 35]. As a result of feeding a nutritionally deprived patient, multiple elements of lean tissue (which is composed of water, mineral, nitrogen, and glycogen) are incorporated, including potassium [36]. In contrast, hypocaloric feeding results in a decreased membrane potential and concentration of intracellular potassium [37]. The events mentioned above suggest that cell ion uptake happens earlier than protein synthesis during nutritional support. In addition, muscle activity is linked to cell energetics and it has been shown that skeletal muscle function can be rapidly altered by undernutrition, without the interference of sepsis, trauma, renal failure and drug administration [38]. The absence of good equipment and standardized expertise has limited its usage. ICU patients present an even more peculiar situation due to clinical conditions such as intubation, use of muscle relaxants and other drugs, hypercapnia, hypoxia and intrinsic muscle disorders. In them, it is difficult to use most of the functional tests mentioned above. However, the assessment of the contraction of the adductor pollicis muscle, in response to an electrical stimulus of the ulnar nerve at the wrist, is a good future possibility for the assessment of nutritional status and for use as an indicator of nutritional repletion [18].

Body Composition Methods

Body composition methods, such as nuclear magnetic resonance, whole body conductance and impedance, neutron activation, hydrodensitometry, and others have been evaluated as nutritional assessment tools in healthy populations and in athletes [39]. Except for a few investigation centers, very little research has been done to prove the utility of these methods in sick patients, and even less in the critically ill. It is extremely difficult to perform these tests in bedridden patients, those who are connected to ventilators, and those who have fluid imbalances. For example, hydrodensitometry, which some consider the gold standard [39] for body composition analysis, would be impossible to perform in ICU patients, as it requires total immersion of the patient in water. Monk et al. [40] used dual-energy X-ray absorptiometry (DEXA), gamma in vivo neutron activation analysis, tritiated water dilution, total body potassium and calorimetry to assess body composition and energy expenditure in a small group of blunt trauma patients. These authors were able to demonstrate the relationship between changes in body compartments and metabolic requirements. As for bioelectrical impedance (BIA),

Chiolero et al. [41] showed that BIA is good for clinical studies in ICU patients, however it is not very accurate for one given patient.

Calorimetry

Calorimetry measures energy expenditure through the analysis of oxygen consumption and carbon dioxide production to reach the respiratory quotient. In the Intensive Care routine, indirect calorimeters are used to measure energy expenditure. Basal energy expenditure (BEE) represents the resting metabolic rate and it is dependent on lean tissue mass and, for this reason, assesses nutritional status indirectly [42]. Calorimetry is influenced by the metabolic status, fever, ambient temperature, and, the thermic effect of food and activity. This test is labor intensive because a steady state is mandatory for accurate results. At least three to five measurements should be done throughout the day to achieve a daily average. Calorimetry is better used as a follow-up tool of nutritional therapy rather than a nutritional status method.

Subjective Global Assessment

Subjective global assessment (SGA), as described by Detsky et al. [43], is a clinical method of assessing the nutritional status of patients, although not initially designed to be used in the ICU setting. It covers various aspects of a patient's nutritional history from body weight changes to functional capacity alterations. SGA presented a good agreement between observers [44, 45] and, therefore, can be used in routine hospital assessment. In addition, SGA has been well correlated when compared to anthropometric measurements. Fiaccadori et al. [46] showed that SGA was validated by anthropomety, morbidity, and mortality, in severely ill patients with Acute Renal Failure. Those patients classified as severely malnourished by SGA presented with a consistent worsening of the traditional objective markers (skinfolds, arm circumferences and albumin) and also remained in the hospital longer. They had significantly more complications (in particular, sepsis and septic shock) and the mortality rate was higher.

Because SGA is a subjective method, it relies on the observer's capacity to collect information from the patient or members of the patient's family, interpret these data, and classify the patient accordingly. Thus, in order to decrease the chances of bias among observers, it is mandatory that all of those willing to perform SGA undergo a process of training.

The following are a few general tips to be followed by those carrying out SGA:

● Performing SGA
  1. Undergo training given by an experienced member of the nutritional team before carrying out SGA
  2. Allow ample time to collect data (even though, most of the times it does not take long).

3. When the patient cannot talk due to clinical conditions such as intubation or severe disease, other members of the family should be called upon to give the information needed.

● Carrying out SGA

1. Loss of body weight. The patient is questioned about his usual weight and any loss of body weight in the last 6 months and in the previous 2 weeks. Patients might not know their usual body weight, in which case the patient should be asked about changes in the fit of their clothes and comments made by relatives or friends.

   – Separating loss of body weight in two periods (6 months and 2 weeks) is important in terms of defining waste as chronic or acute. If a patient reports that weight has been lost in the previous 6 months, but has been stable in the last 2 weeks, the severity of his nutritional status may not be as great as if he had kept losing weight. A patient who has not lost body weight in the previous 6 months, but who has lost more that 10% of his usual weight in the last 2 weeks, is at a greater risk of malnutrition. Body weight loss, in the last 6 months, below 5% is considered mild, between 5%–10% moderated and, above 10% severe [18]. In summary, it is important to quantify weight loss and it is also relevant to identify the pattern of loss in a specific period of time.

2. Altered food intake. The patient should be questioned about his regular eating patterns (type of food used, respecting food groups, number and size of meals) before and after his illness. By doing this, changes in quantity and quality of nutrient intake are assessed providing information on the capacity of achieving protein-energy requirements. For example, a full liquid diet does not reach the patient's daily macro- and micro-nutrient requirements without a supplement.

3. Changes in gastrointestinal symptoms. The presence of diarrhea (more than 3 liquid stools a day), vomiting, nausea and anorexia, if persistent for longer than 15 days, are risk factors for a decrease intake of nutrients, as well as an increase in losses, due to malabsorption (as in the case of diarrhea and vomiting).

4. Functional capacity. The ability of a patient to carry out his routine physical activities in comparison to his ability in the period previous to his illness should be questioned. Malnutrition interferes with muscle function as was mentioned above.

5. The disease and its relation to nutritional requirements. According to the patient's primary diagnosis and/or other illnesses the metabolic demand is altered. The more severe the disease, the higher the stress, and therefore the higher the metabolic requirements. Intensive care patients are usually hypermetabolic.

6. Physical examination. There are four features of the physical examination which are subjectively rated as normal (0), mild (1+), moderate (2+) and severe (3+). The first is the loss of subcutaneous fat, observed at the triceps region and the mid-axillary line at the level of the lower ribs. The second is muscle wasting, which is measured by palpation in the deltoids and quadri-

ceps area. The presence of edema in both ankles and the sacral region, as well as the presence of ascites are evaluated. As long as a co-existing disease, such as renal or hepatic failure, is not present, this edema should be thought of as a consequence of possible nutrition depletion.

7. Nutritional status rank. Based on all of the above features of the history and physical examination, a patient is subjectively ranked as (A) well nourished (B), moderately or suspected malnourished and (C) severely malnourished.

Conclusion

The prevalence of malnutrition in ICU patients has been estimated at 43% [47]. Malnutrition is a consequence of several factors, of which the hypermetabolic milieu is the most important [48]. Thus, the importance of the disease per se and the related catabolic stress as risk factors for the development of malnutrition.

It is difficult to assess the nutritional status of ICU patients, as they use ventilators and various drugs and experience abrupt and significant shifts in water between compartments. However, nutrition therapy is recognized as beneficial to these patients, due to the related complications and mortality associated with malnutrition that might develop throughout their stay in the ICU [3, 4, 49]. In order to receive appropriate nutritional therapy, patients must undergo nutritional assessment. The various methods commonly used to assess the nutritional status of patients have advantages and disadvantages which are summarized in Table 1. These advantages and disadvantages make it difficult to define any one of them as the gold standard for nutritional assessment. However, SGA which was initially described, in surgical patients, as a nutritional assessment technique, has been shown to be easy to perform and highly reliable. SGA assesses different aspects known to be risk factors for malnutrition development, such as alterations in food intake and the metabolic stress of the patient's diagnosis, for example; it should therefore also be used as a tool to assess the nutritional status of ICU patients, either alone or in conjunction with other methods.

Monitoring initial nutritional status is also recommended and extensively described by Powell-Tuck and Goldhill (this volume).

Table 1. Nutritional assessment of critically ill patients: available methods

Method	Characteristics	Drawbacks
Anthropometry	Objective data; inexpensive; loss of body weight has been related to morbidity and mortality	Accuracy of weight loss is not precise; edema alters most measurements; error factors inter and intra observers; data is compared to tables derived from healthy populations
Body composition tests (DEXA, BIA and others)	Define body composition dividing it in compartments; BIA is good for clinical studies in ICU patients, but not very accurate for one given individual	Difficult to perform in ICU patients; mostly expensive
Functional tests	Represent cell ion uptake; linked to cell energetics	Muscle relaxants' and other drugs' interference
Immune tests	Express delayed cutaneous hypersensitivity; inexpensive	Situations that cause anergy influence results
Laboratory tests (albumin, transferrin, prealbumin)	Dependent on liver metabolism; half-lives of 21, 7 and 2 days, respectively; correlation between low concentrations and morbidity and mortality; in acute stress albumin is usually low due to ↑ degradation, transcapillary losses, fluid replacement and ↓ synthesis	Influenced by liver and renal functions; in chronic malnutrition states, blood levels are usually normal; poor tools to assess nutritional deficiencies and measure effectiveness of nutritional support
Nitrogen excretion	Assesses protein metabolism; it estimates daily protein losses with reasonable accuracy; inexpensive	If counterregulatory hormones are -, there will be a protein futile cycle, and the nitrogen balance will be inaccurate; demands good nursing protocols to allow for 24 h urine collections
SGA	Clinical; good sensitivity and especificity; inexpensive; identifies risk factors for malnutrition such as actual diagnosis and evolution, weight changes, altered food intake, malabsorption or losses, functional alterations and physical signs (edema, muscle atrophy, ↓ fat tissue)	Depends on patient's and family's cooperation; it's subjective; demands good training of interviewer; not initially described for ICU patients

References

1. Nightingale JMD, Walsh N, Bullock ME, Wicks AC (1996) Three simple methods of detecting malnutrition on medical wards. J R Soc Med 89:144–148
2. Linn BS (1984) Outcomes of older and younger malnourished and well-nourished patients one year after hospitalization. Am J Clin Nutr 39:66–68
3. Dickhaut SC, Delee J, Page CP (1984) Nutritional status: importance in predicting wound-healing after amputation. J Bone Joint Surg 66:71–75
4. Reinhardt GF, Jyscofski JW, Wilkens DB, Dobrin PB, Mangan JE Jr, Stannard RT (1980) Incidence and mortality of hypoalbuminemic patients in hospitalized veterans. J Parent Ent Nutr 4:357–359
5. Meguid MM (1994) Past, present and future of nutritional support. Nutrition 10: 514S-516 S
6. Reilly HM, Martinequ JK, Moran A, Kennedy H (1995) Nutritional screening – evaluation and implementation of a simple nutrition risk score. Clin Nutr 14:269–273
7. Roubenoff R, Roubenoff RA, Preto J, Balke W (1987) Malnutrition among hospitalized patients. A problem of physician awareness. Arch Intern Med 147:1462–1465
8. Correia, MITD (1999) Assessing the nutritional assessment. NCP 14:142–143
9. Hawley EE, Carden G (1944) The art of science of nutrition, chapter 2. Mosby, St. Louis, pp 25–37
10. Kinosian B, Jeejeebhoy KN (1995) What is malnutrition? Does it matter? Nutrition 11:196S-197 S
11. Jellife DB (1966) The assessment of the nutritional status of the community: with special reference to field surveys in developing regions of the world. World Health Organization monograph. Geneva
12. Waterlow JC (1997) Protein-energy malnutrition: the nature and extent of the problem. Clin Nutr 16:3S-9 S
13. Agradi E, Messina V, Campanella G, Venturini M, Caruso M, Moresco A, et al. (1984) Hospital malnutrition: Incidence and prospective evaluation of general medical patients during hospitalization. Acta Vitaminol Enzymol 6:235–237
14. Bistrian BR, Blackburn GL, Vitale J, Cochran D, Naylor J (1976) Prevalence of malnutrition in general medical patients. JAMA 235:1567–1570
15. McWhirter JP, Pennington CR (1994) Incidence and recognition of malnutrition in hospital. BMJ 308: 945–948
16. Waitzberg DL, Caiaffa WT, Correia MITD (1999) Brazilian survey on hospital nutritional assessment (IBRANUTRI). Rev Bras Nutr Clin 14:123–133
17. Long CL, Schaffel N, Geiger JW, Schiller WR, Blakemore WS (1979) Metabolic response to injury and illness: estimation of energy and protein needs from indirect calorimetry and nitrogen balance. J Parent Ent Nutr 3:452–456
18. Jeejeebhoy KN (1998) Nutritional assessment. Gastroenterology Clinics 27:347–369
19. Stanley KE (1980) Prognostic factors for survival in patients with inoperable lung cancer. J Nat Cancer Inst 65:25–32
20. DeWys WD, Begg C, Lavin PT, Band PR, Bennett JM, Bertino JR et al (1980) Prognostic effect of weight loss prior to chemotherapy in cancer patients. Am J Med 69:491–497
21. Morgan DB, Hill GL, Burkinshaw L, Band PR, Bennett JM, Bertino JR et al (1980) The assessment of weight loss from a single measurement of body weight: the problems and limitations. Am J Clin Nutr 33:2101–2105
22. Frisancho AR (1981) New norms of upper limb fat and muscle areas for assessment of nutritional status. Am J Clin Nutr 34:2540–2545
23. Thuluvath PJ, Triger DR (1995) How valid are our reference standards of nutrition. Nutrition 11:731–733
24. Rady MY, Ryan T, Starr NJ (1998) Perioperative determinants of morbidity and mortality in elderly patients undergoing cardiac surgery. Crit Care Med 26:196–197
25. Apelgren KN, Rombeau JL, Twomey PL, Miller RA (1982) Comparison of nutritional indices and outcome in critically ill patients. Crit Care Med 10:305–307
26. Moshage HJ, Janssen JAM, Franssen JH, Hafkenscheid JC, Yap SH (1987) Study of the molecular mechanism of decreased liver synthesis of albumin in inflammation. J Clin Invest 79:1635–1641

27. Cohen S, Hansen JDL (1962) Metabolism of albumin and gamma-globulin in kwashiorkor. Clin Sci 23:411
28. Fleck A, Raines G, Hawker F, Wallace PI, Trotter J, Ledingham IM et al (1985) Increase vascular permeability: a major cause of hypoalbuminemia in disease and injury. Lancet 1:781–78
29. Rubin H, Carlson S, DeMeo M, Ganger D, Craig RM (1997) Randomized, double-blind study of intravenous human albumin in hypoalbuminemic patients receiving total parenteral nutrition. Crit Care Med 25: 249–252
30. Kuvshinoff BW, Brodsih RJ, McFadden DW (1993) Serum transferrin as a prognostic indicator of spontaneous closure and mortality in gastrointestinal cutaneous fistulas. Ann Surg 217:615–623
31. Bistrian BR (1979) A simple techinque to estimate the severity of stress. Surg Gynecol Obstet 148:675–678
32. Twomey P, Ziegler D, Rombeau J (1982) Utility of skin testing in nutritional assessment: a critical review. J Parent Ent Nutr 6:50–58
33. Buzby GP, Mullen JP, Matthews DC (1980) Prognostic nutritional index in gastrointestinal surgery. Am J Surg 139:160–167
34. Hunt DR. Rowlands BJ, Jonhston D (1985) Hand grip strength- a simple prognostic indicator in surgical patients. J Parent Ent Nutr 9:701–704
35. Christie PM, Hill GL (1990) Effect of intravenous nutrition on nutrition and function in acute attacks of inflammatory bowel disease. Gastroenterology 99:730–736
36. Hill GL, King RFGJ, Smith RC, Smith AH, Oxby CB, Sharafi A et al. (1979) Multi-element analysis of the living body by neutron activation analysis application to critically ill patients receiving intravenous nutrition. Br J Surg 66:868–872
37. Pichard C, Hoshino E, Allard JP, Charlton MP, Atwood HL, Jeejeebhoy KN (1991) Intracellular potassium and membrane potential in rat muscles during malnutrition and subsequent refeeding. Am J Clin Nutr 54:489–498
38. Brough W, Horne G, Blount A, Irving MH, Jeejeebhoy KN (1986) Effects of nutrient intake, surgery, sepsis and long term administration of steroids on muscle function. BMJ 293:983–988
39. Brodie D, Moscrip C, Hutcheon R (1998) Body composition measurement: a review of hydro-densitometry, anthropometry, and impedance methods. Nutrition 14:296–309
40. Monk DN, Plank LD, Franch-Arcas G, Finn PJ, Streat STJ, Hill GL (1996) Sequential changes in the metabolic response in critically injured patients during the first 25 days after blunt trauma. Ann Surg 223:395–406
41. Chiolero R, Gay LJ, Cotting J, Gurtner C, Schutz Y (1992). Assessment of cnages in body water by bioimpedance in acutely ill surgical patients. Intens Care Med 18:322–326.
42. Rocha EEM (1998) Is there place for indirect calorimetry in nutritional assessment. Rev Bras Nutr Clin13:90–100
43. Detsky AS, McLaughlin JR, Baker JP, Jonhston N, Whittaker S, Mendelson RA, Jeejeebhoy KN (1987) What is subjective global assessment of nutritional status? J Parent Ent Nutr 11:8–13
44. Detsky AS, Baker JP, Mendelson RA, Wolman SL, Wesson DE, Jeejeebhoy KN (1984) Evaluating the accuracy of nutritional assessment techniques applied to hospitalized patients: methodology and comparisons. J Parent Ent Nutr 8:153–159
45. Correia MITD, Caiaffa WT, Waitzberg DL (1998) Brazilian national survey on hospital nutritional assessment. Methodology of a multicenter study. Rev Bras Nutr Clin 13:30–40
46. Fiaccadori E, Lombardi M, Leonardi S, Rotelli CF, Tortorella G, Borghetti A (1999) Prevalence and clinical outcome associated with preexisting malnutrition in acute renal failure: a prospective cohort study. J Am Soc Nephrol 10:581–593
47. Giner M, Alessandro L, Meguid M, Gleaon J (1996) In 1995 a correlation between malnutriton and poor outcome in critically ill patients still exists. Nutrition 1996;12:26–29
48. Echenique M, Correia MITD (1998) Advances in nutritional support of the critically ill patient. Rev Bras Nutr Clin13;221–229
49. Naber THJ, Schermer T, Bree A, Nusteling K, Eggink L, Kruimel JW, Bakkeren J, et al. (1997) Prevalence of malnutrition in nonsurgical hospitalized patients and its association with disease complications. Am J Clin Nutr 66:1232–1239

Monitoring Nutritional Support in the Intensive Care Unit

J. Powell-Tuck and D.R. Goldhill

Assessment

Nutritional assessment has been discussed elsewhere in this book. However nutritional monitoring starts with assessment. We shall discuss some aspects briefly by way of introduction. The objectives of assessment are:
- To help decide whether nutritional intervention is indicated and the timing and route of such intervention
- To enable design of an appropriate feed
- To provide baseline measurements for continued monitoring

Assessment might be based upon the subjective global [1] approach or it might include body weight, body mass index, percentage weight loss or other anthropometric measurements. In the context of the intensive care unit body weight and height are often difficult or impossible to obtain and measurements such as the mid arm circumference, which correlates well with BMI, and which predicts outcome in patients admitted through acute services at least as well [58] may prove useful.

To what extent such assessment influences the decision to feed depends upon the clinical indication for ICU admission. Routine admission following major surgery may be for immediate post-operative care only. In the well-nourished patient, feeding, especially by the parenteral route, will not be immediately necessary and may be contraindicated [2, 3]. However for most patients admission to the ICU implies a critical illness and a catabolic state and enteral feeding will, if possible, be instigated early *whatever the nutritional status* of the patient. Nutrition should routinely take fourth priority in the care plan after cardio-respiratory stabilisation, achievement and maintenance of an appropriate circulating volume, and the specific treatment of the underlying condition(s). Nutritional intake needs to start early to correct specific nutrient deficiencies (in the short term) and prevent severe wasting (in the longer term). It should be provided in the simplest safest most cost-effective way acceptable to the patient, their relatives and carers.

An assessment (or guesstimate) of weight is needed in order to calculate approximate energy requirements based upon the Schofield equation, while the Harris Benedict equation demands both height and weight. Such estimates are necessary if the complications of excess energy provision are to be avoided (see below). The information needed can often be obtained from friends or relatives or previous notes.

The purposes of nutritional support are to help achieve:
- Survival and rapid convalescence
- Early metabolic stabilization including the correction of specific nutrient deficiencies
- Preservation of intestinal, immune, respiratory, cardiac and muscle function to prevent complications and optimise survival
- Prevention or treatment of chronic undernutrition and maintenance of lean body mass to speed convalescence

The purposes of monitoring could be said to be the continued assessment of how well these objectives are being met. Importantly, monitoring also has the purpose of preventing the complications of nutritional intervention.

Monitoring

Monitoring Cost-Benefit: Survival and Rapid Convalescence

Audit of ICU results provides overall monitoring of the effectiveness of all the treatments and care the patient receives. Nutritional care is included in this and must, as much as any other treatment, ultimately justify its use and cost by improved results. The effectiveness of nutritional treatment can only be separated from the effect of other interventions by randomised controlled trials which, though difficult to conduct in the context of intensive therapy, are becoming the yardstick by which cost-benefit issues are judged. End points such as mortality rates and length of ICU or hospital stay are increasingly being accepted as the best way to assess effectiveness though they present considerable problems for supportive treatments like nutrition and may demand large scale studies [4, 5] [59].

Monitoring Early Metabolic Stabilization Including the Correction of Specific Nutrient Deficiencies

Deficiencies of water, sodium, potassium, bicarbonate and other specific nutrients are routinely corrected in every ICU. Monitoring the effect of such replacement depends upon the careful recordings of measurements of fluid intake and output. Urine output and CVP measurements will optimise such fluid and electrolyte therapy, while plasma urea and electrolyte and urine electrolyte concentrations require regular checks, sometimes supplemented by measurements of osmolarity. Low urine sodium concentration can be a very useful guide to inadequate sodium provision if renal and cardiac function are normal. High concentrations alert us to the possibility of excess provision or to renal salt-losing states. Regular weighing is not usually practical in the context of the ICU but when possible, using a carefully calibrated and tared weighbed, it provides an excellent means of monitoring day to day fluid accumulation or loss.

The frequency of such checks vary greatly depending upon the clinical condition of the patient but will seldom be less frequent than daily on an Intensive Care Unit. Phosphate and potassium concentrations will need particular attention in the context of refeeding severely undernourished patients in whom the refeeding syndrome presents a threat. Urine and blood glucose monitoring is mandatory during feeding because of the commoness of insulin resistance in this group of patients. Magnesium and zinc depletion may be a particular problem in diarrhoeal states.

Acute deficiencies of specific nutrients may too easily go unrecognised in critical illness. Acute deficiencies of B1 presenting as a lactic acidosis [6], or folic acid presenting as leukopoenia or thrombocytopenia [7], may for example be precipitated by deficient feeds. Monitoring of such vitamins may however be less important than routinely ensuring that feeds contain appropriate amounts. This is especially important in parenteral feeding where most "off the shelf" feeds do not contain vitamins or trace elements.

The detection of iron deficiency and its correction is more problematic. Deficiency is usually detected by the combination of a low serum iron concentration with a high level of tranferrin saturation (total iron binding capacity TIBC). Unfortunately acute illness and undernutrition result in a low TIBC. The alternative measurementof plasma ferritin is also difficult to interpret because it acts as an acute phase reactant rising during acute illness. In practice rapid iron replacement is seldom appropriate in critical illness and some evidence suggests that its sequestration by a high ferritin is a defence mechanism [8].

Precise zinc status monitoring [8] is difficult but clinically we have to rely on the likelihood that severe acute deficiency will be reflected in a low circulating concentration in plasma or leukocytes.

Monitoring the Safety of Enteral Feeding:
The Decision To Use Parenteral Nutrition

Enteral feeding is preferred to the parenteral route because it maintains intestinal mucosal integrity and thereby may reduce bacterial translocation which has been implicated in the aetiology of multiorgan failure. Enteral feeding stimulates gastrointestinal motility and biliary and pancreatic secretions, and reduces the risk of biliary sludge formation.

Enteral nutrition is usually administered to critically ill patients through a naso- or oro-gastric feeding tube. These tubes are passed under direct vision or blindly using a variety of techniques. Less commonly tubes are passed beyond the pylorus. Feed must only be given if there is no doubt that the tube is correctly positioned.

Tube position may be confirmed radiologically by seeing the tip of the tube in the appropriate location on a chest or abdominal X-ray and the position of the tube is monitored by reviewing repeat Xrays which are nearly always necessary for other reasons in ICU patients.

Another commonly used method uses auscultation to listen for air injected through the tube. The auscultation method is unable to accurately determine where the tube lies in the upper gastrointestinal tract. Furthermore auscultation is not always able to identify tubes placed into the lungs. Such techniques should be repeated daily before feeds are administered to monitor tube displacement. The inability to aspirate insufflated air may be useful to confirm transpyloric placement of a feeding tube.

Measuring the pH of feeding tube aspirate may be useful to distinguish between a tube in the stomach and in the small intestine and may also help decide if the tube has been placed into the lungs.

During critical illness intestinal transit is impaired as a result both of paralytic ileus, a response of the intestine to systemic illness, and, in surgical patients, postoperative ileus, in which motor function is impaired in a more organ specific way in response to intra-operative surgical handling. Postoperative ileus is characterised by delayed gastric emptying associated with diminished antral phase III spike activity, somewhat slowed small bowel transit related perhaps to increased frequency of phase III contractions, and colonic distension secondary to loss of aborally propagated spike activity. The abnormality of gastric emptying usually dominates.

The challenge is to provide sufficient enteral nutrition against this background of intestinal motor dysfunction, without exposing the patient to gastro-oesophageal reflux and pulmonary aspiration. Traditionally allowing food or enteral feeding has been delayed until bowel sounds are heard at clinical auscultation and flatus or faeces are passed. Though these are important positive physical signs their absence does not imply that enteral feeding is contraindicated: recent studies have demonstrated the poor correlation of the return of gasto-intestinal motor function with such signs [9]. Some advocate the routine use of jejunal infusions to bypass the delayed gastric emptying but these have a number of disadvantages:

- Reduction in pancreato-biliary secretions
- Negative feedback on gastric emptying and secretion
- Practical difficulties in placing the tubes.
- Complications associated with surgical jejunostomy placement
- A failure of this approach in many studies to demonstrably reduce the complications of reflux and aspiration.

In our practice slow gastric infusion is often used with four hourly aspiration of a medium bore nasogastric tube to ensure that the stomach does not become overfilled with feed or secretions. The technique requires a gastric tube of at least 8Fr and cannot be done with a fine bore tube. The volume of gastric aspirate will be increased when there is poor gastric emptying so that feed remains within the stomach. However aspirating a gastric tube, even one with a large bore, is not a reliable measure of gastric emptying; all the contents may not be aspirated and the stomach physiologically secretes large volumes of gastric juice. This technique has also therefore been criticised [10, 11]. Feed placed directly into the jejunum may also increase the volume of gastric aspirate [12].

A gastric fluid challenge is a refinement of simple gastric aspiration and may be used to give an indication of whether feed can be given gastrically.

A bolus of clear fluid (3–5 ml/kg), is put down the naso-gastric tube and aspirated after 60 min. If the stomach is emptying well then little of the fluid will be aspirated.

There are several more precise methods of measuring gastric emptying, some of which have been used in critically ill patients but which tend to be reserved for research purposes rather than routine use.

Dye Dilution

This technique involves giving a known concentration of dye such as phenol red after a 'meal' is placed into the stomach. The dye is assumed to mix uniformly with the gastric contents. Samples of gastric aspirate are taken and the concentration of the dye measured. The greater the volume of gastric contents the lower the concentration of the dye.

Paracetamol (Acetaminophen) Absorption

This technique relies upon the fact that paracetamol is not absorbed from the stomach but rapidly passes into the blood stream from the small intestine. Several studies have used this technique in critically ill patients [13, 14]. Findings suggest that there is a wide range in gastric emptying in critically ill patients [15]. A dose of paracetamol, typically 1 or 1.5 G, is taken orally or placed down a gastric tube. The plasma concentration of paracetamol is measured at frequent intervals. The peak concentration, time to peak concentration and area under the paracetamol absorption curve indicate the speed with which paracetamol passes out of the stomach into the intestine to be absorbed. This technique is safe and can be repeated daily is necessary. However there is also little information on the kinetics of paracetamol in the critically ill and organ failure and fluid maldistribution may affect the distribution and clearance of paracetamol.

Radionucleotide Scintigraphy

This technique relies on radioactively labelling feed or fluids [16, 17]. The amount of radio-labelled meal remaining in the stomach is determined by an external scanning device, such as a gamma camera or rectilinear scanner. Repeated measurements may be difficult because of the biological half-lives of some of the isotopes used. The equipment is specialised and expensive and there may be additional practical problems using radioactive substances in the intensive care environment.

Ultrasonography

This direct, safe, non-invasive technique involves measurement of a cross-sectional area of the stomach at a fixed reference point. The equipment is relatively expensive, although widely available in most modern hospitals. Although this technique has promise, personal experience suggests that consistent and repeatable measurements are difficult to obtain [18]. With further refinement this method may prove suitable.

X-Ray Measurements

This technique depends on the passage of radio-opaque material from the stomach. The expense and other constraints of radiography mean that repeated assessments are difficult.

Electical Impedance Tomography

This has only recently been refined to the point where it is clinically practical [19]. Electrodes are placed around the upper abdomen in much the same way as electocardiographic electrodes are placed to monitor cardiac rhythm. Not only is this technique non-invasive, it also has the important clinical advantage over previous methods that it quantifies the intragastric volume of standard enteral feeds plus the endogenous gastric secretions. It gives a continuous visual display of the current gastric content volume. Thus the technique, for the first time, offers us the opportunity of continually monitoring what we most need to know while enteral feeds are infused during critical illness. We believe it has promise but, as yet it has not been evaluated in this context.

Aspiration of Enteral Feeding

Aspiration of gastric contents into the lungs is a source of potentially life-threatening pneumonia in the ventilated intensive care patient [20]. Gastric contents will leak around the inflated cuff of most tracheal tubes and this is particularly likely in supine patients. Leakage of colonised subglottic secretions around the cuff is probably the most important risk factor for pneumonia in the intubated patient [21]. Enteral feed contributes to an environment supporting the growth of microorganisms and may provide the route for transmission of gastric organisms to the lower tracheobronchial tree. If large volumes of enteral feed are suctioned from an endotracheal tube or tracheostomy then aspiration has clearly occurred. Several methods for detecting less obvious aspiration have been described.

These include placing the dye methylene blue in the pharynx and looking for blue staining in tracheal secretions. Testing for glucose in the trachea has also been used as a way of detecting aspiration of enteral feed. Unfortunately tracheal aspirates routinely contain high glucose concentrations and neither this method nor looking for methylene blue appears to be reliable for detecting aspiration of feed [22].

pH of Gastric Contents

There is a hypothesis that the organisms associated with infection in critically ill patients, particularly nosocomial pneumonia, originate in the stomach. Normally gastric contents are acidic. In critically ill patients the pH of gastric contents may be higher, either because of treatment with antacids or H2 receptor antagonists, or because of decreased acid secretion.

Bacteria can grow in this non-acid environment whereas normal acidic gastric juices are free from organisms. Measurement of the pH of gastric contents may be useful in controlling gastric colonisation. The pH is best measured with a pH probe placed into the stomach. Alternatively the pH of gastric aspirates can be measured with a pH meter, a pH strip or indicator.

Indications for Parenteral Nutrition

Detailed discussions of the indications for use of the intravenous route of feeding are found in other chapters of this book, but the finding, during attempted enteral feeding, that the feed is accumulating in the stomach, is a reason for finding an alternative approach. Post-pyloric feeding may be chosen or parenteral feeding may be preferable.

Post-pyloric feeding can exacerbate gastric stasis and there may be advantages in monitoring gastric volume during such infusions. It has not been very beneficial in the context of longterm feeding in neurologically impaired patients [23]. Post-pyloric feeding with gastric aspiration can be achieved either by placing a separate intragastric aspiration tube or by using one of the combined tubes which allow gastric aspiration during duodenal or jejunal infusion. Post-pyloric tubes are commonly regurgitated back into the stomach and there may be a place for using a pH monitoring device incorporated into the tube tip which, by indicating a sudden fall in pH, may alert clinicians and nurses to such displacement. Such devices may incidentally also have a role in ensuring that feed is infused intragastically without tube displacement either to oesophagus or duodenum.

When enteral feeding is impossible or clinically otherwise inappropriate, and if feeding is likely to be inadequate for more than 48 h, in the context of an ICU parenteral nutrition is indicated. During such feeding very slow, nutritionally insufficient, enteral feeding is often employed with continued monitoring in an attempt to maintain intestinal mucosal integrity and to encourage return to full enteral feeding at the earliest opportunity.

Monitoring To Prevent the Complications of Nutritional Intervention

Table 1 lists the important complications of parenteral and enteral nutritional support. It is an important part of monitoring to ensure that these complications do not occur or are corrected rapidly. We have already seen for example how the monitoring of gastric aspirates can be used to minimise the risk of oesophageal reflux and pulmonary aspiration.

Routine monitoring for both enteral and parenteral nutrition will include regular measurements of pulse rate, blood pressure, central venous pressure (or inspection of the jugular venous pressure), cardiac rhythm, assessment for oedema or when possible postural hypotension, daily weighing if possible, urine sugar. Chest X-ray confirms positioning of central venous lines and excludes pneumothorax. Such simple monitoring can alert clinicians to diverse problems of

Table 1. Complications of enteral and parenteral nutrition

Enteral nutrition
 Tube placement
  Tracheal placement and infusion
  Intracranial placement in ethmoid fractures
  Pharyngeal or laryngeal trauma
  Precipitation of bleeding in oesophageal disease
  Guide wire perforation of oesophagus or stomach
  Precipitation of vomiting and pulmonary aspiration
  Tube displacement
 Feed Infusion
  Oesophageal infusion and pulmonary aspiration
  Oesophageal reflux and pulmonary aspiration
  Gastric stasis with vomiting and aspiration
  Vomiting during intestinal ileus or obstruction
  Abdominal swelling and discomfort
  Diarrhea
 Metabolic
  Hyperglycemia and glycosuria
  Solute overload and dehydration
  Saline depletion or excess
  Water overload
  Increased carbon dioxide production
  D-lactic acidosis
 Hepatic
  Abnormal liver function tests
Parenteral Nutrition:
 Central line placement
  Pneumothorax
  Hemothorax
  Subclavian artery puncture
  Hematoma
  Extra-venous line placement
 Feed infusion
  Intrapleural or mediastinal infusion
  Cardiac tamponade
  Venous thrombosis
  Septicemia and its sequelae
  Microbial toxin infusion
  Particulate embolus
  Air embolus
  Fat embolus (cracked emulsion)
 Gastrointestinal
  Villous atrophy
  Bacterial and endotoxin translocation
  Gall bladder dilatation and sludging
  Gastric acid stimulation
  Loss of appetite

Table 1. *Continued.*

Hepatic
 Steatosis
 Cholestasis
Metabolic
 Hyperglycemia, glycosuria
 Rebound hypoglycemia
 Solute overload, dehydration
 Saline depletion or overload
 Water intoxication
 Specific nutrient deficiencies: electrolytes, minerals, trace elements (e.g. Zn, Fe, Cr,), vitamins
 Specific nutrient excess: amino acids, lipid, alcohol, xylitol/fructose, vitamin A and D, anticoagulation problems (vitamin K), trace element (e.g. Mn), glucose, water

feeding ranging from excess saline infusion, through metabolic complications such as insulin resistance to malposition of a feeding catheter in the atrium or ventricle.

Blood cultures are obtained at least once weekly in the presence of pyrexia presenting before central venous line placement and are obtained if a new pyrexia develops or if the pattern of an existing pyrexia changes for the worse. Under these circumstances, if line infection is possible, cultures from the line are also obtained using rigorous aseptic technique.

Fluid balance charts are routine and detailed charts are maintained of feeds actually infused. The volume of enteral or parenteral nutrition prescribed may not be given. It is therefore essential to have an accurate record of the volume actually administered. The nutrition should be delivered using an accurate pump or infusor. At regular intervals, usually hourly, a record should be made of the volume delivered. Most modern pumps and infusors will display the volume delivered. This should be compared to the volume set. A record should be made of the time when bottles or bags of feed start and finish. When the bottle or bag has been emptied its volume should be compared to the volume delivered in order to ensure that there is no major discrepancy.

Relevant biochemical monitoring includes assessment of blood sugar, plasma urea and electrolytes, blood gas analysis, liver function tests, calcium, phosphate, magnesium and zinc.

Liver Function Tests

Steatosis and cholestasis are both recognised complications of parenteral feeding [24] and abnormalities have also been associated with enteral. Liver function test which include serum bilirubin, tranaminases, gamma glutamyl transpeptidase, alkaline phosphatase and prothrombin time ratios are checked at minimum once weekly. However the interpretation of abnormality in intensive care patients presents major difficulties because the tests are not specific to nutrition-related problems. Patients on the intensive care unit usually have many other possible explanations for change in liver function ranging from primary liver disease, to circulatory failure, drug exposure and sepsis. Intra-abdominal sepsis is particularly common among those patients with intestinal disorders requiring parenteral feding. Nonetheless abnormalities of liver function or ultrasound findings suggestive of biliary sludging or steatosis can alert nutritionists to extra effort in minimising complications. Thus avoiding energy overload, encouraging some enteral intake, correcting vitamin K deficiency, using antibiotics to reduce intestinal bacterial overgrowth, changing the lipid formulation or adding taurine and/or glutamine to parenteral feeds may all be beneficial in cholestasis, while providing choline may, in addition to careful energy prescription, help steatosis.

Checking Placement of Central Lines for Feeding

In order to prevent cardiac tamponade some believe that the tip of the catheter should be placed proximal to the reflection of the pericardium onto the superior vena cava, a position obtained in practice by checking that the tip of the catheter is placed no lower than 2 cm below a line joining the lower borders of the medial ends of the clavicles on a PA chest Xray [25]. Others have shown that this point becomes unreliable on the AP Xray commonly used in portable Xrays and have suggested that the tip can be placed in the angle formed between the trachea and the right main bronchus on such radiographs [26]. Peres [27] recommends that the tip is placed in the lower superior vena cava close to its junction with the right atrium, because there the catheter is more likely to lie parallel to the wall of the vein whereas the tip may impinge end on to the vessel wall if left more proximal. Of 266 catheters audited by Peres 54 were found to have been placed in the right atrium. In the series of Rutherford et al. the positions of the tips of 100 catheters were checked retrospectively; five were in the right atrium and 53 were below the pericardial reflection on the superior vena cava as judged by the trachea/right main bronchus angle. However, to keep this all in proportion, this paper points out that no record of pericardial tamponade could be found or remembered by staff at their hospital over a 10 year period during which an estimated 10,000 central catheters were used. Various recommendations are made in the literature for the position of central venous feeding catheters which are far fewer numerically than catheters used for pressure monitoring or the infusion of inotropic drugs. Some recommend positioning in the right atrium at least for home parenteral feeding. We prefer the tip to be in the superior vena cava principally because of the potential for an intracardiac catheter to induce arrythmias. Others still prefer the tip to be proximal to the pericardial reflection on the superior vena cava. All such catheters carry the risk of superior vena caval thrombosis – a risk which increases the longer the parenteral feeding continues. Monitoring for this includes clinical inspection of jugular venous pulsation and monitoring flow of the feed.

Respiratory Function and Energy Balance

Some use indirect calorimetry to monitor the adequacy of the energy infusion and to ensure that excess glucose is not infused. Others calculate requirements and do not monitor. There is little excuse for doing neither.

Lipid produces less CO_2 per oxygen consumed than glucose and so some advocate the use of fat inputs of up to 60% of non-protein calories in the short term for patients in respiratory failure. In practice making such adjustments has been shown to be unimportant [28]. Of more importance is to ensure that excess energy, particularly as glucose, is not infused, especially if the patient is retaining CO_2. Though the synthesis of lipid from dietary carbohydrate probably occurs only to a small extent in normal mixed meal eating humans, high carbohydrate loads given continuously by artificial feed can give rise to lipogenesis. The excess energy, rather than the choice of energy substrate is the dominant consideration [28]. Glucose infusion should in general be kept below 4 mg/kg/min to avoid lipogenesis from the glucose infusion producing respiratory quotients above 1 [29] and increased ventilatory drive. Thus glucose infusion rates need monitoring.

During the stress of critical illness there is increased glucose disposal (particularly non-insulin mediated uptake into muscles via the GLUT 1 transporter), increased glucose utilisation, hyperlactataemia, hyperglycaemia with increased gluconeogenesis, decreased glycogen production and insulin resistance (for review see [30]). Under these circumstances excess carbohydrate infusion can induce increased catecholamine drive and result in high CO_2 outputs without the RQ rising above 1 [31].

Monitoring the Nutritional Management of the Critically Ill Obese Patient

Though it has been suggested that severely traumatised obese patients mobilise and oxidise fat poorly with resultant very high urinary nitrogen losses [32], this does not seem to be a problem in obese patients with septic postoperative complications. Two randomised controlled studies from Ohio [33, 34] comparing standard feeds with hypoenergetic isonitrogenous feeds, have suggested that N balance can be as well maintained with hypoenergetic feeds as with feeds containing full requirements for energy. There are times when a hypoenergetic feed can have advantages: it may be more readily infused by peripheral vein, it may result in less hyperglycaemia and hyperinsulinaemia in obese patients for whom insulin resistance may be an increased problem, and may result in less sodium retention. Obese patients may be at particular risk of ventilatory failure and it is clearly important not to drive carbon dioxide production too high. This is one example of a need to monitor urinary nitrogen or urea excretion.

Nitrogen Balance

This is the difference between known nitrogen intake and measured nitrogen loss. A loss indicates tissue catabolism. A negative nitrogen balance of 1 g indicates a loss of 6.25 g protein or about 30 g of hydrated muscle protein. Nitrogen balance can be used to estimate *changes* in body protein content over a period of time and to monitor the adequacy of nitrogen input. Unfortunately accurate measurements of total input and output are difficult in clinical practice. Total output is often estimated from collections of urine alone and from a single metabolite (urea) instead of nitrogen. Whole body protein and tissue rates of synthesis and breakdown can be made using infusions of isotopically labelled amino acids acids. Muscle breakdown can be determined by measuring excretion of 3-methylhistidine, which is released from actin and myosin in skeletal muscle. Four-hour urinary estimations are made after 24–48 h of a meat free diet. The quantity of 4.2 μmol of 3-methylhistidine represents 1 g of mixed muscle protein. These all may give indices of protein turnover but are no more useful than nitrogen balance for monitoring protein intake and metabolism during nutritional support.

Plasma Proteins

Though serum albumin is a useful predictor of surgical outcome, it may not be diminished in undernutrition uncomplicated by disease. Albumin concentration is decreased during infection, in patients with cancer, after burn injury and after trauma or surgery. This well known decrease in albumin concentration during disease is related primarily to increased vascular permeability [35]. While undernutrition may exacerbate disease-related hypoalbuminaemia, albumin concentration primarily reflects a disease process and may be better considered an "index of severity of disease" rather than a strict nutritional indicator, and it is wise to combine its use with some estimate of the acute-phase response such as C-reactive protein or ESR. These same difficulties apply to other plasma proteins which have been as nutritional indicators such as pre-albumin, transferrin and retinol binding protein [36], though these may be more responsive as nutritional indicators because of their shorter turnover time [37].

There was interest in serum fibronectin levels which were said to reflect reticuloendothelial function [38]. In practice serum protein concentrations are so subject to shifts between body fluid compartments and to effects of hemoconcentration/dilution that they are virtually useless in the practical nutritional monitoring of ICU patients though a gradually rising albumin is to sme extent reassuring.

Body Composition

Gain or maintenance of lean body mass is a time-honoured objective of nutritional assessment which may have been given too much emphasis over the maintenance of function in the past in the context of intensive care. Nonetheless it is likely that convalescence will be prolonged if patients emerge from the ICU very wasted. Short term monitoring of body composition is likely to be very inaccurate using the techniques which are routinely clinically practical. Body weight is difficult to measure in critically ill patients and will be confounded by changes in fluid status, especially if there is oedema or ascites. Skinfold measurements can be used for what they are or converted to body density via Durnin and Womersleys [39] and the Siri equations to percent body fat. However body weight is again needed to calculate lean body mass, and lean body mass may be much altered by expansion of the extracellular fluid space. Arm circumference or arm muscle circumference derived using skinfold measurements may be useful, but may be confounded by arm oedema.

Bioelectical Impedance

Bioelectrical impedance is defined as the hindrance to the flow of an alternating current and includes two components, resistance and reactance. Both resistance and reactance can be measured highly reproducibly using an impedance analyser and offer a method of estimating total body water and fat free body mass in healthy adults and children [40] and in patients in whom disturbance of water distribution is not prominent. BIA is affected by variables such as body position, hydration, consumption of food and drink, ambient skin and air temperature, recent physical activity and conductance of the examination table. Good technique requires standardization of these and other variables [41].

Total Body Water Measurement

Total body water reflects lean body mass and is estimated by isotope dilution using D_2O or ^3H_2O. D_2O has been used extensively because it has the same distribution volume as water, is exchanged by the body in a manner similar to water, is non-toxic in tracer amounts, and is measurable with accuracy in blood, urine or saliva. Many different methods of measuring D_2O have been described. An infrared spectrophotometric method using traces doses of D_2O for determination of total body water is a relatively straightforward and inexpensive technique [42]. Measurements can be repeated more frequently if a relatively low dose (about 10 g) D2O is used. In normals lean body mass, kg (LBM) is given by total body water, in litres, 0.73, but such calculations will again be confounded in the critically ill. It may be best to use the total body water measurement as such.

Dexascan

Dual energy X-ray absorptimetry (DEXA) has also been used for the assessment of body composition. This technique is based on the differential attenuation of two transmitted energy photons as they pass through bone and soft tissues. A broad band X-ray generator is used as the source of photons, and the dose incurred is very small. DEXA can be used to estimate the fat free mass in both men and women but is less accurate in the measurement of%fat in men [43, 44]. Reproducibility is good with coefficients of variation usually below 3%. Accuracy assessed for example in comparison with carcase analysis in seven 35–95 kg pigs is good [45] with the regression lines between the two methods of analysis close to the line of identity and there is close correlation between measurements of fat free mass made with DEXA and prompt neutron activation analysis. However systematic differences are found between the three commercial systems available (Lunar, Hologic and Norland) [46]. As with some radiological investigations, the equipment requires movement of the patient to a dedicated unit and has this represents a considerable disadvantage in the contxt of the ICU.

Creatinine/Height Index

Urinary creatinine excretion has been used to estimate lean body mass [47]. The urinary creatinine excretion rate based on body weight has been determined and standardized for ideal body weight as the creatinine height index. On the basis of this normal data one can determine the creatinine excretion appropriate for a healthy individual of a given height.

Total Body Potassium

Potassium is primarily intracellularly distributed and total body potassium is a measure of lean body mass [48]. It can be measured using whole body monitors which detect the radioactivity of the natural radio-isotope ^{40}K. ^{40}K is present in the body as 0.012% of the stable istopes of potassium, ^{39}K and ^{41}K [49]. Factors which deplete potassium concentration in the lean body mass, such as diuretic therapy, diabetes and hyperaldosteronism may limit the interpretation of total body potassium estimations as an index of lean body mass and caution should be applied in the use of this technique as a "gold-standard" for lean body mass. Fat free mass is given by TBK (mmol)/60 in women and TBK/66 in men. Few centres have this equipment and it is not practical for use in critically ill patients.

Exchangeable Sodium/Potassium Ratio

This ratio can be measured using isotope dilution following administration of $^{22}NaCl$ and $^{3}H_2O$ and the exchangeable sodium and potassium expressed as a function of total body water. The ratio is an index of extracellular to intracellular (or body cell) mass. A ratio >1.22 indicates undernutrition. The ratio has been used as prognostic indicator in surgical patients [50].

Prompt Neutron Activation

This technique involves the measurement of the body's contents of potassium, nitrogen, sodium, chlorine, calcium and phosphorus in a whole body radiation counter after irradiation with fast neutrons. From these values, absolute amounts of body fat, protein and minerals are calculated. The equipment is very expensive but the procedure is quick (approximately 40 min) and exposes the subject to a radiation dose which is equal to a chest X-ray [51]. The technique, combined with measurement of total body water can be used to assess the total body content of the six elements; from this multicompartment analysis of body composition becomes possible. For a review the reader is referred to [52].

Measures of Physiological Function and Fatigue

Emphasis has correctly been placed upon physiological assessment of patients as a means to determine their needs for nutritional support. Such measurements vary from immune testing as a guide to the patient's ability to respond to sepsis, through functional tests involving strength and volitional input which might be expected to measure the ability to mobilise (eg arm ergometry, grip strength), to tests independent of volition which test peripheral fatigue/muscle function specifically. Tests of quality of life or "well-being" might fall into this category too. In most patients on the ICU such measures are very difficult to apply.

Immunological Skin Testing

Adequate nutrition is essential for the maintenance of a normal immune system. A toatal lymphocyte count of 800–1200 mm^3 is indicative of moderate protein calorie malnutrition and less than 800 mm^3 indicates severe depletion. Immuno-logical challenge tests can also be used as a test of the cell mediated immune response. Intrdermal injection of a common recall antigen – candida, PPD, strep-tokinase, streptodornase or DNCB – should produce a cutaneous response with-in 24–48 h. Failure to respond indicates an anergic state, but the test may become positive with appropriate nutrition support [53, 54].

Luminal Mucosal pH

An estimate of luminal, gastric or colonic, intramucosal pH (pHi) can be obtained with tonometry. This relies on the ability of carbon dioxide to freely diffuse across its concentration gradient until an equilibrium is reached between the intestinal luminal and intramucosal carbon dioxide tension (PCO2) [55]. Intramucosal pH is calculated by applying the Henderson-Hasselbach equation to a simultaneous determination of arterial plasma bicarbonate and luminal PCO2. In order to mea-sure the luminal PCO2 a balloon, normally filled with saline, is placed into the gut lumen. After an equilibration period the saline is withdrawn and the PCO2 mea-sured. The value of the pHireflects splanchnic tissue oxygenation [56]. Although it seems intuitively reasonable that pHi is a measure of bowel integrity and motility, and therefore the ability to be able to enterally feed a patient, there is no evidence to date that pHi can be used to predict when a patient can be enterally fed. Hypox-ia reduces appetite, increases weight loss alters responses to feeding fasting adap-tation with increases in glucose, lactate, insulin and catecholamine blood concen-trations at the expense of free fatty acid and hydroxybutyrate levels [57]. Moni-toring blood gases and pHi may represent a useful gauge of such metabolic effects.

Conclusion

Intensive care is all about monitoring and nutritional support is intrinsic tio good intensive care. Much of the most important monitoring is of the general status of the patient. As intenxsive care is completed and patients are returned to their routine wards, it is timely to review a complete nutritonal assessment linking it with an appraisal of the patients physical capabilities and ability to swallow and eat. Such appraisals are usually multiprofessional and use the skills of the nurse, physiotherapist, speech therapist and dietitian as well as those of the doctor.

References

1. Baker JP, Detsky AS, Wesson DE, et al. Nutritional assessment: a comparison of clinical judgement and objective measurements. New England Journal of Medicine 1982;306:969–72
2. Brennan MF, Pisters PWT, Posner M, Quesada O, Shike M. A prospective randomized trial of total parenteral nutrition after major pancreatic resection for malignancy. Annals of Surgery 1994;220:436–444
3. Veterans affairs total, parenteral nutrition cooperative study group. Perioperative total parenteral nutrition in surgical patients. New England Journal of Medicine 1991;325:525–32
4. Griffiths RD, Jones C, Palmer TE. Six-month outcome of critically ill patients given glutamine-supplemented parenteral nutrition. Nutrition 1997;13:295–302
5. Powell-Tuck J, Jamieson CP, Bettany GEA, et al. A double blind, randomised controlled trial of glutamine supplementation in parenteral nutrition. Gut 1999;45:82–88
6. Anonymous. Lactic acidosis traced to thiamine deficiency related to nationwide shortage of multivitamins for total parenteral nutrition – United States,1997. MMWR Morb Mortal Wkly Rep 1997;46:523–8
7. Ibbotson RM, Colvin BT, Colvin MP. Folic acid deficiency during intensive therapy. British Medical Journal 1975;ii:145
8. Thurnham DI. Micronutrients and immune function: some recent developments. Journal of Clinical Pathology 1997;50:887–91
9. Goldhill DR., Toner CC, Tarling MM, Baxter K, Withington PS, R. W. Double-blind, randomized study of the effect of cisapride on gastric emptying in critically ill patients. Critical Care Medicine 1998; 25:447–51
10. McClave SA, Snider HL, Lowen CC, et al. Use of residual volume as a marker for enteral feeding intolerance: prospective blinded comparison with physical examination and radiographic findings. Journal of Parenteral and Enteral Nutrition 1992;16:99–105
11. Lin HC, van Citters GW. Stopping enteral feeding for arbitrary gastric residual volume may not be physiologically sound: results of a computer simulation model. Journal of Parenteral and Enteral Nutrition 1997;21:286–9
12. Chendrasekhar A. Jejunal feeding in the absence of reflux increases nasogastric output in critically ill trauma patients. American surgeon 1996;62:887–888
13. Hu OY, Ho ST, Wang JJ, Ho W, Wang HJ, Lin CY. Evaluation of gastric emptying in severe, burn-injured patients. Critical Care Medicine 1993;21:527–531
14. Goldhill DR., Toner CC, Tarling MM, Baxter K, Withington PS, R. W. Double-blind, randomized study of the effect of cisapride on gastric emptying in critically ill patients. Critical Care Medicine 1998; 25:447–51
15. Tarling MM, Toner CC, Withington PS, Baxter MK, Whelpton R, Goldhill DR. A model of gastric emptying using paracetamol absorption in intensive care patients. Intensive Care Medicine;23:256–260
16. Ott L, Young B, Phillips R, et al. Altered gastric emptying in the head-injured patient: relationship to feeding intolerance. Journal Neurosurgical Research 1991;74:738–742
17. Spapen HD, Duinslaeger L, Diltoer M, Gillet R, Bossuyt A, Huyghens LP. Gastric emptying in critically ill patients is accelerated by adding cisapride to a standard enteral feeding protocol: results of a prospective, randomized, controlled trial. Critical Care Medicine 1995;23:481–5
18. Goldhill DR, White SA, Owen NO, Hately W. Ultrasonographic measurement of gastric emptying in volunteers: assessment of technique and effect of low dose dopamine. British Journal of Anaesthesia 1997;79:136P

19. Wright JW. The effect of intraluminal content on gastrointestinal motility in man. [PhD]: Nottingham, 1995. 337 p

20. Pingleton S.K. Aspiration of enteral feeding in mechanically ventilated patients: how do we monitor? Critical Care Medicine 1994;22:1524–1525

21. Rello J, Sonora R, Jubert P, Artigas A, Rue M, Valles J. Pneumonia in intubated patients: role of respiratory airway care. American Journal of Respiratory and Critical Care Medicine 1996;154:111–115

22. Torres A, Serra-Batlles J, Ros E, et al. Pulmonary aspiration of gastric contents in patients receiving mechanical ventilation: the effect of body position. Annals of Internal Medicine 1992;116:540–3

23. Lazarus B, Murphy J, Culpepper L. Aspiration associated with long-term gastric versus jejunal feeding: a critical analysis of the literature. Archives of Physical Medicine & Rehabilitation 1990; 71 (1):46–53

24. Quigley E, Marsh M, N, Shaffer J, L, Markin R, S,. Hepatobiliary complications of total parenteral nutrition. Gastroenterology 1993;104:286–301

25. Greenall MJ., Blewitt RW., McMahon MJ. Cardiac tamponade and central venous catheters. British Medical Journal 1975; 2 (5971):595–7

26. Rutherford J, Merry AF, Occleshaw CJ. Depth of central venous catheterization: an audit of practice in a cardiac surgical unit. Anaesthesia & Intensive Care. 1994;22 (3):267–71

27. Peres P. Positioning central venous catheters-a prospective survey. Anaesthesia & Intensive Care. 1990;18 (4):536–9,

28. Talpers S, Romberger DJ, Bunce SB, Pingleton SK. Nutritionally associated increased carbon dioxide production. Excess total calories vs high proportion of carbohydrate calories. Chest 1992;102 (2):551–5

29. Guenst JM, Nelson LD. Predictors of total parenteral nutrition-induced lipogenesis. Chest 1994;105:553–9

30. Mizock B. Alterations in carbohydrate metabolism during stress: a review of the literature. American Journal of Medicine 1995;98:75–84

31. Askanazi J, Carpentier YA, Elwyn DH, et al. Influence of total parenteral nutrition on fuel utilization in injury and sepsis. Annals of Surgery 1980;191:40–6

32. Jeevanandam M, Young DH, Schiller WR. Obesity and the metabolic response to severe multiple trauma in man. Journal of Clinical Investigation 1991;87:262–9

33. Burge JC, Goon A, Choban PS, Flancbaum L. Efficacy of hypocaloric total parenteral nutrition in hospitalized obese patients: a prospective, double-blind randomized trial. Journal of Parenteral and Enteral Nutrition 1994;18:203–7

34. Choban PS, Burge JC, Scales D, Flancbaum L. Hypoenergetic nutrition support in hospitalized obese patients: a simplified method for clinical application. American Journal of Clinical Nutrition 1997;66:546–50

35. Fleck A, Raines G, Hawker f, et al. Increased vascular permeability: a major cause of hypoalbuminaemia in disease and injury. Lancet 1985;i:781–4

36. Ingenbleek Y, Van Den Schrieck HG, De Nayer P, De Visscher M. Albumin, transferrin and the thyroxine-binding prealbumin/retinol-binding protein (TBPA-RBP) complex in assessment of malnutrition. Clinica Chimica Acta 1975;63:61–7

37. Shetty PS, Watrasiewicz KE, Jung RT, James WP. Rapid-turnover transport proteins: an index of subclinical protein-energy malnutrition. Lancet 1979;2:230–2

38. McKone TK, Davis AT, Dean RE. Fibronectin. A new nutritional parameter. American surgeon 1985;51 (6):336–9,

39. Durnin J, V, G,A, Womersley J. Body fat assessed from total body densityand its estimation from skinfold thicknesses: measurements in 481 men and women aged from 16–72 years. British Journal of Nutrition 1974;32:77–97

40. Houtkooper LB, Going SB, Lohman TG, Roche AF, Van Loan M. Bioelectrical impedance estimation of fat-free body mass in children and youth: a cross-validation study. Journal of Applied Physiology: Respiratory, Environmental, Exercise Physiology. 1992;72 (1): 366–73

41. Anonymous. Biolelectrical impedance analysis in body composition measurement: National Institutes of Health Technology Assessment Conference statement. American Journal of Clinical Nutrition 1996;64 (3 Suppl):524S-532 S

42. Lukaski HC, Johnson PE., et al. A simple, inexpensive method of determining total body water using a tracer dose of D2O and infrared absorption of biological fluids. American Journal of Clinical Nutrition 1985; 41:363–70

43. van Loan M, Mayclin PL. Body composition assessment: dual-energy X-ray absorptiometry (DEXA) compared to reference methods. European Journal of Clinical Nutrition 1992;46 (2):125-30

44. Clark R, Kuta JM, Sullivan JC. Prediction of percent body fat in adult males using dual energy X-ray absorptiometry, skinfolds, and hydrostatic weighing. Medicine & Science in Sports & Exercise 1993;25 (4):528–35

45. Svendsen O, L, Haarbo J, Hassager C, Christiansen C. Accuracy of body composition by dual-energy X-ray absorptiometry in vivo. American Journal of Clinical Nutrition 1993;57:605–8

46. Laskey M, A. Dual X-ray absorptiometry and body composition. Nutrition 1996;12:45–51

47. Forbes GB, Bruining GJ. Urinary creatinine excretion and lean body mass. American Journal of Clinical Nutrition 1976;29 (12):1359–66

48. Alleyne GA, Viteri F, Alvarado J. Indices of body composition in infantile malnutrition: total body potassium and urinary creatinine. American Journal of Clinical Nutrition 1970;23 (7):875–8

49. Hawkins T, Goode AW. The determination of total-body potassium using a whole-body monitor. Physics in Medicine & Biology. 1976;21 (2):293–7

50. Tellado J, M, Garcia-Sabrido J, L, Hanley J, A, Shizgal H, M, Christou N, V,. Predicting mortality based on body composition analysis. Annals of Surgery 1989;209:81–87

51. Hill GL, McCarthy ID, Collins JP, Smith AH. A new method for the rapid measurement of body composition in critically ill surgical patients. 1978; 65 (10):732–5

52. Heymsfield S, B, Wang Z, Baumgartner R, N, Dilmanian F, A, Ma R, Yasumura S. Body composition and ageing: a study by in vivo neutron activation analysis. Journal of Nutrition 1993;123 (2 Suppl):432–7

53. Cerra FB, Lehman S, Konstantinides N, Konstantinides F, Shronts EP, Holman R. Effect of enteral nutrient on in vitro tests of immune function in ICU patients: a preliminary report. Nutrition 1990;6:84–7

54. Cerra FB, Lehmann S, Konstantinides N, et al. Improvement in immune function in ICU patients by enteral nutrition supplemented with arginine, RNA, and menhaden oil is independent of nitrogen balance. Nutrition 1991;7:193–9

55. Doglio GR, Pusajo JF, Egurrola MA, et al. Gastric mucosal pH as a prognostic index of mortality in critically ill patients. Critical Care Medicine 1991;19:1037–1040

56. Gutierrez G, Palizas F, Doglio G, et al. Gastric intramucosal pH as a therapeutic index of tissue oxygenation in critically ill patients. Lancet 1992;339:195–199

57. Pison CM, Chauvin C, Perrault H, et al. In vivo hypoxic exposure impairs metabolic adaptations to a 48 h fast in rats. European Respiratory Journal 1998;12 (3):658–65

58. Vlaming S, Biehler A, Chattopadhyay S, Jamieson C, Cunliffe A, Powell-Tuck J. Nutritional status of patients on admission to acute services of a London teaching hospital. Proceedings of the Nutrition Society 1999;58:119A

59. Takala J, Ruokonen E, Webster NR, Nielsen MS, Zandstra DF, Vundelinckx G, et al. Increased mortality associated with growth hormone treatment in critically ill adults. New England Journal of Medicine 1999;341:785–92

Nutritional Effects on Respiratory and Muscle Dysfunction in Intensive Care Unit Patients

K.N. Jeejeebhoy

Introduction

Patients receiving intensive care develop progressive muscle wasting and weakness. The causes of wasting are multiple, however malnutrition is one of the factors which can contribute to muscle dysfunction. In addition, these patients may have difficulty in ventilation. Part of this difficulty is related to weakness or dysfunction of the respiratory muscles. In this review it is proposed to indicate how malnutrition can influence muscle function and how nutrition support can be used to improve muscle and respiratory function.

Hitherto, malnutrition has been equated with the presence of wasting and weight loss. However, malnutrition starts when the nutrient intake of the individual does not meet the requirements for day-to-day living and activity. The initial effects are metabolic and do not affect the clinical status because there are compensatory changes which counteract the lack of nutrition. Subsequently, hypocaloric feeding was shown to result in weakness and muscle dysfunction prior to wasting by Keys et al. [1]. Subsequently, because nutrient intake is insufficient to meet the catabolic turnover of tissues, there is loss of mass. However, the loss of mass reduces the metabolic requirements and ultimately the degree of tissue wasting reduces the metabolic requirements to equal the reduced intake. At this point a new equilibrium is restored but at a lower body mass. Hence, functional changes are one of the earliest consequences of malnutrition and as will be shown subsequently are restored before any increase in body weight. In addition loss of function or its restoration is an outcome in itself. For example if a person is thinner, it may even be beneficial or may result in weakness. However, weakness and fatigue are always detrimental to quality of life and may even be life threatening when it involves respiratory muscles.

Effect of Malnutrition on Body Composition and Muscle Function

Lack of nutrient intake results in a loss of body fat and lean tissue [1] and hitherto the effects of nutritional depletion and repletion with refeeding have been judged by changes in body composition, especially of lean tissue. One of the elements responding to nutrient intake is body potassium, which has been used as an index of body cell mass [2], the metabolically active component of the lean tissue. In contrast to body nitrogen, body potassium responds rapidly to feeding by both oral [3] and intravenous routes [4]. These changes have been interpreted as being due to changes in lean mass. However the early restitution of body potassium without a rise in body nitrogen indicates that cell ion uptake occurs earlier than protein synthesis with nutritional support. In support of this conclusion it has been shown, using ion selective electrodes, that hypocaloric feeding results in a fall in muscle membrane potential and in the concentration of intracellular ionic K^+[5]. The changes were specifically related to nutrient deprivation as they could not be reversed by potassium supplementation per se. Since five molecules of ATP are required for the incorporation of one molecule of amino acid into protein, and 77% of the free-energy change of ATP hydrolysis is used to maintain the Na-K gradient across the cell membrane, and energy intake limits nitrogen retention, these findings suggest that nutritional support initially alters cell energetics rather than mass.

Z band degeneration and calcium accumulation with hypocaloric feeding in humans at a time when body weight and total body nitrogen are within the normal range [6]. These myofibrillar effects are related to changes in cell energetics.

In order to understand how malnutrition influences muscle function it is necessary to examine the effects of nutrient deprivation on individual parameters of muscle function and studies which define the mechanisms underlying these changes.

Assessment of Muscle Function in the ICU

Traditionally, muscle performance is assessed by tests which involve voluntary movement such as fatigue during endurance exercise, rapidity and force of isometric contraction and grip strength. These measurements cannot be done in ICU patients and therefore methods which involve stimulated muscle function have to be used which do not depend on voluntary effort. In order to study critically ill patients it was necessary to develop a method which did not require the cooperation of the patient and was not non-specifically affected by sepsis, drugs, trauma, surgical intervention and anesthesia. In order to do this we selected the approach taken by Edwards [7] to study muscle fatigue. It consisted of measuring the contraction of the adductor pollicis muscle in response to an electrical stimulus of the ulnar nerve at the wrist. When the nerve is stimulated at the above site with unidirectional square wave pulses lasting only 50–70 μs at a range of frequencies from 10–100 Hz, there is a progressive increase in force with a maximal attained at 50 Hz. The plotted results constitute a force-frequency curve. In addition when the nerve is stimulated at 20 Hz for 2 s and then the stimulus is switched off, the muscle relaxes and the rate of this relaxation can be measured.

Force Frequency Curve (Ratio of Low Frequency Force to High Frequency Force)

As muscle is stimulated with increasing rate of stimuli ranging from 10–100 Hz, the force of contraction in the human adductor pollicis muscle rises. However, in muscle from malnourished humans the force at 10 Hz (F10) remains normal but the increase of force with increasing frequency of stimuli to 100 Hz (F100) does not occur. Thus the F10/F100 ratio rises in malnutrition (Fig. 1).

Relaxation Rate

Muscle relaxation is an intrinsic property of muscle which is very constant. Muscle relaxation is an exponential function and therefore the absolute rate of relaxation depends upon the maximal force developed during stimulated contraction (Fig. 2). To obtain the rate constant of relaxation, Edwards has expressed the rate as the % of maximal force lost per 10 ms. To understand the significance of slow relaxation it is necessary to understand that muscle stimulation results in calcium efflux from the endoplasmic reticulum into the cytosol. The rise in cytosolic calcium causes muscle to contract. Muscle relaxation occurs because calcium is pumped against a concentration gradient back into the endoplasmic reticulum. This is an energy demanding process. In malnourished muscle relaxation is markedly slow. Since relaxation depends on detachment of myosin cross-bridges following binding with ATP [8], its rate is likely to be altered by factors governing ATP hydrolysis, or acto-myosin interactions.

Force of Maximal Contraction

Grip strength has been widely used in the evaluation of nutritional status. It has been shown to predict the development of complications in malnourished patients [9]. The equivalent function in ICU patients is the force of maximal contraction at 50 Hz.

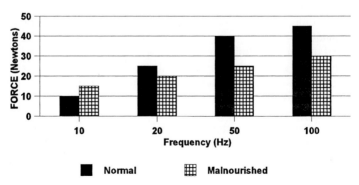

Fig. 1. Force frequency

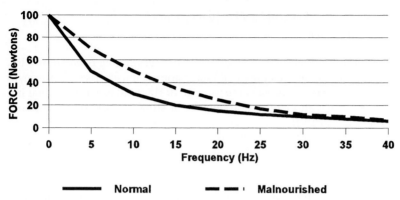

Fig. 2. Relaxation

Mechanism of Changes
in Muscle Function Due to Malnutrition

Why does this happen in the nutritionally deprived patient or animal? In order to answer this question, it is necessary to examine the effects of muscle pH and availability of substrate, as well as Cell energetics.

pH and Substrate Availability

Glycogen deficiency is not a cause of altered skeletal muscle function (SMF) [10]. Fatty acids are abundant in the starved state and are unlikely to be limiting. Furthermore malnutrition alters muscle pH minimally [11].

Muscle Cell Energetics

Studies using ^{31}P-NMR (nuclear magnetic resonance spectrosopy) have given insight into the effect of protein-energy malnutrition on skeletal muscle function. ATP production is under feedback control from ATP consumption. The ADP is a regulator of both glycolysis and mitochondrial oxygen consumption. Mitochondrial oxygen consumption increases with a rise in ADP levels thus increasing the rate of ATP production from ADP. Chance et al. [12] have shown that with increasing work load the phosphorus (Pi) to phosphocreatine (PCr) ratio, which is proportional to FADP rises until Pi/PCr approximates 1.0. Then the relationship between Pi/PCr and muscle work alters so that a marked change in the ratio is associated with but a small increase in work. Experimentally the flattening of the curve of the relation between work and Pi/PCr ratio is associated with fatigue. At this point a further rise in ADP levels will not stimulate mitochondrial oxygen consumption. In order to assess the effects of malnutrition changes in the ATP, PCr and Pi were evaluated.

Muscle Energetics in the Resting State

In this study [11] control rats (CONT) were fed chow ad libitum. The CONT was compared to another group subjected to chronic undernutrition by a week of hypocaloric feeding (HYPO). These HYPO rats were fed 25% of CONT calories until they lost 20% of their initial weight. A group of HYPO rats were refed ad libitum for a week and restudied. In all groups we measured levels of ATP, CrP, Pi and pH, using a combination of NMR and biochemical analysis. In addition, free Mg^{2+}, free ADP and free energy change of ATP hydrolysis were calculated.

The ATP levels in muscle were unchanged by hypocaloric feeding or by refeeding the malnourished animal. On the other hand there was a marked fall in PCr with hypocaloric feeding which was restored by refeeding. The pH fell by 0.04 but the intracellular magnesium were normal. Based on these data the free ADP levels (FADP) levels were significantly increased and the free energy change of ATP hydrolysis was significantly reduced.

Significance of the Observed Changes in Malnourished Resting Muscle

Muscle biopsy data in critically ill septic subjects showed lower phosphagens [13], similar to those seen in HYPO rats described above. The findings are similar to those related to hypocalorically fed rats in the present study. The fall in PCr and rise in free ADP have been noted in fatigue [14]. However, there are major differences. In fatigue there is a significant fall in pH (to below 7.0), and a rise in Pi. In malnutrition the Pi was not significantly different from controls, therefore changes in Pi concentration could not be the cause of the change in the force frequency curve and relaxation rate seen in malnourished muscle. The fall in PCr and rise in free ADP could be due to a change in fiber type because change in fiber type is associated with changes in ATP and Pi levels which was not seen in malnutrition [15]. The changes are more likely to be due to a loss of muscle PCr relative to total Creatine, resulting in a relative loss of energy reserve. Since ADP is rapidly translocated into the mitochondria and phosphorylated to ATP, a rise in the ADP and fall PCr with normal ATP and Pi levels are consistent with deficient oxidative phosphorylation in mitochondria. To confirm this hypothesis the effect of malnutrition on the rate of rephosphorylation of ATP during muscle relaxation after a brief contraction was studied [16].

Effect of Stimulation on Energetics in Malnutrition

The free phosphorus level (Pi) increases after stimulation of muscle due to ATP hydrolysis required to provide energy for contraction. During relaxation the Pi is used by mitochondria to rephosphorylate ADP to ATP by aerobic oxidation. Therefore the fall in Pi levels after stimulation was observed in Control (CONT) and hypocalorically (HYPO) fed animals. The feeding regimens are similar to those described above [11]. The rate of fall in Pi was significantly slower in

HYPO as compared with CONT rats and was restored to the control level by refeeding. The data are consistent with a reduction of oxidative phosphorylation due to mitochondrial dysfunction and not due to a change in fibre type or anoxia for reasons discussed below. Similar changes have been observed in mitochondrial myopathies [17]. Although the reduced PCr could be due to a rise in the proportion of oxidative type I fibers noted to occur in malnutrition, the slow recovery of the PCr/Pi ratio noted herein is not consistent with this possibility. Type I fibers with a high oxidative activity show a very rapid post-exercise recovery of the PCr/Pi ratio. It is not due to anoxia as the muscle pH did not fall. While muscle lactate measured at the end of the experiment was significantly higher in HYPO muscles, the difference could not be due to anoxia as it was similarly raised in the unstimulated limb and was not increased by stimulation. It may be speculated that a mildly raised lactate level unchanged by stimulation (with resultant increase in oxygen consumption) may be due to a change in muscle NAD/NADH ratio. On the other hand there is clear evidence that the rate of ADP rephosphorylation is reduced with malnutrition [16]. The cause of the mitochondrial abnormality remains speculative, however in previous human studies we showed that hypocaloric feeding with 400 kcal/d for 2 weeks resulted in vacuolation of mitochondria observed by electron microscopy in muscle biopsies [6].

Relationship of Changed Muscle Energetics in Malnutrition to Function

Dawson et al. [14] found a linear correlation between the relaxation rate and the Delta G_{ATP}. The Delta G_{ATP} is the free energy transferred for muscle contraction per mole of ATP. They found that Delta G_{ATP} changed as relaxation slowed. We have shown both these changes in skeletal muscle during malnutrition [3][11]. Since muscle relaxation is caused by uptake of calcium into the lateral cisternae of the sarcoplasmic reticulum, the total force available to drive Ca^{2+} into the sarcoplasmic reticulum during relaxation is:

$$-(dG/d\,E)_{total}=-(dG/dE)_{ATP}-n\,(dG/dE)_{Ca} \tag{1}$$

Also the work required to pump a mole of calcium into the sarcoplasmic reticulum is:

$$(dG/dE)_{Ca}=2.58 \ln [\text{free } Ca^{2+}] \text{ in}/[\text{free } Ca^{2+}] \text{ out Kj mol}^{-1} \tag{2}$$

Since the hydrolysis of 1 mol of ATP results in the uptake of 2 mol of Ca^{2+} therefore $n=2$. Substituting Eq. 2 into Eq. 1. When $-(dG/d\,E)_{total}=0$ and calcium distribution is in eqilibrium then:

$$(dG/d)_{ATP}=5.98 \ln [\text{free } Ca^{2+}] \text{ in}/[\text{free } Ca^{2+}] \text{ out}$$

Rearranging the equation:

$$[\text{Free } Ca^{2+}]_{in}/[\text{Free } Ca^{2+}] \text{ out}=e^{(dG/dE)ATP/5.9} \tag{3}$$

In the equation dG/dE is the free energy change in the system. $(dG/dE)_{ATP}$ is the energy given by ATP hydrolysis and $(dG/dE)_{Ca}$ is the energy required for calcium movement into the sarcoplasmic reticulum in order to relax muscle. The $(dG/dE)_{total}$ needs to be in balance to drive calcium back and relax muscle. Hence small changes in dG/dE of ATP (change in the free-energy change of ATP hydrolysis) may have profound effects on the regulation of free cytosolic calcium. There is a rise in muscle calcium in malnourished rats. Abnormal energetics of hypocaloric muscle may increase cytosolic calcium because the steep electrochemical gradient for calcium across the sarcolemma makes the entry of calcium into the cell a passive process and calcium efflux requires energy. The energy for calcium efflux requires ATP hydrolysis by the CaMgATPase system and by Na exchange (the exchanged Na has to be pumped out of the cell by Na-K ATPase). Jackson et al. noted that muscle fatigue was associated with Z band degeneration; which could be avoided by excluding calcium from the medium [18]. These findings in suggest that calcium accumulation may injure hypocaloric muscle and reduce mitochondrial function.

Direct Measurement of the Effect of Malnutrition and Refeeding on Mitochondrial Energetics

Since the ^{31}P-NMR studies showed that muscle function abnormalities in malnutrition are likely to be the result of mitochondrial dysfunction resulting in reduced oxidative phosphorylation, studies were performed to measure the effect of malnutrition on enzyme complexes controlling oxidative phosphorylation. In hypocalorically fed rats there was a significant fall in Complex I, II and III but not complex IV. These changes were specifically reversed by feeding protein [19]. Of greater interest was the finding that the changes in muscle were mirrored in blood mononuclear cells [19]. In humans with malnutrition mitochondrial complex abnormalities were demonstrated [20] and were corrected by refeeding [21]. In Table 1, the standard nutritional assessment is compared to changes in mitochondrial complex activity on D0 (prefeeding) and D7 (1 week refed) and D14 (2 weeks refed) in malnourished patients. It is clear that complex I activity is reduced in malnourished patients and is restored before other parameters.

Summary of Functional Mechanisms

The above data show that malnutrition has profound effects at the membrane level changing the energetics of the sodium pump as well as changes in calcium kinetics affecting muscle function. The central problem appears to be limitation of aerobic and anaerobic energy production. The energetic changes are then responsible for altered function and changes in cell composition. For example the estimation of lean body mass by total body potassium probably reflects alteration in the sodium-potassium pump energetics rather than an actual change in lean tissue per se. Therefore the demonstration of the effects and treatment of malnutrition should be based on functional considerations.

Table 1. Effect of feeding on mononuclear cell mitochondrial complex (from [21])

	Weight	BMI	LBM	kcal/kg	Albumin	Complex I	Citrate S
D0	47.2	17.3	34.4	14.6	26	1.7	19
	(10.5)	(3.6)	(8.1)	(12.3)	(7)	(0.9)	(11.3)
D7	47.3	17.3	33.7	30.4*	26	2.6**	29.2*
	(9.8)	(3.2)	(6.1)	(14.7)	(4)	(1.4)	(13.9)
D14	45.3	16.3	33.6	42.4*	25	2.6**	22.9***
	(10.6)	(3.6)	(6.0)	(11.6)	(2)	(1.1)	(11.6)

*$P<0.01$, **$P<0.03$ and ***$P=0.02$ vs D0 (Wilcoxon test).

Muscle Function in Different Clinical Conditions Relevant to ICU Patients

Effect of Malnutrition on Skeletal Muscle Function

A number of studies have shown that SMF can be altered by nutrient deprivation and restored by refeeding [22–24]. In order to determine the effect of nutrition on muscle function in a model of pure protein-energy malnutrition in the human, anorexia nervosa was studied. In the anorexic patient there was a marked increase of the F10/F100 ratio (ratio of the force at 10 Hz to 100 Hz) and a slowing of muscle relaxation [3] Feeding reversed these changes over a period of 8 weeks [3] before restoration of body nitrogen or weight. These findings have been confirmed in normal subjects starved for 48 h [25]. However, because the muscle function abnormality did not correlate with body composition, and acutely starved subjects returned to normal soon after feeding, the authors concluded that muscle function did not diagnose "malnutrition" but was an index of "muscle energetics". As explained above, the their data actually shows that muscle function is a sensitive index of food deprivation and occurs before any change in body composition and is restored by feeding. Similarly, recently in dialysis patients [26] Fahal et al. found that "The only significant predictor of loss of muscle strength and abnormality of relaxation in this study was the nutritional state". In patients with chronic obstructive lung disease (COPD), the force-frequency and relaxation (as described above) of the sternomastoid muscle was abnormal and was restored by refeeding [27]. These effects are nutritional and not influenced by trauma [28], sepsis and steroid administration [29]. In critically ill malnourished patients measurement of the force of contraction at 50 Hz (F50) increased by a mean of 50% in 11 patients within 3 weeks of nutrition support using TPN [29] at a time when there was no change in arm muscle circumference, triceps skin fold and serum albumin. Christie and Hill [30] also showed that nutritional support improves muscle, including diaphragmatic function before any increase in body protein or body mass. Finally Windsor and Hill [31] demonstrated that the functional effects of nutrition are more important than subnormal body protein as an index of surgical risk.

Effect of Malnutrition on Respiratory Muscle Function

Malnutrition has been shown to have significant effects on the diaphragm [32, 33] and it has been shown that the functional effects of malnutrition on the diaphragm are disproportionately greater than the wasting of this muscle [34]. In a patient with anorexia with 50% weight loss there was severe dysfunction of respiratory muscle function which was restored by refeeding [35]. In malnourished COPD patients respiratory muscle strength was reduced and was corrected by refeeding [27].

Effect of the Deprivation
of Specific Nutrients on Muscle Function

The effect of low plasma levels of potassium, magnesium and phosphorus are well known and can be corrected by normalizing plasma levels. On the other hand specific nutrient effects have been shown on muscle function. In elderly human volunteers Castaneda et al. [36] found that reduced protein intake without a reduction in total energy intake (specific protein deficiency) significantly reduced muscle function as defined above as well as the grip strength. Zince deficiency does not alter force but does reduce work capacity [37].

Conclusions and Future Developments

In the ICU anthropometric measurements, immune function and plasma proteins are not an index of malnutrition. Despite its disadvantages the data given above show that it is specific for malnutrition and not altered by trauma or sepsis. It is indicative of critical diaphragmatic function and responds early to feeding. It is specifically influenced by protein refeeding. These features make it appropriate for ICU patients. Since the mechanism of abnormal muscle function is abnormal mitochondrial function, direct assessment of mitochondrial function as indicated above in lymphocytes [21] may be the way of the future.

References

1. Keys A, Brozek J, Henschel A, Mickelsen O, Taylor HL (1950) The Biology of Human Starvation. Vol I and II. Minneapolis, University of Minnesota Press.
2. Moore FD, Olesen KH, McMurrey JD, Parker HV, Ball MR, Boyden CM (1963) The body cell mass and its supporting environment. Philadelphia: WB Saunders
3. Russell DMcR, Prendergast PJ, Darby PL, Garfinkel PE, Whitwell J, Jeejeebhoy KN (1983) A comparison between muscle function and body composition in anorexia nervosa: the effect of refeeding. Am J Clin Nutr 38: 229–237
4. Almond DJ, King RFGJ, Burkinshaw L (1987) Potassium depletion in surgical patients: Intracellular cation deficiency is independent of loss of body protein. Clin Nutr. 6:45–50
5. Pichard C, E Hoshino, JP Allard, MP Charlton, HL Atwood, KN Jeejeebhoy (1991) Intracellular potassium and membrane potential in rat muscles during malnutrition and subsequent refeeding. Am J Clin Nutr 54:489–498

6. Russell, DMcR, PM Walker, LA Leiter, et al. (1984) Metabolic and structural changes in skeletal muscle during hypocaloric dieting. Am J Clin Nutr 39: 503–513
7. Edwards RHT. (1978) Physiological analysis of skeletal muscle weakness and fatigue. Clin. Sci. Mol. Med. 54:463–470
8. Lymn RW, Taylor EW (1971) Mechanism of adenosine triphosphate hydrolysis by actomyosin. Biochemistry 10:4617–4624, 1971
9. Klidjian AM, Foster KJ, Kammerling RM, Cooper A, Karran SJ (1980). Relation of anthropometric and dynamometric variables to serious post-operative complications. Br. Med. J. 2:899–901.
10. Russell, DMcR, HL Atwood, JS Whittaker, et al. (1984) The effect of fasting and hypocaloric diets on the functional and metabolic characteristics of rat gastrocnemius muscle. Clin Sci 67:185–194
11. Pichard C, C Vaughan, R Struk, RL Armstrong, KN Jeejeebhoy (1988) The effect of dietary manipulations (fasting, hypocaloric feeding and subsequent refeeding) on rat muscle energetics as assessed by nuclear magnetic resonance spectroscopy. J Clin Invest 82: 895–901
12. Chance B, Eleff S, Leigh JS (1981) Mitochondrial regulation of phosphocreatine, phosphate ratios in exercised human muscle: a gated ^{31}P NMR study. Proc Natl Acad Sci USA 78:6714–6718
13. Liaw KY, Askanazi, J, Michelson, CB, et al. (1980) Effect of injury and sepsis on high-energy phosphate in muscle and red cells. J. Trauma 20: 755–759
14. Dawson MJ, Gadian DG, Wilkie DR (1980) Mechanical relaxation rate and metabolism studied in fatiguing muscle by phosphorus nuclear magnetic resonance. J Physiol (Lond) 299:465–484, 1980
15. Meyer RA, Brown TR, Kushmerick, MJ (1985) Phosphorus nuclear magnetic resonance of fast- and slow-twitch muscle. Am. J. Physiol. 248: (Cell Physiol. 17):C279-C287
16. Mijan de la Torre A, Madapallimattam A, Cross A, Armstrong RL, Jeejeebhoy KN. (1993) Effect of fasting, hypocaloric feeding, and refeeding on the energetics of stimulated rat muscle as assessed by nuclear magnetic resonance spectroscopy. J Clin Invest 92: 114–121
17. Argov Z, Maris J, Damico L, et al. (1987) Bioenergetic heterogeneity of human mitochondrial myopathies as demonstrated by in vivo phosphorus magnetic resonance spectroscopy. Neurology 37:257–262
18. Jackson MJ, Jones DA and Edwards RHT (1984) Experimental skeletal muscle damage: nature of calcium-activated degenerative process. Eur J Clin Invest 14:369–374
19. Briet F and Jeejeebhoy KN. (1999) Effect of Hypocaloric feeding and refeeding on muscle and mononuclear cell mitochondria in enterally fed rat. Gastroenterology. 116:A541
20. Briet F. Twomey C and Jeejeebhoy KN. (1999) Refeeding increases mitochondrial complex activity in malnourished patients. Evidence for a sensitive nutritional marker. Gastroenterology 116:A541
21. Twomey C and Jeejeebhoy KN. (1999) Impaired lymphocyte mitochondrial complex activity in malnourished patients with significant weight loss. Gastroenterology 116:A582
22. Lopes J, DMcR Russell, J Whitwell, KN Jeejeebhoy (1982) Skeletal muscle function in malnutrition. Am J Clin Nutr 36:602–610
23. Russell, DMcR, LA Leiter, J Whitwell, EB Marliss, KN Jeejeebhoy (1983) Skeletal muscle function during hypocaloric diets and fasting: a comparison with standard nutritional assessment parameters. Am J Clin Nutr 37: 133–138
24. Berkelhammer CH, LA Leiter, KN Jeejeebhoy, et al. (1985) Skeletal muscle function in chronic renal failure: an index of nutritional status. Am J Clin Nutr 42: 845–854
25. Shizgal HM, Vasilevsky CA, Gardiner PF, Wang WZ, Tuitt DA, Brabant GV. (1986) Nutritional assessment and skeletal muscle function. Am J Clin Nutr 44:761–71
26. Fahal IH, Bell GM, Bone JM, Edwards RH. Physiological abnormalities of skeletal muscle in dialysis patients. (1997) Nephrol Dial Transplant 12:119–27
27. Efthimiou J Fleming J, Gomes C, Spiro SG. (1988)The effect of supplementary oral nutrition in poorly nourished patients with chronic obstructive pulmonary disease. Am Rev Respir Dis 137:1075–82

28. Assessment of involuntary muscle function in patients after critical injury or severe sepsis. Finn PJ; Plank LD; Clark MA; Connolly AB; Hill GL. JPEN J Parenter Enteral Nutr 1996 Sep-Oct;20 (5):332–7
29. Brough W, Horne G, Blount A, Irving MH, Jeejeebhoy KN. (1986) Effects of nutrient intake, surgery, sepsis, and long term administration of steroids on muscle function. Br Med J 293: 983–988
30. Christie PM, Hill GL (1990) Effect of intravenous nutrition on nutrition and function in acute attacks of inflammatory bowel disease. Gastroenterology 99:730–736
31. Windsor JA, Hill GL (1988) Weight loss with physiologic impairment: A basic indicator of surgical risk. Ann Surg 207:290–296
32. Fraser, IM, DMcR Russell, S Whittaker, et al. (1984) Skeletal and diaphragmatic muscle function in malnourished chronic obstructive lung disease. Am Rev Respir Dis 129: A269
33. Dureuil B, Viires N, Veber B, Pavlovic D, et al. (1989) Acute diaphragmatic changes induced by starvation in rats. Am J Clin Nutr 49:738–44
34. Dureuil B; Matuszczak Y. (1998) Alteration in nutritional status and diaphragm muscle function. Reprod Nutr Dev 38:175–80
35. Ryan CF; Whittaker JS; Road JD. (1992) Ventilatory dysfunction in severe anorexia nervosa. Chest 102:1286–8
36. Elderly women accommodate to a low-protein diet with losses of body cell mass, muscle function, and immune response. Castaneda C; Charnley JM; Evans WJ; Crim M. Am J Clin Nutr 1995 Jul;62 (1):30–9
37. The effects of zinc depletion on peak force and total work of knee and shoulder extensor and flexor muscles. Van Loan MD; Sutherland B; Lowe NM; Turnlund JR King JC. Int J Sport Nutr 1999 Jun;9 (2):125–35

Perioperative Nutrition

N. Cano

Introduction: Goals of Perioperative Nutrition

Malnutrition in surgical patients is associated with delayed wound healing and increased risk of morbidity and mortality. The main goal of perioperative nutrition is to reduce the incidence of postoperative complications, the length of postoperative hospitalization and operative mortality. Additional goals are to decrease the effects of disease and surgery-related malnutrition on body composition, organ functions and subsequent patient performance.

Since the beginning of artificial nutrition, surgery has been the main indication of this therapy despite the lack of data demonstrating its beneficial effects. A 1987-meta-analysis of 11 randomized or quasi-randomized available trials concluded that the routine use of perioperative parenteral nutrition (PN) in unselected surgical patients was not justified but may be helpful in high-risk subgroups of these patients [1]. The routine use of PN in surgical patients was further questioned after the Veterans affairs study, which demonstrated, in a 395-patient randomized series, that the rates of major complications during the first 30 days after surgery were similar in PN and control patients, as were the overall 90-day mortality rates [2]. Since this study, several recommendations from scientific societies have addressed the use of nutritional support in surgical patients [3–7]. Because of the prognostic impact of protein stores and immune function, recent studies were devoted to new nutritional substrates and to hormone therapies which may be of interest according to their protein-sparing or immune effects. This brief review considers nutritional and metabolic features in pre and postoperative phases as well as the nutritional support modalities and indications.

Preoperative Nutritional Status

Prevalence of Malnutrition and Relationships with Postoperative Outcome

Approximately 40% of candidates to general and vascular surgery present with malnutrition. The influence of malnutrition on postoperative outcome has been reported in major but not minor surgery and may be more pronounced in elderly [3]. The association of malnutrition with postoperative morbidity and mortality was demonstrated in general surgery [2], digestive surgery [8], non-cancer patients [9] and cancer patients [10]. Moreover, the severity of postoperative complications was reported to be related to the degree of preoperative malnutrition [2]. It must be underlined that malnutrition most often reflects the severity of the underlying disease and the occurrence of underlying-disease complications. Hence, in selected populations such as patients with gastrointestinal cancer, multivariate analysis failed to demonstrate an independent effect of malnutrition on postoperative outcome [10]. This can explain the limits of the nutritional support impact on postoperative evolution.

Nutritional Assessment

In surgical patients, predictive value of postoperative complications is a criteria of first importance for selecting nutritional parameters, and subsequently for indicating nutritional support. Among anthropometric parameters, loss of body weight appeared as the most useful for predicting postoperative complications. A weight loss ≥20% clearly indicates poor postoperative outcome. The rapidity of weight loss constitution is correlated with its predictive value: a weight loss ≥10% within a 6-month period or a weight loss ≥5 kg during the 3 preoperative months are considered as indicators of higher incidence of major postoperative complications [3]. It was further demonstrated that patients with weight loss ≥10% and physiologic impairment such as hypoalbuminemia, abnormal skeletal muscle or respiratory muscle function, were at increased risk of postoperative complications (primarily septic) and longer hospital stay [11]. Indicators of protein malnutrition appeared as the best predictors of complications both in medical and surgical patients. A prospective study of 218 digestive-surgery patients showed that, among 15 tested variables, serum albumin <35 g/l, transferrin <1.74 g/l and prealbumin <0.12 g/l had the highest predictive values of postoperative complications. In this study, prealbumin was the most performant prognostic indicator (positive predictive value 43%, negative predictive value 87%) [12]. The predictive value of hypoalbuminemia was confirmed in larger series [13], the cut-off for increased risk varying from 30 g/l to 35 g/l. Promising studies showed the ability of hand-grip dynamometry for screening patients at risk [14]. Bioelectrical impedance analysis (BIA), was demonstrated to be useful for predicting postoperative complications in selected patients [15]. The subjective global assessment (SGA) [16], including anamnesis and clinical examination data, make it possible to classify patients into 4 categories: normal nutritional status, mild, moderate and severe malnutrition. When used by trained nutritionists, this index was shown to be useful for predicting postoperative complications and for indicating nutritional support [2].

During routine preoperative assessment, weight loss and plasma proteins appear as simple and useful indices for identifying severely malnourished patients [3]. The Nutrition Risk Index [NRI; (1519 ×serum albumin g/l)+41.7 (current weight/usual weight)] [2] takes into account body mass variations and serum albumin. NRI <83.5 was demonstrated to be a pertinent indice for selecting severely malnourished patients in whom nutritional support is required [2]. These patients can also be identified by a weight loss >20% with a serum albumin <33 g/l or a weight loss >10% with a serum albumin <28 g/l [17].

Nutrient Metabolism in Surgical Patients

Nutrient metabolism during surgery depends on preoperative patient condition and surgery-induced metabolic changes.

Preoperative Metabolic Status

Malnutrition, Perioperative Starvation

Fuel stores in healthy adults are given in Table 1. Total or partial starvation has been defined by daily intakes ≤60% of theoretical requirements [3]. In normal subjects, endocrine and metabolic adaptation makes it possible to tolerate prolonged starvation without compromising survival [18]. After 2–3 days of starvation, glucose needs are mainly satisfied by gluconeogenesis from amino acids released by protein degradation (approximately 75 g of protein/day, i.e. 300 g of muscle). Then, the increase in fat utilization and ketogenesis is associated with a decrease in gluconeogenesis, and proteolysis falls at 20–30 g/day. Surgical stress markedly impairs these adaptative mechanisms and increases protein losses. Thus, tolerance to starvation depends on preoperative nutritional status, length of perioperative starvation, and intensity of agression. Preoperative feeding can be altered by underlying disease, hospitalization, and preoperative investigations. Postoperative starvation is usually longer in digestive than in non-digestive surgery. In non-malnourished patients, during elective and non-complicated surgery, a starvation of 7–14 days is usually believed not to compromise the outcome [3–5, 19].

Cancer

Abnormal nutrient metabolism induces decreased efficacy of nutritional support in cancer patients [10]. Energy expenditure is often elevated according to tumor types. Moreover, while normal subjects adapt to starvation by decreasing their energy expenditure, this adaptative response is lacking in cancer patients. Carbohydrate metabolism is characterized by increased glucose turnover, increased gluconeogenesis, and insulin resistance for glucose. Depletion of fat stores is usual and associated with hypertriglyceridemia and inconstantly with increased glycerol and fatty acid turnover. Protein turnover and muscle protein breakdown increase while nitrogen balance decrease. These metabolic disturbancies appear to be due to systemic inflammatory response to cancer, mediated by macrophage activation and cytokine production, as in other inflammatory states (see below). As glutamine is avidly consumed by rapidly dividing cells, special attention was devoted to glutamine metabolism in tumor bearing animals and in cancer patients [10]. In animals but not in humans, tumors can behave as 'glutamine trap'. In humans, the main finding is that muscle protein depletion is associated with a reduction of muscle and arterial glutamine concentrations and decreased ability of muscle to produce glutamine. The subsequent decrease in glutamine availability may alter glutamine-consuming cell function, particularly in immune system and gut.

Liver Failure

In liver transplant candidates, hypermetabolism and body cell mass/body mass ratio less than 35% were shown to independently predict postoperative mortality [15]. Hypermetabolism is found in one third of stable cirrhotic patients [20]. Energy metabolism is further characterized by peripheral resistance to insulin concerning non-oxydative glucose metabolism, accelerated metabolism of starvation, decreased liver and muscle glycogen storage and increased gluconeogenesis [7, 21]. Endogenous and exogenous lipid are normally oxidized during liver failure. Increased protein turnover and decreased albumin synthesis were demonstrated during cirrhosis [7].

Nutritional and Metabolic Effects of Surgery

Similarly to various stimuli such as trauma or infection, major surgery induce a systemic inflammatory response of varying intensity. Mobilization of fuel stores and gluconeogenesis are stimulated by the release of catecholamines, cortisol, glucagon and growth hormone as well as by insulin-resistance. Interleukin-1 and tumor necrosis factor are responsible for an increase in muscle protein catabolism and a decrease in protein synthesis, and interleukin-6 for acute-phase protein synthesis in the liver [22]. Endocrine changes in stress conditions were recently reviewed [23]. They are characterized by a down regulation of hypothalamo-pituitary-thyroid axis and low plasma T3 concentrations. Both the liver and damaged territories adapt to stressful signals. Cytokines suppress the synthesis of prealbumin causing the drop of retinol-binding protein. The subsequent release of increased amounts of thyroxine and retinol in free form strengthens the effects of cytokines. Moreover, thyroxine-binding globulin, corticosteroid-binding globulin, and IGF-binding-protein-3 degradation allows the occurrence of peak

Table 1. Fuel stores in healthy female (60 kg body weight) and male (70 kg body weight; from [18, 57, 58])

Fuel stores	Female			Male		
	kg	% body weight	kcal	kg	% body weight	kcal
Fat	19	31.7	176,700	16	22.8	148,800
Protein	8.6	14.3	36,120	10.1	14.4	42,400
Glycogen	0.4	0.1	1600	0.5	0.1	2000

endocrine and mitogenic influences at the site of inflammation [23]. This adaptative situation is associated with hyperthermia, weight loss and hypoalbuminemia. Increased protein catabolism and hypermetabolism vary with the intensity of stress and are responsible for a decreased response to nutritional support. The prolongation of such a metabolic state results in severe protein depletion. EN but not PN was reported to attenuate both endocrine and metabolic responses to stress [18]. Regional anesthesia, particularly epidural, may also decrease the extent of the metabolic response to surgery [18].

Nutritional Support

Expected Effects of Conventional Nutritional Support

Recent meta-analyses and reviews evaluated prospective randomized controlled trials (PRCT) of perioperative PN and enteral nutrition (EN) [4, 5, 24–26]. In the largest PRCT of preoperative PN [2], patients were randomized to receive 7–15 days or no preoperative nutrition and were followed for 3 months after surgery. Overall mortality was similar in the two groups and infectious complications were more frequent in PN group (14.1% vs 6.4%, $P<0.01$). Study of patients subgroups showed that PN was only beneficial in severely malnourished patients and reduced non-infectious complications (5% vs 43%, $P<0.05$). Meta-analysis of 13 trials confirmed theses data, showing that a 10% reduction of complications can be expected from preoperative PN in malnourished patients [5]. Meta-analysis of 9 trials concluded that routine postoperative PN in malnourished patients not receiving preoperative nutrition results in a 10% increase of complication rate, without change in mortality. Perioperative EN is less documented than PN. Only two PRCTs studied preoperative EN as compared with standard oral diet. Complication rates tended to be lower in EN patients, the difference between groups being significant in one study [5]. Data supporting the use of postoperative EN are more substantial. Meta-analysis of four PRCTs of early jejunal tube feeding, in patients with gastrointestinal cancers, did not show obvious change in postoperative morbidity and mortality [5]. Since then, PRCTs in patients operated for intestinal resection [27] or intestinal perforation and peritonitis [28] showed that early postoperative EN significantly reduced complication rates. Moreover, EN at the opposite of standard intravenous fluid, avoided the occurrence of increased intestinal permeability [27]. In depleted elderly women after repair of femoral neck, both supplementary nasogastric EN [29] and oral supplements [30] were shown to accelerate independent motility, and to shorten in-hospital stay.

Pharmaconutrition, Anabolic Agents

Protein sparing is critical to body structure and function and thereby to surgical patient outcome [31]. Because of the limited impact of conventional nutritional support in improving protein sparing, new nutritive agents aimed to preserve lean body mass and immune function were developed, leading to the concept of pharmaconutrition. In stress and cancer patients, because of the depletion of muscle protein stores, glutamine is considered as a conditionally essential amino acid [10]. Trials on glutamine-enriched PN during bone marrow transplantation led to inconstant benefits [32, 33]. In critically ill patients, a PRCT of glutamine-containing PN showed an improvement of survival at 6 months [34]. During abdominal surgery, glutamine-enriched PN was shown to improve nitrogen balance and muscle glutamine content [31]. Two PRCTs in major abdominal surgery [35, 36], showed that glutamine-enriched PN shortened hospital stays and improve immune status and nitrogen balance. These studies demonstrate that glutamine-enriched PN enables to improve outcome in surgical and critically ill patients and may be cost-saving [34]. 'Immunonutrition' was recently developed in cancer patients, using the immunomodulating properties of omega-3 fatty acids, immunostimulating effect of arginine and its metabolite, NO, and nucleotides. During major surgery for upper gastrointestinal malignancies, a PRCT showed that fish oil-enriched EN as compared with standard EN induced a 50% decline in gastrointestinal complications and infections [37]. In digestive cancer patients, a PRCT of perioperative EN supplemented with arginine, omega-3 fatty acids and nucleotides (Impact®) showed an increase in phagocytosis ability, intestinal microperfusion, intestinal mucosa oxygen metabolism and postoperative levels of nitric oxide, and a decrease in plasma concentrations of C-reactive protein [38]. A PRCT of Impact® vs standard EN, given 7 days before and 7 days after surgery, was conducted in 206 digestive cancer patients and showed significant reduction of postoperative infections and length of hospitalisation with immunonutrition [39]. Similarly, in patients with head and neck cancers, perioperative Impact® but not standard formula, significantly reduced infection rate [40]. Comparison of 14-day perioperative and 7-day postoperative administrations of Impact® in gastric cancer patients showed that perioperative but not postoperative administration of Impact ameliorated host defense mechanisms and inflammatory response, and improved plasma prealbumin [41]. Similar poor effects of postoperative immunonutrition were reported in two other PRCTs [42, 43]. At the opposite, in another PRCT in gastrointestinal cancer patients, early postoperative Impact significantly reduced the frequency of late infectious and wound complications together with treatment costs [44].

Anabolic agents such as testosterone and anabolic steroid have been proposed many years ago in order to improve the nitrogen sparing effect of nutritional support [31]. It was reported that recombinant growth hormone (rGH) associated with low protein and calorie intake can maintain nitrogen balance, and that IGF1 can improve both protein anabolism and immune functions [31]. Recent PRCTs of rGH during surgery for ulcerative colitis [45, 46] or cancer [47] showed improvements in lean body mass conservation, protein kinetics and muscle function. However, to our knowledge, no PRCT demonstrated benefit of GH or IGF1 administration in terms or reduction of postoperative complications, length of hospitalization or mortality.

Routes for Nutritional Support

Main indications concerning the routes for nutrition are given in Table 2. Few comparative studies of preoperative EN and PN have been performed [5]. Some authors estimate that more data on preoperative EN are required before recommending its routine use [5, 25]. There is however an increasing agreement for a preferential use of EN [3, 4, 6, 17, 19]. EN, using polymeric nutritive mixtures, is usually given through nasogastric tube or, when long-term refeeding is expected, through perendoscopic gastrostomy [3]. The association of EN and PN is often necessary to achieve nutritional goals in the early postoperative period. Due to the 10% complication rate of PN [5], the preferential use of EN, when patient tolerate it, is admitted. After upper gastrointestinal tract surgery, jejunostomy enables an earlier refeeding than nasogastric tube. Recent PRCTs compared standard EN and PN after major hepatic, gastric or pancreatic surgery [48–50]: no significant difference in nutritional parameters or complication rates was found. In one study [50], side effects of early EN were recorded in 22.7% of the patients: abdominal distension 9%, abdominal cramps 6%, diarrhea 6%, emesis 2%, displacement of jejunustomy 1%. Only 6.3% did not reach the nutritional goal. EN was cheaper than PN. In patients without documented malnutrition, prophylactic jejunostomy was associated with high rates of catheter-related, infectious and respiratory complications, and its benefit/risk ratio is still questioned [31]. The frequency of severe complications of postoperative EN have been estimated at 2% [51]. In a PRCT of cyclic vs continuous EN after pancreatoduodenectomy [52], cyclic EN induced shorter period of EN, faster return to normal diet and shorter hospital stay. Continuously high CCK levels could explain prolonged time until normal diet is tolerated during continuous EN. Few but encouraging results have been achieved with oral supplementation following gastrointestinal surgery [53].

Nutritional Supply in Surgical Patients

General Principles

Table 2 gives general principles for nutritional supply in the perioperative period according to consensus data [3, 4]. It is generally admitted that preoperative nutrition should be given for 7–10 days. Longer preoperative nutrition support would increase risk of nosocomial infection [24, 25]. Postoperative nutritional support length should not be less than 7 days [17].

Systemic Inflammatory Response

In order to avoid overfeeding, consensual recommendations are to ensure energy support equivalent to energy expenditure [6, 54]. Usual needs vary from 20 kcal/kg/day in non-malnourished patients to 35 kcal/kg/day in malnourished or severely stressed patients. Fat should not exceed 30% of non-protien energy supply. Standard fat emulsions are usually given. Medium chain triglycerides are well tolerated and may be useful in selected circumstances. According to

Table 2. General guidelines for perioperative nutritional support. EN is enteral nutrition and PN, parenteral nutrition

Energy supply [3]	25–35 kcal/kg body weight/day Carbohydrates: 50%–70% Fat: 30%–50%, long chain triglycerides
Nitrogen supply [3, 4]	Preoperative nutrition: 0.15–0.25 g nitrogen/kg body weight/day Postoperative nutrition: 0.25–0.3 g nitrogen/kg body weight/day
Electrolytes and micronutrients [3]	Increased requirement for phosphorus and magnesium Vitamins: A, B1, B6, C, E and folate Trace elements: zinc, selenium
Route for nutrition [3]	EN should be used in patients who are able to tolerate it. According to the type of surgical procedure, EN can be given through: (a) Nasogastric tube, particularly in preoperative feeding and after non-digestive surgery (b) Surgical jejunostomy, after upper gastrointestinal tract surgery (c) Gastrostomy, most often perendoscopic in long term feeding PN should be used when EN is not tolerated or unsufficient to ensure nutritional needs. Central venous access is most often used, particularly when the nutritive mixture exceeds 800 mosm/l

the severity of the stress nitrogen support should vary from 0.25 g/kg/day to 0.35 g/kg/day. No benefit was demonstrated for nutritional supplies higher than 0.35 g/kg/day. In severely ill patients glutamine-enriched PN can be proposed.

Cancer

Because most of data concerning perioperative nutrition were obtained in cancer patients, general guidelines have to be applied in these patients. More specifically, promising data recently emerged concerning glutamine-enriched PN and perioperative EN supplemented with arginine, omega-3 fatty acids and nucleotides: both regimens have been proven to reduce postoperative complications and the length of in-hospital stay.

Liver Failure

Nutritional support has been shown to be of interest both during liver resections, by reducing septic complications and maintaining liver function [55] and during transplantation, by improving nitrogen balance and reducing length of artificial ventilation [56]. Recommended energy supply in transplant patients is 1.3×calculated energy expenditure with fat constituting 35%–50% of non-protein calories. Usual nitrogen supply varies from 0.2–0.25 g nitrogen/kg body weight/day. No advantage of branched-chain amino acid-enriched solutions was demonstrated. Parenteral nutrition should only by used when enteral feeding is not possible [7].

Indications of Nutritional Support

Figure 1 gives the French Consensus Group recommendations [3]. Preoperative nutrition was only recommended in severely malnourished patients undergoing major surgical procedures. Postoperative nutritional support was recommended in severely malnourished patients, patients with expected postoperative starvation superior to 7 days, and patients with complications responsible for stress or prolonged starvation. When indicated, postoperative nutrition must be initiated within the 48 postoperative hours [17]. These recommendations were consistent with recommendations from other groups [4, 5].

Conclusions

Present data underline the limits of perioperative nutritional support. Using conventional PN, only preoperative nutrition in severely malnourished patient candidate to major surgical procedure was demonstrated to be of clinical benefit. During the postoperative phase, only EN was shown be beneficial in selected conditions. Nutritional support is usually recommended in patients with highly catabolic state or prolonged starvation, despite no clear benefit was demonstrated. New substrates such as glutamine and 'immunonutrients', aimed to enhance protein sparing and immune function, were demonstrated to be beneficial in selected conditions. A clear and consensual definition of patients elligible for such treatment, taking into account their cost/benefit ratio, is required before their routine use is recommended.

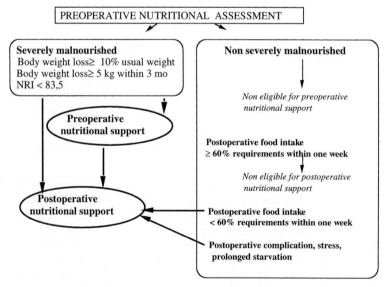

Fig. 1. French Consensus Group [3] recommendations for indicating perioperative nutritional support

References

1. Detsky AS, Baker JP, ORourke K, Goel V (1987) Perioperative parenteral nutrition: a meta-analysis. Ann Intern Med 107:195–203
2. Veterans Affairs Total Parenteral Nutrition Cooperative Study Group (1991) Perioperative total parenteral nutrition in surgical patients. N Engl J Med 324:525–532
3. Conférence de consensus: Nutrition artificielle periopératoire en chirurgie programmée de l'adulte: recommandations du Jury (1995) Nutr Clin Métabol 9 (suppl 1):13–22
4. Consensus statement Italian Society of Parenteral and Enteral nutrition: Perioperative nutrition: the rationale fot nutritional support (1996) Clin Nutr 15:155–156
5. Klein S, Kinney J, JeeJeebhoy K et al. (1997) Nutritional support in clinical practice: review of published data and recommendations for future research directions. JPEN 21:133–156
6. Cerra FB, Benitez MR, Blackburn GL et al. (1997) Applied nutrition in ICU patients. A consensus statement of the American College of Chest Physicians. Chest 111:769–778
7. Plauth M, Merli M, Kondrup J et al. (1997) ESPEN guidelines for nutrition in liver disease and transplantation. Clin Nutr 16:43–55
8. Detsky AS (1987) Predicting nutrition-associated complications for patients undergoing gastrointestinal surgery. N Engl J Med 11:440–446
9. Warnold I, Lundholm K (1984) Clinical significance of preoperative nutritional status in 215 noncancer patients. Ann Surg 199 (3):299–305
10. De Blaauw I, Deutz NEP, Von Meyenfeldt MF (1997) Metabolic changes in cancer cachexia – first of two parts. Clin Nutr 16:169–176
11. Windsor JA, Hill GL (1988) Weight loss with physiologic impairment: a basic indicator of surgical risk. Ann Surg 207:290–296
12. Pettigrew RA, Hill GL (1986) Indicators of surgical risk and clinical judgement. Br J Med 73:47–51
13. McClave SA (1992) Differenciating subtypes (hypoalbuminemic vs marastic) of protein-calorie malnutrition: incidence and clinical significance in a university hospital setting. JPEN 16:337–342
14. Klidjian AM (1982) Detection of dangerous malnutrition. JPEN 6:119–121
15. Selberg O, Böttcher J, Tusch G, Pichlmayr R, Henkel E, Müller MJ (1997) Identification of high- and low-risk patients before liver transplantation: a prospective cohort study of nutritional and metabolic parameters in 150 patients. Hepatology 25:652–657
16. Detsky AS, Baker JP, Mendelson RA, Wolman SL, Wesson DE, Jeejeebhoy KN (1984) Evaluating the accuracy of nutritional assessment techniques applied to hospitalized patients: methodology and comparisons. JPEN 8:153–159
17. Boulétreau P, Chambrier C (1998) La nutrition artificielle periopératoire en chirurgie programmée de l'adulte. In: Leverve X, Cosnes J, Erny P, Hasselmann M (eds) Traité de Nutrition Artificielle de l'Adulte, troisième partie: Pathologie, Editions Mariette Guéna, Paris, pp 693–704
18. Chioléro R (1995) Conséquences de l'acte chirurgical sur l'état nutritionnel. Nutr Clin Métabol 9 (suppl 1):45–52
19. McClave SA, Snider HL, Spain DA (1999) Preoperative issues in clinical nutrition. Chest 115:64S-70 S
20. Müller MJ, Böttcher J, Selberg O et al. (1999) Hypermetabolism in clinically stable patients with liver cirrhosis. Am J Clin Nutr 69:1194–1201
21. Cano N, Leverve XM (1997) Influence of chronic liver disease and chronic renal failure on nutrient metabolism and undernutrition. Nutrition 13:381–383
22. Gabay C, Kuschner I (1999) Acute-phase proteins and other systemis responses to inflammation. N Engl J Med 340:448–454
23. Ingenbleek Y, Bernstein L (1999) The stressful condition as a nutritionally dependent adaptative dichotomy. Nutrition 15:305–320
24. Heyland DK, MacDonald S, Keefe L, Drover JW (1998) Total parenteral nutrition in the critically ill patient: a meta-analysis. JAMA 280:2013–2019

25. Torosian MH (1999) Perioperative nutrition support for patients undergoing gastrointestinal surgery: critical analysis and recommendations. World J Surg 23:565–569
26. Waitzberg DL, Plopper C, Terra RM (1999) Postoperative total parenteral nutrition. World J Surg 23:560–564
27. Carr CS, Ling KD, Boulos P, Singer M (1996) Randomised trial of safety and efficacy of immediate postoperative enteral feeding in patients undergoing gastrointestinal resection. BMJ 312:869–871
28. Singh G, Ram RP, Khanna SK (1998) Early postoperative enteral feeding in patients with nontraumatic intestinal perforation and peritonitis. J Am Coll Surg 187:142–146
29. Bastow MD, Rawlings J, Allison S (1983) Benefits of supplementary tube feeding after fractured neck of the femur. Br Med J 187:1589–1592
30. Delmi M, Rapin CH, Bengoa JM, Delmas PD, Vasey H, Bonjour JP (1990) Dietary supplementation in elderly patients with fractured neck of the femur. Lancet 335:1013–1016
31. Wilmore DW (1999) Postoperative protein sparing. World J Surg 23:545–552
32. Ziegler TR, Young LS, Benfell Kea (1992) Clinical and metabolic efficacy of glutamine-supplemented parenteral nutrition after bone marrow transplantation. Ann Intern Med 116:821–828
33. Schloerb PR, Skikne BS (1999) Oral and parenteral glutamine in bone marrow transplantation: a randomized, double-blind study. JPEN 23:117–122
34. Griffiths RD, Jones C, Palmer TEA (1997) Six-month outcome of critically ill patientsgiven glutamine supplemented parenteral nutrition. Nutrition 13:295–302
35. Morlion BJ, Stehle P, Wachter Pea (1998) TPN with glutamine dipeptide after major abdominal surgery. Ann Surg 227:302–308
36. Powell Tuck J (1999) Total parenteral nutrition with glutamine dipeptide shortened hospital stays and improved immune status and nitrogen economy after major abdominal surgery. Gut 44:155
37. Kenler AS, Swails WS, Driscoll D et al. (1996) Early enteral feeding in postsurgical cancer patients. Fish oil structured lipid-based polymeric formula versus a standard polymeric formula. Ann Surg 223:316–33
38. Braga M, Gianotti L, Cestari A, Vignali A, Pellegatta F, Dolci A, Di Carlo V (1996) Gut function and immune and inflammatory responses in patients perioperatively fed with supplemented enteral formulas. Arch Surg 131:1257–1265
39. Braga M, Gianotti L, Radaelli G et al. (1999) Perioperative immunonutrition in patients undergoing cancer surgery: results of a randomized double-blind phase 3 trial. Arch Surg 134:428–433
40. Snyderman CH, Kachman K, Molseed L et al. (1999) Reduced postoperative infections with an immune-enhancing nutritional supplement. Laryngoscope 109:915–921
41. Braga M, Gianotti L, Vignali A, Di Carlo V (1998) Immunonutrition in gastric cancer surgical patients. Nutrition 14:831–835
42. Heslin MJ, Latkany L, Leung D et al. (1997) A prospective, randomized trial of early enteral feeding after resection of upper gastrointestinal malignancy. Ann Surg 226:567–580
43. McCarter MD, Gentilini OD, Gomez ME, Daly JM (1998) Preoperative oral supplement with immunonutrients in cancer patients. JPEN 22:206–211
44. Senkal M, Mumme A, Eickhoff U et al. (1997) Early postoperative enteral immunonutrition: clinical outcome and cost-comparison analysis in surgical patients. Crit Care Med 25:1489–1496
45. Jensen MB, Kissmeyer Nielsen P, Laurberg S (1998) Perioperative growth hormone treatment increases nitrogen and fluid balance and results in short-term and long-term conservation of lean tissue mass. Am J Clin Nutr 68:840–846
46. Kissmeyer Nielsen P, Jensen MB, Laurberg S (1999) Perioperative growth hormone treatment and functional outcome after major abdominal surgery: a randomized, double-blind, controlled study. Ann Surg 229:298–302
47. Berman RS, Harrison LE, Pearlstone DB, Burt M, Brennan MF (1999) Growth hormone, alone and in combination with insulin, increases whole body and skeletal muscle protein kinetics in cancer patients after surgery. Ann Surg 229:1–10

48. Shirabe K, Matsumata T, Shimada M et al. (1997) A comparison of parenteral hyperalimentation and early enteral feeding regarding systemic immunity after major hepatic resection-the results of a randomized prospective study. Hepatogastroenterology 44:205–209
49. Sand J, Luostarinen M, Matikainen M (1997) Enteral or parenteral feeding after total gastrectomy: prospective randomised pilot study. Eur J Surg 163:761–766
50. Braga M, Gianotti L, Vignali A, Cestari A, Bisagni P, Di Carlo V (1998) Artificial nutrition after major abdominal surgery: impact of route of administration and composition of the diet. Crit Care Med 26:24–30
51. Beau P (1995) Nutrition entérale pré et post opératoire en chirurgie réglée de l'adulte: techniques, avantages et inconvénients. Nutr Clin Métabol 9 (suppl 1):133–138
52. van Berge Henegouwen MI, Akkermans LM et al. (1997) Prospective, randomized trial on the effect of cyclic versus continuous enteral nutrition on postoperative gastric function after pylorus-preserving pancreatoduodenectomy. Ann Surg 226:677–685
53. Keele AM, Bray MJ, Emery PW, Duncan HD, Silk DB (1997) Two phase randomised controlled clinical trial of postoperative oral dietary supplements in surgical patients. Gut 40:393–399
54. Conférence de consensus: Nutrition de l'agressé: recommandations du jury (1998) Nutr Clin Metab 12:229–237
55. Fan ST, Lo C-M, Lai ECS, Chu K-M, Liu C-L, Wong J (1994) Perioperative nutritional support in patients undergoing hepatectomy for hepatocellular carcinoma. N Engl J Med 331:1547–1552
56. Reilly J, Mehta R, Teperman L et al. (1990) Nutritional support after liver transplantation: a randomized prospective study. JPEN 14:386–391
57. Heymsfield SB, Waki M, Kehayias J et al. (1991) Chemical and elemental analysis of humans in vivo using improved body composition models. Am J Physiol 261:E190–198
58. Moore F (1959) Metabolic care of the surgical patient. Philadelphia

Perioperative Nutrition in Elective Surgery

S.P. Allison

Introduction

Mortality and morbidity following most elective surgical procedures are now fairly low and relate mainly to underlying cardiorespiratory function and associated disease. It is inherently unlikely therefore that nutritional support will make a difference except among those with significant antecedent malnutrition, or prolonged inability to eat normally in the postoperative period. Again, the demonstration that measures of undernutrition correlate with postoperative complications suggest, but do not prove, that nutritional intervention will improve clinical outcome. Early studies of perioperative nutritional support contented themselves with showing improved nitrogen balance and weight gain, although in the short term the latter is largely due to an accumulation of water. In the last 20 years, however, studies have focused on the more important issues of improvements in function, reduced complications, more rapid convalescence, and shorter hospital stay.

Perioperative management, like other branches of medicine, has been a victim of fashion and is still influenced by outdated concepts which have been discredited by evidence. Perioperative nutrition is no exception. The process of patient assessment and clinical decision-making will be reviewed, as will the indications for perioperative feeding, the modalities used, and the components of feeds.

Our thinking in this field has been dominated by the metabolic response to injury, the consequences of starvation and the question to what extent and at what point these affect clinical outcome and demand some form of intervention. In his Treatise on the Blood, Inflammation and Gunshot Wounds in 1794, John Hunter [1] crystallised the paradox, saying: "Impressions are capable of producing or increasing natural actions, and are then called stimuli; but they are likewise capable of producing too much action, as well as depraved, unnatural, or what we commonly call diseased actions". In the 1920s, Cuthbertson [2] described the increased metabolic rate and negative nitrogen balance which accompany inflammation, injury or surgery, and his ideas were elaborated by Moore [3] and others in the 1950s and 60's. The mechanism of neuroendocrine and cytokine mediation of these responses has been elaborated over the last 50 years. Cuthbertson divided the response to injury into the ebb, or shock, phase, followed by the flow, or catabolic, phase. To this concept Moore added the subsequent anabolic or convalescent phase, when lost tissue is re-formed. The tendency to retain salt and water with surgery and anesthesia was described as early as 1903 [4], but defined in the perioperative period by Coller et al. [5] in 1944 and Wilkinson [6] in 1952. Moore [3] subsequently coined the terms 'sodium retention' and 'sodium diuresis' phase to coincide with the flow and convalescent phase of the metabolic response, and showed that the return of the ability to excrete an excess salt and water load is one of the heralds of convalescence. The functional consequences of starvation and weight loss owe much to the seminal studies of Keys [7] and colleagues in the 1940s and 50's, showing the gradual impairment of mental and physical function which accompanies weight loss of more than 10% in an individual with initially normal body composition. The relationship between starvation and weight loss, and impaired function and clinical outcome has been studied extensively by Hill and colleagues [8–10] showing impaired wound healing, diminished muscle and respiratory function, mental depression, and impaired immune response when loss of total body protein exceeds 20% (correlating approximately with 15% weight loss).

Jeejeebhoy [11, 12] has also emphasised the assessment of function in the diagnosis of malnutrition and as a measure of the response to nutritional support.

Cuthbertson showed, as have others since, that nutritional support, however aggressively administered, is unable to reverse the catabolic process, although it may remove the element of starvation and therefore limit negative energy and protein balance. The idea that all patients undergoing surgery might benefit from aggressive perioperative nutritional support has given way to a much more conservative, selective and targeted approach. Hyperalimentation in an attempt to force the flow phase of injury into anabolism has been shown to be unsuccessful and hazardous. Instead, improvements in surgery, anesthesia and perioperative management have been designed to minimise the stressful stimulus to catabolism, thereby slowing the wasting process to the point where much less feed is required to meet metabolic requirements. We are now more concerned to avoid metabolic, fluid and electrolyte overload perioperatively, increasing food intake as the convalescent or anabolic phase begins and mobilisation allows resynthesis of lean mass.

Measurement of Malnutrition

This subject has been confused by the introduction of so-called nutritional indices [13] which mix measures of disease severity, such as serum albumin [14], with more specific nutritional parameters like weight loss. Such indices are valid predictors of the risk of postoperative complications and should therefore be termed "risk" rather than "nutritional" indices. The nutritional component should be considered separately, and should include measures of function [15] since low/normal anthropometric indices may be compatible with normal health [8–12]. The literature suggests that a combination of Body Mass Index, a history of more than 5% involuntary weight loss in the previous 3 months, a poor appetite with diminished food intake, and muscle weakness measured by hand dynamometry [15], will identify those patients whose clinical outcome is likely to be impaired by undernutrition, and in whom nutritional intervention may have specific benefits. In the postoperative period, Meguid and colleagues [16] have introduced the concept of inadequate oral nutrient intake period, or IONIP. In combination with other risk factors, patients who were unable to meet 60% of their requirements orally by the 7th to 10th day had an increased complication rate and it is suggested that they receive nutritional support by whatever means is practicable.

Evidence for Benefit from Treatment

Attempts to meet the whole patients' nutritional requirements in the immediate perioperative period, especially by parenteral nutrition (PN), have had mixed success [17]. Indeed, the Veterans' Administration Trial [18] of PN in the pre- and postoperative period showed more infectious complications in the treated than the controls (Table 1). Such treatment, therefore, has the capacity to do harm as well as good. In a sub-set of patients who were more severely malnourished preoperatively, there was a significant reduction in mechanical complications postoperatively and a trend towards some improvement in infectious complications. Similarly, the Maastricht trial [19] of perioperative nutrition showed no benefit, but also no harm in those who were previously malnourished, although among those who had lost more than 10% of their body weight, there was a reduction in postoperative abdominal sepsis with both enteral (EN) and parenteral nutrition (PN) (Table 2). A recent meta-analysis of perioperative feeding [20] (Fig. 1) concluded that there was no benefit, and indeed possible harm, from the routine use of short periods of postoperative PN, whereas there appeared to be some benefit when this was given perioperatively to patients with severe antecedent malnutrition (Fig. 2).

The idea that EN is more effective, cheaper and has fewer complications than PN is based largely on animal studies and the hypothesis that EN reduces bacterial translocation and beneficially affects gut-associated lymphatic tissue [21]. As a recent review by Lipman [22] points out, however, the evidence in support of this in man is inconclusive, certainly as regards elective surgery, although in specific instances, such as major trauma [23] or liver transplantation [24], the evidence is stronger [25]. In examining the evidence, we need to bear in mind not just the route of administration of feed, but its content. Feed given by the parenteral route results in the administration of larger volumes of salt and water, larger amounts of glucose with consequent hyperglycemia, higher amounts of energy, and an entirely different profile of fat and amino acids. Outcome may therefore be determined as much by the content and amount of the feed as by the route of administration. There may also be advantages in some cases for a combination of the two. Parenteral nutrition may be given peripherally by short cannulae changed daily or via pediatric PVC or sialastic cannulae which may last for 1–2 weeks. In the absence of peripheral access or for long periods of feeding, central line feeding is preferred.

Early enteral feeding postoperatively has a long pedigree [26], and a recent study by Beier-Holgersen [27] with hypocaloric, small volume, nasojejunal feeding postoperatively, showed reduced postoperative infections. One-sixth of her patients were described as malnourished preoperatively. Two other studies [28,

Table 1. Results of the Veterans Administration Trial (1991): degree of malnutrition (Nutrition Risk Index, percentages)

Major complications	Borderline	Mild	Severe
Infectious			
\TPN group	12.5	14.4*	15.8
\Control group	9.1	3.7	21.4
Noninfectious			
\TPN group	12.5	20.0	5.3**
\Control group	23.6	19.4	42.9

*$P=0.004$, **$P=0.03$

Table 2. Results of the Maastricht trial (1992): postoperative complication rates in patients with total parenteral nutrition (TPN) or total parenteral nutrition (TEN) and in depleted and non-depleted controls (percentages in patients with >10% weight loss; 25% of study population)

	TPN ($n=18$)	TEN ($n=13$)	Depleted ($n=11$)	Control Nondepleted ($n=8$)
Anastomotic leakage	5.5	15.4	27.3	25
Intra-abdominal sepsis	0*,**	15.4*,**	36.4*,**	25*
Other sepsis	0	7.6	18.2	0

* $P<0.05$, TPN vs TEN vs depleted vs nondepleted
, $P<0.05$, TPN+TEN vs depleted

29] of early postoperative enteral feeding were, however, negative. These differing results may well have been influenced by the demography of the population studied, the proportion of those previously malnourished, technical aspects of the feed and other factors such as analgesia and blood loss. Enteral feeding bypasses the cephalic phase of the eating process and is theoretically therefore inferior to oral feeding, because the 1500 ml of saliva produced daily in response to food not only has an important digestive function but contains a formidable array of anti-bacterial agents and immunoglobulins [25].

In two studies from Silk's group [30, 31], oral supplements given from the fifth or sixth postoperative day to patients undergoing moderate to major gastrointestinal surgery increased energy and protein intake, resulted in less weight loss, and were associated with improved muscle function, fewer infections, and shorter hospital stay. The average preoperative weight loss in these studies, however, was over 7%, suggesting that the study population contained a high proportion of malnourished individuals. Hessov's group [32] examined the effects of post-discharge oral supplements in the community, and showed improved weight gain but no benefits in terms of functional outcome. In contrast, Pennington's group [33]

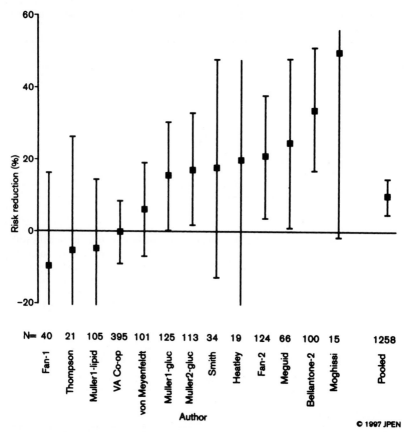

Fig. 1. Prospective randomized controlled trials evaluating the effect of preoperative total parenteral nutrition (TPN) on postoperative complications. The mean increase or decrease in postoperative complications, with 95% confidence intervals, are shown for each study. Values above 0 indicate a decrease in complications associated with the use of TPN; those below 0 indicate an increase in complications. When the 95% confidence intervals are above or below 0 the differences in postoperative complications between the group receiving TPN and the control group are statistically significant. The pooled analysis of these trials found a 10% decrease (an overall decrease from 40% to 30%) in postoperative complications in patients who received preoperative TPN. Published with permission

selected patients with BMI <20, triceps skinfold or mid-arm muscle circumference less than the 15th percentile on admission, and/or a weight loss of more than 5% during the operative period. The provision of oral supplements following discharge in this group of patients not only produced greater weight gain, but improved function and lessened infections as measured by the number of antibiotic prescriptions.

The use of probiotics is a growing area of interest [25]. The idea that there are 'good' bacteria such as Lactobacillus Plantarum or Rudei which may protect the host from invasion by pathogenic bacteria is not new but, in combination with

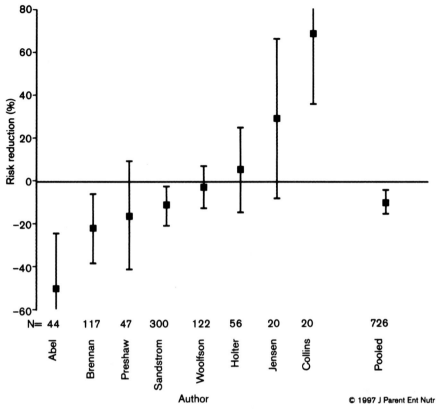

Fig. 2. Prospective randomized controlled trials evaluating the effect of early postoperative total parenteral nutrition (TPN) (without preoperative TPN) on postoperative complications. The mean increase or decrease in postoperative complications, with 95% confidence intervals, are shown for each study. Values above 0 indicate a decrease in complications associated with the use of TPN; those below 0 indicate an increase in complications. When the 95% confidence intervals are above or below 0 the difference in postoperative complications between the group receiving TPN and the control group are statistically significant. The pooled analysis of these trials found a 10% increase (an overall increase from 30% to 40%) in postoperative complications in patients who received postoperative TPN. Published with permission

appropriate substrates may contribute to improved outcome in the future. We are beginning to reach the limits of antibiotic efficacy and the concept of gut recontamination rather than decontamination has attractive possibilities.

Recent studies from Sweden and Denmark [34–37] suggest that short periods of pre- and postoperative starvation may not be as harmless as we have imagined, and that sending patients to surgery in a metabolically starved condition increases insulin resistance and negative nitrogen balance and impairs outcome. Ljungqvist's group, in Stockholm, have shown that the giving of an oral glucose load the night before surgery and 2 h before operation is not only well-tolerated, but results in diminished postoperative insulin resistance, reduced catabolism, improved function, and even shorter hospital stay. These studies indicate that it may be useful to manipulate metabolism with small doses of substrate given in hypocaloric amounts, at a time when aggressive attempts to meet full nutritional requirements may even be harmful.

Conventional surgical management with nasogastric suction, an intravenous drip and systemic opiates, has also been challenged. Wara and Hessov [37] showed that patients undergoing colorectal surgery fed orally from the first post-operative day, without gastric suction of intravenous fluids, had a better nutritional intake, an earlier return of gastrointestinal function, no more vomiting, and no increase in complications. These findings are supported by a meta-analysis of 26 trials [38], which concluded that routine nasogastric decompression is not supported in the literature by scientific evidence. This analysis also found that fever, atelectasis and pneumonia were significantly less common in patients managed without a nasogastric tube, and that only one patient in 20 really required such a tube. Patients are more likely to need a nasogastric tube following upper GI surgery, but the use of such tubes in small bowel and colorectal surgery has largely been abandoned by some Scandinavian centres. This approach is facilitated by the postoperative use of 4 days of low thoracic epidural analgesia, which unlike systemic opiates does not interfere with return of gastrointestinal function, combined with aggressive mobilisation and oral intake from the first postoperative day [39]. These measures result in preservation of gastrointestinal and muscle function, as well as more rapid convalescence and earlier discharge from hospital.

Salt and Water Balance

The giving of water and electrolytes is inseparable from the administration of feed by whatever route, and it is therefore pertinent to consider this in relation to perioperative nutrition. Both chronic malnutrition and the response to surgery are associated with the inability to excrete an excess salt and water load, and relative expansion of the extracellular fluid volume [3, 7]. Surgical patients are, therefore, easily overloaded by the injudicious administration of salt and water with undesirable clinical consequences. Starker et al. [40] showed that among malnourished patients receiving preoperative PN, those who retained fluid and developed hypoalbuminemia had more postoperative complications than those who achieved a diuresis and a rise in serum albumin. Similar results have been reported by Sitges-Serra's group [41]. Salt and water overload may have several deleterious effects that impair clinical outcome. The serum albumin concentration is diluted by approximately 1 g/l for every litre of salt and water retained [42]. This may be associated with delayed return of gastric and small bowel function [43]. Respiratory function may also be impaired, and postoperative respiratory complications increased, as well as heart failure precipitated in susceptible individuals [41]. Interstitial edema develops, interfering with wound healing. It is also important to remember that 5% dextrose administration has important effects on electrolyte as well as water balance, not only causing hypophosphatemia and hypokalemia, but enhancing renal sodium reabsorption [44].

Although some degree of salt and water overload may be an unavoidable consequence of fluid resuscitation in shock, its profligate use in the postoperative period may impair recovery and in some cases be dangerous. A balance needs to be struck between avoiding salt and water depletion and pre-renal failure on the one hand, and overload on the other. These problems may be monitored by changes in weight and serum albumin, and prevented or treated by restricting glucose, water and sodium intake to levels which maintain balance. Careful consideration of requirements for salt and water should play as much part in the design of feeds as those for energy and. protein [42].

Design and Content of Feeds

The broad principles governing the design of feeds in nutritional support remain the same whether oral, enteral or parenteral. In patients who are depleted preoperatively, and in whom some degree of repletion is desired, the full daily requirements need to be met, plus an additional amount for tissue gain. An intake of 35 kcalories per kilogram with half the non-protein energy from fat and half from carbohydrate will meet the requirements of most patients in this circumstance. Between 1.2 and 1.5 g protein per kilogram may also suffice. Care should be taken not to overload the patient with salt and water, and that a full complement of minerals and micronutrients are supplied. Any specific deficits of electrolytes, minerals or micronutrients should be made up. It is not uncommon, for example, for patients with severe Crohn's disease to have deficiencies in zinc, magnesium and selenium, as well as some vitamins. In the well-nourished patient, the avoidance of the metabolic consequences of starvation may be achieved by giving very small amounts of glucose, with or without protein, in the immediate preoperative period. In the early postoperative phase, it is desirable to avoid energy and protein overload. Good results have been obtained using hypocaloric feeds with 20 kcal/kg and 1 g/kg of protein. In patients with prolonged postoperative gastrointestinal failure, it is necessary to meet the full requirements, which are very similar to those used for the preoperative depleted patient. Following elective surgery it is rarely necessary to exceed 30 kcal/kg, although in the convalescent and anabolic phase, higher levels of energy and protein are well tolerated. Although there is good evidence for benefit from special substrates and immune-enhancing diets in other circumstances, there is no evidence to support their use in the patient undergoing elective surgery. There is also no evidence to support other than whole protein defined formula diets for enteral use.

Nutritional Support in Elective Surgery

Patients undergoing elective surgery should be screened for malnutrition by a combination of simple anthropometric measurements, with recording of percentage involuntary weight loss (more than 5% in the previous 3 months), food intake and appetite, combined with some functional measurements such as hand dynamometry. Serum albumin and/or prealbumin should be recorded, not for nutritional reasons so much, but as a measure of the severity of underlying disease and a predictor of surgical risk. There is evidence that avoidance of the endocrine and metabolic changes associated with fasting reduces the metabolic response to surgery and improves outcome. This can be achieved with a glucose drink administered the night before and 2 h prior to surgery. Routine "drip and suck" regimens are outmoded in most cases, apart from some patients undergoing upper gastrointestinal surgery. Better results are achieved by aggressive, early oral feeding combined with epidural analgesia and early and vigorous mobilisation. There is evidence that early oral feeding with supplements may improve outcome, even among patients without prior malnutrition. Among those with prior malnutrition, oral supplementation during the convalescent phase and post-discharge may not only increase weight but also accelerate functional recovery. Among those without prior malnutrition, there is no evidence of benefit from oral supplements post-discharge. The evidence concerning perioperative artificial nutrition is to some extent conflicting, although the position is clearer than it was. Perioperative enteral or parenteral nutrition has been shown to be of benefit only in patients with prior malnutrition, and may even be harmful in some patients who are well-nourished on admission. Early postoperative enteral nutrition using jejunal tubes may be of benefit, particularly where prior malnutrition exists. Parenteral nutrition is the treatment of gastrointestinal failure, as dialysis is the treatment of renal failure and ventilation the treatment of respiratory failure. In cases of severe gastrointestinal disease, with preoperative malnutrition, it is probably beneficial to give two to 3 weeks of preoperative nutritional support, although this will depend on other factors such as the urgency of surgical intervention.

Conclusion

With prolonged postoperative complications which prevent adequate oral or enteral nutrition, parenteral feeding is of benefit and may be life saving, with good long-term survival [45]. In the acute inflammatory phase of illness, or the early postoperative period, a conservative regimen should be employed, with avoidance of any overload, particularly of energy, glucose, salt and water. Some of the reported ill effects of parenteral nutrition may be directly related to these factors rather than to the route of administration per se. When feeding is indicated, the enteral route is probably to be preferred if this is technically possible. In many cases, a combination of parenteral and enteral feeding is appropriate depending on the clinical situation and the phase of illness. In the hands of an expert team, parenteral nutrition has few complications and should be used unhesitatingly where necessary. High complication rates are unacceptable and an indication for staff retraining and reorganisation [17].

Nutritional support cannot compensate for deficiencies in other aspects of management, and must be seen as part of an optimal package of care based on published evidence, which in some cases poses a challenge to some conventional surgical and anesthetic practices.

References

1. Hunter J (1794) A Treatise on the Blood, Inflammation and Gunshot Wounds. G Nichol
2. Cuthbertson DP (1932) Observations on the disturbance of metabolism produced by injury to the limbs. Q J Med 1:233–246
3. Moore FD (1959) The Metabolic Care of the Surgical Patient. Saunders, Philadelphia
4. Pringle H, Maunsell RCB, Pringle S (1905) Effects of ether anaesthesia on renal activity. BMJ 2:942
5. Coller FA, Campbell KN, Vaughan AH et al. (1944) Postoperative salt intolerance. Ann Surg 119:533
6. Wilkinson AW, Billing BH, Nagy C et al. (1949) Excretion of chloride and sodium after surgical operations. Lancet 1:640
7. Keys A, Brozek J, Henschel A (1950) The Biology of Human Starvation. University of Minnesota Press, Minneapolis
8. Hill GL (1992) Body composition research: Implications for the practice of clinical nutrition. JPEN 16:197–218
9. Hill GL (1992) Disorders of Nutrition and Metabolism in Clinical Surgery. Churchill Livingstone, Edinburgh
10. Vernon DR, Hill G (1998) The relationship between tissue loss and function: recent developments. Current Opinion in Clinical Nutrition and Metabolic Care 1:5–8
11. Jeejeebhoy KN (1988) Bulk or bounce – the object of nutritional support. J PEN 12:539–549
12. Jeejeebhoy KN (1988) The Functional Basis of Assessment. In: Kinney JM, Jeejeebhoy KN, Hill GL, Owen OE (eds) Nutrition and Metabolism in Patient Care. WB Saunders, pp 739–751
13. Mullen JL, Buzby GP, Waldman TG, Gertner MH, Hobbs CL, Rosatao EF (1979) Prediction of operative morbidity and mortality by preoperative nutritional assessment. Surg Forum 30:80–82
14. Fleck A (1988) Plasma proteins as nutritional indicators in the perioperative period. In: Allison SP, Kinney JM (eds) Perioperative Nutrition. Brit J Clin Pract 42: Suppl 63:20–24
15. Klidjian AM, Foster KJ, Kammerling RM, Cooper A, Karran SJ (1980) Relation of anthropometric and dynamometric variables to serious postoperative complications. Br Med J ii: 899–901
16. Meguid MM, Campos ACL, Meguid V, Debonis D, Terz JJ (1988) IONIP, a criterion of surgical outcome and patient selection for perioperative nutrition support. Br J Clin Pract 42: Suppl 63:8–14
17. Allison SP (1992) The uses and limitations of nutritional support. Clin Nutr 11:319–330
18. Veterans Affairs Total Parenteral Nutrition Study Group (1991) Perioperative total parenteral nutrition in surgical patients. New Engl J Med 325:525–532
19. Von Mayenfeldt MF, Meijerink WJHJ, Rouflart MMJ, Buil-Maassen MTHJ, Soeters PB (1992) Perioperative nutritional support: a randomised clinical trial. Clin Nutr 11:180–186
20. Satyanarayana R, Klein S (1998) Clinical efficacy of perioperative nutrition support. Current Opinion in Clinical Nutrition and Metabolic Care 1:51–58
21. Silk BA, Green CJ (1998) Perioperative nutrition: parenteral versus enteral. Current Opinion in Clinical Nutrition and Metabolic Care 1:21–27
22. Lipman TO (1998) Grains or veins: Is enteral nutrition really better than parenteral nutrition? A look at the evidence. JPEN 22:167–182
23. Kudsk KA, Croece MA, Fabian TC, Minaid G, Tolley EA, Poret HA et al. (1992) Enteral versus parenteral feeding. Ann Surg 215:503–513
24. Sharpe MD, Pukil J, Lowndes R et al. (1995) Early enteral feeding (EEF) reduces incidence of early rejection following orthotopic liver transplantation. Joint Congress of Liver Transplantation (Abstract), London
25. Bengmark S (1998) Progress in perioperative enteral tube feeding. Clin Nutr 17:145–152
26. Abbott WO, Rawson AG (1939) Tube for use in postoperative care of gastroenterostomy patients. JAMA 112:2414

27. Beier-Holgersen R, Boesby S (1996) Influence of postoperative enteral nutrition on postsurgical infections. GUT 39:833–835
28. Heslin MJ, Latkany L, Leung D et al. (1997) A prospective randomized trial of early enteral feeding after resection of upper GI malignancy. A prospective randomized trial of early enteral feeding after resection of upper GI malignancy. Ann Surg 226:567–580.
29. Watters JM, Kirkpatrick SM, Norris SB, Shamji FM, Wells GA (1997) Immediate postoperative enteral feeding results in impaired respiratory mechanics and decreased mobility. Ann Surg 226 (3): 369–377
30. Rana SK, Bray J, Menzies-Gow N et al. (1992) Short term benefits of postoperative oral dietary supplements in surgical patients. Clin Nutr 11:337–344
31. Keele AM, Bray MJ, Emery PW, Silk DBA (1996) A randomised controlled clinical trial of postoperative oral dietary supplements in surgical patients. JPEN 19: Suppl 1, 215
32. Jensen MB, Hessov I (1997) Randomization to nutritional intervention at home did not improve postoperative function, fatigue or well-being. Br J Surg 84:113–118
33. Beattie AH, Prack AT, Baxter JP, Pennington CR (1999) The change in nutritional status after surgery: the influence of oral supplements. Clin Nutr 18: Suppl 1:19–20
34. Hessov I, Ljungqvist O (1998) Perioperative oral nutrition. Current Opinion in Clinical Nutrition and Metabolic Care 1:29–33
35. Thorell A, Nygren J, Ljungqvist O (1999) Insulin resistance: a marker of surgical stress. Current Opinion in Clinical Nutrition and Metabolic Care 2:69–78
36. Ljungqvist et al. (1999) (unpublished).
37. Wara P, Hessov I (1985) Nutritional intake after colorectal surgery; a comparison of a traditional and a new postoperative regimen. Clin Nutr 4:225–228
38. Cheatham ML, Chapman WC, Key SP et al. (1995) A meta-analysis of selective versus routine nasogastric decompression after elective laparotomy. Ann Surg 221:469–478
39. Henriksen MG, Hansen HV, Hessov I (1999) Early oral nutrition after elective colorectal surgery. Influence of balanced analgesia and enforced mobilization. Nutrition (in press)
40. Starker PM, Lasala PA, Askanazi J et al. (1986) Influence of preoperative total parenteral nutrition upon morbidity and mortality. Surgery, Gynaecology and Obstetrics 162:569–574
41. Sitges-Serra A, Guzman FA (1998) Fluid and sodium problems in perioperative feeding: What further studies need to be done? Current Opinion in Clinical Nutrition and Metabolic Care 1: 9–14
42. Lobo DN, Bjarnason K, Field J, Rowlands BJ, Allison SP (1999) Changes in weight, fluid balance and serum albumin in patients referred for nutritional support. Clin Nutr 18:197– 201
43. Mecray PM, Barden RP, Ravdin IS (1937) Nutritional edema: its effect on the gastric emptying time before and after gastric operations. Surgery 1:53–64

Nutrition Support in Blunt and Penetrating Torso Trauma

M.M. McQuiggan and F.A. Moore

Introduction

Over the past 25 years, clinical studies have provided convincing evidence that early nutritional support benefits stressed surgical patients by preventing acute protein malnutrition [1–3]. Additionally, enteral nutrition, when compared to parenteral [4–6], has been demonstrated to be the preferred route of substrate delivery. Moreover, recent basic and clinical investigation offers the prospect that the benefits of traditional nutrition support can be amplified by supplementing specific nutrients that impart pharmacological immune-enhancing effects [7–22]. The focus of this chapter is to define optimal nutrition following major torso trauma and to describe a systematic method to deliver nutrition care in the ICU.

Early Nutritional Support is Beneficial

Background

In the late 1970s, multiple organ failure (MOF) had emerged as a major clinical problem in Trauma ICUs and uncontrolled infection was identified to be a primary risk factor [23]. Soon thereafter, persistent hypercatabolism with secondary protein malnutrition and delayed immunosuppression were recognized to be prominent features of this syndrome [3]. Based on the collective work of a variety of investigators, the following paradigm was proposed [1–3] (see Fig. 1). Persistent hypercatabolism dominates the metabolic response to major trauma. Endogenous amino acids are mobilized for the acute phase response, gluconeogenesis and energy production. At first, these amino acid demands are met by skeletal muscle proteolysis. Eventually, this "autocannibalism" progressively erodes crucial visceral structure elements as well as circulating proteins. The resulting acute protein malnutrition is associated with cardiac, pulmonary, hepatic, gastrointestinal and immunologic dysfunction. In essence, subclinical multiple organ dysfunction evolves as the patient becomes progressively more immunocompromised. Delayed infection then extends hypermetabolism that eventuates into fulminant MOF.

PERSISTENT HYPERCATABOLISM

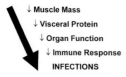

↓ Muscle Mass
↓ Visceral Protein
↓ Organ Function
↓ Immune Response
INFECTIONS

MULTIPLE ORGAN FAILURE

Fig. 1. Metabolic response to trauma

Thus, it became widely accepted that persistent hypercatabolism was an important co-factor for MOF. The natural question then was whether provision of early nutritional support in high risk trauma patients could improve outcome.

Clinical Investigation

A prospective randomized trial (PRCT) was conducted to investigate the potential benefits of early postinjury nutritional support [2]. Over a 30-month period ending November 1983, 75 (20%) of 371 injured patients requiring emergency laparotomy had an Abdominal Trauma Index (ATI) >15 and, were enrolled. The control group (n=31) received conventional 5% dextrose crystalloids (approximately 2L/day) intravenously during the first 5 postoperative days, and then TPN was started if they could not tolerate oral intake (29% ultimately received TPN). The early fed group (n=32) had a needle catheter jejunostomy (NCJ) placed at laparotomy and infusion of an elemental, low-fat diet (Vivonex HN) was begun within 12 h postoperatively and advanced to goal at 72 h. As expected, the early fed group had significantly better cumulative nitrogen balance measured on days 4 and 7. More importantly, the early fed patients developed significantly fewer major septic complications [3 (9%) all abdominal abscesses versus 9 (29%) in controls with 7 abdominal abscesses and 2 pneumonia].

Similar results were observed in a PRCT [1] performed at the Shriners' Burn Institute in Cincinnati, Ohio, Eighteen children with a burn size 40% of body surface area were randomized to a high protein diet (25% of total calories as protein) or a standard isocaloric protein diet (15% protein). The diets were primarily delivered by the enteral route and supplemental TPN was used as needed. Both groups were comparable with respect to demographic data and burn size and the frequency of inhalation injury. Patients randomized to the high protein diet had significantly fewer bacteremic days (8% vs. 11%), significantly fewer days on antibiotics (72% vs 83%), and had a significantly lower mortality (0% vs. 44%).

Enteral is the Preferred Route of Substrate Delivery

Background

In the early 1970s, total enteral nutrition (TEN) was preferred over total parenteral nutrition (TPN) because it was cheaper, safer and more convenient. Futhermore, it was believed that critically ill patients could not utilize exogenous nutrients early after a stressful insult and that the gut was a dormant organ. Thus, TEN was delayed until the gut was clearly functioning. By the late 1970s, a better understanding of resuscitation and stress metabolism provided the rationale for earlier nutrition. Since TPN was more widely available, safer, and central venous access had become routine in ICU patients, TPN became the preferred mode of support in severely injured patients. However, research in the1980s suggested that TEN was physiologically superior to TPN because substrates delivered enterally are better utilized [24]. Additionally, TEN compared to TPN prevents gut mucosal atrophy, attenuates the stress response, maintains immunocompetence, and preserves gut flora [25–29]. Finally, in the 1990s, clinical studies suggested that TPN by itself may be harmful. Three prospective trials of perioperative TPN have demonstrated that patients randomized to TPN (compared to no nutritional support) had higher postoperative infectious morbidity [30–32].

Clinical Investigation

Over the past decade, a series of studies specifically designed studies to determine whether TEN compared to TPN offered a clinical outcome advantage have been performed. Table 1 summarizes the results of two early PRCTs performed in patients with torso trauma [4, 5]. Both demonstrated a reduction in major septic complications in patients randomized to TEN. Table 2 summarizes the results of a subsequent meta-analysis of eight PRCTs confirming a reduction in septic morbidities with TEN [6].

New "Immune-Enhancing" Diets Offer Additional Clinical Benefits

Background

Despite tremendous advances in patient care, late infections continue to be an unsolved problem. In large part, these infections occur due to failure of local and systemic host defenses. While exact causes of late immunosuppression are not clear, it is believed to occur as a result of dysfunctional regulation of inflammation (see Fig. 2). A traumatic insult precipitates early systemic hyperinflammation, i.e., SIRS; the amplitude and duration (generally 3–5 days) depends on the magnitude of the initial insult. As time proceeds, certain components of this early hyperinflammation are endogenously down-regulated to prevent unnecessary, potentially auto-destructive inflammation. The resulting delayed immunosuppression, however, sets the stage for secondary infections.

Table 1. Septic morbidity of TEN vs. TPN study groups (from [4, 5])

Moore et al. [4]		TEN (n=29)		TPN (n=30)
Major infections				
Abdominal abscess	1	1 patient	2	6 patients[a]
Pneumonia	0	(13%)	6	(20%)
Minor Infections				
Wound	3		1	
Catheter	0	4 patients	2	5 patients
Urinary	0	(14%)	1	(17%)
Other	1		2	
Kudsk et al. [5]		n=51		n=45
Major infections				
Abscess	2	8 patients	8	17 patients[a]
Pneumonia	6	(14%)	14	(38%)
Minor infections				
Line sepsis	1	4 patients	6	10 patients
Wound	3	(8%)	4	(22%)

TEN, total enteral nutrition; TPN, total parenteral nutrition.
[a]$p < .05$.

Table 2. Meta-analysis of 8 PRCT'S comparing TEN vs. TPN in which septic outcome was assessed: number of septic events (from [4])

Moore et al. [4]		TEN (n=118)		TPN (n=112)
Abscess	5		7	
Pneumonia	6	19 patients	14	39 patients[a]
Bacteremia	1	(16%)	6	(35%)
Line sepsis	0		7	
Other	12		13	

TEN, total enteral nutrition; TPN, total parenteral nutrition.
[a]$p < .05$.

While various strategies have been proposed and tested to modulate this dysfunctional inflammatory response, the most promising approach to date has been the delivery of specific nutrients that exert pharmacologic immune-enhancing effects. Glutamine is acknowledged to be the preferred fuel of the enterocyte and is thought to stimulate lymphocyte and monocyte functions [7]. Arginine promotes collagen synthesis required in wound healing and increases the number of total lymphocytes as well as the proportion of helper T cells. Additionally, arginine is the chief precursor of nitric oxide synthesis and has been shown to enhance delayed cutaneous hypersensitivity and lymphocyte blastogenesis [8]. Traditional enteral products contain a high proportion of plant-derived omega-6 polyunsaturated fatty acid (PUFA). However, diets with a low omega-6 PUFA and high fish-oil derived omega-3 PUFA content are known to suppress the synthesis of cytokines that exhibit potent inflammatory activities, e.g., TNF alpha and Il-1beta [9, 33]. Finally, exogenous nucleotides may be necessary in stressed states to maintain rapid cell proliferation and responsiveness [10].

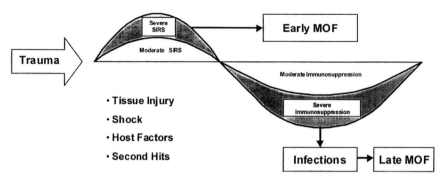

Fig. 2. Dysfunctional regulation of inflammation

Clinical Investigation

Recently, "immune-enhancing" enteral formulas supplemented with one or more of the above mentioned nutrients have become commercially available and are being tested by a number of investigators [11–22, 34, 35]. In this era of evidence-based medicine, these data are becoming increasingly difficult to dismiss. To date, there are at least 13 published PRCTs where an immune enhancing diet (IED) is compared to a standard enteral diet (SED) and where the outcome was a prede-termined endpoint (see Table 3). Of these 13 PRCTs, six demonstrated improved outcome, five were highly suggestive of improved outcome, and two did not demonstrate any advantage.

Five of these PRCTs were performed in trauma patients [14, 15, 18, 22, 34]. The first trauma study by Brown, et al. [14] was a single-institution trial. Thir-ty seven polytrauma patients (ISS 28±3 IED; 34±3 SED ns) were randomized to receive either the study IED ($n=19$), a noncommercial product enriched with arginine, omega-3 fatty acids and beta-carotene, or an isonitrogenous control SED ($n=18$), Osmolite HN with ProMod. The IED patients experienced signifi-cantly fewer delayed infections (total 3:1 pneumonia, 1 UTI, 1 bacteremia) than those who received the SED (total 10: 7 pneumonia, 1 wound infection, 1 UTI, 1 sinusitis).

The second trauma study was conducted by Moore et al. [15] and was a multi-center PRCT. Ninety eight patients were randomized to receive the study IED ($n=51$), a polymeric formula enriched with glutamine, arginine, omega-3 fatty acids and nucleotides (Immun-Aid) or the control SED ($n=47$), an elemental diet (Vivonex TEN) which contains glutamine. The entry criteria were an ATI of 18–40 or Injury Severity Score (ISS) of 16–45 (excluding major head injuries: GCS<8). Because of the higher nitrogen content of the IED formula, the study group received more nitrogen than the SED group (day 7: study=0.34gm nitrogen/kg/day vs. control=0.16 g/kg/day). After 7 days of feeding, patients receiving the study diet compared to the control diet experienced significantly greater increases in total lymphocytes, T-lymphocytes, T-helper, and B-lympho-cyte cells. In regards to clinical outcome, days of mechanical ventilation (mean=1.9 vs. control=5.3), ICU stay (5.3 vs. 8.6) and hospital stay (14.6 vs. 17.2)

Table 3. Assessment of patient outcome in 13 prospective, randomized controlled trials comparing immune-enhancing diets (*IED*) versus standard enteral diets (*SED*)

Reference	Year	Patient type	n	IED	SED	Isonitrogenous	Results with IED	Improved outcome
Gottschlich [11]	1990	Burns	50	Noncommercial study formula	Osmolite+Promote or Traumacal	Yes	↓ WI ↓ LOS	Yes
Daly [13]	1992	GI surg	77	Impact	Undisclosed Control diet	No	↓ WC ↓ Inf	Yes
Brown [14]	1994	Trauma	37	Noncommercial Study formula	Osmolite HN +ProMod	Yes	↓ Inf	Yes
Moore [15]	1994	Trauma	98	Immun-Aid	Vivonex TEN	No	↓ IAA ↓ MOF	Yes
Bower [16]	1995	Mixed ICU	296	Impact	Osmolite HN	No	Subsets ↓ Inf ↓ LOS	? Yes
Daly [17]	1995	GI cancer	60	Impact	Traumacal	Yes	↓ WC ↓ Inf ↓ LOS	Yes
Kudsk [18]	1996	Trauma	35	Immun-Aid	Promote+Casec	Yes	↓ ABT ↓ Inf ↓ LOS ↓ Costs	Yes
Senkel [19]	1997	GI Surg	154	Impact	Undisclosed Control Diet	Yes	Subsets ↓ Inf	? Yes
Mendez [34]	1997	Trauma	43	Noncommercial Study formula	Osmolite HN +ProMod	Yes	↑ ARDS	No
Saffle [35]	1997	Burns	50	Impact	Replete	Yes	–	No
Braga [20]	1998	GI cancer	154	Impact	Undisclosed Control diet	Yes	↓ SS subsets ↓ Inf ↓ LOS	? Yes

Reference	Year	Patient type	n	IED	SED	Isonitrogenous	Results with IED	Improved outcome
Atkinson [21]	1998	Mixed ICU	369	Impact	Undisclosed Control diet	Yes	Subsets ↓ Vent Days ↓ LOS	? Yes
Weimann [22]	1998	Trauma	32	Impact	Undisclosed Control diet	Yes	↓ SIRS ↓ MOF	? Yes

WI, wound infection; GI, gastrointestinal; Surg, surgical; WC, wound complication; LOS, length of stay; Inf, infections; IAA, intra-abdominal abscess; MOF, multiple organ failure; ABT, antibiotics; SS, sepsis score; SIRS, systemic inflammatory response syndrome.
Osmolite, Ross Laboratories, Columbus, OH; Promote, Ross Laboratories, Columbus, OH; Traumacal, Mead Johnson, Evansville, IN; Impact, Novartis, Minneapolis, MN; ProMod, Ross Laboratories, Columbus, OH; Immun-Aid, McGaw, Irvine, CA; Vivonex TEN, Novartis, Minneapolis, MN; Casec, Mead Johnson, Evansville, IN; Replete, Nestle, Deerfield, IL.

were all less in patients receiving the IED, but these differences did not reach statistical significance. The key clinical finding was that the study group had significantly fewer intra-abdominal abscesses (IED=0% vs. SED=11%) and a significantly lower incidence of MOF (IED=0% vs. SED=11%).

The third trauma study by Kudsk et al. [18], was a single institution PRCT that addressed the issue of an isonitrogenous control diet. Thirty five severely injured trauma patients (ATI>25 or ISS>21) were randomized to receive the study IED, Immun-Aid or the control SED (n=17), an isonitrogenous blend of Promote with Casec. Nitrogen intake was similar (average daily: IED=.23 vs. SED 0.23 g nitrogen/kg/day). The key clinical finding (similar to the previous study) was that the patients who received the IED had significantly fewer intraabdominal abscesses [IED=1 (6%) vs. SED=6 (35%]. There was also a significant reduction in therapeutic antibiotic use (3 vs. 7 days) and hospital stay (7 vs. 18 days).

The fourth trauma study was conducted by Mendez et al. [34] and was a single institution PRCT. Forty three patients were randomized to receive the study IED (n=22), a noncommercial formula enriched with omega-3 fatty acids L-arginine, taurine and trace elements (selenium, chromium, molybdenum) or the control SED (n=21), which was an isonitrogenous blend of Osmolyte HN supplemented with ProMod. The entry criteria were trauma patients with an ISS >13 admitted to the ICU. Both groups received similar nitrogen intakes (average: IED=0.24 vs. SED=0.22 g of nitrogen/kg/day). While there were no significant differences in patient outcome, the IED group appeared to have longer mechanical ventilation, ICU, and hospital days. A major confounding variable in the evaluation of outcome is that more of the IED patients developed ARDS [10 (45%), of which 7 (70%) were early onset prior to study enrollment] than did the SED patients [4 (19%), of which 3 (75%) were early onset].

The fifth trauma study was conducted by Weimann et al. [22] and was a single institution study. Thirty two patients were randomized to receive the study IED (n=16), a polymeric diet enriched with arginine, Omega-3 fatty acids, and nucleotides (Impact) or an isonitrogenous control diet (n=16). Both groups also received supplemental TPN. The entry criteria were trauma patients with an ISS >20. The primary endpoints were SIRS and MOF defined by a standard scoring system. The IED patients experienced significantly fewer overall days of SIRS (IED=8.3±6.3 vs. SED=13.3±6.7 days) and had significantly lower MOF scores.

Nonocclusive Small Bowel Necrosis

With wider application of enteral nutrition in ICU patients, nonocclusive small bowel necrosis (NOBN) has emerged as a devastating complication. The incidence among patient populations described is <0.5%; however, the mortality is high at 70%. While gut hypoperfusion due to incomplete resuscitation is commonly stated to be the prelude, our experience indicates that NOBN is a delayed event in ICU patients who require progressively more high acuity care [37]. Most are tolerating TEN and then experience a setback, e.g., refractory ARDS, acute renal failure, or pneumonia. All of our patients with NOBN were receiving polymeric formulas (which are used in 95%–97% of patients); although, other centers have reported similar phenomenom with elemental feedings. Consistent clinical monitoring failed to detect this entity early in its course. Gastric tonometer measurement of regional CO_2 ($PrCO_2$) may emerge as an objective indicator to discontinue enteral feeding.

Practice Guideline Development and Implementation

As a result of the above clinical evidence, a practice guideline was devised at our university-affiliated teaching hospital. The guideline was presented to a multidisciplinary group for their input to enhance acceptance [36]. When insufficient evidence existed, expert opinion was used to derive specific guidelines.

Patient Selection for Early Nutrition Support

Potential candidates are identified within the first day of ICU admission. The criteria are: (a) major head injuries (abnormal head CT scan plus a Glasgow Coma Score <8); (b) major trauma (significant injuries to two or more body regions); (c) major abdominal trauma (ATI >18); (d) major upper gastrointestinal surgery that precludes oral intake for >5 days; (e) 2nd or 3rd degree burns >20% total body surface area; (f) chronically malnourished, and (g) significant comorbid disease including lung disease (COPD requiring bronchodilators or steroids), liver disease (admission bilirubin >2.5 mg%, history of hepatic encephalopathy, or cirrhosis), kidney disease (chronic renal disease requiring dialysis or renal transplant), active malignancy and diseases of immune dysfunction.

Enteral Formula Selection

Immune Enhancing Diet

These formulas are polymeric products which contain additional glutamine, arginine, fish oil and nucleotides. They are used for patients sustaining major chest and abdominal trauma who are at known risk for septic complications and MOF. Usage is limited to a ten-day period and thereafter a polymeric, high protein formula is used. Criteria for the use of these specialty formulas are listed in Table 4.

Elemental Formulas

These formulas contain free amino acids, short chain peptides, and a minimal amount of fat. Criteria for use include: (a) patients who have been enterally fasted for 8 days, (b) acute pancreatitis, (c) short gut, (d) high output distal ileal or colonic fistula, and e) persistent diarrhea >48 h while on polymeric formula.

Table 4. Criteria for using immune enhancing enteral formulas

---

Combined flail chest/pulmonary contusion requiring prolonged mechanical ventilation

Major abdominal trauma defined by an Abdominal Trauma Index >18.

Major gastrointestinal surgery for carcinoma

Two or more of the following:

- >6 units blood transfusion requirement in first 12 h
- Major pelvic fracture (e.g. acetabular, vertical shear, "open-book" fracture)
- Two or more long bone fractures

Polymeric High-Protein Formula

Polymeric formulas contain intact protein, carbohydrate and a normal fat load. Their protein content is 50% greater than standard polymeric formulas. Usage is indicated in patients who do not meet the criteria for immune-enhancing diets but have normal digestive and absorptive capacity of the GI tract, and are believed to have increased nitrogen requirements. Higher protein formulas were selected as our "default" feeding with the thought that positive nitrogen balance is more critical than positive caloric balance. Criteria include: (a) major torso trauma; (b) major head injuries; (c) major upper GI surgery; (d) obese patients with moderate calorie need, but high protein needs; and e) patients undergoing continuous venous-venous hemodialysis (CVVHD).

Renal Failure Formula

These polymeric formulas are concentrated (2 kcal/cc) and contain reduced sodium, potassium and phosphorous loads. They are used in patients with acute renal failure requiring intermittent hemodialysis.

Total Parenteral Nutrition

TPN is used with increasing rarity in our patient population. Over 85% of our high risk patients ultimately tolerate enteral nutrition and do not require TPN. Indications for TPN include (a) massive small bowel resection [38], (b) high output fistulae, (c) documented intolerance to enteral feeding protocol (see Table 4), and (d) perceived high risk for NOBN including active shock resuscitation, use of high dose alpha-agonists, prCO2>90, and intermittent hemodialysis with hemodynamic instability. Continued usage of TPN is re-evaluated daily to limit overutilization. National guidelines for utilization of parenteral nutrition are published periodically [39].

Our support protocol guidelines dictate implementation of TPN on ICU day 8 if <60% of nutrient needs are being delivered enterally. Routine perioperative usage of parenteral nutrition in surgical patients has no demonstrated outcome advantage [30]. Standard amino acids are the only solutions employed due to the lack of evidence of enhanced clinical outcomes with highly priced, specialized formulas [40].

Enteral Access

Impaired gastric emptying is common in mechanically ventilated, critically ill patients [41]. Because early gastric feeding is not well tolerated in our patient population, we have developed a protocol to ensure that jejunal access is obtained early postinjury (see Fig. 3). NCJ is our preferred method of access in those patients who require an early laparotomy [42]. If an abbreviated laparotomy is required (e.g. unstable patient with dilutional coagulopathy), the NCJ can be placed during a subsequent operation, usually within the first 48 h after injury. For critically injured patients who do not undergo early laparotomy, enteral access is obtained by endoscopic placement of an 8-French nasobiliary tube in the first 36 h after injury [43, 44] by the ICU Procedure Team at the bedside [45]. This NJ tube can be used indefinitely, but, if the need for long term access becomes

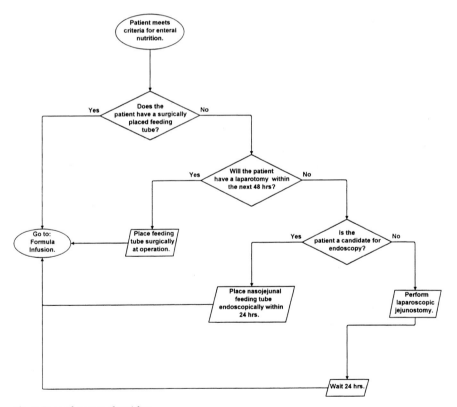

Fig. 3. Enteral access algorithm

apparent, it will be converted into a jejunal extension tube through a percutaneous endoscopic gastrostomy (PEG-J).

Infrequently, a patient may require enteral access yet, upper gastrointestinal endoscopy is contraindicated. In such patients a jejunostomy tube can be easily placed intraoperatively using laparoscopy [46].

Feeding Tube Maintenance

Physician and nurse responsibilities for care of the feeding tube, site maintenance, and tube removal are clearly delineated. A list of drugs that are suitable for delivery via a small bore feeding tube was compiled. Minimizing inappropriate drug delivery through the tubes, as well as routine tube flushing with 20 cc of water every 6 h, increases tube life. Still, the main weakness of the small bore jejunal tubes is the tendency to become occluded with formula. The long NJ tubes require replacement while NCJs can sometimes be disimpacted by flushing with a TB syringe. Kinking of the NCJ as it is passed through the abdominal wall is another cause of occlusion. This can be remedied by withdrawing the NCJ several centimeters.

Formula Advancement

Following shock resuscitation and after jejunal access has been established, full strength formula is infused at 15 cc per hour and advanced every 12 h in 15 cc increments, if there are no moderate or severe symptoms of intolerance. Once the rate of 60 cc hourly is achieved, the rate of formula infusion is advanced every 24 h until the goal specified by the dietitian is achieved.

Monitoring and Managing GI Tolerance

Enteral tolerance parameters are assessed and documented on an enteral tolerance flowsheet every 12 h by the bedside ICU nurse. Vomiting, cramping, distention, abdominal girth, tenderness, diarrhea and nasogastric output are recorded. The flowsheet is reviewed on morning and afternoon rounds by the team. The decision to advance the feeding per protocol, therefore, is based on the objective data. Table 5 provides management guidelines for stratified levels of enteral tolerance.

Directing the Nutritional Regimen

Protocol patients are evaluated by the ICU registered dietitian (RD) within 72 h of admission. The RD (a) confirms that the indications and formula selection are consistent with the protocol, (b) serves as an expert resource for the bedside nurse and physicians, (c) determines the ultimate infusion goal based on stress

Table 5. Managing enteral intolerance

Indicator	Severity	Definition	Treatment
Vomiting	Occurrence	1–4× times/12 h	Place NG suction catheter. Check existing NG function. Decrease rate by 50% if vomiting persists and notify primary team
Abdominal distentionand/or cramping, tenderness (if detectable)	Mild	Hx and/or PE	Maintain TF infusion rate. Repeat exam q 6 h. If indicators remain mild, advance TF per protocol
	Moderate	Hx and/or PE	Stop TF infusion. Order AP KUB supine X-ray. Assess for small bowel obstruction. If SBO, notify primary team. Place gastric tonometer NG catheter. Replace existing NG catheter if not tonometer. If PrCO$_2$ >70 and gap>30 notify primary team. Reexamine in 6 h
	Moderate >24 h or severe	Hx and/or PE	Stop TF infusion. Set IV fluid infusion rate at 250 cc/h. Notify primary team: consider CBC, lactate, ABGs, Chem7, CT scan abdomen
Diarrhea	Mild	1–2× per shift or 100–200 cc/12 h	Increase TF infusion rate per protocol
	Moderate	3–4× per shift or 200–300 cc/12 h	Maintain TF infusion rate. Reassess in 6 h: if mild or moderate, advance or maintain rate as per protocol
	Severe	>4× per shift or >300 cc/12 h	Decrease TF infusion rate by 50%. Give Lomotil 10 cc q6 h via feeding tube. Review medication profile: note antibiotics, prokinetic agents, sorbitol-containing elixirs. Stool studies: fecal leukocytes, toxin assays. If persists >48 h change to elemental TF
High NG output	Measured	>800 cc/12 h	Check existing X-ray for post-pyloric placement of feeding tube. If >48 h since last X-ray, order KUB. If not post-pyloric, notify primary team. Check NG aspirate for glucose. If glucose present notify primary team

level, anthropometric and clinical data, and (d) identifies the cases that merit discussion at weekly multidisciplinary nutrition rounds.

Total kilocalorie goals are initially set at 30 kcal/kg in normal weight patients, 20–25 kcal/kg of adjusted weight in obese individuals, and 40 kcal/kg in marasmic patients. Protein is targeted at 1.5–1.75 g/kg. The goals are continually refined based on clinical data, nitrogen balance, prealbumin and indirect calorimetry measurements.

Computerized Protocol

In concept, early enteral nutrition is a logical process based on specific patient requirements, currently accepted clinical measures of nutritional status, and integrated clinician knowledge of a patient's requirements, status and clinical course. Unfortunately, in practice, this process is difficult to implement. Its timely administration is often delayed for a variety of reasons (e.g. failure to obtain enteral access, need for secondary operations) as well as the lack of training and experience of the bedside clinicians.

To address this issue, we are developing a computerized protocol to enhance implementation of the practice guideline for early enteral nutrition [47, 48]. Based on our experience with the use of a computerized protocol for management of mechanical ventilation of patients with ARDS, we believe that a computerized protocol is feasible and offers a number of advantages compared to standard practice [49].

The process of early postinjury enteral nutrition is being described based on expert clinician (RD and intensivist) leadership, ongoing literature review, and working group consensus. The near term goal of protocol development is complete description of the process as detailed clinical flow chart logic, and implementation in the ICU according to agreed logical process rules. The long term goal is computerization of the clinical protocol logic to provide an automated standardized protocol to direct clinical decision making for the individual patient, and to record decision making, clinical status and progress. Ongoing modification and refinement of the protocol logic according to clinical findings, consensus, and incorporation of new monitors and techniques is intended.

Conclusions

(a) Early nutritional support offers clinical outcome benefits for patients sustaining major torso trauma. (b) The enteral route is preferred over the parenteral route. (c) Immune-enhancing formulas offer additional benefits over standard enteral formulas in severely injured patients. (d) Development of a multidisciplinary practice guideline for early enteral nutrition is a reasonable method to establish detailed consensus as to who will benefit from early enteral support, the type of access to pursue, guidelines for formula selection, monitoring, and management of intolerance, and the means to monitor the effectiveness of support. This guideline also serves as a teaching tool for multiple disciplines and computerization will enhance its efficient implementation in the complex ICU environment.

Acknowledgements. This work is supported by the National Institutes of Health Grant RO-1 GM559571-01.

References

1. Alexander JW, Macmillian BG, Stinnett JD, et al: Beneficial effects of aggressive protein feeding in severely burned children. Ann Surg 1980; 192 (4):505–517
2. Moore EE, Jones TN: Benefits of immediate jejunal feeding after major abdominal trauma – a prospective randomized study. J Trauma 1986; 26:874–883
3. Cerra FB: Hypermetabolism, organ failure, and metabolic support. Surgery 1987;101 (1):1–11
4. Moore FA, Moore EE, Jones, TN, McCroskey, BL, Peterson VM: TEN versus TPN following major abdominal trauma – reduced septic morbidity. J Trauma 1989; 29 (7):916–922
5. Kudsk KA, Croce MA, Fabian TC, et al: Enteral versus parenteral feeding: Effects on septic morbidity following blunt and penetrating abdominal trauma. Ann Surg 1992; 215 (5):503–511
6. Moore FA, Feliciano DV, Andrassy RJ, et al: Early enteral feeding, compared with parenteral, reduces postoperative septic complications – The results of a meta-analysis. Ann Surg 1992, 2169 (2):172–183
7. Wilmore DW, Shabert, JK.: Role of glutamine in immunologic responses. Nutrition 1998;14 (7–8):618–626
8. Barbul A, Lazarou SA, Efron DT, Wasserbrug HL, Efrom G et al: Arginine enhances wound healing and lymphocyte immune responses in humans. Surgery 1990; 108 (2):331–336
9. Alexander JW, Saito H, Trocki O, Ogle CK, et al: The importance of lipid type in the diet after burn injury. Ann Surg 1986; 204 (1):1–8
10. Van Buren CT, Kulkarni AD, Fanslow WC, Rudolph FBet al: Dietary nucleotides, a requirement for helper/inducer T lymphocytes. Transplantation 1985; 40 (6):694–697
11. Gottschlich MM, Jenkins M, Warden GD, et al: Differential effects of three enteral dietary regimens on selected outcome variables in burn patients. JPEN 1990;14 (3):225–236
12. Cerra FB, Lehman S, Konstantinides N, et al: Improvement in immune function in ICU patients by enteral nutrition supplemented with arginine, RNA and menhaden oil is independent of nitrogen balance. Nutrition 1991; 7 (3):193–199
13. Daly JM, Liberman MD, Goldfine J, et al: Enteral nutrition with supplemental arginine, RNA and omega-3 fatty acids in patients after operation: Immunologic, metabolic and clinical outcome. Surgery 1992;112 (1):56–67
14. Brown RO, Hunt H, Mowatt-Larssen CA, Wojtysiak SL, Henningfield MF, Kudsk KA Comparison of specialized and standard enteral formulas in trauma patients. Pharmacotherapy 1994; 14 (3):314–320
15. Moore FA, Moore EE, Kudsk KA, et al. : Clinical benefits of an immune-enhancing diet for early postinjury enteral feeding. J Trauma 1994; 37 (4):607–615
16. Bower RH, Cerra FB, Bershadsky B, et al: Early enteral administration of a formula supplemented with arginine, nucleotides, and fish oil in intensive care unit patients: Results of a multicenter, prospective, randomized clinical trial. Crit Care Med 1995; 23 (3):436–449
17. Daly JM, Weintraub FN, Shou J, Rosato EF, Lucia M: Enteral nutrition during multimodality therapy in upper gastrointestinal cancer patients. Ann Surg 1995; 221 (4):327–338
18. Kudsk KA, Minard G, Croce MA, et al: A randomized trial of isonitrogenous enteral diets following severe trauma: An immune-enhancing diet reduces septic complications. Ann Surg 1996; 224 (4):531–540

19. Senkal M, Mumme A, Eickhoff U, et al: Early postoperative enteral immunonutrition: Clinical outcome and cost-comparison analysis in surgical patients. Crit Care Med 1997;25 (9)1489–1496

20. Braga M, Gianotti L, Vignali A, Gestari A, Bisagni P, Carlo Vet al: Artificial nutrition after major abdominal surgery: Impact of route of administration and composition of the diet. Crit Care Med 1998;26:24–30

21. Atkinson S, Sieffert E, Bihari D: A prospective, randomized, double-blind, controlled clinical trial of enteral immunonutrition in the critically ill. Crit Care Med 1998; 26 (7):1164–1172

22. Weimann A, Bastian, L, Bischoff WE: Influence of arginine, omega-3 fatty acids and nucleotide-supplemented enteral support on systemic inflammatory response syndrome and multiple organ failure in patients after severe trauma. Nutrition 1998;14 (2):165–72

23. Fry DE, Pearlstein L, Fulton RL, Polk HC: Multiple system organ failure: The role of uncontrolled infection. Arch Surg 1980; 115 (2):136–140

24. McArdle AH, Palmason C, Morency I, Brown RA: A rationale for enteral feeding as the preferable route for hyperalimentation. Surgery 1981; 90:616–623

25. Mochizuki H, Trocki O, Dominioni L, Brackett KA, Joffe SN, Alexander JW: Mechanism of prevention of postburn hypermetabolism and catabolism by early enteral feeding. Ann Surg 1984; 200: 297–310

26. Kudsk KA, Carpenter G, Peterson SR, Sheldon GF: Effect of enteral and parenteral feeding in malnourished rats with hemoglobin – E. coli adjuvant peritonitis. J Surg Res 1981;31 (2):105–110

27. Alverdy J, Chi HS, Sheldon GF: The effect of parenteral nutrition on gastrointestinal immunity: The importance of enteral stimulation. Ann Surg 1985; 202 (6):681–684

28. Lowry SF: The route of feeding influences injury responses. J Trauma 1990; 30 (12 Suppl):S10–15

29. Kudsk KA, Li J, Renegar KB: Loss of upper respiratory tract immunity with parenteral feeding. Ann Surg 1996; 223 (6):629–35

30. Veterans Affair Total Parenteral Cooperative Study Group: Perioperative total parenteral nutrition in surgical patients. N Engl J Med 1991;325 (8):525–532

31. Sandstrom R, Drott C, Hyltander A, et al: The effect of postoperative intravenous feeding (TPN) on outcome following major surgery evaluated in a randomized study. Ann Surg 1993; 217 (2):185–195

32. Brennan MF, Pisters PWT, Posner M, Quesada O, Shike M: A prospective randomized trial of total parenteral nutrition after major pancreatic resection for malignancy. Ann Surg 1994; 220 (4):436–441

33. Bell SJ, Mascioli EA, Bistrian BR, Babayan VK, Blackburn GL: Alternative lipid sources for enteral and parenteral nutrition: long and medium-chain triglycerides, structured triglycerides, and fish oils. J Am Diet Assoc 1991 91 (1):74–8

34. Mendez C, Jurkovich GJ, Garcia I, Davis D, Parker A, Maier RV: Effects of an immune-enhancing diet in critically injured patients. J Trauma 1997;42 (5):933–940

35. Saffle JR, Wiebke G, Jennings K, Morris SE, Barton RG: Randomized trial of immune-enhancing enteral nutrition in burn patients. J Trauma 1997;42:793–800

36. Clemmer TP, Spuhler VJ.: Developing and gaining acceptance for patient care protocols. New Horizons 1998; 6 (1):12–19

37. Marvin RG, McKinley BA, McQuiggan MM, Cocanour CS, Moore FA: Nonocclusive bowel necrosis in critically ill trauma patients receiving enteral nutrition manifests no reliable clinical signs for early detection. Am J Surg (in press)

38. Dudrick SJ, Latifi R, Fosnocht DE: Management of the short bowel syndrome. Surg Clin No Am 71 (3):625–43

39. ASPEN (1993) Guidelines for the use of parenteral and enteral nutrition in adult patients. JPEN 17 (4 Supp):1SA-26SA

40. Heyman MB: General and specialized parenteral amino acid formulations for nutrition support. J Am Diet Assoc 1990;90 (3):401–8:411–416

41. Heyland DK, Tougas G, King D, Cook DJ: Impaired gastric emptying in mechanically venti-lated, critically ill patients. Intensive Care Med 1996;22 (12):1339–44
42. Myers JG, Page, CP, Steward, RM, Schwesinger WH, Sirinek KR, Aust JB:Complications of needle catheter jejunostomy in 2,022 consecutive applications. Amer J Surg 1995;170 (6):547–550
43. Coates NE, MacFadyen BV: Endoscopic jejunal access for enteral feeding. Am J Surg 1995; 169 (6):627–628
44. Reed RL, Eachempati SR, Russell MK, Fahkry C: Endoscopic placement of jejunal feeding catheters in critically ill patients by a push technique. J Trauma 1998;45 (2):388–393
45. Marvin RG, Moore FA, Cocanour CS, et al: Implementation of a procedure team improves utilization and reduces cost for critically ill patients in the ICU. J Trauma 1998; 44:425
46. Duh QY, Way LW: Laparoscopic jejunostomy using T-fasteners as retractors and anchors. Arch Surg 1993; 128 (1):105–108
47. Morris AH: Algorithm based decision making. Principles and Practice of Intensive Care Monitoring. Tobin MJ (Ed). New York, McGraw-Hill,1997:1355–1381
48. East TD, Morris AH, Wallace CJ, et al: A strategy for development of computerized critical care decision support systems. Int J Clin Mon it Comput 1992;8 (4):263–269
49. Morris AH: Protocol management of adult respiratory distress syndrome. New Horizons 1993; 1 (4):593–602

Nutritional Support in Neurologic Injury

A.P. Borzotta

Introduction

Neurologic injuries severe enough to require admission to a critical care unit include blunt and penetrating trauma and cerebrovascular accidents. Such patients will require the physician's attention to nutritional support for weeks to months before they are able to resume adequate spontaneous oral intake. Traumatic brain injury induces systemic metabolic changes marked by hypermetabolism, hypercatabolism, the acute phase response, decreased immunocompetence and altered gastrointestinal function. Stroke patients are usually elderly, 6%–31% have pre-existing nutritional deficits [1–3], and undernutrition often worsens during the hospital stay [3, 4]. Unfortunately, limited information exists concerning the acute metabolic changes due to stroke, a situation resembling the state of knowledge concerning metabolism and nutritional support of brain injured patients circa 1980. The ability to self-feed may be affected by paralysis of limbs, cognitive deficits, and dysphagia. These problems can be identified in the ICU and anticipated to be part of the patient's long-term course [5].

In both brain injury and stroke, the clinical impact of inadequate or improper nutritional support is measured in terms of decubiti, pneumonia, mortality, prolonged rehabilitation and possibly diminished cognitive recovery. While there are insufficient data to support a nutritional treatment standard [6], appropriate use of guidelines requires understanding how systemic changes are related to the severity of injury, the different stages of recovery, the utilization of substrates and the choice of a route of delivery. This chapter will define the metabolic effects of traumatic brain injury and stroke, review information on protein and energy substrate utilization in neurotrauma, examine the rationales for different routes of nutrient delivery, and discuss the impact of feeding on neurologic outcome.

The Metabolic Response to Severe Brain Injury

Brain injury induces an acute-phase response manifested by fever, leukocytosis, negative nitrogen balance, increased synthesis of acute-phase proteins, and altered serum mineral levels [7]. These responses are not solely attributable to multiple injury, craniotomy, steroid therapy, patient movement, infections or nutritional support. Multiple mediators interact, including cytokines, counter-

regulatory hormones, and sympathetic hyperactivity. The subject has been extensively reviewed [8, 9].

The cytokines interleukin-1 (IL-1), interleukin-6 (IL-6) and tumor necrosis
factor (TNF) have important roles in the metabolic response to brain injury. IL-1
is produced by brain glial cells as well as monocytes, and is found in injured portions of the brain in experimental head injury in rats [8]. IL-1 causes fever, accelerated synthesis of acute phase reactants, neutrophilia, and altered peripheral
muscle protein metabolism. Compared to systemic administration, intracere-
broventricular delivery of IL-1 has enhanced biological potency, suggesting that
there is a unique site of action for cytokines within the brain. Interleukin-1 and
interleukin-6 (IL-6) levels are elevated in ventricular fluid following brain injury,
and plasma IL-6 levels remain significantly increased for weeks [9]. These data
strongly indicate both local and systemic roles for brain-injury related cytokine
release.

Brain injury causes increased levels of blood and urine catecholamines, blood
glucagon and blood cortisol. The increases are inversely related to the severity of
brain injury, as defined by the Glasgow Coma Scale score [10], paralleling the clinical observation of an inverse relationship of hypermetabolism and GCS [8, 9, 11].
Feldman et al. [10] found a significant positive association between catecholamine excretion, elevated measured resting energy expenditure (MREE) and
negative nitrogen balance. By the end of the second week postinjury, negative
nitrogen balance was more closely associated with urinary cortisol excretion.
When given as part of brain injury management, methylprednisolone increases
nitrogen excretion up to 30% compared to no steroid treatment but does not
increase metabolic rates [12].

The influence of sympathetic hyperactivity in the hypermetabolic state of
brain injury is deducible from the elevated catecholamine levels in patients with
decerebrate posturing [11], the reduction of MREE either by treatment with the
beta blocking drug propranolol [13] or induction of barbiturate coma [14]. Thus,
neuroendocrine influences, cytokines, the severity of injury and certain therapies
jointly shape the metabolic response to brain injury, which changes over time.

Nutritional Requirements

Caloric Requirements in Severe Traumatic Brain Injury

Head injury increases energy expenditure an average of 40% above predicted
basal energy expenditure (BEE), varying from 130%–250% of that expected [6, 7,
11, 15, 16]. The wide variation is due to age, gender, spontaneous motor activity or
posturing, fever, severity of injury, therapies, and changes in the systemic
response to injury over time. In children and adolescents, the increases range
from 110%–176%, similar to changes in adults [17]. Hypermetabolism increases
with lower Glasgow Coma Scale scores [10, 11, 15], posturing, and time postinjury,
peaking in 2 weeks but lasting for 5 weeks or more (Fig. 1). Several authors [6, 8,
9, 14] have shown that either neuromuscular blockade or barbiturate induced
coma decreases energy expenditure to between 100% and 125% of predicted BEE.

While random or localizing movements do not significantly alter energy expenditure, posturing increases caloric utilization by 20% [10].

BEE can be estimated to begin writing a nutritional prescription. The Harris-Benedict equation for basal energy expenditure (BEE) is the usual starting point for estimation, requiring only gender, age, height and weight for calculation:
- Males: BEE=66.5+(13.8×weight [kg])+(5×height [cm]) – (6.8×age)
- Females: BEE=655+(9.6×weight [kg])+(1.8×height [cm]) – (4.7×age)

The BEE must be multiplied by a stress factor to estimate the calories needed or resting metabolic expenditure (RME): 1.4 is recommended [6]. Clifton et al. published a nomogram based upon a multiple regression analysis of 312 measurements over 2 weeks in 57 patients, which incorporates Glasgow Coma Scale score, heart rate and day since injury [15]:
- GCS equal to or less than 7:db/spp%RME=152–14 (GCS)+0.4 (HR)+7 (DSI)
- GCS greater than 7:db/spp%RME=90–3 (GCS)+0.9 (HR).

However, Sunderland and Heilbrun [18] found that 42% of such calculated values were outside the range of 75%–125% of values measured by indirect calorimetry, representing a significant risk for overfeeding or underfeeding. They concluded that indirect calorimetry should be the standard for the precise determination of caloric needs [6, 18].

Indirect calorimeters are bedside devices which measure oxygen consumption through a ventilator circuit or by using a hood in free-breathing patients. Based upon the known caloric yield of consuming 1 l oxygen, the calorimeter yields a value, termed measured resting energy expenditure (MREE). These devices are not universally available, and require skilled technical support and some inter-

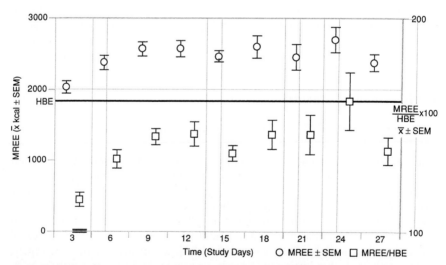

Fig. 1. Energy profile: ENT and TPN combined. *Circles* combined MREE data from 59 patients with severe head injury randomized to enteral or TPN feeding within 72 h of admission. It averages 2600 kcal/day by day 9, persisting for 4 weeks. The MREE/BEE is about 1.45

pretation of values before the MREE is applied. Brief measurements are as reliable as 24 h measurements in stable patients [19], but episodes of fever, agitation or posturing will increase the actual energy expenditure beyond that measured at rest, requiring an adjustment in the prescribed calories to be delivered. Some centers add 10% to the MREE to compensate for interruptions in the delivery of enteral feeding.

Caloric Requirements After Stroke

Data is limited. Davalos et al. [20] used indirect calorimetry to determine MREE in 46 patients with an acute stroke. Normally nourished patients required 1580–1706 kcal a day, while malnourished patients had an admission MREE of 1064 kcal which rose to 1680 kcal/d in 1 week. Nutritional parameters deteriorated despite feeding an excess of calories compared to MREE, indicating the existence of a moderately hypercatabolic state following cerebrovascular accident.

Protein Requirements

Nitrogen losses increase steadily after brain injury, peaking in the second week and remaining elevated throughout hospitalization [7, 11, 16, 21] (Fig. 2). Deutschman et al. reported decreasing excretion after only 7 days, but those patients were not fed [22]. Multi-system injuries slightly but not significantly increase nitrogen excretion [16, 22]. Nitrogen losses are rarely balanced by pro-

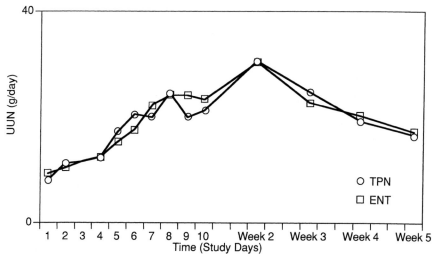

Fig. 2. Urine urea nitrogen (UUN) excretion. Nitrogen losses following severe brain injury are 10 g/day on admission, doubling in little over 1 week and reaching a peak of 30 g/day in 2 weeks postinjury, in a group of aggressively fed patients (nitrogen replacement goal of UUN+4 g nitrogen, or 2.5 g protein/kg/day)

tein feeding, although intake up to 2.2 g/kg/day is more effective than 1.5 g/kg/day [24]. This is due to an increase in the percentage of calories derived from protein after head injury from 10%–15% to values as high as 30% [21]. Increasing the percentage of total calories derived from protein from 14%–22% improves nitrogen balance [25]. While these losses are not diminished by nonprotein calories, even when intake is double the BEE [26], nitrogen balance is enhanced by providing adequate energy substrate.

Branched chain amino acid enriched TPN promotes positive nitrogen balance compared to a standard formula [27], but numerous studies in other areas of illness have not shown an important clinical benefit of branched chain amino acids. Administration of growth hormone to immobilized patients with head injury or spinal cord injury increases transferrin and albumin levels, but does not improve nitrogen balance [28].

Routes of Delivery

Total Parenteral Nutrition

Nutritional support by intravenous infusion can be started almost immediately after resuscitation. The concern that hyperosmolar solutions may potentiate cerebral edema was prospectively studied in 96 patients randomized within 48 h postinjury to receive either TPN or NG feeding [29]. No difference was found in peak daily intracranial pressure (ICP), the frequency of failure of standard therapy to control ICP, peak serum osmolality, or mortality. Peak serum glucose was higher with TPN for the first 2 weeks, compared to enteral feeding.

It is known that hyperglycemia at the time of admission worsens neurologic outcome. Peak blood glucose levels above 200 mg/dl in the first 24 h postinjury are associated with less favorable Glasgow Outcome Scale scores at 18 days, 3 months and 1 year [30]. In a mild cortical impact animal model of brain injury, glucose administration increased injury only when a secondary ischemic insult was introduced. When ischemia occurs at the time of impact in a severe contusion model, existing hyperglycemia worsened injury, but postinjury glucose infusion had no effect on contusion volume [31]. The conclusion can be drawn that TPN is safe and effective for the early introduction of nutritional support. However, early combined TPN-enteral feeding had no beneficial effect on nitrogen balance compared to TPN alone [32]. TPN-related hyperglycemia developing some time after admission may still be deleterious, especially if associated with hypotension, increased ICP or other causes of brain ischemia. Further data are needed regarding these late associations.

Enteral Nutritional Support

It is essential to read the literature on enteral nutritional support with close regard to the actual site of deposition of nutrients, which may be usefully characterized as prepyloric (gastric) or postpyloric (jejunal). Prepyloric feeding routes includes nasogastric (NG) tubes and all forms of gastrostomy, while postpyloric feeding includes percutaneous gastrojejunostomy, operative and laparoscopic jejunostomy. Duodenal feeding through nasoduodenal tubes can be achieved, but the tubes are plagued by dislodgement into the stomach and some reflux of feedings [8]. The distinctions are important because of the gastrointestinal changes brought on by brain injury. Lower esophageal sphincter pressure is diminished allowing increased gastroesophageal reflux for at least 1–2 weeks postinjury [33]. Gastric atony is not universal, but is severe enough to preclude effective gastric feeding in half of patients for up to 11 days [34]. Some greater success with NG feeding can be achieved if gastric residual volumes of 200 ml are accepted, but there is theoretically an increased risk of aspiration.

Gastrostomy tubes can be placed during laparotomy, by laparoscopic methods, percutaneously under either fluoroscopic (PFG) or endoscopic (PEG) control. All avoid the nuisance of a transnasal tube, the need for nasal septal bridles or repeated insertion and chest radiographs, and interruptions in feeding. A smaller tube can be passed within the gastrostomy tube into the proximal jejunum (PEGJ). Some kits allow simultaneous gastric decompression, while others fully occupy the gastric tube lumen.

An essential technique to maintain long-term small-bore jejunal tube patency is to irrigate it every 3 days with the following recipe: 30 ml water+1 pancreatic enzyme tablet+1 bicarbonate tablet, allowing 10 ml to stay in the tube 10 min until the total is used. This has completely done away with tube blockage at our institution.

Since 40%–85% of brain injured patients will continue to need enteral feeding after hospital discharge [16, 35], ICU decision making should take into account the long-term course of care. PEG allows increased feeding efficiency compared to NG tubes [36] and the improved nutrient delivery is associated with improved neurologic function in stroke patients [37]. Gastrostomy tube feeding is often preferred to nasogastric tubes by extended care facilities [38]. Although Hiebert et al. [39] found that continuous gastric feeding reduces the risk of distention and aspiration, Cogan et al. [40] found no difference between continuous and intermittent gastric feeding. An essential point in the transition from continuous to intermittent feeding may be the rate of delivery of the feeding bolus. Rapid infusions decrease lower esophageal sphincter pressure and are associated with scintigraphic reflux up to the sternal notch not seen with slower infusions [41]. Both gastric and jejunal feeding tolerance may be altered by sepsis, electrolyte imbalance, opiates and barbiturate coma. Careful surveillance for increased gastric residuals, abdominal distention or cramp must occur in the face of altered drug therapy or onset of complications.

Nutrient Administration and Outcome

Morbidity and Mortality Outcomes After Traumatic Brain Injury

Little attention was paid to the early nutritional support of brain injured patients until the 1980s. Rapp et al. [42] randomly assigned 38 severely head injured patients to receive TPN or NG tube feedings. Over the 18-day study period, TPN patients received a mean of 1750 kcal/day and 10.2 g N/day, reaching their target levels in 7 days. The NG group's mean intake was 685 kcal/day and 4.0 g N/day, with a significant number failing to tolerate feedings for over a week. This study, essentially a comparison of hypocaloric TPN versus early starvation, is important for showing that the consequence of severe undernutrition is an increased mortality rate: eight died in the NG group and none in the TPN group. Seven deaths were due to sepsis, indicating the deleterious role of delayed nutritional support on immunocompetence.

In a small study concerned with the effect of timing of nutritional support upon immune function, nine head injured patients began TPN early (day 1) or late (day 5). After a week, the early group had increased CD4 cells, CD4-CD8 ratios and T-lymphocyte response to mitogens [43]. While an early start seems important, total calories delivered is also key. Hoyt et al. [44] began nutrition within 48 h postinjury, but the feedings were hypocaloric (mean <1300 kcal/day) and all patients remained anergic to a battery of skin antigen tests. Lymphocyte function was depressed in terms of CD4 expression and mitogen stimulation [44].

Hadley and associates [45] randomized 45 patients to initiate TPN or NG feeding within 48 h of injury. Caloric balance (146% of BEE) was achieved slowly: 9 days for TPN and 12 for the NG group. Although average nitrogen intake was higher in the TPN group (13.1 gN/d vs. 11.4 gN/d; $P<0.01$), no difference occurred in serum albumin levels, weight loss, or infectious morbidity. In a prospective, randomized comparison of TPN versus NG feeding in 51 head-injured patients, the NG group benefited from refinements in enteral nutritional delivery, but 36% still crossed over to parenteral support by day 7 postinjury due to gastroparesis [29]. The TPN group received significantly more prescribed calories (75.6% vs. 59%; $P=0.02$) and protein (1.35 vs. 0.91 g protein/kg/day; $P=0.004$). The groups did not differ in serum albumin, lymphocyte count or delayed hypersensitivity skin test responses, mortality or infectious morbidity. However, the 11 patients who did not tolerate NG feedings for a week had a significantly higher incidence of septic shock. Delay of a week or longer before starting some kind of nutritional support is clearly associated with increased infectious morbidity and death.

The minimum caloric intake to preclude such complications is less clear. In a post hoc analysis of ten patients by Waters et al. [46], those receiving a mean of 38% of MREE had no greater infectious morbidity than those receiving 91% of MREE. In a recent study of 59 patients randomized to start either TPN or jejunal feeding within 72 h of injury, nutrient delivery was pushed to a target rate of 120% of MREE within 60 h of onset of feeding. Delivered calories and protein were equivalent, and no differences in infectious morbidity were found [16]. Together, these studies indicate that nutritional support begun within 48–72 h of injury by either the parenteral or jejunal route, delivering a minimum of 40% of MREE and at least 1 g N/kg/day by the seventh post injury day, will reduce septic morbidity compared to delayed and/or inadequate feeding. Goals of 140% BEE for calories and 1.5 gN/kg/day can be reliably achieved using either TPN or jejunal feeding within the same time frame.

Neurological Outcomes After Traumatic Brain Injury

Several studies report improvements in neurologic recovery associated with early, adequate nutritional support. Young et al. [29] found that earlier onset of feeding and better delivery of planned substrate support by TPN compared to NG feeding resulted in a more rapid increase in GCS scores at 18 days and higher scores at 3 months but not at 6 or 12 months of follow-up. In a small series of ten patients, those with lesser caloric deficits also had better neurologic outcomes [46]. We prospectively assessed cognitive recovery in 23 patients randomized to TPN and 36 to jejunal feeding, and found significantly higher Western Neurosensory Stimulation Profile scores at discharge, and a trend ($P=0.07$) toward higher Rancho los Amigos scores in the enterally fed group [47]. The difference was not related to infection rates, delivery of calories or nitrogen, or injury severity. A possible explanation lay in a greater delivery of certain micronutrients in the enteral formulation compared to the parenteral formulation: one was zinc. Young et al. [48] prospectively randomized 68 patients with severe head injuries to receive standard (2.5 mg) or supplemental (12 mg) zinc. Although serum zinc concentrations did not differ, and the supplemented group had higher urine zinc excretion, there appeared to be net zinc retention in the supplemented group. By analysis of covariance, the supplemented group had a significantly higher mean GCS score on day 28 compared to the standard group. However, Choi and Koh [49] warn that zinc may contribute to neuronal death in ischemic and other forms of brain injury.

The studies suggest that early, aggressive nutritional support, particularly feeding into the gastrointestinal tract, may favorably influence cognitive recovery. The role of micronutrients requires study using more refined cognitive tests than GCS or GOS.

Morbidity and Mortality Outcome After Stroke

Information is much more limited concerning the influence of nutritional support on outcomes in stroke patients, particularly during the critical illness phase of stroke. Just as in head injury prior to the late 1980s, there seems to be a tolerance for starvation and/or inadequate feeding of stroke patients. This tolerance effects both short-term, acute hospitalization results and the long-term rehabilitation of stroke patients.

Norton et al. [38] randomized 30spp comatose patients 14 days after acute stroke to NG or gastrostomy tube feedings. Gastrostomy fed patients showed greater improvement in serum albumin levels (+0.3 vs. –0.9 g/dl; $P<0.03$), midarm circumference (+1 vs. –3 cm; $P<0.03$), weight gain (2.2 vs. -2.6 kg; $P<0.03$), and lower six-week mortality (13% vs. 57%; $P<0.05$). Finally, 37% of gastrostomy fed patients were discharged home, compared to none fed by NG tube. The differences were felt to be due to a reduction in aspiration induced bronchopneumonia and more consistent delivery of nutrients via gastrostomy. In a retrospective review of 52 patients, those fed within 72 h of admission had a hospital length of stay of 20.1 ± 12.9 days, compared to 29.8 ± 20 days ($P=0.036$) in those fed later by

Nyswonger and associates [1]. Earlier feeding continued to influence length of stay for patients admitted to a rehabilitation program (18 vs. 25.3 days) or an extended care facility (23.2 vs. 34.7 days). Increased length of stay was associated with pneumonia, ventilator dependence, urinary tract infections, and decubitus ulcers needing operation, all variables influenced by nutritional support. In 1998, Gariballa et al. [50] randomized 42 acute ischemic stroke inpatients without dysphagia to receive sip supplementation within 1 week of admission. Energy intake was significantly greater in the supplemented group (1807 vs 1084 kcal/day; $P<0.001$), as was protein intake (65.1 vs 44.1 g/day; $P<0.001$). There was a trend to lower mortality in the supplemented group at 3 months (10% vs 35%; $P=0.127$), and clinically modest but statistically significant better serum albumin and iron levels.

In a retrospective look at 37 patients receiving percutaneous gastrostomy a median of 26 days after stroke (range 12–131), Wanklyn et al. [51] found a high incidence of complications, and only 12 patients survived more than 3 months. These poor results are likely related to early experience with PEG and progressive malnutrition due to excessive delay in securing enteral access. Park et al. [52] randomized 40 stable patients with neurological dysphagia to receive gastric feeding via NG or PEG tubes. Treatment failure occurred in 94% of NG fed patients (tube displacement×3, blockage, failure to place, patient refusal) versus none of PEG patients. NG fed patients received significantly less prescribed feeding (55% vs. 93%; $P<0.001$), and tolerated the tube less well (mean 5.2 days vs. 28 days). When acute stroke patients enter a rehabilitation program, the most potentially modifiable outcome relating to length of stay and functional outcome is malnutrition [5]. Attention to nutritional support during the acute hospitalization for stroke will likely reduce morbidity, positively influence the patient's speed of recovery, timeliness of discharge and later course in a rehabilitation program [3]. These hypotheses need to be demonstrated in clinical studies in stroke patients.

Dysphagia, Aspiration, and Routes of Delivery

Head injured and stroke patients may have trouble swallowing and/or inadequate protective airway reflexes. Oropharyngeal dysphagia within 3 days of stroke is associated with significantly increased risk of chest infection [53]. Although most patients recover within a week, mortality increases if swallowing problems are present, even without an altered level of consciousness [53]. In a prospective study of three levels of speech therapist intervention for stabilized, alert but dysphagic stroke patients, DePippo et al. [54] found no significant difference between the groups in the incidence of pneumonia, dehydration or calorie-nitrogen deficit. Limited patient and family instruction regarding diet modification and compensatory swallowing techniques was as effective as therapist control of diet and daily training sessions. Although often mentioned as a standard assessment tool in dysphagia [55], studies of videofluoroscopy did not find that it added useful information to bedside assessment by therapists [53, 54].

Pneumonia may follow aspiration of oral secretions, gastric juice or tube feedings. It is often difficult to distinguish among them, even with use of dyed tube feedings or glucose testing of tracheal secretions. This difficulty in definition and recognition is part of the reason reported rates of aspiration vary from 2% to 95% [55]. Lower rates of pneumonia are found in some [30] but not all [16, 45] comparisons of TPN to enteral feeding in brain injured patients. Traumatic brain injury decreases lower esophageal sphincter tone for up to 2 weeks, permitting gastroesophageal reflux [33]. The presence of an NG tube will also increase gastroesophageal reflux [41]. Coupled with delayed gastric emptying, which may take 7–14 days to return to normal [8, 34, 42, 45], it seems logical to reduce the risk of aspiration pneumonia by avoiding intragastric delivery of feedings by any route. No episodes of gastroduodenal reflux followed percutaneous gastrojejunostomy in one multicenter study [56]. Compared to gastric feeding, significantly fewer pneumonias occur after PEGJ in patients with brain injury [57] or critical illness [58]. PEGJ can be safely done within three postinjury days, causing no significant acute or sustained increase in intracranial pressure [59]. Table 1 summarizes the advantages and disadvantages of parenteral and enteral access routes for nutritional support.

Conclusions

Nutritional support should begin within 72 h of admission following severe brain injury, and probably in stroke patients rendered paraplegic, dysphagic or in those with pre-existing malnutrition (Fig. 3). The preferred route is percutaneous endoscopic gastrojejunostomy due to its safety, high success rate, durability and adaptability over time. When gastric motility resumes and protective airway reflexes return, the jejunal catheter can be removed, allowing either continuous or bolus intragastric feeding. This system is useful for weeks to years (the later requiring device changes, perhaps to skin level gastrostomy buttons). It is usually not necessary to begin nutritional support with TPN, to combine TPN and enteral feeding, or to delay PEGJ except for clarification of immediate survivability.

The energy substrate goal should be 140% of estimated BEE (Harris-Benedict equation×1.4) or, whenever available, directed by indirect calorimetry at regular intervals. The nitrogen goal should be a minimum of 1.5 g protein/kg/day, and may be increased to as much as 2.5 g protein/kg/day as directed by weekly urine urea nitrogen measurements. There is no clear data supporting the use of any particular formulation of TPN or enteral feedings in brain injury or stroke. Last, we recommend that continuous jejunal feeding via PEGJ be coupled with early tracheostomy and that reintroduction of oral feeding be under the guidance of a speech therapist.

Table 1. Selecting a route for nutrition support (LES lower esophageal sphincter)

Route	Advantage	Disadvantage
Parenteral	Easy to initiate Advance to goal in <48 h Highly protocolized	Pneumothorax Catheter sepsis Expensive Gut disuse/bacterial translocation? Acalculous cholecystitis
Oral diet	Low cost Full digestive processes Maintains gut integrity	Delayed weeks–months Limited by dysphagia Requires full physical and cognitive integration
Nasogastric tubes	Low cost Universally available Accepts all diets Maintains gut integrity	Requires gastric emptying Pharyngeal dysfunction Alters LES function Pulmonary feeding Dislodgment problems Patient discomfort/refusal
Nasoduodenal tubes	Low cost Does not require gastric emptying (as for NG tubes)	Displacement to stomach (as for NG tubes)
Gastrostomy	Multiple techniques for placement Bypasses pharynx and LES Good patient tolerance	Wound dehiscence Local infections No definite decrease in aspiration rates Dislodgement
Jejunostomy	Bypasses pharynx, LES and pylorus Uninterrupted delivery of nutrients Does not require gastric emptying Less aspiration pneumonia Good patient tolerance	Operating room procedure Wound dehiscence Local infections Tube blockage Dislodgement
Percutaneous endoscopic gastrojejunostomy	Bedside procedure (as for jejunostomy)	Local infections Displacement to stomach Tube blockage

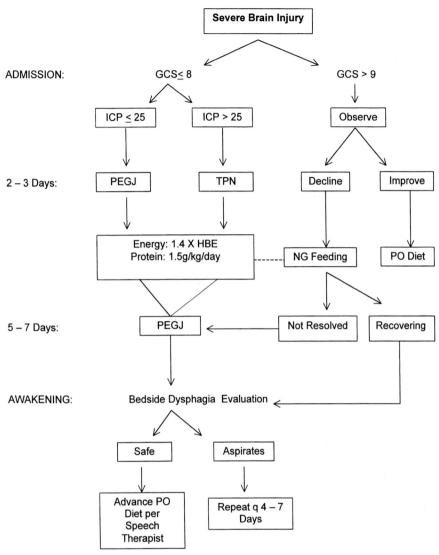

Fig. 3. Algorithm outlining the acute and long-term nutritional support of patients with severe brain injury. Initiation of feeding should begin within 72 h postinjury, preferably by PEGJ, although many physicians are more comfortable using TPN for patients with elevated ICP. Less injured patients who decline should have a definitive support decision made by the end of the first postinjury week. As patients awaken, swallowing safety should be assessed prior to initiation of oral feeding, and enteral feeding should be decreased until patients demonstrate a defined capacity to take in adequate nourishment

References

1. Bullock R, Chesnut RM, Clifton G et al. (1996) Nutritional support of brain-injured patients J Neurotrauma 13:721–729
2. Nyswonger GD, Helmchen RH (1992) Early enteral nutrition and length of stay in stroke patients J Neurosci Nsg 24:220–223
3. Axelsson K, Asplund K, Norberg A, Alafuzoff I (1988) Nutritional status in patients with acute stroke Acta Med Scand 224:217–224, 1988
4. Davalos A, Ricart W, Gonzalez-Huix F, Soler S et al. (1996) Effect of malnutrition after acute stroke on clinical outcome Stroke 27:1028–1032
5. Unosson M, Ek A-C, Bjurulf P, von Schenck H, Larsson J (1994) Feeding dependence and nutritional status after acute stroke Stroke 25:366–371
6. Finestone HM, Greene-Finestone LS, Wilson ES, Teasell RW (1996) Prolonged length of stay and reduced functional improvement rate in malnourished stroke rehabilitation patients Arch Phys Med Rehabil 77:340–345
7. Young B, Ott L, Norton J et al. (1985) Metabolic and nutritional sequelae in the non-steroid treated head injury patient Neurosurgery 17:784–791
8. Ott L, McClain C, Young B (1989) Nutrition and severe brain injury Nutrition 5:75–79
9. Young B, Ott L, Yingling B, McClain C (1992) Nutrition and brain injury J Neurotrauma 9:S375–383
10. Feldman Z, Contant CF, Pahwa R et al. (1993) The relationship between hormonal mediators and systemic hypermetabolism after severe head injury J Trauma 34:806–812
11. Robertson CS, Clifton GL, Grossman RG (1984) Oxygen utilzation and cardiovascular function in head-injured patients Neurosurgery 15:307–314
12. Robertson CS, Clifton GL, Goodman JC (1985) Steroid administration and nitrogen excretion in the head injured patient J Neurosurgery 63:714–718
13. Chiolero RL, Beitenstein E, Thorin D et al. (1989) Effects of propranolol on resting metabolic rate after severe head injury Crit Care Med 17:328-
14. Gadisseux P, Ward JD, Young HF (1984) Nutrition and the neurosurgical patient J Neurosurgery 60:219–232
15. Clifton GL, Robertson CS, Choi SC (1986) Assessment of nutritional requirements of head-injured patients J Neurosurg 64:895–901
16. Borzotta AP, Pennings J, Papasadero B et al. (1994) Enteral versus parenteral nutrition after severe closed head injury J Trauma 37:459–468
17. Phillips R, Ott L, Young BA, Walsh J (1987) Nutritional support and measured energy expenditure of the child and adolescent with head injury J Neurosurg 67:846–851
18. Sunderland PM, Heilbrun MP (1992) Estimating energy expenditure in traumatic brain injury: Comparison of indirect calorimetry with predictive formulas Neurosurg 31:246–253
19. Weekes E, Elia M (1996) Observations on the patterns of 24-h energy expenditure changes in body composition and gastric emptying in head-injured patients receiving nasogastric tube feeding J Parent Enter Nutr 20:31–37
20. Davalos A, Ricart W, Gonzalez-Huix F et al. (1996) Effect of malnutrition after acute stroke on clinical outcome Stroke 27:1028–1032
21. Clifton GL, Robertson CS, Grossman RG, Hodge S, Foltz R and Garza C (1984) The metabolic response to severe head injury J Neurosurg 60:687–696
22. Deutschman CS, Konstantinides FN, Raup S, Thienprasit P, Cerra FB (1986) Physiological and metabolic response to isolated closed-head injury J Neurosurg 64:89–98
23. Fell D, Benner B, Billings A, Siemens R, Harbison B and Newmark SR (1984) Metabolic profiles in patients with acute neurosurgical injuries Crit Care Med 12:649–652
24. Twyman D, Young AB, Ott L, Norton JA, Vivins BA (1985) High protein enteral feedings: A means of achieving positive nitrogen balance in head injured patients J Parenter Enter Nutr 9:679–684
25. Clifton GL, Robertson CS, Constant CF (1985) Enteral hyperalimentation in head injury J Neurosurg 62:186–193

26. Bivins BA, Twyman DL, Young AB (1986) Failure of nonprotein calories to mediate protein conservation in brain-injured patients J Trauma 26:980–986

27. Ott LG, Schmidt JJ, Young AB et al. (1988) Comparison of administration of two standard intravenous amino acid formulas to severely brain-injured patients Drug Intelligence Clin Pharm 22:763–768

28. Behrman SW, Kudsk KA, Brown RO, Vehe KL, Wojtysiak SL (1995) The effect of growth hormone on nutritional markers in enterally fed immobilized trauma patients J Parenter Enter Nutr 19:41–46

29. Young BA, Ott L, Haack D et al. (1987) Effect of total parenteral nutrition upon intracranial pressure in severe head injury J Neurosurg 67:76–80

30. Young B, Ott L, Twyman D et al. (1987) The effect of nutritional support on outcome from severe head injury J Neurosurg 67:668–676

31. Cherian L, Goodman JC, Robertson CS (1998) Effect of glusocse administration on contusion vlume after moderate cortical impact injury in rats J Neurotrauma 15:1059–1066

32. Hausmann D, Mosebach O, Caspari R, Lippoldt R, Schafer TG (1987) Effects of steroid on nitrogen loss and plasma amino acid profiles after head injury J Parenter Enter Nutr 11:10 S (abstract)

33. Saxe JM, Ledgerwood AM, Lucas CE, Lucas WF (1994) Lower esophageal sphincter dysfunction precluded safe gastric feeding after head injury J Trauma 37:581–584

34. Norton JA, Ott LG, McClain C et al. (1988) Intolerance to enteral feeding in the brain-injured patient J Neurosurg 68:62–66

35. Akkersdijk WL, Roukema JA, vd Werken C (1998) Percutaneous endoscopic gastrostomy for patients with severe cerebral injury Injury 29:11–14

36. Wicks C, Gimson A, Vlavianos P et al. (1992) Assessment of the percutaneous endoscopic gastrostomy feeding tube as part of an integrated approach to enteral feeding Gut 33:613–616

37. Allison MC, Morris AJ, Park RH, Mills PR (1992) Percutaneous endoscopic gastrostomy tube feeding may improve outcome of late rehabilitation following stroke J R Soc Med 85:147–149

38. Norton B, Homer-Ward M, Donnelly MT, Long RG, Holmes GKT (1996) A randomised prospective comparison of percutaneous endoscopic gstrostomy and nasogastric tube feeding after acute dysphagic stroke BMJ 312:13–16

39. Hiebert JM, Brown A, Anderson RG et al. (1981) Comparison of continuous versus intermittent tube feedings in adult burn patients J Parenter Enter Nutr 5:73–75

40. Cogan R, Weintraub J (1989) Aspiration pneumonia in nursing home patients fed via gastrostomy tubes Am J Gastroenterol 84:1509–1512

41. Hamaoui E (1995) (editorial) Gastroesophageal reflux during gastrostomy feeding J Parenter Enter Nutr 19:172–173

42. Rapp RP, Young B, Twyman D et al. (1983) The favorable effect of early parenteral feeding on survival in head-injured patients J Neurosurg 58:906–912

43. Sacks GS, Brown RO, Teague D, Dickerson RN, Tolley EA, Kudsk KA (1995) Early nutrition support modifies immune function in patients sustaining severe head injury J Parenter Enter Nutr 19:387–392

44. Hoyt DB, Ozkan AN, Hansbrough JF et al. (1990) Head injury: An immunologic deficit in T-cell activation J Trauma 30:759–767

45. Hadley MN, Grahm TW, Harrington T, Saxhiller WR, McDermott MK and Posillico DB (1986) Nutritional support and neurotrauma: A critical review of early nutrition in forty-five acute head injury patients Neurosurg 19:367–373

46. Waters DC, Dechert R, Bartlett R (1986) Metabolic studies in head injury patients: A preliminary report Surgery 100:531–534

47. Borzotta AP, Osborne A, Bledsoe F et al. (1993) Enteral nutritional support enhances cognitive recovery after severe closed head injury Surgical Forum 44:29–31

48. Young B, Ott L, Kasarskis E et al. (1996) Zinc supplementation is associated with improved neurologic recovery rate and visceral protein levels of patients with severe closed head injury J Neurotrauma 13:25–34

49. Choi DW and Koh JY (1998) Zinc and brain injury Annu Rev Neurosci 21:347–375
50. Gariballa SE, Parker SG, Taub M. Castleden CM (1998) A randomized, controlled, single-blind trial of nutritional supplementation after acute stroke J Parenter Enter Nutr 22:315–319
51. Wanklyn P, Cox N, Belfield P (1995) Outcome in patients who require a gastrostomy after stroke Age and Ageing 24:510–514
52. Park RH, Allison MC, Lang J et al. (1992) Randomised comparison of percutaneous endoscopic gastrostomy and nasogastric tube feeding in patients with persisting neurological dysphagia BMJ 304:1406–1409
53. Smithard DG, O'Neill PA, Park C et al. (1996) Complications and outcome after acute stroke: Does dysphagia matter? Stroke 27:1200–1204
54. DePippo KL, Holas MA, Reding MJ, Mandel FS, Lesser ML (1994) Dysphagia therapy following stroke: a controlled trial Neurology 44:1655–1660
55. Kirby DF and DeLegge MH (1997) Enteral nutrition and the neurological diseases. In: Rombeau JL and Rolandelli RH (eds) Clinical Nutrition: Enteral and Tube Feeding 3rd edn WB Saunders Co, Philadelphia pp 286–299
56. DeLegge MH, Duckwork F, McHenry L, Foxx-Orenstein A, Craig RM, Kirby DF (1995) Percutaneous endoscopic gastrojejunostomy: A dual center safety and efficacy trial J Parenter Enter Nutr 19:239–243
57. Grahm TW, Zadrozny DB, Harrington T (1989) The benefits of early jejunal hyperalimentation in the head-injured patient Neurosurg 25:729–735
58. Montecalvo MA, Steger KA, Farber HW et al. (1992) Nutritional outcome and pneumonia in critical care patients randomizewd to gastric versus jejunal tube feedings Crit Care Med 20:1377–1387
59. DeBoisblanc M and Borzotta AP (1997) ICP monitoring during percutaneous endoscopic jejunostomy (PEJ) early after severe head injury (in) Proceedings, Tenth International Symposium on Intracranial Pressure and Neuromonitoring in brain injury Abstract PO-1-001

Nutritional Support of the Severely Burned Patient

S.E. Wolf, A.P. Sanford, and D.N. Herndon

Introduction

Advances in treatment of burns have caused marked decreases in mortality. In 1952, 50% of young patients would be predicted to die with a 50% TBSA burn [1], whereas in today's top burn units, almost any size burn in a young patient would be predicted to survive (Table 1) [2]. The treatment advances have been in the areas of resuscitation, wound closure, infection control, and support of the hypermetabolic response to trauma. In regards to hypermetabolism and nutritional treatments, weight losses of greater than 30% were common among burn patients prior to the advent of continuous enteral nutritional support. These losses were at least partly responsible for high mortality rates associated with moderate and large size burns [3]. With modern treatments, weight losses after burn can be prevented.

Nutritional support of the hypermetabolic response to injury has been extensively studied with severe burns often used as the model. Reasons for their use are several. Burned patients have a quantifiable injury based on the total body surface area burned (TBSA), and burn size is proportional to increases in oxygen consumption [4], urinary nitrogen losses [5], and weight loss [6]. Energy expenditure can also be estimated by the TBSA burn [7, 8]. Thus, the metabolic responses to severe burn are predictable, providing a model to prospectively test nutritional interventions on outcomes.

Table 1. Burn mortality (LD%50): the numbers are the %TBSA burn at which 50% of patients would be expected to die

		Age Groups (years)			
	n	0–14	15–44	45–64	>65
Bull and Fisher (1942–1952)	2807	49	46	27	10
Bull (1967–1970)	1922	64	56	40	17
Curreri and Abston (1975–1979)	1508	77	63	38	23
SBI/UTMB (1980–1997)	2164	98	70	46	19

Significant improvements have occurred over time, particularly in the younger age groups.

Pathophysiology

Once the severely burned have been resuscitated, wound closure is accomplished. Unfortunately, even using relatively rapid closure techniques, increased metabolic rate up to 100% over predicted resting energy expenditure persists throughout the acute hospitalization for up to 9 months after discharge [5, 65]. Muscle catabolism ensues and glucose flow increases 2–3 times normal [10], leaving patients who are weak, without reserves to rehabilitate rapidly.

Energy expenditure increases are driven by the inflammatory response to the wound which produces pro-inflammatory cytokines (tumor necrosis factor-α, interleukin-1, interleukin-6), prostaglandins, and other inflammatory mediators. These mediators become systemic when the burn size exceeds 20% of the TBSA [11]. Xanthine oxidase activity increases in response to burn wounds, which result in increased production of oxygen free radicals and distant organ lipid peroxidation. Levels of naturally occurring antioxidants such as vitamin E are decreased due to consumption [12].

The pain response associated with the wound activates the limbic system directly. Fear, emotion, and thalamic relay of peripheral nociceptive stimuli alter the thermoregulatory setpoint in the hypothalamus to result in hyperthermia. As patients strive to reach the higher setpoint, shivering and futile substrate cycling with production of high energy phosphate bonds increase to provide heat. Efforts to reduce energy requirements by increasing ambient temperature limit the absolute degree of hypermetabolism, but do not abolish it (Fig. 1) [4, 5].

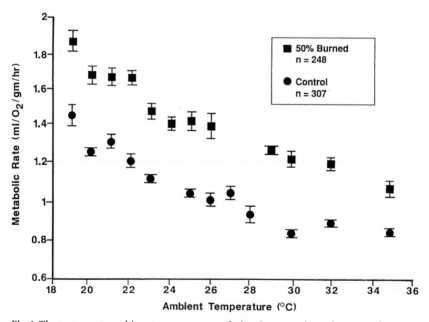

Fig. 1. The response to ambient temperature regulation. Increases in environmental temperature decrease metabolic needs for heat production as measured by oxygen consumption

Inflammatory and neural stimuli cause the hypothalamus to initiate the release systemic catabolic hormones, including the catecholamines, glucagon, and cortisol (Fig. 2). Catecholamines are elevated two to ten fold in proportion to burn size [13], and cortisol is elevated ten fold with a loss of circadian rhythm [14]. These hormones stimulate glycogenolysis, gluconeogenesis, proteolysis, and free fatty acid release through stimulation of hormone-sensitive lipoprotein lipase. When these three hormones are infused into normal volunteers, the hypermetabolic response is mimicked, resulting in nitrogen loss and hyperglycemia [15]. However, the complete response including proteolysis and acute phase protein production was elicited only with the concomitant induction of inflammation [16].

Substrate for gluconeogenesis is provided from the glycerol backbone of degraded triglycerides and from proteolysis-liberated amino acids. Most of the available body protein for this process is located in the active musculature, resulting in loss of lean body mass as the catabolic process continues [17]. Lactate and alanine are important intermediates that are released in proportion to the extent of injury [18]. Glutamine, the most prevalent amino acid in muscle, is also released in massive quantities to deplete muscle stores to 50% of previous concentrations [19]. This depletion appears to occur in the first 48 h after injury (unpublished data). Phenylalanine is also released from muscle in a disproportionate rate [20].

Catecholamines remain elevated until wound closure is complete, providing a shift from the thyroid axis to the sympathoadrenal axis for metabolic control. Glucagon also remains elevated while active forms of thyroid hormone decrease and inactive forms increase. The thyroid gland maintains its sensitivity to thyroid stimulating hormone [21]. This condition is referred to as the "sick euthyroid" state.

In burned patients, a substrate cycle exists when opposing non-equilibrium reactions catalyzed by differing signals are active simultaneously [22]. Substrate is utilized to produce high energy phosphate bonds, which are broken to resynthesize the substrate. No net increase or decrease in substrate is accomplished, with the only result being an increase in heat generation, thus the term "futile substrate cycling". One such example is the glucose-lactate-glucose metabolic

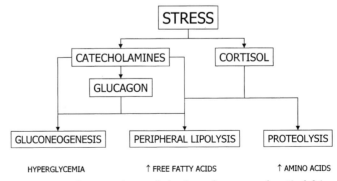

Fig. 2. The endocrine stress response. Increases in catecholamines, glucagon, and cortisol drive mobilization of energy substrate

sequence known as the Cori cycle. This sequence is highly active in burned patients, with the production of lactate and pyruvate from glucose in the periphery which is converted back to glucose in the liver by gluconeogenesis. Gluconeogenic amino acids, such as alanine and glutamine, are also used in such a cycle to produce glucose. Glucose is the preferred fuel for healing cells, such as leukocytes and fibroblasts [23]. Intuitively, if supplemental glucose was provided at a sufficient rate to provide energy substrate for the wound, these cycles could be inhibited. However, burned patients are unable to metabolize glucose when the rate of infusion exceeds 4 mg/kg/min, with the proposed mechanism being oversaturation of the metabolic pathways in the liver. Lipids and proteins are then utilized to meet the remaining metabolic requirements [10, 24]. These may come from endogenous sources.

The protein catabolic effects of burn on the muscle have been extensively studied. Protein synthesis and protein breakdown in the muscle are simultaneously stimulated after severe burn, however, protein breakdown in stimulated to a greater extent [25]. Therefore, the principal defect is an accelerated rate of protein breakdown with a failure of compensatory synthesis [26]. The result is net amino acids efflux from the cells and a negative nitrogen balance. The response was not simply due to prolonged enforced bed rest [27]. Similar to the findings with glucose, it was found that nutritional support with protein and amino acid intake levels several times higher than the normal requirement failed to completely reverse net protein catabolism [28].

Nutritional Support

Metabolic Needs

Caloric intakes required by burned patients can be estimated based on an analysis of energy expenditure. Total energy expenditure (TEE) is composed of calories expended for basal metabolism in addition to calories expended during activity, and can be measured accurately by direct calorimetry. This measurement is made by determining heat elaborated while a subject is placed in a sealed insulated chamber, which is not generally possible in these critically ill patients. Indirect calorimetry, which takes advantage of the stoichiometric relationship between oxygen consumption and carbon dioxide production during respiratory gas exchange, is another method which can be used to measure energy expenditure. This measurement assumes a steady state, and therefore is only practicable at rest during constant feeding or in the post-absorptive state. By the measurement of gas exchange, equations are calculated that provide an estimate of resting energy expenditure (REE). Total energy expenditure is estimated by the addition of an activity factor.

A novel method using stable isotopic techniques to measure total energy expenditure have been made in burned patients. In these studies using doubly-labeled water (^2H_2O and $H_2{}^{18}O$), the fate of the labeled hydrogen follows the kinetics of water flux alone while the labeled oxygen follows that of water and of CO_2 during equilibration with free hydrogen ion through carbonic anhydrase.

Measurements of the differences in turnover in water (urine) and CO_2 (expired gases) over a prolonged period gives an estimate of total CO_2 production. Because the measures are made over time, a relative steady state is reached and thus TEE is estimated. When these measurements were made in burned children during convalescence and compared to REE by indirect calorimetry, it was found that TEE exceeded measured REE by a factor of $1.18+0.17$ ($r^2=0.92$). The highest TEE measured in the subjects was $1.4\times$ REE [7]. Therefore, to meet the needs of all the children measured in this study, $1.4\times$ REE exogenous calories would be required [7, 8].

Resting energy expenditure can be estimated without measurement by using the Harris-Benedict equation. This formula, which was developed using direct calorimetric measurements of normal adults [29], uses sex and total body surface area (height and weight) as the independent variables to determine predicted basal energy expenditure (PBEE). Burned patients have the addition of TBSA burned and time after burn as independent variables significantly affecting energy expenditure [8]. The following equation, then can predict the caloric intake required to meet the TEE of 95% of severely burned children: $\text{TEE}=(1.55\times\text{PBEE})+(2.39\times\text{PBEE}^{0.75})$. In most cases, this is close to $2\times$ PBEE for burns greater than 40% TBSA.

Although mobile metabolic carts to measure indirect calorimetry are ideal, expense and maintenance needs preclude their routine use in most units. For these reasons, several formulas have been devised to calculate caloric requirements in their absence (Table 2). One is to multiply the basal energy expenditure determined by the Harris-Benedict formula by 2 in burns over 40%, assuming a 100% increase in total energy expenditure as defined above. Other commonly used calculations include the Curreri formula, which calls for 25 kcal/kg/day plus 40 kcal/% TBSA burned/day. This formula provides for maintenance needs in addition to the caloric needs related to the burn wounds [30]. This formula was devised as a regression from nitrogen balance data in severely burned adults and may actually overestimate needs over the entire hospitalization, as the measurements were made only over the first 20 days after injury. This study was also done in an era when much of the burn wound was left intact until definitive coverage could be made, which differs from current techniques of early total excision. Caution should also be exercised in the elderly, who have lower metabolic rates. A separate formula based on similar measurements has been devised for this population (20 kcal/kg+40 kcal/%TBSA burned) [31].

Table 2. Caloric formulas for severely burned patients

Age group	Estimated daily caloric needs
Infants (0–12 months)	2100 kcal/TBSA+1000 kcal/TBSA burned
Children (1–12 years)	1800 kcal/TBSA+1300 kcal/TBSA burned
Adolescents (12–18 years)	1500 kcal/TBSA+1500 kcal/TBSA burned
Adults (19–65 years)	25 kcal/kg+40 kcal/TBSA burned
Elderly (>65 years)	20 kcal/kg+40 kcal/TBSA burned

In children, formulas based on body surface area are more appropriate because of the greater body surface area per kilogram. The following formulas were devised based on caloric intake required to maintain body weight over the course of acute hospitalization for differing age groups (Table 2) [6, 32, 33]. These changes with age are based on the body surface area alterations that occur with growth. If these intakes are not maintained, weight loss ensues which is associated with increased length of hospital stay (Table 3).

Monitoring Nutritional Support

Once a dietary intake has been selected, the patient should be monitored to ensure adequate provision of calories. These monitors are generally laboratory measurements of organ function and protein synthetic capacity (Table 4). Abnormalities in these exams should lead to a re-evaluation of the nutritional prescription.

Dietary Composition

The composition of the nutritional supplement is also important. The optimal dietary composition contains 1–2 g/kg/day of protein, which provides a calorie to nitrogen ratio at around 100:1 with the above suggested caloric intakes. This amount of protein will provide for the synthetic needs of the patient, thus sparing to some extent the proteolysis occurring in the active muscle tissue. Higher protein delivery (2–3 g/kg/day) may be required in infants who have greater renal losses. Recent evidence also suggests that even higher protein intakes may spare muscle protein [34].

Non-protein calories can be delivered either as carbohydrate or as fat. Carbohydrates have the advantage of stimulating endogenous insulin production, which may have the beneficial effects on muscle and the burn wounds as an anabolic hormone. Recent data suggests that glucose is the preferred fuel during burn induced hypermetabolism [35], and thus exogenous delivery should be based on carbohydrates. We also have as yet unpublished data that revealed an improvement in net balance of amino acids across the leg when a carbohydrate based diet with 2.3% fat was given compared to an isonitrogenous isocaloric diet with an identical protein source containing 40% fat. This effect was presumably via a stimulation of endogenous insulin production. Furthermore, the addition of a fat load to the liver after severe burn may in fact be deleterious. It was recently shown that almost all of the fat transported in VLDL after severe burn is derived from peripheral lipolysis and not from de novo synthesis of fatty acids in the liver from dietary carbohydrates, even on a high carbohydrate diet [36]. Therefore, the role of de novo synthesis fatty acid synthesis as the cause of fatty liver demonstrated in severely burned patients [37] might be minor in comparison to the load provided by peripheral lipolysis. Additional fat to deliver non-carbohydrate calories would then only tax an already overloaded system. We recommend a diet that delivers non-protein calories in the form of carbohydrate. Of course, essential fatty acids must be given to avoid fatty acid deficiency.

Table 3. Comparison of severely burned children meeting calculated caloric needs to those who did not

	Patients meeting predicted caloric needs	Patients not meeting predicted needs
% kcal met	100±7	78±6*
% Weight change	2±2	−16±5*
Length of hospital stay (days)	39±10	80±46
Predicted weight loss (kg)	-0.1±1	−8±5*
Actual weight loss (kg)	0.8±1	−8±5*

*$P<0.05$.

Table 4. Monitoring nutritional support

Measurements	Frequency	Comments
Serum electrolytes	Daily until stable	Common abnormalities in Na^+, K^+, Cl^-, Ca^{2+}, Mg^{2+}, and PO_4
BUN and serum creatinine	Daily until stable, then weekly	
Liver profile	3× per week	
Glucose	Daily	May require exogenous insulin to maintain euglycemia
Albumin, prealbumin, transferrin, or retinol binding protein	Weekly production	Indicators of constitutive protein
Resting energy expenditure	Weekly	Caloric needs=REE× 1.4

Vitamins and Minerals

Several vitamins are required by healing cells to function properly. Among the most important is vitamin C, which is required for collagen cross-linking. The anti-oxidant effects of vitamin during resuscitation have been recently shown to inhibit wound conversion from partial thickness to full-thickness, and decrease resuscitation requirements [38]. Vitamin A is known to be the most commonly depleted vitamin, which is important in collagen synthesis and maturation and T-lymphocyte function [39]. The B vitamins have been shown to increase skin strength and fibroblastic content in scar tissue [40, 41].

Zinc and selenium also play a role in the treatment of burned patients. Zinc deficiency impairs the rate of wound re-epithelialization and lessens the gain in wound strength through impaired amino acid utilization [42]. Urinary zinc losses increase after burn [43] with decreased levels in plasma and skin. Selenium is required for glutathione peroxidase enzyme activity, and is known to be diminished with the use of topical silver preparations [44]. Given that we know these vitamins and minerals are important in wound healing, adequate supplementation should be provided in the diet when possible.

Nutritional Delivery

In patients with greater than 40% total body surface area, lean body mass is reduced 25% over the first 4 weeks when patients are fed only from hospital trays. For these reasons, burn patients are generally fed via either enteral catheters of by parenteral means. Parenteral nutrition may be given in isotonic solutions through peripheral catheters, or with hypertonic solutions in central catheters. In general, the caloric demands of burn patients prohibit the use of peripheral parenteral nutrition. Total parenteral nutrition (TPN) delivered centrally in burned patients has been associated with increased complications and mortality [45]. In this study, patients receiving TPN had a higher mortality rate that was associated with septic events and relative immunosuppression [46] compared to another group fed enterally with whole milk (Fig. 3). For this reason, TPN should be reserved only for those patients who cannot tolerate enteral feedings.

Enteral feeding via transpyloric tubes is recommended, and should be started during resuscitation. Studies have shown that burn-induced ileus can be subverted with this technique with delivery of total caloric needs within 3 days without complications [47]. Early feedings are also associated with a reduction in the hypermetabolic response to burn [48]. Gastric erosions can occur later in the course, which can be avoided by partial gastric feedings to buffer the stomach. Not all patients can tolerate enteral feedings, however, and this clinical finding has been associated with increased septic morbidity not necessarily related to the gut [49].

Nutritional Adjuncts

Even with adequate provision of calories and protein to meet calculated needs, hypermetabolism and proteolysis persist, although somewhat abated [28, 50]. For these reasons, investigators have been searching for complementary therapies to further reduce the ravages of catabolism. The inflammatory response that was alluded to in the pathophysiology section is likely to be of teleologic benefit during resuscitation and progressing to the "flow phase" of the response to injury. However, the prolonged catabolism that persists weeks to months even after the wounds are healed are clearly detrimental, with loss of lean body mass and the strength to rehabilitate. It is catabolism during this phase that is targeted. The greatest demonstrable loss takes place in muscle.

Accelerated net protein catabolism after injury can persist for months. The principal defect is an accelerated rate of protein breakdown with a failure of compensatory synthesis [26], resulting in a negative net nitrogen balance at the cellular level. Therefore, net efflux of amino acids out of the muscle cell is favored (Fig. 4). Pharmacologic strategies then must address the relative decrease in protein synthesis and increase in amino acid efflux.

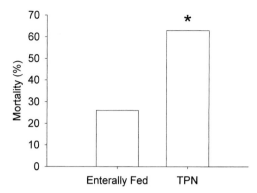

Fig. 3. Mortality increases with TPN. Patients fed an enteral diet had a lower mortality rate compared to those receiving TPN

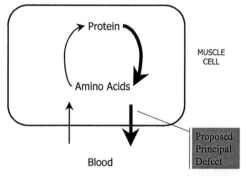

Fig. 4. The muscle cell during burn hypermetabolism. Protein breakdown is increased relative to protein synthesis with an efflux of amino acids from the cell. The principal defect lies in the transport of amino acids out of the cell instead of reutilization in stimulated protein synthesis

A class of drugs called the anabolic hormones have been shown to affect amino acid kinetics in the muscle after severe burn [51]. These can be broken into 3 broad categories according to their structure and mechanism of action: growth factors, androgenic steroids, and catabolic hormone antagonists.

The growth factors consist of proteins that have mitogenic and protein synthesis stimulating properties. The best studied of this group in burns include growth hormone (GH), insulin-like growth factor-I (IGF-1), and insulin. GH has been shown to accelerate donor site wound healing [9, 52], improve muscle protein synthesis [53], decrease albumin requirements [54], and decrease length of hospital stay in severely burned children. Growth hormone treatment in severely burned adults showed improvements in mortality and wound healing [55, 56]. The effects on muscle appeared to be as a stimulant of muscle protein synthesis [53]. IGF-1 has been shown to improve protein oxidation [57], however this study was hampered by the hypoglycemic effects of the drug. Recent studies using IGF-

1 in combination with its principal binding protein IGF binding protein-3 (IGF-BP-3) did not have these hypoglycemic effects while stimulating net protein synthesis in the muscle of both burned children [58] and burned adults [59]. The effect appeared to be related to a more efficient utilization of amino acids within the cell without affecting inward amino acid transport. The net result was a decrease in outward amino acid transport and thus improved protein net balance. IGF-1/IGFBP-3 treatment in adults may be hampered by the development of peripheral neuropathies. Perhaps the best anabolic growth factor is insulin. Treatment with insulin for 5 days at high doses (6 μU/kg/min) resulted in significant improvements in net protein synthesis. In this study, it was found that insulin increased both protein synthesis and protein breakdown in the muscle cells with a greater increase in synthesis. It also stimulated inward transport of amino acids from the blood [25]. It is this combination of the increase in protein synthesis and increase in inward transport of amino acids which is likely to cause the greatest anabolic effects in muscle. One caveat to this study was the high requirements of glucose to maintain euglycemia, to say nothing of the clinical diligence required to avert complications. Another study using lower doses of insulin required no additional glucose above calculated nutritional needs while showing similar improvements in net protein synthesis. However, the effect on inward transport of amino acids was lost [60].

The androgenic steroid class consists of such compounds as oxandrolone and testosterone. Both of these agents have been used in burned patients with success. Oxandrolone has been shown to improve strength in rehabilitating burn patients [61], and another study showed an improvement in wound healing and hospitalization time [62]. We have unpublished data to suggest that these effects are related to increases in protein synthesis without changes in protein breakdown, resulting in a decrease in amino acids efflux from the cell. We have similar data on the effects of testosterone.

The final class of drugs consist of antagonists to the catabolic hormones, primarily the catecholamines and cortisol. Propranolol is a non-specific competitive antagonist to β-catecholamine receptors which has been shown to decrease myocardial work in burned children when given in doses to diminish tachycardia associated with burn by 25% [63]. Responses to cold stress and isoproterenol challenge were preserved during treatment indicating cardiac responsiveness was maintained [64]. Propranolol has also been shown to decrease peripheral lipolysis, and perhaps diminish the development of fatty liver in the severely burned [36]. Recent unpublished data suggests that propranolol treatment over the hospital course decreases resting energy expenditure and improves protein kinetics in the muscle by decreasing protein breakdown.

Cortisol antagonists, including ketoconazole which inhibits the synthesis of cortisol by the adrenal and the potent abortifacient RU-486 which also serves as a competitive antagonist to the glucocorticoids, may have a role in improving nutritional parameters in burned patients by decreasing the cortisol signal. These studies are only now beginning to get underway.

Summary

Severe burns represent one of the best models for the study of hypermetabolism and catabolism after injury. Energy expenditure and dietary provisions for this patient population have been extensively studied, resulting in the current burn feeding formulas. Further work into the signals for the response and treatments in addition to the diet may provide further therapeutic measures that could be instituted to improve the outcomes of these patients.

Reference

1. Bull JP, Fisher AJ (1949) A study in mortality in a burn unit: standards for the evaluation for alternative methods of treatment. Ann Surg 130:160–173
2. Wolf SE, Rose JK, Desai MH, Mileski JH, Barrow RE, Herndon DN (1997) Mortality determinants in massive pediatric burns: an analysis of 103 children with greater than 80% TBSA burns (70% full-thickness). Ann Surg 225:554–569
3. Newsome TW, Mason AD, Pruitt BA (1973) Weight loss following thermal injury. Ann Surg 178:215–217
4. Herndon DN, Wilmore DW, Mason AD, Pruitt BA (1974) Development and analysis of a small animal model stimulating the human postburn hypermetabolic response. J Surg Res
5. Wilmore DW, Long JM, Mason AD, Skreen RW, Pruitt BA (1974) Catecholamines: mediators of the hypermetabolic response in thermally burned patients. Ann Surg 180:280–290
6. Hildreth MA, Herndon DN, Desai MH, Broemeling LD (1990) Current treatment reduces calories required to maintain weight in pediatric patients with burns. J Burn Care Rehabil 11:405–409
7. Goran MI, Peters E.J, Herndon DN, Wolfe RR (1990) Total energy expenditure in burned children using the doubly labeled water technique. Am J Physiol 259:E576-E585
8. Goran MI. Broemeling LD, Herndon DN, Peters EJ, Wolfe RR (1991) Estimating energy requirements in burned children: a new approach derived from measurements of resting energy expenditure. Am J Clin Nutrition 54:35–40
9. Herndon DN, Barrow RE, Kunkel KR, Broemeling LD, Rutan RL (1990) Effects of recombinant human growth hormone on donor site healing in severely burned children. Ann Surg 212:424–431
10. Wolfe RR, Herndon DN, Jahoor F, Miyoshi H, Wolfe M (1987) Effect of severe burn on substrate cycling by glucose and fatty acids. N Eng J Med 317:403–408
11. Michie H, Wilmore DW (1990) Sepsis, signals, and surgical sequelae: a hypothesis. Arch Surg 125:531–535
12. LaLonde C, Nayak U, Hennigan J, Demling RH (1997) Excessive liver oxidant stress causes mortality in response to burn injury combined with endotoxin and is prevented with antioxidants. J Burn Care Rehabil 18:187–192
13. Becker RA, Vaughan GM, Goodwin CW, Mason AD, Pruitt BA (1980) Plasma norepinephrine, epinephrine, and thyroid hormone interactions in severely burned patients. Arch Surg 115:439–443
14. Vaughan GM, Becker RA, Allen JP, Goodwin CW, Mason AD, Pruitt BA (1982) Cortisol and corticotrophin in burned patients. J Trauma 22:263–273
15. Bessey PQ, Watters JM, Aoki TT, Wilmore DW (1984) Combined hormonal infusions stimulate the metabolic response to injury. Ann Surg 200:264–280
16. Watters JM, Bessey PQ, Dinarello CA, Wolff SM, Wilmore DW (1986) Both inflammatory mediators and endocrine mediators stimulate the host response to sepsis. Arch Surg 121:179–190
17. Stinnett JD, Alexander JW, Watanabe C, et al. (1982) Plasma and skeletal muscle amino acids following severe burn injury in patients and experimental animals. Ann Surg 195:75–89

18. Aulick H, Wilmore DW (1979) Increased peripheral amino acid release following thermal injury. Surgery 85:560–565
19. Clowes GHA, Randell HT, Cha CJ (1980) Amino acid and energy metabolism in septic and traumatized patients. JPEN 4:195–203
20. Herndon DN, Wilmore DW, Mason AD, Pruitt BA (1978) Abnormalities of phenylalanine and tyrosine kinetics: significance in septic and non-septic patients. Arch Surg 113:133–135
21. Vaughan GM, Becker RA, Unger RH, et al. (1985) Nonthyroidal control of metabolism after burn injury – possible role of glucagon. Metab 34:637–641
22. Muller MJ, Meyer N, Herndon DN, Abston S (1995) Nutritional support for the burned patient. In: Latifi R, Dudrick SJ (eds) Surgical Nutrition: Strategies in Critically Ill Patients. pp103–121
23. Falcone PA, Caldwell MD (1990) Wound metabolism. Clin Plast Surg 17:443–456
24. Jahoor F, Shangraw RE, Miyoshi H, Wallfish H, Herndon DN, Wolfe RR (1989) Role of insulin and glucose oxidation in mediating protein catabolism of burns and sepsis. Am J Physiol 257:E323-E331
25. Sakuri Y, Aarsland AA, Chinkes DL, Nguyen TT, Pierre EJ, Wolfe RR, Herndon DN (1996) Anabolic effects of insulin in burned patients. Ann Surg 222:283–297
26. Jahoor F, Desai MH, Herndon DN, Wolfe RR (1988) Dynamics of protein metabolic response to burn injury. Metab 37:330–337
27. Shangraw RE, Stuart CA, Prince MJ, Peters EJ, Wolfe RR (1988) Insulin responsiveness of protein metabolism in vivo following bedrest in humans. Am J Physiol:E548-E558
28. Shaw JHF, Wolfe RR (1989) An integrated analysis of glucose, fat, and protein metabolism in severely traumatized patients: studies in the basal state and the response to total parenteral nutrition. Ann Surg 209:63–72
29. Harris JA, Benedict FG (1919) Biometric studies of basal metabolism in man. Carnegie Institution of Washington 270
30. Curreri PW (1978) Nutritional support of burn patients. World J Surg 2:215–222
31. Adams MR, Kelly CH, Luterman A, Curreri PW (1987) Nutritional requirements of patients with major burns. J Am Diet Assoc 65:415–417
32. Hildreth MA, Herndon DN, Desai MH, Duke MA (1989) Caloric needs of adolescent patients with burns. J Burn Care Rehabil 10:523–526
33. Hildreth MA, Herndon DN, Desai MH, Broemeling LD (1993) Caloric requirements of patients with burns under one year of age. J Burn Care Rehabil 14:108–112
34. Biolo G, Tipton KD, Klein S, Wolfe RR (1997) An abundant supply of amino acids enhances the metabolic effect of exercise on muscle protein. Am J Physiol 273:E122-E129
35. Gore DC, Wolfe RR, Wolf SE, Herndon DN (1999) Glucose kinetics and plasma concentrations in severely burned adults. J Trauma (in press)
36. Aarsland AA, Chinkes DL, Wolfe RR, et al. (1989) Beta-blockade lowers peripheral lipolysis in burn patients receiving growth hormone. Rate of hepatic very low density lipoprotein triglyceride secretion remains unchanged. Ann Surg 223:777–789
37. Wolf SE, Barrow RE, Herndon DN (1996) Growth hormone and IGF-1 therapy in the hypercatabolic patient. Bailliere's Clin Endo Metab 10:447–463
38. Tanaka H, Matsuda H, Shimazaki S, Hanumadas M, Matsuda T (1997) Reduced resuscitation fluid volume for second-degree burns with delayed initiation of Ascorbic acid therapy. Arch Surg 132:158–161
39. Barbul A, Regan MC (1993) Biology of wound healing. In: Fischer JE (ed) Surgical Basic Science. Mosby, St. Louis, pp 67–89
40. Grenier JF, Aprahamian M, Genot C, Dentinger A (1982) Pantothenic acid efficiency on wound healing. Acta Vitaminol Enzymol 4:81–85
41. Lakshmi R, Lakshmi AV, Bamji MS (1989) Skin wound healing and riboflavin deficiency. Biochem Med Metab Biol 42:185–191
42. Prasad AS (1986) Clinical, endocrinological, and biochemical effects of zinc deficiency. J Clin Endocrinol Metab 3:567–589
43. Larson DL, Maxwell R, Abston S (1970) Zinc deficiency in burned children. Plast Reconstr Surg 46:13–21

44. Boosalis MG, Solem LD, Ahrenholz DH, McCall JT, McClain CJ (1986) Serum and urinary selenium levels in thermal injury. Burns 12:236–240
45. Herndon DN, Barrow RE, Stein M, et al. (1989) Increased mortality with intravenous supplemental feeding in severely burned patients. J Burn Care Rehabil 10:309–313
46. Herndon DN, Stein M, Rutan TC (1987) Failure of TPN supplementation to improve liver function, immunity, and mortality in thermally injured patients. J Trauma 27:195–198
47. McDonald WS, Sharp CW. Deitch EA (1991) Immediate enteral feeding is safe and effective. Ann Surg 213:177–183
48. Mochizuki H, Trocki O, Dominioni L., Brackett KA, Joffe SN, Alexander JW (1984) Mechanism of prevention of post-burn hypermetabolism and catabolism by early enteral feeding. Ann Surg 200:297–310
49. Wolf SE, Jeschke MG, Rose JK, Desai MH, Herndon DN (1997) Enteral feeding intolerance: An indicator of sepsis associated mortality in burned children. Arch Surg 132:1310–1314
50. Streat SJ, Beddoe AH, Hill GL (1987) Aggressive nutritional support dies not prevent protein loss despite fat gain in septic intensive care patients. J Trauma 27:262–266
51. Ramzy PI, Wolf SE, Herndon DN (1999) Current status of anabolic hormone administration in human burn injury. JPEN (in press)
52. Gilpin DA, Barrow RE, Rutan RL, Broemeling LD, Herndon DN (1994) Recombinant human growth hormone accelerates wound healing in children with large cutaneous burns. Ann Surg 223:14–25
53. Gore DC, Honeycutt D, Jahoor F, Wolfe RR, Herndon DN (1991) Effect of exogenous growth hormone on whole-body and isolated-limb protein kinetics in burned patients. Arch Surg 126:38–43
54. Ramirez RJ, Wolf SE, Barrow RE, Herndon DN (1998) Growth hormone therapy in burns: a safe therapeutic approach. Ann Surg 228:439–448
55. Knox J, Demling R, Wilmore DW, Sarraf P, Santos A (1995) Increased survival after major thermal injury: the effect of growth hormone therpy in adults. J Trauma 39:526–532.
56. Singh KP, Prasad AS, Chari PS, Dash J (1998) Effect of growth hormone therapy in burn patients on conservative treatment. Burns 24:733–738
57. Cioffi WG, Gore DC, Pruitt BA, Carrougher G, Guler HP, McManus WF (1994) Insulin-like growth factor-1 lowers protein oxidation in patients with thermal injury. Ann Surg 220:310–319
58. Herndon DN, Ramzy PI, Debroy MA, et al. (1999) Muscle protein catabolism after severe burn: effects of IGF-1/IGFBP-3 treatment. Ann Surg 229:713–722
59. Debroy MA, Wolf SE, Xhang XJ, et al. (1999) Anabolic effects of insulin-like growth factor in combination with insulin-like growth factor binding protein-3 in severely burned adults. J Trauma (in press)
60. Ferrando AA, Chinkes DL, Wolf SE, Matin S, Herndon DN, Wolfe RR (1999) A submaximal dose of insulin promotes net skeletal muscle protein synthesis in patients with severe burns. Ann Surg 229:11–18
61. Demling RH, Desanti L (1997) Oxandrolone, an anabolic steroid, significantly increases the rate of weight gain in the recovery phase after major burns. J Trauma 43:47–51
62. Demling RH (1999) Comparison of the anabolic effects and complications of human growth hormone and the testosterone analog, oxandrolone, after severe burn injury. Burns 25:215–221
63. Minifee PK, Barrow RE, Abston S, Herndon DN (1989) Improved myocardial oxygen utilization following propranolol infusion in adolescents with postburn hypermetabolism. J Paed Surg 24:806–811
64. Honeycutt D, Barrow RE, Herndon DN (1992) Cold stress response in patients with severe burns after beta blockade. J Burn Care Rehabil 13:181–186
65. Milnor, OA, Cioffi CG, Mason AD, Mc Manus WF, Pruitt BA. A longitudinal study of resting energy expenditure in thermally injured patients. J Trauma 1994, 37:167–70

Liver Function: Alteration and Insufficiency

X.M. Leverve and M.-A. Piquet

Role of Liver in Nutritional Homeostasis

Liver is the major organ in the control of the metabolic and nutritional home-ostasis. Indeed, it plays a determinant role in all main macronutrient pathways, i.e. carbohydrates, lipids and proteins [1]. It is also implicated in micronutrient metabolism: vitamins and trace elements. Due to several specific and high metabolic capacities, liver is also involved in the metabolism and excretion of many exogenous compounds or toxic substances. This chapter focuses on a brief review of some of the main features of liver metabolism and on the relationships between liver diseases and nutritional status and support.

General Aspects of Liver Metabolism

The prominent role of liver in whole-body metabolism is related to three main functions: synthesis, storage and metabolism.

A unique capacity of metabolite synthesis is one of the major features of liver metabolism. This capacity concerns glucose at first since liver possesses the whole enzymatic machinery permitting to synthesise this vital compound from various substrates including other carbohydrates (glycerol, fructose, sorbitol, etc.) and amino acids and also to release it after hydrolysis by glucose 6-phosphatase [2]. Liver is also a very potent organ in non-essential fatty acid and amino acid synthesis [2].

The storage capacity concerns essentially the glucose in the form of glycogen-macromolecules, although in some special circumstances and to a much less extent triglycerides and proteins can also be concerned. It is also one of the main organs for the storage of vitamins, and for almost all trace elements.

The metabolic capacity concerns several pathways including those permitting to transform nutrients after intestinal absorption and metabolism. More-over, liver has a unique role in the metabolism of poisons and xenobiotics. This property is linked to conjugation capacities and to a specific peroxidative pathway (cytochrome P 450) [3]. Liver is also specifically involved in degradation and excretion of endogenous compounds like cholesterol, bilirubin, ammonia and most of the essential amino acids, branched-chain excepted [2]. Ammonia, coming from protein catabolism, is excreted as a non-toxic molecule, via the urea cycle, a specific hepatic pathway (but see below) linked to pH homeostasis.

The portal drainage is essential for the specific metabolism of exogenous nutrients. Indeed, every hydrophilic substrate from oral route enters the body after a first pass through liver. This explains the hepatic metabolism of carbohydrates and proteins in fed state. Conversely, hydrophobic substrates, like triglycerides, are not absorbed via the blood stream and the portal vein to the liver but via the lymphatic vessels. Thus, these metabolites escape the liver first-pass and are delivered directly into the general circulation. This anatomical peculiarity is of major importance in the liver ability to modulate substrate delivery to peripheral tissues both in quantitative (amount of glucose delivered) or qualitative (blood composition of amino acid) aspects (see Fig. 1).

The liver is constituted by two distinct organs since two different populations of cells, periportal and perivenous cells, are working in concert [4]. Hence, the synergistic result of this metabolic compartmentation is of great importance in both physiology and pathology. Such co-operation has been shown for several sub-

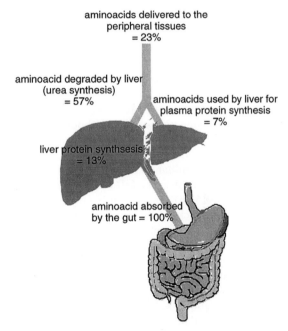

aminoacids delivered to the
peripheral tissues
= 23%

aminoacid degraded by liver
(urea synthesis)
= 57%

aminoacids used by liver for
plasma protein synthesis
= 7%

liver protein synthsesis
= 13%

aminoacid absorbed
by the gut = 100%

Fig. 1. Role of liver in the remodelling of amino acid mixture after gut absorption. Liver is very active in amino acid metabolism (deamination and transamination) and protein synthesis. Thirteen percent of amino acids provided by intestine after an experimental proteic meal are directly used by the liver and 7% for plasma protein synthesis. Hence, liver handles nearly 20% of the total amino acid load for protein synthesis and as much as 57% are degraded to urea. Hence, only 23% of the total amino acid load are delivered to the peripheral tissues. Such large waste is compensated by a major qualitative advantage: by removing amino acids in excess liver is able to remodel the composition and to release tto peripheral tissues the most adapted mixture. (From [25])

strates and pathways (glucose and amino acids for instance) [4]. Moreover, the balance between ureagenesis (achieved in periportal cells) and the glutamine synthesis (in perivenous cells) is probably of great physiological significance in the role of liver in pH homeostasis ([5] and see below).

A *large capacity of "cellular recruitment"* explains the considerable capacity of liver metabolic adaptation. This large anatomic and functional reserve of liver is clear when considering the good metabolic tolerance of large liver resection [6]. Furthermore, when considering lactate homeostasis, liver clearance capacity is high and a large increase in blood lactate is probably more often due to decreased consumption rather than increased production [7, 8].

Liver and Fed-Fasted Alternation

The liver is the key organ in the management of fed or fasted states, and liver metabolic adaptation is of major importance to face the peculiar condition of long term fasting [1, 9]. Adipose tissue also plays a determinant role in concert with liver in this alternation, the metabolic orchestration being conducted by insulin. In fed state, insulin is high and the main body fuel is represented by glucose oxidation, carbohydrates being present in large amounts in the meal. High insulin concentration favours glycogen synthesis, lipid storage and prevents lipid oxidation. Conversely, in the post-absorptive period, substrate concentrations and insulin decrease progressively and the metabolic picture is opposite: glucose is less oxidised since it must be either synthesised from amino acids or released from glycogen, while fatty acids represent the major oxidisable substrate directly or through ketone pathway [1]. Although the actual energetic storage contained by liver is limited (less than 100 g glycogen), it is a pivotal organ in fasting adaptation due to its ability to synthesise glucose and ketone bodies, these later becoming the dominant oxidative substrates in long term fasting. If glycogen can be found in almost every cell (including red blood cells [10]), liver (75 g) and muscle (100–150 g) excepted, it is only present in a very limited amount. Moreover, muscle is lacking glucose 6-phosphatase activity, and therefore it is believed to be not capable of net glucose release. Hence, muscle glycogen is used only as substrate supplier for muscle contraction and not for sustaining blood glucose levels except in very peculiar conditions [11]. Gluconeogenesis from lactate or amino acids is depending of the presence of a key enzyme: phospho*enol*pyruvate carboxykinase (PEPCK). Classically, this enzyme is present in significant amount only in liver and in kidney [2]. Therefore in long term fasting, kidney is capable of net glucose synthesis and release since this organ also contains glucose 6-phosphatase as in liver. This renal source of glucose may represent up to 30% of total glucose production after a long period of fasting [12]. The lack of PEPCK activity in other tissues has been recently questioned and some evidences have been reported in favour of a significant gluconeogenic capacity in muscle cells [13]. Conversely to long-chain fatty acid β-oxidation, ketone body oxidation is a ubiquitous pathway present in every mitochondrion-containing cells (including brain), and ketogenesis is a liver specific pathway powerfully inhibited by insulin [1, 2]. Beside starvation in adult, ketone body metabolism plays a crucial role at birth, since liver is not ready for gluconeogenesis. Indeed foetal PEPCK activity is lacking, the maternal liver being responsible for glucose synthesis for both mother and foetus. Since insulin is a powerful inhibitor of PEPCK transcription a profound drop in blood glucose at birth is necessary to permits the initiation of first time PEPCK transcription by new-born liver. At this time, the newborn brain is protected by ketone bodies. This explains why fatty acids are the most adequate substrates at this period of life and the major importance of triglyceride storage during the last months of pregnancy [14].

Liver and Lipid Metabolism

Although liver is not an important organ for lipid storage in healthy conditions, it must be underlined that, together with adipose tissue, it is very efficient in fatty acid synthesis, esterification and triglyceride synthesis [1, 15]. Indeed endothelial cells from liver capillaries are rich in hepatic lipase, enzyme responsible for lipoprotein triglyceride and phospholipid hydrolysis, permitting thus a very active fatty acid uptake by liver cells. Moreover, plasma membranes of hepatocytes are rich in apoprotein-E receptors leading to a very active uptake of intermediary-density lipoproteins (IDL). Finally, liver is the unique organ able to synthesise the apoprotein B100, main determinant factor in VLDL secretion [16]. Hence, due to all of these properties, liver is very active and crucial for whole body lipid metabolism: fatty acid uptake, triglyceride synthesis and export to the peripheral tissues as VLDL. Beside its role in triglyceride metabolism, liver is also a prominent organ in cholesterol homeostasis: (a) it is the most efficient organ for cholesterol synthesis, (b) it is the only organ able to excrete cholesterol in the bile with a highly regulated entero-hepatic recycling and (c) it is responsible for the synthesis of cholesterol-acyl transferase, permitting the esterification of cholesterol in HDL. This latter property being essential for reverse cholesterol transport to the liver [17]. Hence liver is the main organ responsible for the subtle tuning of cholesterol homeostasis, essential component for cellular membrane physiology.

Liver and Protein Metabolism

The liver has two important functions in protein metabolism: (a) the synthesis of several vital proteins and (b) due to very active amino acid metabolism [1, 18] it modulates amino acid composition delivered to the peripheral tissues in the fed state [19, 20].

The liver has a unique role in the synthesis of specific proteins. It is one of the most active tissues in protein synthesis and with the exception of immuno-globulines, all circulating proteins present in the blood are synthesised by the liver. Due to specific changes according the nutritional status and the presence or not of an inflammatory response, two groups of plasma proteins originating from the liver has been opposed. Among the group of "nutritional proteins", albumin and transthyretin (or prealbumin) has long been recognised while many others are also influenced by the nutritional status (i.e. transferrin, TBG, SBG, etc.). Plasma concentration of nutritional proteins is affected by undernutrition but inflammatory response and liver failure decrease it as well. In order to discriminate between nutritional of inflammatory origins, it was proposed to assess simultaneously the inflammatory proteins orosomucoid and C reactive protein, which are increased by stress or inflammatory response [21]. Some years ago, Ingenbleek and Carpentier have proposed the Prognostic Inflammatory and Nutritional Index (PINI) which is: [C reactive protein (mg/l)×orosomucoid (mg/l)/[albumin (g/l)×transthyretin (mg/l] [22]. In healthy subjects, its value is very closed to one while it is between 0–10 at low risk; 11–20 at moderate; 21–30 at severe risk of complications and 31–40 at life threatening risk. It must be emphasised that, as originally proposed by the authors, the PINI is a risk index of postoperative complications. Although, classically albumin is viewed as a typical "nutritional protein" with a depressed synthesis in inflammatory or stress states, recent findings have challenged this point of view in severe head-trauma patients [23]. In fact, many of our knowledge on protein metabolism in vivo are obtained from the determination of the static concentrations of plasma protein instead of dynamic synthesis rate. In the reported study, the very significant decrease in albumin concentration was due to a major enhancement of peripheral albumin catabolism despite a large increase in its synthesis rate [23]. The meaning of such an active albumin catabolism in these severe illnesses and the tissues involved in this phenomenon are not known as yet.

Protein degradation in liver is also a major mechanism since the protein content of this organ, determined by the balance between synthesis and breakdown, is probably more dependent of breakdown rate than of synthesis change [24]. Conversely to muscle, the other main organ in quantitative protein metabolism, where protein breakdown is mainly achieved by non-lysosomal pathways (i.e. ATP-ubiquitin-proteasome pathway or calpains) and regulated by hormones and cytokines [25], in liver the main pathway for protein catabolism is the lysosomal autophagy, which is mainly regulated by amino acid concentrations. It has been shown that in several physiological or pathological conditions the protein content was indeed modulated by large changes in the rate of protein breakdown [26].

Liver modulates the amino acid mixture delivered to peripheral tissues after gut absorption [18–20, 27, 28]. This mechanism of extreme importance permits the liver to play a determinant role in the efficiency of alimentary protein use and therefore on whole body protein economy (Fig. 1). Moreover, because of this property, liver failure as well as chronic acidosis (due to either renal or pulmonary failures) strongly impair protein metabolism, leading to a decrease in dietary protein efficiency and thus to an increase in protein requirement to avoid protein malnutrition.

This specific role of liver is based on: (a) channelling of hydrophilic substrate (including amino acids) toward the liver by portal flow, (b) active deamination and transamination permitting to modify the primitive amino acid composition (c) regulation of urea cycle activity by pH. Urea synthesis rises almost immediately during protein absorption indicating an increased rate of amino acid catabolism. As a result, the amino acid mixture in hepatic vein significantly differs from that of portal blood with branched-chain amino acid enrichment [37, 39]. Liver ammonia metabolism can be orientated either to urea cycle or to glutamine synthesis [5]. Although the first pathway occurs in periportal cells and has both ammonia and bicarbonate as substrate in an equimolar proportion, the second is located in perivenous cells and does not consume any bicarbonate. Hence, remodelling of amino acid mixture by liver is depending on (a) urea cycle capacity (periportal cell mass, i.e. liver function), (b) pH homeostasis (metabolic acidosis inhibits urea cycle and activates glutaminase activity while alkalosis does the opposite) and (c) metabolic co-ordination between periportal and perivenous cells. Recently the role of liver in glutamine synthesis has been challenged since the balance of glutamine across the liver is closed to zero. It is believed that in fact the muscle mass is the main source of glutamine [29]. This may explain the effect of chronic acidosis on muscle protein mass. The role of urea cycle in bicarbonate metabolism explains the occurrence of metabolic alkalosis in the case of a severe impairment of urea synthesis (cirrhosis for instance) and its bad prognosis value.

Liver and Inter-Organ Cooperation

Although, liver has a large variety of specific functions some of this specific functions can be shared by other organs. Urea synthesis is a good example of a specific function of the liver: periportal hepatocytes are the only cells containing the whole enzymatic machinery required for achieving the complete urea cycle pathway [2, 29]. However, many tissues, including muscle and brain for instance, contain arginase which cleaves arginine into urea and ornithine. Hence, if liver is undoubtedly required for urea synthesis from ammonia and bicarbonate, arginine cleavage, last step of urea synthesis can be achieved in other tissues. Indeed, it has been shown in patients suffering from chronic renal failure that brain was the main organ for urea production [30, 31]. Hence although in this condition, urea comes actually from the brain, its synthesis from ammonia would not have been possible in the absence of liver metabolism. This is clearly confirmed, as seen above, by the fact that urea production collapses in end-stage liver cirrhosis.

Hence, even when the metabolic activity of a given organ is assessed by arterio-venous differences, such inter-organ co-operation can be completely missed. Therefore it is not possible to simply answer to the question of which organ is responsible for urea synthesis in this case: it is the result of an inter-organ metabolic co-operation.

Interrelationships Between Liver Disease and Nutritional Status

Effects of Malnutrition on Liver Morphology and Function

Protein-energy malnutrition may affect liver morphology and function and the importance of protein in the maintenance of normal structure and function of liver is prominent. Selective protein depletion can produce fatty liver and fibrosis in experimental animals, but data are less convincing in humans, although enlarged fatty liver and occasionally fibrosis are observed in kwashiorkor in children. In most cases, providing an adequate diet reverses morphologic alterations of the liver. Considering liver functions, quantitative tests such as aminopyrine or indocyanine-green clearance show an improvement when cirrhotic patients are treated with nutritional support [32]. Nevertheless, these functional tests are not able to identify patients who will respond to nutritional intervention: they are global indicators of liver functional impairment not able to differentiate between malnutrition- or disease-induced liver malfunction [33].

Effects of Chronic Liver Disease on Nutrition and Metabolism

Malnutrition is a common finding in patients with chronic liver disease. Using anthropometric criteria, prevalence of malnutrition ranges from 20%–60%, and increases with the severity of the disease assessed by Child score [34, 35]. Since alcoholism is frequently associated with poor nutritional status, it has been suggested that patients with alcoholic cirrhosis were more malnourished than patients with cirrhosis from other aetiologies [34].

Pathogenesis of Malnutrition

The pathogenesis of malnutrition is multifactorial (Table 1). A decreased dietary intake is a predominant factor and is correlated with the severity of liver disease [36]. Anorexia and nausea, present in more than 50% of patients [37], and frequent hospitalisations with dietary restrictions required by complications such as ascites or encephalopathy are responsible for this. Digestion and absorption of nutrients are impaired because of a decrease in bile acid secretion due to hepatocellular insufficiency. This is particularly severe in primary biliary cirrhosis. Furthermore, pancreatic insufficiency and enteropathy are frequently associated in

Table 1. Pathogenesis of malnutrition in chronic liver disease

Factors	Mechanisms
Decreased dietary intake	Anorexia, nausea due to liver disease Dietary restrictions, hospitalizations
Impaired nutrient digestion and absorption	Cholestasis Pancreatic insufficiency Enteropathy
Increased energy expenditure	Complications Increased gluconeogenesis
Metabolism alterations	Protein breakdown Insulin resistance "Accelerated starvation"

alcoholic patients. Moreover, substrate metabolism also is affected in patients with chronic liver disease.

Inasmuch as energy expenditure is concern, data of the literature are conflicting because of differences in the mass used for calculation (actual or ideal "dry" body mass). However, it was demonstrated that cirrhotic patients have increased resting energy expenditure when expressed per unit of lean body mass, which is further enhanced by progress of the severity of the disease [38]. However, increased basal requirement may be counterbalanced by reduced physical activity [33]. The increased energy expenditure during chronic liver disease can be explained by complications, by acute hepatic failure [39], and also by changes in substrate metabolism.

On the one hand, liver fibrosis reduces hepatic glycogen stores, and consequently gluconeogenesis is stimulated to maintain glycemia in the post absorptive state. Since the energy cost of gluconeogenesis is higher than that of glycogenolysis, stimulation of gluconeogenesis is responsible for a part of increased resting energy expenditure. Despite the increase in gluconeogenesis, hepatic glucose production rate is sometimes low [40], explaining hypoglycemia which occurs especially during acute hepatic failure. On the other hand, insulin resistance, which is a constant finding in hepatic insufficiency, leads to impaired glucose tolerance and to alteration of substrate metabolism. Hence, the preferred fuel substrate is altered in cirrhosis. As shown by calorimetric studies after an overnight fast [38], 75% of energy metabolism are provided by fat oxidation in cirrhotics compared to 35% for control subjects. Therefore, liver cirrhosis should be considered as an "accelerated starvation disease", with early recruitment of alternative fuels [41]. Consequently, extended period of starvation must be avoided in patients with cirrhosis.

Protein turnover in stable chronic liver disease has been found to be normal or increased, but when expressed per unit of lean body mass, protein breakdown appears to be accelerated [38, 42]. In complicated cirrhosis, protein catabolism is stimulated because of release of cytokines, and protein requirements are increased in such patients [33]. Beside protein degradation, synthesis is also affected. Maximum rate of urea synthesis decreases by 50% during chronic liver disease. This leads to hyperamoniemia, elevated amino acidemia with predominance of aromatic amino acids, and metabolic alkalosis in the case of major hepatic failure as seen above. The enhancement of the ratio of aromatic/branched-chain amino acids is one of the factors possibly involved in the pathogenesis of hepatic encephalopathy.

Impact of Malnutrition on Prognosis

Malnutrition worsens the prognosis of patients with cirrhosis. In short-term studies, the presence of malnutrition significantly decreased the survival [43]. Although, malnutrition is correlated to the severity of the liver disease, multivariate analysis have shown that nutritional parameters are independent predictors of survival in both compensated [44] and decompensated [36] cirrhotic patients. Moreover, nutritional support is efficient in decreasing mortality [45] and morbidity [46] in patients with chronic liver disease.

Nutritional Support in Liver Disease

Assessment of Nutritional Status

It is difficult in patient with liver disease, as it is the case in ICU patients, because of extracellular fluid retention. Mass and body mass index are inaccurate in presence of ascites or oedema. Circulating concentrations of plasma proteins, such as albumin and prealbumin, are affected by both liver disease [47] and inflammatory state. Bioelectric impedance is of little value in presence of ascites [48], unless using segmental measurements [49]. Despite the fact that creatine is synthesised by the liver, urinary creatinine excretion, which is correlated to muscle mass, seems usable in liver disease [50]. Since direct methods such as in vivo neutron activation or isotopic dilution are generally not available, anthropometry (mid-arm circumference and triceps skinfold) is widely used and permits to increase the sensitivity of detection of malnutrition as compared to subjective assessment [34]. It must be emphasised that a reliable evaluation of the spontaneous nutrient intake allows selection of patients at high risk. Indeed, spontaneous nutrient intake is correlated to mortality [36] and to response to nutritional support [45].

Goals of Nutritional Support

The main objective of nutritional support is to treat malnutrition and to fulfil energy and protein requirements. Such nutritional supplementation is rational since malnutrition is a prognostic factor of mortality [36, 43]. On the other hand, nutritional support should not worsen or when possible to improve hepatic encephalopathy. The exact pathogenesis of hepatic encephalopathy in patients with chronic liver disease has not yet been fully explained, but most of hypothesis imply nutritional factors [51]. The mechanism of encephalopathy is an alteration of neurotransmission due to either neurotoxins or false neurotransmitters. In this way, ammonia produced by dietary protein catabolism or by bacteria as well as short-chain fatty acids are neurotoxic. Moreover, synthesis of false neurotransmitters from aromatic amino acids is enhanced in cirrhotic patients. Other nutritional factors such as zinc deficiency, polyunsaturated fatty acids deficiency or manganese excess, have been suggested. The main role of nutrients in the pathophysiology of hepatic encephalopathy implicates nutrition and diet as an important part of the treatment of this entity.

Access for Artificial Nutrition: Enteral or Parenteral?

If oral supplementation is inadequate or impossible, artificial nutrition is required. Nutrition should then be provided by enteral route, and parenteral nutrition should only be used when enteral feeding is not possible or impracticable [33]. Indeed, enteral route preserve gut structure and prevent bacterial translocation. It has been clearly demonstrated that morbidity of enteral nutrition was lower than that of parenteral nutrition [52]. Coagulopathy or oesophageal varices are not an absolute contraindication to prolonged placement of nasoenteric tubes [53, 54]. However, performing percutaneous endoscopic gastrostomy in cirrhotic patient is difficult and dangerous because of ascites and portal hypertension. There is no general agreement as to whether enteral feeding should be intermittent or continuous, but extended period of starvation must be avoided in patients with cirrhosis because of the behaviour of "accelerated starvation".

General Requirements and Recommendation

The European Society of Parenteral and Enteral Nutrition (ESPEN) recently published guidelines for nutrition in liver disease [33] (Table 2). Assessment of energy requirements is difficult in cirrhosis, because measured energy expenditure has been found very variable from one patient to the other. When measurement of energy expenditure is not possible, available data suggest a recommended intake of 25–30 kcal/kg ideal weight/day non-protein energy in clinically stable cirrhosis, and 35–40 kcal/kg ideal weight/day in complicated cirrhosis (infection, bleeding, malnutrition) [33, 45]. For parenteral nutrition, energy should be provided by glucose and fat in a ratio of 65–50: 35%–50% of non-protein calories. Clearance of fat emulsions is usually normal in cirrhotic patients.

Because of increased protein catabolism and decreased efficiency of oral protein metabolism, patients with stable cirrhosis appear to have increased protein requirements of 1.2 g/kg ideal weight/day to maintain nitrogen homeostasis as opposed to 0.8 g/kg/day in normal individuals. In case of malnutrition or acute complications (encephalopathy excepted), protein requirements increase to 1.5 g/kg ideal weight/day [33]. Micronutrient deficiencies are frequent in cirrhosis, but no data on requirements are available in this patient group.

Specific Aspects

Nutrition in Cirrhosis with Encephalopathy

Malnutrition *per se* is a possible cause of encephalopathy, and an adequate nutritional support with standard protein intake can counteract low grade encephalopathy [45]. However, a number of authors have proposed to decrease even to suppress protein intake in order to decrease blood ammonia. In fact, suppressing exogenous protein intake has no advantage, because it is counterbalanced by endogenous protein catabolism. But protein restriction to 0.5 g/kg/day resulted sometimes in improvement of encephalopathy, leading to the definition of "protein intolerant" patients [55]. Protein restriction should be used only transiently, and after exclusion of other precipitating causes of encephalopathy such as gastrointestinal bleeding or infection. Adequate nutrition should be reinstituted after a few days. If encephalopathy recurs, patient is considered as proven protein intolerant, and qualitative changes in protein intake may be helpful [33].

Table 2. Recommendations of the 1997 ESPEN Consensus Group

Clinical condition	Non-protein energy (kcal/kg/day)	Protein or amino acids (g/kg/day)
Compensated cirrhosis	25–35	1.0–1.2
Complications		
Inadequate intake	35–40	1.5
Malnutrition		
Encephalopathy I, II	25–35	Transiently 0.5 then 1.0–1.5; if protein intolerant: vegetable protein or BCAA supplement
Encephalopathy III, IV	25–35	0.5–1.2; BCAA enriched solution

For calculations ideal body weight should be used.

A diet predominantly composed of vegetable proteins improves nitrogen balance and hepatic encephalopathy as compared to animal protein diet [55]. Enhanced gut motility, modifications in colonic microflora and changes in hormonal response due to fibre component of these vegetable diets are likely to account for these therapeutic effects. Nevertheless, these patients are frequently anorectic and therefore they have difficulties to eat bulky vegetable diets in the adequate amounts to meet daily nutrient requirements, moreover these diets are not adapted to artificial nutrition.

Branched-chain amino acids (BCAA) enriched formula may be more interesting. BCAA's inhibit competitively the transport in the brain of aromatic amino acids, which are precursor of false neurotransmitters. An overview and a meta-analysis suggested that an oral [56] or parenteral [57] supplementation maintain nitrogen balance without worsening mental state, but most of the authors [57, 58] conclude that the superiority on conventional amino acid mixtures or alimentary proteins is not definitely proved. More and better designed studies are needed to definitely prove or disprove the role of this treatment. In view of the relevant cost of BCAA, BCAA supplementation should be used only in proven protein intolerant patients to achieve adequate nitrogen intake [33].

Nutrition in Liver Transplantation

Malnutrition is not a contraindication to transplantation but may negatively affect outcome. The effect of preoperative nutritional support has not been studied, but early postoperative nutrition is clearly beneficial following liver transplantation in terms of morbidity. Nutritional requirements are not different from those of other surgical patients [33]. Kaliemia and magnesemia should be especially monitored because of the treatment by ciclosporine.

Effect of Nutritional Support on Outcome

Nutritional intervention increases survival in cirrhotic patients with complications leading to low spontaneous dietary intake [45]. Controlled trials in cirrhotic patients show that nutritional support decreases sepsis [46], postoperative [59] and post-transplantation [60] complications, and hospitalization frequency [61]. Liver function [54], as well as hepatic encephalopathy [45, 56, 57] may improve.

Artificial Nutrition in Fulminant Hepatic Failure

Fulminant hepatitis combines acute hepatocellular insufficiency and stress state. It is unknown whether such patients are able to suitably metabolise fat or amino acids. An important aspect of the management is the need for very close monitoring of blood glucose levels to prevent hypoglycaemia due to decrease in glycogen stores and impairment of gluconeogenic pathways. It is useless and even dangerous to infuse more than 5 mg/kg/min glucose, because capacity of oxidation of this substrate is limited by stress state and non-oxidised glucose enter in lipogenesis pathway leading to steatosis. In patients with cerebral oedema, serum osmolality should be monitored, because after glucose metabolised, the excess free water may potentially contribute adversely to brain swelling. Phosphate and magnesium supplementations are frequently necessary.

Perspectives in Pharmacological Nutrition

Further studies are required to provide pharmacological or nutritional ways to improve spontaneous dietary intake, hepatic encephalopathy and metabolic alterations in cirrhotic patients, or to decrease alcohol or virus toxicity. The role of branched-chain amino acids in encephalopathy remains to be definitely proved. Other specific nutrients will be probably developed. For example, utility of polyunsaturated fatty acids in hepatic encephalopathy, phospholipids in alcoholic hepatitis or vitamin E in chronic viral hepatitis remains to be assessed.

References

1. Frayn K. Metabolic Regulation: a Human Perspective. London: Portland Press; 1996
2. Newsholme EA, Leech AR, editors. Biochemistry for the Medical sciences. Chichester, U.K.: John Wiley and Sons; 1990
3. Grant DM. Detoxification pathways in the liver. J Inherit Metab Dis 1991;14 (4):421–30
4. Jungermann K, Kietzmann T. Zonation of parenchymal and nonparenchymal metabolism in liver. Annu Rev Nutr 1996;16:179–203
5. Haussinger D, Lenzen C, Soboll S. Acid-base regulation of hepatic glutamine degradation. Contrib Nephrol 1988;63:161–6
6. Chiolero R, Tappy L, Gillet M, Revelly JP, Roth H, Cayeux C, et al. Effect of major hepatectomy on glucose and lactate metabolism. Ann Surg 1999;229 (4):505–13
7. Levraut J, Ciebiera JP, Chave S, Rabary O, Jambou P, Carles M, et al. Mild hyperlactatemia in stable septic patients is due to impaired lactate clearance rather than overproduction. Am J Respir Crit Care Med 1998;157 (4 Pt 1):1021–6

8. Leverve XM, Mustafa I, Péronnet F. Pivotal role of lactate in aerobic metabolism. In: Vincent JL, editor. Yearbook of intensive care and emergency medicine. Berlin: Springer-verlag; 1998. p. 588–96

9. Cahill GF. Starvation in man. New England Journal of Medecine 1970;282:668–75

10. Moses SW, Bashan N, Gutman A. Glycogen metabolism in the normal red blood cell. Blood 1972;40 (6):836–43

11. Wicklmayr M, Dietze G. On the mechanism of glucose release from the muscle of juvenile diabetics in acute insulin deficiency. Eur J Clin Invest 1978;8 (2):81–6

12. Schoolwerth AC, Smith BC, Culpepper RM. Renal gluconeogenesis. Miner Electrolyte Metab 1988;14 (6):347–61

13. Ryan C, Radziuk J. Muscle glyconeogenesis during recovery from a prolonged swim in rats. Am J Physiol 1994;267 (2 Pt 1):E210–8

14. Pegorier JP, Garcia-Garcia MV, Prip-Buus C, Duee PH, Kohl C, Girard J. Induction of ketogenesis and fatty acid oxidation by glucagon and cyclic AMP in cultured hepatocytes from rabbit fetuses. Evidence for a decreased sensitivity of carnitine palmitoyltransferase I to malonyl- CoA inhibition after glucagon or cyclic AMP treatment. Biochem J 1989;264 (1): 93–100

15. Hellerstein MK, Schwarz JM, Neese RA. Regulation of hepatic de novo lipogenesis in humans. Annu Rev Nutr 1996;16:523–57

16. Yao Z, McLeod RS. Synthesis and secretion of hepatic apolipoprotein B-containing lipoproteins. Biochim Biophys Acta 1994;1212 (2):152–66

17. Lagrost L. Regulation of cholesteryl ester transfer protein (CETP) activity: review of in vitro and in vivo studies. Biochim Biophys Acta 1994;1215 (3):209–36

18. Felig P. Amino acid metabolism in man. Annu Rev Biochem 1975;44:933–55

19. Elwyn DH, Parikh HC, Shoemaker WC. Amino acid movements between gut, liver, and periphery in unanesthetized dogs. Am J Physiol 1968;215 (5):1260–75

20. Elia M, Folmer P, Schlatmann A, Goren A, Austin S. Amino acid metabolism in muscle and in the whole body of man before and after ingestion of a single mixed meal. Am J Clin Nutr 1989;49 (6):1203–10

21. Bonnefoy M, Ayzac L, Ingenbleek Y, Kostka T, Boisson RC, Bienvenu J. Usefulness of the prognostic inflammatory and nutritional index (PINI) in hospitalized elderly patients. Int J Vitam Nutr Res 1998;68 (3):189–95

22. Ingenbleek Y, Carpentier YA. A prognostic inflammatory and nutritional index scoring critically ill patients. Int J Vitam Nutr Res 1985;55 (1):91–101

23. Mansoor O, Cayol M, Gachon P, Boirie Y, Schoeffler P, Obled C, et al. Albumin and fibrinogen syntheses increase while muscle protein synthesis decreases in head-injured patients. Am J Physiol 1997;273 (5 Pt 1):E898–902

24. Scornik OA, Howell SK, Botbol V. Protein depletion and replenishment in mice: different roles of muscle and liver. Am J Physiol 1997;273 (6 Pt 1):E1158–67

25. Attaix D, Taillandier D, Temparis S, Larbaud D, Aurousseau E, Combaret L, et al. Regulation of ATP-ubiquitin-dependent proteolysis in muscle wasting. Reprod Nutr Dev 1994;34 (6):583–97

26. Mortimore GE, Poso AR. Intracellular protein catabolism and its control during nutrient deprivation and supply. Annu Rev Nutr 1987;7:539–64

27. Deferrari G, Garibotto G, Robaudo C, Sala M, Tizianello A. Splanchnic exchange of amino acids after amino acid ingestion in patients with chronic renal insufficiency. Am J Clin Nutr 1988;48 (1):72–83

28. Tizianello A, De Ferrari G, Garibotto G, Robaudo C. Amino acid metabolism and the liver in renal failure. Am J Clin Nutr 1980;33 (7):1354–62

29. Meijer AJ, Lamers WH, Chamuleau RA. Nitrogen metabolism and ornithine cycle function. Physiol Rev 1990;70 (3):701–48

30. Tizianello A, de Ferrari G, Garibotto G, Gurreri G, Bruzzone M. Cerebral and hepatic urea synthesis in patients with chronic renal insufficiency. Proc Eur Dial Transplant Assoc 1978;15:500–5

31. Deferrari G, Garibotto G, Robaudo C, Ghiggeri GM, Tizianello A. Brain metabolism of amino acids and ammonia in patients with chronic renal insufficiency. Kidney Int 1981;20 (4):505–10
32. Mezey E, Caballeria J, Mitchell MC, Pares A, Herlong HF, Rodes J. Effect of parenteral amino acid supplementation on short-term and long- term outcomes in severe alcoholic hepatitis: a randomized controlled trial. Hepatology 1991;14 (6):1090–6
33. Plauth m, Merli m, Kondrup J, Weimann A, Ferenci p, Müller M. ESPEN guidelines for nutrition in liver disease and transplantation. Clin nutr 1997;16:43–55
34. Nutritional status in cirrhosis. Italian Multicentre Cooperative Project on Nutrition in Liver Cirrhosis. J Hepatol 1994;21 (3):317–25
35. Roggero P, Cataliotti E, Ulla L, Stuflesser S, Nebbia G, Bracaloni D, et al. Factors influencing malnutrition in children waiting for liver transplants. Am J Clin Nutr 1997;65 (6):1852–7
36. Mendenhall CL, Moritz TE, Roselle GA, Morgan TR, Nemchausky BA, Tamburro CH, et al. A study of oral nutritional support with oxandrolone in malnourished patients with alcoholic hepatitis: results of a Department of Veterans Affairs cooperative study. Hepatology 1993;17 (4):564–76
37. Achord JL. Malnutrition and the role of nutritional support in alcoholic liver disease. Am J Gastroenterol 1987;82 (1):1–7
38. McCullough AJ, Tavill AS. Disordered energy and protein metabolism in liver disease. Semin Liver Dis 1991;11 (4):265–77
39. Schneeweiss B, Pammer J, Ratheiser K, Schneider B, Madl C, Kramer L, et al. Energy metabolism in acute hepatic failure. Gastroenterology 1993;105 (5):1515–21
40. Petrides AS, DeFronzo RA. Glucose metabolism in cirrhosis: a review with some perspectives for the future. Diabetes Metab Rev 1989;5 (8):691–709
41. Owen OE, Reichard GA, Jr., Patel MS, Boden G. Energy metabolism in feasting and fasting. Adv Exp Med Biol 1979;111:169–88
42. Cano N, Leverve XM. Influence of chronic liver disease and chronic renal failure on nutrient metabolism and undernutrition. Nutrition 1997;13 (4):381–3
43. Merli M, Riggio O, Dally L. Does malnutrition affect survival in cirrhosis? PINC (Policentrica Italiana Nutrizione Cirrosi). Hepatology 1996;23 (5):1041–6
44. Moller S, Bendtsen F, Christensen E, Henriksen JH. Prognostic variables in patients with cirrhosis and oesophageal varices without prior bleeding. J Hepatol 1994;21 (6):940–6
45. Kondrup J, Muller MJ. Energy and protein requirements of patients with chronic liver disease. J Hepatol 1997;27 (1):239–47
46. Hasse JM, Blue LS, Liepa GU, Goldstein RM, Jennings LW, Mor E, et al. Early enteral nutrition support in patients undergoing liver transplantation. JPEN J Parenter Enteral Nutr 1995;19 (6):437–43
47. Merli M, Romiti A, Riggio O, Capocaccia L. Optimal nutritional indexes in chronic liver disease. JPEN J Parenter Enteral Nutr 1987;11 (5 Suppl):130S-4 S
48. Campillo B, Bories PN, Pornin B, Devanlay M. Influence of liver failure, ascites, and energy expenditure on the response to oral nutrition in alcoholic liver cirrhosis. Nutrition 1997;13 (7–8):613–21
49. Schloerb PR, Forster J, Delcore R, Kindscher JD. Bioelectrical impedance in the clinical evaluation of liver disease. Am J Clin Nutr 1996;64 (3 Suppl):510S-4 S
50. Pirlich M, Selberg O, Boker K, Schwarze M, Muller MJ. The creatinine approach to estimate skeletal muscle mass in patients with cirrhosis. Hepatology 1996;24 (6):1422–7
51. Perney P, Pomier-Layrargues G. [Hepatic encephalopathy. Physiopathology and treatment]. Gastroenterol Clin Biol 1994;18 (12):1069–76
52. Moore FA, Feliciano DV, Andrassy RJ, McArdle AH, Booth FV, Morgenstein-Wagner TB, et al. Early enteral feeding, compared with parenteral, reduces postoperative septic complications. The results of a meta-analysis. Ann Surg 1992;216 (2):172–83
53. Cabre E, Gonzalez-Huix F, Abad-Lacruz A, Esteve M, Acero D, Fernandez-Banares F, et al. Effect of total enteral nutrition on the short-term outcome of severely malnourished cirrhotics. A randomized controlled trial. Gastroenterology 1990;98 (3):715–20

54. Kearns PJ, Young H, Garcia G, Blaschke T, O'Hanlon G, Rinki M, et al. Accelerated improvement of alcoholic liver disease with enteral nutrition. Gastroenterology 1992;102 (1):200–5.
55. Mullen KD, Weber FL, Jr. Role of nutrition in hepatic encephalopathy. Semin Liver Dis 1991;11 (4):292–304
56. Fabbri A, Magrini N, Bianchi G, Zoli M, Marchesini G. Overview of randomized clinical trials of oral branched-chain amino acid treatment in chronic hepatic encephalopathy. JPEN J Parenter Enteral Nutr 1996;20 (2):159–64
57. Naylor CD, O'Rourke K, Detsky AS, Baker JP. Parenteral nutrition with branched-chain amino acids in hepatic encephalopathy. A meta-analysis. Gastroenterology 1989;97 (4):1033–42
58. Eriksson LS, Conn HO. Branched-chain amino acids in the management of hepatic encephalopathy: an analysis of variants. Hepatology 1989;10 (2):228–46
59. Fan ST, Lo CM, Lai EC, Chu KM, Liu CL, Wong J. Perioperative nutritional support in patients undergoing hepatectomy for hepatocellular carcinoma. N Engl J Med 1994;331 (23):1547–52
60. Reilly J, Mehta R, Teperman L, Cemaj S, Tzakis A, Yanaga K, et al. Nutritional support after liver transplantation: a randomized prospective study. JPEN J Parenter Enteral Nutr 1990;14 (4):386–91
61. Hirsch S, Bunout D, de la Maza P, Iturriaga H, Petermann M, Icazar G, et al. Controlled trial on nutrition supplementation in outpatients with symptomatic alcoholic cirrhosis. JPEN J Parenter Enteral Nutr 1993;17 (2):119–24

Nutritional Support in Acute Respiratory Failure

X. Leverve, D. Barnoud, and C. Pichard

Introduction

Mechanical ventilation is applied to at least half of intensive care patients to treat respiratory failure with or without lung injury. Ventilator-dependence refers to the need of a patient for prolonged support by a ventilator, which is the case in approximately 15% of ICU patients [1]. Patients with trauma, burns, sepsis, acute respiratory distress syndrome (ARDS) and multiple organ dysfunction (MODS) present a hypermetabolic and catabolic state leading to extensive endogenous protein breakdown and major loss of muscle mass, including respiratory muscles. As a result, these patients are prone to respiratory muscle fatigue and/or failure, leading to unsuccessful weaning attempts from the ventilator [2]. In chronic obstructive pulmonary disease (COPD) patients requiring mechanical ventilation, weaning from the ventilator can be extremely difficult, due to the additive effects of chronic malnutrition, increased work of breathing, increased load on inspiratory muscles, hypoxia and hypercapnia [3, 4].

This chapter focuses on nutritional strategies in attempting to reduce muscle catabolism and to correct malnutrition while avoiding the pitfalls of excessive or inappropriate substrate administration. Pathophysiology of chronic and acute nutritional disorders in the different group of patients with respiratory failure will be first reviewed, then the basics of nutritional assessment and monitoring, and finally the specific aspects of their nutritional management.

Metabolic and Nutritional Consequences of Respiratory Failure

The relationships between respiratory failure and metabolic disturbances are complex and three groups of patients could be individualised. In the first group the nutritional depletion is the consequence of a COPD and the nutritional status appears to be prominent on the prognosis [5, 6]. The second group consists in acutely ill patients in which acquired undernutrition, among other factors (hypophosphatemia [7], hypocalcemia [8], hypomagnesemia [9], post-surgery pain, etc.), could be a cause of ventilatory dependence or weaning difficulties [10]. In the last group, a non-adequate nutritional support containing too high caloric intakes might delay the weaning by itself.

Infection or inflammatory status are probably the most common feature of patients with respiratory failure and/or need for mechanical ventilation. This fact has a major importance since it is now well recognised that acute or chronic inflammation results in a marked loss of lean body mass with nutritional consequences [11, 12]. From a clinical point of view, bronchial infection is the leading cause of acute respiratory failure in COPD. Therefore denutrition of these patients is the consequence of both pre-existing nutritional depletion and acute insult. Severe pneumonia, due to direct invasion of lung parenchyma by bacteria or viruses, is a very catabolic illness and a prolonged ventilatory support is often associated with a significant denutrition. Non-infectious lung injury is frequent in trauma and shock and the inflammatory response is responsible for metabolic consequences.

Denutrition in Chronic Respiratory Failure

A significant proportion of patients with chronic pulmonary diseases is malnourished and this nutritional depletion contributes to the deterioration of the clinical status and to the prognosis. Indeed it has been reported that 60% of hospitalised COPD patients exhibit a 10% decrease in body weight and a 20% decrease in body weight can be documented in 25% of these patients [13]. Moreover, when hospitalised for acute respiratory failure, 60% of COPD patients present a 20% loss of body weight [14]. The most severe nutritional deficits are observed in patients requiring mechanical ventilation [3]. Nutritional depletion appears to predominate in patients with emphysema "pink puffer type" compared to those with chronic bronchitis "blue bloater type" [4]. Muscle wasting is responsible for a depressed respiratory muscle function, which is significantly related to the outcome of the patients as independent parameter [5]. Malnutrition and loss of body weight is the consequence of a chronic negative energy balance, related to decreased nutritional intakes, increased energy expenditure or both. It can be due to the underlying disease but also to coinciding pathologies. Insufficient nutritional intake has been evoked but some studies have demonstrated that in the majority of COPD patient's nutrient intake is largely adequate to meet their needs [3, 15]. Several studies have shown increased energy expenditure in underweight COPD patients compared to COPD patients with normal weight or to underweight non-COPD patients [16]. This finding being possibly attributed to the increased work of breathing imposed by obstructive disease and emphysema, which rises further during episodes of respiratory failure [4]. Moreover, during acute episodes of respiratory tract infection, energy expenditure could further increase due to the added work of breathing [17]. In addition there is a decrease in nutritional intakes and intestinal absorption as consequence of hypoxia [18] and of inflammatory status [11, 12]. Indeed, it has been shown that TNF was significantly higher in undernourished as compared to obese COPD patients [11]. The link between inflammatory status and nutritional defect (type, severity and reversibility) is probably a general feature, which is found in many other undernourished states such as liver, renal and heart failures. The situation is even further complicated by the fact that the metabolic adaptation to fasting appears to be impaired by hypoxia in animal studies [19]. These patients have only a minor chance to fully regain their weight loss after such an episode, since hypercaloric nutrition, which is necessary for anabolism, increases in fact their energy expenditure disproportionately, due to an elevated thermic effect of nutrients compared to malnourished non-COPD patients [20]. Thus, a precarious equilibrium exists between energy expenditure and nutritional intake in most stable COPD patients with a risk of depletion. The balance is frequently shifted towards increased catabolism and insufficient intake during infectious episodes, and the restoration of body weight is limited, thereby inducing a progressive loss of fat and lean body mass over the years.

Metabolic Alteration in Acute Illnesses

Since the pioneer work by Sir David Cuthbertson it is known that post-trauma patients, as all other acute illnesses, present an integrated neuroendocrine catabolic response involving several hormones and cytokines [21]. Conversely to the initial description with two successive phases: "ebb" phase and "flow" phase, in patients with sepsis or ARDS without initial trauma, the "ebb phase" is absent, and the increased metabolic activity, characteristics of the "flow" phase, is present from the beginning. This metabolic response affects carbohydrate, lipid and protein metabolisms and the classical increase in 24-h energy expenditure exceptionally exceeds 35 kcal/kg BW/day.

Blood glucose is usually elevated due to both an increased liver gluconeogenesis and a relative impairment in glucose utilisation [22, 23]. In fact, the clearance of glucose actually increases in septic patients compared to normal volunteers but insulin effect is decreased [23]. The association of hyperglycemia with insulin resistance is a prominent feature of the metabolic response to acute disease [23]. To some extent, the increase in blood glucose concentration could be viewed as adaptive since it allows to increase glucose metabolism in tissues depending on its concentration (macrophage, endothelium and immune or inflammatory cells) at the expense of insulin-dependent tissues like muscle and adipocytes. Indeed, under physiological conditions, *i.e.* in absence of insulin resistance, a similar increase in blood glucose concentrations accompanied with a physiological insulin response would result in a large uptake of glucose in skeletal muscle and adipose tissue. Therefore the development of insulin resistance avoids such wastage and allows a preferential use of glucose produced from aminoacids released from muscle breakdown in the insulin-independent tissues thus excluding adipose tissue and non-injured muscles. The elevated levels of counter-regulatory hormones such as glucagon, cortisol, and catecholamines (endogenous and exogenous) contributes to increase glucose production and to antagonise the effects of insulin [22]. Furthermore, inflammatory cytokines released during sepsis have been shown to interfere with substrate metabolism. For instance, TNF-infused to rats induces a large increase in glucose production and uptake, as well as an inability of insulin to suppress hepatic glucose production and enhance glucose uptake by peripheral tissues [24].

Lipids represent the main fuel for oxidative metabolism during acute stress such as that found in sepsis and trauma. The discrepancy between increased carbohydrate turnover and increased lipid oxidation in acute situation is only apparent since the main feature of carbohydrates is to recycle (Cori's and Felig's cycles for instance). Indeed in the case of recycling, liver energy expenditure from lipid oxidation plays an important role in energy homeostasis [25]. The lipids used as fuel in the various tissues are provided by the release of free fatty acids from adipocyte, as a result of the stimulation of hormone-sensitive lipase by glucagon and catecholamines. It is of interest to note that diaphragm contains a higher proportion of lipids than skeletal muscle [26]. Different patterns of changes in lipid metabolism have been described. Classically, an increase in plasma triglycerides is observed while cholesterol is either unaffected or decreased. The high triglyceride concentration plasma is linked to an increase in VLDL concentrations resulting from both an enhancement in the rate of synthesis by the liver, and a decrease in clearance due to an inhibition of lipoprotein lipase [27]. Despite a decreased lipolytic activity, exogenous lipids are well-metabolised. A possible role of triglyceride-rich particles in the defence against endotoxins has been emphasised in preventing mortality from sepsis in a model of severe sepsis in rats [28].

Protein metabolism is strongly affected in acutely ill patients the overall picture being that of a redistribution of priorities between organs (liver *versus* muscles) or different pathways (enhancement of liver "inflammatory-protein" synthesis and decrease in "nutritional-protein"). Nonetheless, it must be noted that the view of a depressed "nutritional protein" synthesis during acute catabolic states has been recently challenged, albumin synthesis being shown to increase in patients after major head injury while plasma concentration was low [29]. The large increase in protein turnover associated with a hypercatabolic state results in increased nitrogen losses and a negative nitrogen balance [30]. As result of protein breakdown, large quantities of amino acids are released in the blood stream. Although the composition of this mixture roughly reflects the aminoacid proportion of muscle content, there is some exceptions: asparagine, aspartate, serine, and branched-chain amino acids (BCAA: leucine, isoleucine, valine), which are released in reduced proportions, while alanine and glutamine are released in higher proportions. Emphasise have been made recently concerning certain amino acids which may serve specific purposes, whether as fuel or intracellular regulatory mechanisms. Three examples of this are arginine, glutamine and BCAAs. Arginine, NO precursor, has been shown to be an immunomodulator substance, which improves resistance to infection in animal models and human studies. Glutamine appears to be a key oxidative fuel for the gastro-intestinal tract, as well as a regulating factor in skeletal muscle protein breakdown. Glutamine serves as a regulator of renal acid-base balance, fuel for the immune-response cells, in particular macrophages, and also as a key substrate for intestinal mucosal cells [31]. Approximately 50% of the BCAAs released by skeletal muscles proteolysis are oxidized directly by these same muscles. It has also been suggested that BCAAs could serve as a preferential fuel substrate during sepsis, when glucose and lipid oxidations are decreased, although this point remains controversial.

The net increase in protein breakdown leads to increase urinary nitrogen losses, whose magnitude parallels the increase in metabolic rate. Urinary nitrogen losses during acute stress reach 20–30 g/70 kg/day, with a mean value of 15 g/70 kg/day, i.e. considerably higher than the 12 g/70 kg/day of the initial fasting state. It must be noted that 20 g urinary nitrogen is roughly equivalent to the breakdown of 135 g protein, i.e. 500 g muscle tissue. Since, as discussed above, most of this protein comes from skeletal muscle, a prolonged hypermetabolic phase obligatory and rapidly results in alterations of skeletal muscle structure and function.

Clinical Consequences of Undernutrition on Pulmonary Function and Weaning

Prolonged hypermetabolic state with a high level of protein catabolism will necessarily lead to severe consequences involving several organ and functions among them the immune disorders are of major relevance. Lethal issue of theses metabolic consequences may eventually occur and it has long been known that death due to extreme malnutrition is frequently related to infectious lung disease and respiratory failure [32]. Hence, interaction between malnutrition and acute respiratory failure is complex: acute lung disease induces acute malnutrition, which requires a specific approach, while respiratory failure is often the consequence of a chronic malnutrition. In such cases, treatment of the pulmonary disease is frequently unsuccessful in absence of nutritional support. But conversely, correction of the nutritional status requires a long period of time during which respiratory support must be maintained involving a concomitant risk of specific nosocomial complications such as pneumonia.

One of the key factors in prolonged ventilator-dependency is respiratory muscle function. After the treatment of the underlying disease has been successfully achieved, weaning from the ventilator may cause tachypnea, rapid shallow breathing and alterations in blood gases indicating an insufficient spontaneous breathing [33]. This is often the case when the hypermetabolic phase has been severe or prolonged. Such impairment in respiratory muscle function is often the consequence of the severe skeletal muscle protein breakdown during the acute phase further amplified by muscle atrophy due to prolonged immobilisation and by the use of muscle relaxants [34]. Indeed acute myopathy or neuromyopathy can occur, following the prolonged use of muscle relaxants, either alone or in association with corticosteroids [35]. Moreover, a critical illness polyneuropathy has been described in sepsis and MODS. Thus, skeletal muscle loss and dysfunction in many patients having undergone a protracted course of hypermetabolic illness leading can be a major cause of long post-ICU rehabilitation. However, an even more crucial point is the impact of muscle loss on respiratory muscles, particularly the diaphragm. An autopsy study by Arora and Rochester showed that the loss of diaphragmatic mass related malnutrition is proportional to the atrophy incurred by the non-respiratory muscles [36]. Furthermore the decrease in respiratory muscle strength is out of proportion to the loss of body weight and diaphragmatic mass: respiratory muscle strength decreased by 60% (both on inspiratory and expiratory muscles) and maximal voluntary ventilation by 50% in malnourished patients (30% below ideal weight) as compared with healthy age-matched controls [37]. This suggests that, besides the loss of contractile mass, the muscle remaining has become myopathic as it can be suggested by the reported lowering of intracellular energy and potassium stores [38]. However, these data do not stem from ICU patients, and extrapolation to this particular population must be cautious.

The capacity to sustain indefinite spontaneous unassisted tidal breathing is dependent on three factors: a- the level of central respiratory drive, b- the capacity of the respiratory muscle pump, and c- the workload on the respiratory muscles [39]. Interstitial oedema, reduced lung compliance, bronchoconstriction, left ventricular failure, hyperinflation, intrinsic positive end-expiratory pressure, and added load due to the endotracheal and the ventilator circuit factors is often encountered in patients recovering from hypermetabolic condition. All these factors participate to the increased load on respiratory muscles and therefore may worsen the weaning difficulties [40]. Likewise, central respiratory drive is often elevated in patients during weaning trials [33]. Hence, the combination of increased load and central drive leads to a rise in the work of breathing when ventilatory support is withdrawn. This increased work of breathing can lead to fatigue of the respiratory muscles weakened by the prolonged catabolic phase [2]. Fatigue of the respiratory muscles invariably leads to progressive respiratory insufficiency and failure to wean from the ventilator. Since the risk of nosocomial pneumonia increases by approximately 1–3% per day of mechanical ventilation [41], protracted ventilator dependency can lead to further muscle loss through hypermetabolic septic episodes, the ultimate chances of successful weaning becoming slimmer with each new episode.

Ventilator Dependence in COPD Patients

Weaning difficulties are also often encountered in COPD patients undergoing acute exacerbation. However, pre-existing undernutrition with loss of diaphragm mass and strength adds to problems described above. In these patients, inspiratory muscle workload is increased while the diaphragm is placed in adverse working conditions [40]. The result is an increased work of breathing and an increased risk of muscle fatigue [2, 4]. This situation is worsened during weaning from the ventilator, due to the fact that the workload placed on respiratory muscles increases, often dramatically, when mechanical ventilatory support is reduced [42]. Furthermore, any decrease in perfusion or oxygenation, such as can occur in ICU patients will influence unfavourably respiratory muscle energy reserves, and lower the threshold of fatigue [2].

Nutritional Assessment

Evaluation of nutritional state is the first important step to detect pre-existing malnutrition and to monitor the efficacy of nutritional support. Anthropometric measurements such as skinfold thickness and arm circumference are of little interest, if any, in severe ICU patients because of difficult access of measurement sites (phlebitis, burns, wound dressings, supine position), large and rapid changes in body hydration-state and absence of validation in this setting [43]. Body composition can be evaluated by bioelectrical impedance analysis (BIA). Although BIA is a rapid, safe and non-invasive technique, which can be performed at the bedside, providing valuable information on the degree of protein-calorie malnutrition and overall hydration [43], it is less reliable in ICU [44]. Serum protein level is a poor indicator of nutritional status in critically ill patients [22].

Determination of total urinary nitrogen excretion permitting to calculate nitrogen balance is a useful method to assess protein turnover [43] as well as the impact of nutritional support. Although it must be noted that nitrogen loss are often underestimated leading to an overestimation of the nitrogen balance, it remains the is most useful way in ICU patients to monitor the magnitude of protein breakdown, and the beneficial effects of nutritional or hormonal interventions [43].

The determination of the level of the nutritional requirements is an important step for conducting a nutritional support. Although in most cases, it is estimated that at rest, males require 25–30 non-protein kcal/kg/day, and females 20–25 non-protein kcal/kg/day the use of the Harris-Benedict equation might lead to a better definition of the energy needs: Basal energy expenditure:

- Men: 66+[13.7× body weight (kg)]+5× height (cm)]–[6.8× age (years)]
- Women: 65.5+[9.6× body weight (kg)]+[1.7× height (cm)]–[4.7× age (years)]

However, in ICU patients, the predictions might not always be accurate, depending on the underlying disease state among many other factors. Indirect calorimetry, which consists of measuring oxygen consumption ($\dot{V}O_2$) and CO_2 production ($\dot{V}CO_2$) is more accurate, but sometimes data are difficult to interpret in ICU patients.

Techniques for Nutritional Support in Acute Lung Disease

During the hypermetabolic phase of the critical illness, nutritional support should provide sufficient fuel for the raised metabolic activity, while minimising excessive protein breakdown and muscle wasting. But, to wean the patient from the ventilator, the main rule is to give the best chance of successful weaning. This implies to avoid excessive caloric intakes while promoting anabolism and reconstruction of muscular mass if possible.

Enteral Versus Parenteral Feeding?

The two available routes for feeding are enteral and parenteral. It is widely accepted that enteral feeding should be preferred whenever possible. Indeed, bypassing the gut induces deleterious structural and functional changes of the intestinal mucosal barrier. In normal human volunteers, total jejunal mucosal thickness and villous cell counts were decreased after 14 days of total parenteral nutrition. This was accompanied by intracellular oedema, and increased intestinal permeability [45]. Enteral feeding reversed these changes. On the contrary, in critically ill patients, enteral nutrition over a ten-day period has been shown to improve normal absorption and to reduce abnormal mucosal permeability [46]. This favourable effect results from various factors, such as the stimulation of epithelial cell metabolism by direct contact with nutrients, the increase in mucosal blood flow, and the secretion of enterotrophic gastrointestinal hormones such as gastrin and enteroglucagon. Therefore preventing mucosal atrophy and permeability increase is probably an important goal. In critically ill patients, enteral nutrition is frequently and erroneously delayed because of prolonged gastric emptying and regurgitation of enteral feeds. As a result of the delay in enteral feeding, a worsening of the negative nitrogen balance and further weight loss can occur [47]. Consequently, enteral feeding should begin as early as possible, not necessarily with the goal of providing total support, but with that of exerting the beneficial effects on the gut outlined above, which can be attained with even small amounts of enteral feeding [48]. Decreased gastroduodenal motility is a frequent finding in ICU patients, whose aetiology is multifactorial [49] therefore, enteral nutrition should be administered at a low rate (20 ml/h, 24 h/day). Gastric emptying can be enhanced by the administration of prokinetic agents such as cisapride [50] and residue should be measured twice a day. Alternatively, naso-duodenal tubes can be used, since they bypass the slow emptying stomach. However, duodenal positioning of the tube is difficult to maintain, and tolerance (diarrhea) to substantial amounts of nutrients is often lower when they are administered distal to the stomach. During this time, partial enteral feeding should be combined with parenteral nutrition to insure adequate protein-caloric intake. Intravenous feeding is traditionally associated with the complications of central venous catheterization, such as arterial puncture, pneumothorax, air emboli, and catheter-related infections. However, many of the ICU patients discussed here are equipped with such catheters for purposes other than nutrition, and using the parenteral route probably does not contribute to added risk. Nonetheless, an increased infection rate has been repeatedly documented in ICU patients receiving parenteral feeding [48]. In such acutely ill patients, intravenous nutrition should be infused continuously over a 24-h period, and not in a cyclic fashion. Indeed, continuous infusion results in a lower thermogenic effect and CO_2 production as well as improved energy balance.

Carbohydrate Versus Fat?

Glucose is an obligatory fuel for various organs, such as the central nervous system, erythrocytes, and immune cells, as well as in wound and tissue repair. The minimum daily requirement for normal subjects is approximately 200 g/day, which is roughly equivalent to the 2 mg/kg/min glucose produced by hepatic gluconeogenesis [51]. Above this amount, whether glucose or fat should be given, as fuel has been the subject of controversy. Glucose exceeding 4 mg/kg/min is certainly responsible for several side effects, some being possibly very deleterious [52]. Hyperglycemia due to the peripheral resistance to glucose uptake, as discussed previously, is frequent and could be responsible for intra- and extracellular dehydration. Moreover, when glucose intakes exceed total oxidative capacity, stimulation of hepatic lipogenesis increases liver metabolic cost and might lead to acute steatosis. The increased CO_2 production exacerbates the pathological ventilatory limitation due to the underlying disease, which is a serious pitfall in the nutritional care of such patients. The increase in CO_2 production can be the consequence of several factors: (a) glucose oxidation results in a higher CO_2 formation as compared to lipids (the respiratory quotient is 1 versus 0.7 for lipids); (b) high glucose is responsible for catecholamine release leading to a further increase in metabolic rate; and (c) lipogenesis is associated with an energy cost associated with a high respiratory quotient (above 1). Most of the time, the rise in CO_2 production has only little effects in the majority of mechanically ventilated patients [1] but it might be a problem when weaning is difficult especially in the presence of respiratory muscle weakness. Indeed, the increased minute ventilation necessary to clear excess CO_2 can be sufficient to result in respiratory muscle fatigue and weaning failure [2]. Nevertheless, it should be remembered that total caloric load is responsible for increased CO_2 production rather than the proportion of glucose versus lipids. Indeed, as shown by Talpers et al. CO_2 production did not change when carbohydrate/lipid ratio are ranging from 40%–75% during isocaloric administration, but rose markedly as total caloric intake are up to 200% of the resting energy expenditure [53]. It has been reported that lipid emulsions when administered rapidly (i.e. 500 ml of 20% lipid emulsion over 8 h) may induce a worsening of hypoxemia in patients with sepsis-associated acute respiratory failure and high levels of venous admixture [54]. However this problem can be avoided when lipids are administered slowly, over a 24-h period, and below 0.5 mg/kg/min [52]. Thus, in acute respiratory failure, lipids could represent between 30 and 40% of the non-protein caloric requirements. Some studies have shown that lipid emulsions containing medium-chain triglycerides could have beneficial effects, due to the lack of carnitine requirement for oxidation [55]. However, this metabolic feature is true only in liver and the precise place of MCT in nutritional strategies for patients with lung injury remains to be determined [52].

Minimising protein loss is also an important goal. If providing adequate oxidative fuel permits to avoid excessive protein oxidation, several studies have shown that this is far from sufficient. Indeed, besides the deleterious effects seen above, administration of generous caloric intakes (2370 kcal/day, as 50% glucose/50% fat) and high amino-acid via a parenteral route for 10 days in septic patients is insufficient to prevent protein loss while body fat stores increased. Similar findings have been recently observed in postoperative patients. When comparing hypo-, iso-, and hypercaloric nutritional regimens in non-surgical patients with multiple organ failure, it was found that if the latter two prevented protein catabolism both increased energy expenditure. Providing amino acids in sufficient quantities could play a role in sparing endogenous protein by substituting exogenous for endogenous fuel as well as substrate for the synthesis of acute phase proteins. Because of the high rate of protein catabolism, protein should be administered at doses above the standard 1 g/kg/day recommended in normal individuals. Besides quantitative aspects, qualitative mixture of aminoacid is equally important. Unfortunately, the composition of currently used amino acid solutions presents some degree of imbalance in the face of the metabolic challenges involved [31]. The use of BCAA, which present the advantages of being readily usable in peripheral metabolic processes and also participate in protein catabolism regulation, could thus contribute to enhance nitrogen retention when given in higher amount than those already present in most nutrition formulas. However, this point remains to be clarified through further trials. The stimulatory effect of BCAAs on the central respiratory drive probably accounts for the increased ventilatory response to CO_2 documented in response to protein infusion [1]. Whether this is beneficial or not is controversial, but in patients with respiratory muscle weakness, this could be deleterious, by increasing the risk of respiratory muscle fatigue [2]. Glutamine is a special aminoacid whose use is now widely accepted. Promising results of improved nitrogen balance and reduced muscle catabolism in patients after bone marrow transplantation and elective abdominal surgery prompted further investigations in ICU patients whose favourable results on survival has been demonstrated [56]. Finally, glutamine, has demonstrated favourable effects on maintaining gut integrity during stress and enhancing immune cell function

The third point to discuss is how promote muscle anabolism. Muscle protein synthesis can be stimulated by hormonal manipulations. Human growth hormone (hGH) is clearly the most powerful of the anabolic hormones, together with IGF-1, insulin, and testosterone. hGH is a 22,000-kDa protein, normally secreted by the anterior pituitary, which can be obtained by biosynthesis, exerts most of its effects through the action of IGF-1 produced in the liver. Several studies in ICU patients have demonstrated beneficial effects on protein anabolism, and nitrogen balance after severe burns, sepsis and major surgery. hGH can help maintain a positive nitrogen balance even in the presence of hypocaloric feeding, which could prove beneficial in some patients in which the excessive CO_2 production and increased energy expenditure induced by iso- or hypercaloric feeding might be avoided. However, even though these favourable results on nitrogen balance are promising, it should be remembered that the ultimate goal is to improve muscle mass and function, thereby shortening weaning from the ventilator. Unfortunately, there is little data to support this. In a prospective, randomised controlled trial a positive effect on nitrogen balance of hGH was found but without significant improvement in peripheral muscle force, respiratory muscle endurance or weaning times [57]. Consequently, and considering the high cost of hGH therapy, further trials should address the issue of which patients are most apt to benefit from this treatment. Very recently, in a multicenter large trial an increased mortality has been found to be associated with growth hormone treatment in critically ill adults [58]. Although the mechanism of such effect is not clear this finding is probably of major importance for future studies with growth hormone.

Electrolyte and trace element administration is an important aspect of nutritional management. In this particular group of patients with respiratory failure and undernutrition, the importance of potassium, magnesium and phosphorous must be stressed since they play a major role for optimising muscle cell function [38]. Hence, careful attention should be placed on repletion and supplementation with micronutrients during nutritional support.

Conclusion and Practical Approach

In clinical practice, energy intake of patients with acute respiratory insufficiency should match energy expenditure. Direct measurement of resting energy expenditure by indirect calorimetry is ideal when possible, if not the use of Harris and Benedict equation permits to estimate this value. As seen above energy expenditure exceeds only rarely 35 kcal/kg/d. Except for very rare situation, the proportion of fat and carbohydrates should be around 30:70 as it is the case most usually. This leads to intakes of 15–18 kcal/kg/d as carbohydrates and 6–8 kcal/kg/d as lipids. Newer trends advocating carbohydrate/fat proportions of 35/65 should be reserved to clinical trials, or to difficult weaning with high deadspace ventilation. The protein content should be approximately 1.2 g/kg/day, increased to 1.5 g/kg/day in patients with very high levels of metabolic stress or during refeeding after extensive catabolism. Protein intake should not exceed 1.8 g/kg/day.

References

1. Takala J (1993) Nutrition and metabolism in acute respiratory failure, In: D. Wilmore and Y. Carpentier, Metabolic support of the critically ill patient, Springer-Verlag: Berlin, Heidelberg, New York. p 390–406
2. Roussos C, Zakynthinos S (1996) Fatigue of the respiratory muscles. Intensive Care Med 22: 134–155
3. Fiaccadori E, Del Canale S, Coffrini E, et al. (1988) Hypercapnic-hypoxemic chronic obstructive pulmonary disease (COPD): influence of severity of COPD on nutritional status. Am J Clin Nutr 48: 680–685
4. Jounieaux V, Mayeux I (1995) Oxygen cost of breathing in patients with emphysema or chronic bronchitis in acute respiratory failure. Am J Respir Crit Care Med 152: 2181–2184
5. Schols AM (1997) Nutrition and outcome in chronic respiratory disease. Nutrition 13: 161–3
6. Schols AM, Slangen J, Volovics L, Wouters EF (1998) Weight loss is a reversible factor in the prognosis of chronic obstructive pulmonary disease. Am J Respir Crit Care Med 157: 1791–7
7. Aubier M, Murciano D, Lecocguic Y, et al. (1985) Effect of hypophosphatemia on diaphragmatic contractility in patients with acute respiratory failure. N Engl J Med 313: 420–4
8. Aubier M, Viires N, Piquet J, et al. (1985) Effects of hypocalcemia on diaphragmatic strength generation. J Appl Physiol 58: 2054–61
9. Dhingra S, Solven F, Wilson A, McCarthy DS (1984) Hypomagnesemia and respiratory muscle power. Am Rev Respir Dis 129: 497–8
10. Arora NS, Rochester DF (1982) Effect of body weight and muscularity on human diaphragm muscle mass, thickness, and area. J Appl Physiol 52: 64–70
11. Di Francia M, Barbier D, Mege JL, Orehek J (1994) Tumor necrosis factor-alpha levels and weight loss in chronic obstructive pulmonary disease. Am J Respir Crit Care Med 150: 1453–5
12. Pouw EM, Schols AM, Deutz NE, Wouters EF (1998) Plasma and muscle amino acid levels in relation to resting energy expenditure and inflammation in stable chronic obstructive pulmonary disease. Am J Respir Crit Care Med 158: 797–801
13. Hunter A, Carey M, Larsh H (1981) The nutritional status of patients with chronic obstructive plumonary disease. Am Rev Respir Dis 124: 376–381
14. Driver A, McAlevy M, Smith J (1982) Nutritional assessment of patients with chronic obstructive pulmonary disease and acute respiratory failure. Chest 82: 568–571
15. Schols A, Soeters P, Mostert R, Saris W, Wouters E (1991) Energy balance in chronic obstructive pulmonary disease. Am Rev Resp Dis 143: 1248–1252

16. Schols AM, Soeters PB, Mostert R, Saris WH, Wouters EF (1991) Energy balance in chronic obstructive pulmonary disease. Am Rev Respir Dis 143: 1248–52
17. Field S, Kelly S, Macklem P (1982) The oxygen cost of breathing in patients with cardiorespiratory disease. Am Rev Respir Dis 126: 9–13
18. Schols A, Mostert R, Cobben N, Soeters P, Wouters E (1991) Transcutaneous oxygen saturation and carbon dioxide tension during meals in patients with chronic obstructive pulmonary disease. Chest 100: 1287–92
19. Pison CM, Chauvin C, Perrault H, et al. (1998) In vivo hypoxic exposure impairs metabolic adaptations to a 48 h fast in rats. Eur Respir J 12: 658–65
20. Goldstein S, Askanasi J, Weissman C, Thomashow B, Kiney J (1987) Energy expenditure in patients with chronic obstructive pulmonary disease. Chest 91: 222–224
21. Voerman HJ, Groeneveld AB, de Boer H, et al. (1993) Time course and variability of the endocrine and metabolic response to severe sepsis. Surgery 114: 951–9
22. Kinney J (1995) Metabolic responses of the critically ill patient. Crit Care Clin 11: 569–585
23. Shangraw R, Jahoor F, Wolfe R, Lang C (1996) Pyruvate dehydrogenase inactivity is not responsible for sepsis-induced insulin resistance. Crit Care Med 24: 566–574
24. Lang C, Dobrescu C, Bagby G (1992) Tumor necrosis factor impairs insulin action on peripheral glucose disposal and hepatic glucose output. Endocrinology 130: 43–52
25. Leverve X (1998) Metabolic and nutritional consequences of chronic hypoxia. Clin Nutr 17: 241–51
26. Bazzy AR, Akabas SR, Hays AP, Haddad GG (1988) Respiratory muscle response to load and glycogen content in type I and II fibers. Exp Neurol 101: 17–28
27. Meraihi Z, Lutz O, Scheftel JM, et al. (1991) Decreased lipolytic activity in tissues during infectious and inflammatory stress. Nutrition 7: 93–7; discussion 98
28. Read TE, Grunfeld C, Kumwenda Z, et al. (1995) Triglyceride-rich lipoproteins improve survival when given after endotoxin in rats. Surgery 117: 62–7
29. Mansoor O, Cayol M, Gachon P, et al. (1997) Albumin and fibrinogen syntheses increase while muscle protein synthesis decreases in head-injured patients. Am J Physiol 273: E898–902
30. Hasselgren PO, Pedersen P, Sax HC, Warner BW, Fischer JE (1988) Current concepts of protein turnover and amino acid transport in liver and skeletal muscle during sepsis. Archives of Surgery 123: 992–999
31. Fürst P, Stehle P (1993) Are we giving unbalanced amino acid solutions?, In: D. Wilmore and Y. Carpentier, Metabolic support of the critically ill patient, Springer-Verlag: Berlin, Heidelberg, New York. p. 119–136
32. Helweg-Larsen P, Hoffmeyer H, Kieler J, et al. (1952) Famine diseases in German concentration camps. Complications and sequels. Acta Medica Scandinavica 144 suppl: 274
33. Tobin M, Perez W, Guenther S, et al. (1986) The pattern of breathing during successful and unsuccessful trials of weaning from mechanical ventilation. Am Rev Respir Dis 134: 1111–1118
34. Duchateau J, Hainaut K (1987) Electrical and mechanical changes in immobilized human muscle. J Appl Physiol 62: 2168–2173
35. Watling S, Dasta J (1994) Prolonged paralysis in intensive care unit patients after the use of neuromuscular blocking agents: a review of the litterature. Crit Care Med 22: 884–893
36. Arora N, Rochester D (1982) Effect of chronic obstructive pulmonary disease on diaphragm muscle dimensions. Am Rev Respir Dis 123: A176
37. Arora NS, Rochester DF (1982) Respiratory muscle strength and maximal voluntary ventilation in undernourished patients. Am Rev Respir Dis 126: 5–8
38. Pichard C, Vaughan C, Struk R, Armstrong R, Jeejeebhoy K (1988) Effect of dietary manipulation (fasting, hypocaloric feeding and subsequent refeeding) on rat muscles energetics as assessed by nuclear magnetic resonance spectroscope. J Clin Invest 82: 895–901
39. Goldstone J, Moxham J (1991) Weaning from mechanical ventilation. Thorax 46: 56–62
40. Rossi A, Polese G, Brandi G, Conti G (1995) Intrinsic positive end-expiratory pressure. Intensive Care Med 21: 522–536

41. George D (1995) Epidemiology of nosocomial pneumonia in intensive care unit patients. Clin Chest Med 16: 29–44
42. Annat G, Viale J, Dereymez C, et al. (1990) Oxygen cost of breathing and diaphragmatic pressure-time index. Measurement in patients with COPD during weaning with pressure support ventilation. Chest 98: 411–414
43. Manning E, Shenkin A (1995) Nutritional assessment in the critically ill. Crit Care Clin 11: 603–634
44. Chioléro RL, Gay LJ, Cotting J, Gurtner C, Schutz Y (1993) Assessment of changes in body water by bioimpedance in acutely ill surgical patients. Critical Care Medicine 18: 322–326
45. Buchman A, Moukarzel A, Bhuta S, et al. (1995) Parenteral nutrition is associated with intestinal morphologic and functional changes in humans. JPEN 19: 453–460
46. Hadfield R, Sinclair D, Houldsworth P, Evans T (1995) Effects of enteral and parenteral nutrition on gut mucosal permeability in the critically ill. Am J Respir Crit Care Med 152: 1545–1548
47. Weekes E, Elia M (1996) Observations on the patterns of 24-h energy expenditure changes in body composition and gastric emptying in head-injured patients receiving nasogastric tube feeding. JPEN 20: 31–37
48. Zaloga G, Black K, Prielipp P (1992) Effect of rate of enteral nutrient supply on gut mass. JPEN 16: 39–42
49. Dive A, Moulart M, Jonard P, Jamart J, Mahieu P (1994) Gastroduodenal motility in mechanically ventilated critically ill patients: a manometric study. Crit Care Med 22: 441–447
50. Spapen H, Duinslaeger L, Diltoer M, et al. (1995) Gastric emptying in critically ill patients is accelerated by adding cisapride to a standard enteral feeding protocol: results of a prospective, randomized, controlled trial. Crit Care Med 23: 481–485
51. Long C, Kinney J, Geiger J (1976) Nonsuppressibility of gluconeogenesis by glucose in septic patients. Metabolism 25: 193–201
52. Wojnar M, Hawkins W, Lang C (1995) Nutritional support of the septic patient. Crit Care Clin 11: 717–733
53. Talpers S, Romberger D, Bunce S, Pingleton S (1992) Nutritionally associated increased carbon dioxide production: excess total calories vs. high proportion of carbohydrate calories. Chest 102: 551–555
54. Venus B, Smith R, Patel C, Sandoval E (1989) Hemodynamic and gas exchange alterations during Intralipid infusion in patients with adult respiratory distress syndrome. Chest 95: 1278–1281
55. Weissman C, Chioléro R, Askanasi J, et al. (1988) Intravenous infusion of a medium-chain triglyceride-enriched lipid emulsion. Crit Care Med 16: 1183–1190
56. Griffiths RD (1997) Outcome of critically ill patients after supplementation with glutamine. Nutrition 13: 752–4
57. Pichard C, Kyle U, Chevrolet J, et al. (1996) Lack of effects on muscle function of recombinant growth hormone in patients requiring prolonged mechanical ventilation: a prospective randomized controlled study. Crit Care Med 24: 403–413
58. Takala J, Ruokonen E, Webster NR, et al. (1999) Increased mortality associated with growth hormone treatment in critically ill adults [see comments]. N Engl J Med 341: 785–92

Nutrition Support in Pancreatitis

S.A. McClave and H.L. Snider

Introduction

The principles of nutritional therapy in the patient with acute pancreatitis have changed dramatically over the past several years. In other disease processes similar to pancreatitis, providing nutritional support to patients, particularly by the enteral route, improves outcome compared to patients who receive no nutritional therapy [1]. Acute pancreatitis is characterized by a catabolic hypermetabolic stress state, commonly producing deterioration of nutritional status. Retrospective evidence suggests that failure to provide nutritional support worsens outcome [2]. We are now better at defining which patients with acute pancreatitis need aggressive nutritional therapy [3–6]. In pancreatitis, route of nutritional support has been shown to impact patient outcome [7, 8]. Failure to maintain gut integrity correlates to worsening overall severity of illness and increased likelihood for complications [8]. We now have a better understanding of the physiologic principles involved in the stimulation of the pancreas and the factors which exacerbate the disease process of pancreatitis. The emphasis of nutritional therapy is gradually shifting from eliminating all stimulation of the pancreas while providing parenteral nutrients, to reducing stimulation to subclinical levels while providing enteric feeding through a nasojejunal tube, thus maintaining gut integrity.

Pathophysiology

Pancreatitis causes a systemic immunoinflammatory response to a localized process of autodigestion of the gland, initiated by premature activation of proteolytic digestive enzymes [9–11]. Although the trigger event which initiates the process is not well defined, the initial step involves co-localization of digestive enzyme zymogens and lysosomal hydrolase cothepsin B, which promotes the conversion of trypsinogen to trypsin [12]. The premature activation and release of trypsin into the cytoplasm of the acinar cell generates the primary injury [12]. Following this initial insult to the acinar cell, an amplification process ensues with release of cytokines, inflammatory mediators, and an aggressive inflammatory cell recruitment [12]. It is this amplification process that results in the systemic manifestations of the disease process and accounts for the overall morbidity and mortality [13]. The peak of inflammatory cytokine production occurs 24–36 h after the onset of the pain. The onset of severe systemic manifestations and distant organ failure usually present 2–4 days after the peak of cytokine production [13]. The overall severity of pancreatitis has been linked clinically to a number of factors including the levels of cytokines generated (interleukin-1, 6 and 8, as well as tumor necrosis factor) [13], the presence of necrosis on computerized tomography (CT) scan [14, 15], infection within the gland [16, 17], failure of at least one distant organ [14], and the route of nutritional support [8]. The localized focus of inflammation or necrosis within the gland generates a primary stress response. The degree to which the process is provoked or attenuated relates in part to the status of gut integrity [18]. Impaired gut integrity can act as a secondary focus generating additional stress responses of its own.

A key problem in acute pancreatitis is the production and release of proteolytic enzymes which autodigest the gland [12]. Reducing the stimulation and secretion of these enzymes to some subclinical level has seemed important in the past to halting or reversing the disease process. Understanding the issues related to stimulation of the pancreas is important to the clinician. Most stimulation of the pancreas occurs in response to gut luminal agents [19]. Studies in both animals and humans indicate that nutrients infused by the parenteral route result in little or no stimulation of the pancreas [20]. Any exacerbation of pancreatitis in patients on TPN is invariably associated with the occurrence of hypercalcemia [21] or hypertriglyceridemia [22]. Level of the gastrointestinal (GI) tract into which nutrients are infused may be the biggest factor in whether or not the pancreas is stimulated [23]. There are three phases of pancreatic stimulation – the cephalic, gastric, and intestinal phases (Fig. 1). A variety of different stimulants are involved at each level, including neurovagal stimulation, chemical stimulation from gastric acid and various food sources, mechanical stimulation from gastric distention, and hormonal stimulation from the release of gastrin, CCK, and secretin [23].

The higher the level of the GI tract into which nutrients are infused, the greater the number of factors that are invoked and a resultant greater response in pancreatic secretion. The quality and characteristics of the nutrients infused into the gut have a variable effect on stimulation of the gland (Fig. 2) [23]. At one end of the spectrum with the highest degree of stimulation is fat, with long chain fatty acids having more stimulation than medium chain triglycerides. Carbohydrate infusion results in the least stimulation of the pancreas (compared to protein and fat) [24]. Hyperosmolar nutrients may lead to greater stimulation than isosmolar agents [24]. A spectrum of stimulation exists from the oral to jejunal level of feeding and from long chain fatty acid to carbohydrate in composition (Fig. 3). Feeding infused low enough into the jejunum may result in minimal stimulation and may even lead to increased inhibition of pancreatic secretion from agents such as bile acids, rising pH, luminal proteases, and hormones such as pancreatic polypeptide and peptide YY [23]. In patients with severe pancreatitis, it is important to avoid as many stimulatory factors as possible, and thus nutritional management may require the infusion of an odorless isosmolar elemental formula (which is nearly fat free with protein in the form of individual amino acids) down low into the jejunum [24]. A patient with mild pancreatitis may tolerate a greater number of stimulatory factors and tolerate the same formula ingested orally [24].

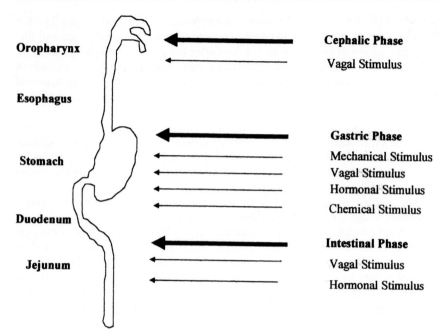

Fig. 1. Stimulatory phases for pancreatic exocrine secretion

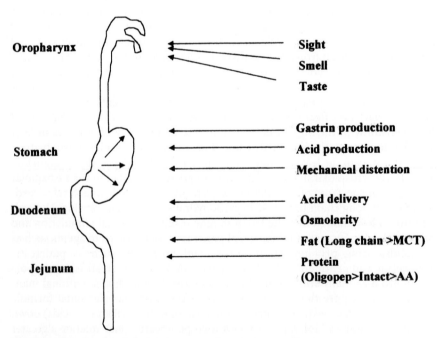

Fig. 2. Specific stimulatory factors in pancreatic exocrine secretion

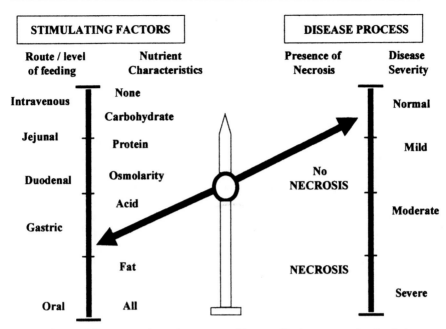

Fig. 3. Balance of disease severity and spectrum of factors affecting pancreatic stimulation

In the past, the goal of therapeutic management was to reduce pancreatic secretion to unstimulated basal levels, a principal that was applied universally regardless of degree of severity of pancreatitis. This practice succeeded in relief of pain only and never was proven to impact patient outcome [25]. Additional efforts to reduce pancreatic stimulation in prospective randomized controlled trials, including nasogastric aspiration, hormonal therapy (somatostatin, glucagon, calcitonin), and pharmacologic agents (cimetidine, anticholinergic drugs), have failed to show any effect on patient outcome [26, 27]. Exacerbation of pain with refeeding often may be tolerated without incident, and only in a small percentage of cases does a true exacerbation of the disease process develop [28]. The degree to which pancreatic secretion should be suppressed to achieve resolution of the disease process is not known. There are three components to pancreatic exocrine secretion, volume, bicarbonate, and protein enzyme output, each having its own independent stimulatory factors. Because protein enzymes are most responsible for autodigestion of the gland, strategies which reduce enzyme output but maintain volume and bicarbonate output may be adequately resting the gland [29]. Ironically, pancreatic secretion is almost abolished at the peak of inflammation and has been shown to take up to several months to return to normal following an exacerbation [27, 30, 31]. Reducing stimulation to some subclinical level may be adequate to allow the disease process to resolve, and eliminating secretion to unstimulated basal levels may not be required.

There is good evidence now in humans that loss of gut integrity with prolonged gut disuse (particularly with use of TPN) has been associated with decreased height and transformation in villous morphology [32]. In animals, intestinal permeability is dramatically increased. In humans, gut disuse is associated with increased exposure to endotoxin and decreased antioxidant capacity [8]. Failure to use the GI tract causes loss of gut integrity and worsens the stress response associated with pancreatitis [8]. With loss of gut integrity, the gut can act as the "motor" of the multiple organ failure sepsis (MOFS) syndrome, exacerbating the stress response generated by an immune system already primed by pancreatic inflammation [18]. Prolonged increases in C Reactive Protein levels, hyperglycemia, and APACHE II scores, with slower resolution of overall toxicity and the systemic inflamatory response syndrome (SIRS) were seen in one study in the control group placed on TPN and gut rest, compared to the study group who received enteral nutrients via nasojejunal feeding [8].

Loss of gut integrity may allow bacteria of gut origin to infect the gland by translocation of bacteria via intestinal lymphatics, by portal vein (which may then migrate to the common bile duct and eventually back to the pancreatic duct), or by direct migration into the pancreatic bed via colonic micro-perforations [25]. In animals, intestinal bacteria were shown to contaminate inflamed pancreatic tissue [25]. Gut decontamination in rats with antibiotics decreased the rate of positive cultures from mesenteric lymph nodes and reduced the mortality rate from experimentally induced pancreatitis [33]. In humans, 60% of phlegmons and infected pseudocysts were shown in one study to be culture positive for gram negative coloforms, again suggesting an enteric source for pancreatic infection [34].

Patient Selection

The key issue in the nutritional assessment of patients with acute pancreatitis is to differentiate mild from severe disease (Table 1). Mild acute pancreatitis may be defined by 2 Ranson criteria, an APACHE II score of ≤9, and absence of necrosis on dynamic CT scan [5, 6]. Patients with mild pancreatitis represent approximately 80% of the admissions for acute pancreatitis. During the first 48 h of admission the APACHE II score should be expected to decrease by 1 point [4, 5, 14]. The likelihood for these patients developing complications of multiple organ failure during their hospitalization is <8% and their mortality rate is close to 0% [3, 4]. Their chance of successfully advancing to oral diet within 7 days is 81% [35]. The likelihood for relapse of pancreatitis with early advancement to PO diet is low at <12% [28]. This group of patients does not need aggressive artificial nutritional support.

Severe pancreatitis on the other hand may be defined by ≥3 Ranson criteria, an APACHE II score of ≥10, and evidence of pancreatic necrosis on CT scan [5, 6]. Patients with severe pancreatitis have a likelihood of developing multiple organ failure of approximately 38% and an associated mortality rate of 19% [3]. Their chance for relapse of the pancreatitis with early advancement to PO diet is 35% [28], and their likelihood for successfully achieving advancement to PO diet within 7 days is close to 0% [35]. This group of patients needs aggressive nutritional support. These patients are most likely to show improved outcome if gut access is

Table 1. Differentiating mild from severe acute pancreatitis

Parameters	Mild	Severe
Admissions	80.0%	20.0%
Ranson criteria	≤2	≥3
APACHE II score	≤9	≥10
Δ APACHE II (48 h)	↓ by 1	↑ by 3
Pancreatic necrosis	No	Yes
Compications	7.7%	38.0%
Mortality	0.0%	19.3%
PO died by 5 d	81.0%	0.0%

attained and the enteral route of feeding is utilized. Compared to use of TPN, enteral feeding in this group of pancreatitis patients may be expected to result in more rapid resolution of the systemic inflammatory response and greater reduction in disease severity [8, 36].

Practical Application

In patients with severe pancreatitis, the timing of nutritional support differs depending on the route of provision. If enteral access can be achieved in patients with severe pancreatitis, a nasoenteric tube should be placed and feeding initiated within 48 h of admission. Although tubes may be placed radiographically, use of endoscopy affords the opportunity to clip the distal end of the tube to the mucosa (which can be done without the use of fluoroscopy or transfer of the patient to the radiology suite). A pediatric colonoscope is better than the shorter gastroscope and the more flexible enteroscope for placement of the nasojejunal tube. Placement of a bridle around the nasal septum, using a small 5 french neonatal feeding tube is encouraged to secure the proximal end of the tube. Bedside techniques are successful only in placing the tube past the pylorus, but cannot be relied upon for placing the tube at or below the Ligament of Treitz. If nausea or vomiting is prominent on admission, a nasoenteric aspirate/feed tube should be placed to allow simultaneous decompression of the stomach through the gastric port while nutrients are infused through the jejunal port into the small bowel.

While the optimal composition of formula is not known, the choice of formula may be of greater importance when pancreatitis is more severe. Unfortunately, comparison of formulas in humans with acute pancreatitis has not been studied. If feeding is infused low enough in the GI tract, any formula may be adequate in reducing pancreatic stimulation to subclinical levels. The formula with the greatest theoretical advantage for reducing pancreatic secretion would be a true elemental formula, which is nearly fat free, with protein comprised entirely of individual amino acids. In a gut luminal environment devoid of pancreatic enzymes, however, semi-elemental formulas (in which protein is in the form of small peptides and fat is mainly in the form of medium chain triglycerides) have been shown to be associated with greater absorption, are well tolerated, and thus may be an acceptable alternative [36, 37, 38]. Patients with pancreatitis on nasoenteric feeds need to be monitored closely, watching for evidence of nausea, vomiting, abdominal distention, and diarrhea. Residual volumes aspirated from a tube placed into the jejunum should be low (generally <10 cc) [36]. Residual volumes which exceed 25–50 cc should raise suspicion that the tube in the small bowel may have migrated back to the stomach or proximal duodenum. Rarely an exacerbation of the systemic inflammatory response (with increasing fever and white blood cell count) may be the only sign that the tube has migrated proximally [36]. Persistent pain, which is not appreciably worse, and minor fluctuations in the amylase and lipase, may be expected in the patient on jejunal feeds. Only a sustained exacerbation of abdominal pain and increase in pancreatic enzymes should alert the clinician to the possibility of intolerance. The first step with evidence of intolerance is to confirm tube position. Rarely a patient with the tube at or below the Ligament of Treitz will show evidence of intolerance with infusion of luminal nutrients. The vast majority of patients on jejunal feeds tolerate the feeding well with gradual resolution of the disease process. Ileus is surprisingly a minimal problem and in one prospective study occurred in only 31% of patients with severe pancreatitis (resulting in a decrease in the rate of infusion for 2–4 days, but not requiring complete cessation of feeding) [8]. Diarrhea occurs infrequently in acute pancreatitis, but becomes more of a problem with enteral feeding in patients with chronic or long-term complications such as pseudocyst, ascites, or fistula.

The necessity of using the parenteral route affects the timing of nutritional support in a different manner. For patients with severe pancreatitis, in whom there is inability to gain enteral access or there is clearcut intolerance to enteral feeds (Fig. 4), provision of parenteral nutrition support may need to be delayed. Early TPN when compared to no nutritional therapy, even in patients with mild pancreatitis, was associated with worsening outcome, as evidenced by a high rate of catheter-related sepsis, and a longer length of hospitalization (by 6 days) [35]. Because of the possibility of exacerbating the stress response [18], it may be appropriate to withhold TPN for 5 days to allow the peak inflammatory response to abate. Achieving intravenous fluid resuscitation, correcting electrolyte abnormalities, and providing analgesia are more important during this time. After this period, patients expected to remain NPO for an additional 5–7 days should have a central line placed and TPN started. A mixed fuel regimen should be used, keeping the fat composition to <15%–30% of the total calories, to avoid the immunosupressant effects of long chain fat [1]. The TPN should be advanced slowly, controlling the glucose to levels <150–200 mg/dl (an insulin drip should be used readily to control glucose levels). The likelihood of glucose intolerance is in the range of 60%–80%, and resultant hyperglycemia may only exacerbate the likelihood for nosocomial infection and catheter-related sepsis [39]. The likelihood of fat intolerance is only 12%–15% [40]. Serum triglyceride levels should be monitored and kept ≤ 400 mg/dl. Caloric requirements should be measured by indirect calorimetry, if possible, to avoid overfeeding. Serum calcium levels should be monitored to avoid hypercalcemia which can exacerbate pancreatitis [21].

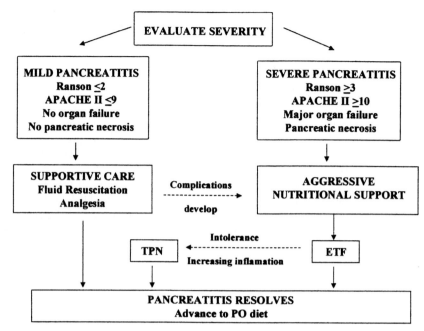

Fig. 4. Algorithm for nutritional support in pancreatitis

The decision to advance to oral clear liquids should be based on resolution of abdominal pain and nausea/vomiting, and a decrease in amylase and lipase over the preceding 48 h (but not necessarily to normal levels). The nasojejunal tube should be kept in place in case there is evidence of intolerance upon advancement to oral diet [36]. Relapse of pancreatitis upon advancement to oral diet should be avoided, as the length of hospitalization may be prolonged 2–3 fold with inappropriate early advancement and disease exacerbation [28]. Advancement to oral diet should be delayed in patients who show evidence of pancreatic necrosis on CT scan, pain duration of >6 days, and lipase levels which remain elevated three times the normal level, as these are all factors associated with relapse upon early advancement [28]. Factors not associated with relapse include maximal amylase levels, C reactive protein levels, presence of fluid collections, pancreatic calcifications, dilated pancreatic duct, and need for surgery [28].

Patients who have mild pancreatitis should receive IV fluid recussitation, correction of serum electrolytes, and analgesic support. Only if these patients fail to achieve oral diet by 5–7 days or develop a complication, should they be evaluated for nasoenteric feeding.

Influence of Complications

The development of complications arising from pancreatitis, including pseudocyst, fluid collections, fistulas, or ascites, is not a contraindication to enteral feeding [24, 41, 42]. In the absence of clear-cut intolerance, nasoenteric feeding or even feeding through a percutaneous endoscopic gastrostomy/jejunostomy tube may be well tolerated. In poorly controlled, mostly retrospective case series, patients with chronic complications of pancreatitis (who otherwise experienced an exacerbation of symptoms with advancement to oral diet) were able to tolerate nasogastric and occasionally oral feedings with elemental formulas [41, 42]. Many of the patients managed on enteral feeding had become intolerant of TPN or had developed complications of intravenous access and were advanced to enteral feeds out of necessity. Diarrhea is usually a more frequent problem in patients with chronic complications of pancreatitis, than in patients with an acute exacerbation of pancreatitis [43, 44].

The need for surgical intervention to manage hemorrhagic or infectious complications of pancreatitis is not an automatic indication for TPN, and ironically provides an opportunity to achieve surgically placed e nteral access. An early 1970 study by Lawson (published when TPN was just being developed) stressed the need for placement of a jejunal tube at the time of major surgical operations for complications of pancreatitis [45]. Kudsk reiterated these recommendations in 1990 [46].

Future Direction

Over time, clinicians will gain greater experience with use of the enteral route of feeding in patients with pancreatitis. The timing of feeding will be better defined both for the early enteral feeding, and for the delayed parenteral feeding in those patients in whom enteral feeding is not feasible. The optimum composition of formulas with regard to the percentage of carbohydrate and fat, the specific form of fat and protein in the formula, and whether use of supplemental enzymes promote better tolerance, may all be delineated. Tolerance of enteral feedings will be better defined and techniques to promote tolerance in patients with pancreatitis will be developed. Additional pharmacologic agents to help attenuate the stress response, such as platelet activating factor antagonists or leukotriene inhibitors, may be useful adjuncts to therapy designed to maintain gut integrity. Overall, efforts in nutritional therapy for the patient with pancreatitis will shift to reducing stimulation of pancreatic secretion to subclinical levels, reducing the associated stress response, maintaining gut integrity, and avoiding iotrogenic complications.

References

1. McClave SA, Snider HL, Spain DA (1999) Preoperative Issues in Clinical Nutrition. Chest 115:64–70 S
2. Sitzmann JV, Steinborn PA, Zinner MJ, et al. (1989) Total Parenteral Nutrition and Alternate Energy Substrates in Treatment of Severe Acute Pancreatitis. Surg Gynecol Obstet 168:311–317
3. Wilson C, Heath DI, Imrie CW (1990) Prediction of Outcome In Acute Pancreatitis: A Comparative Study of APACHE II, Clinical Assessment and Multiple Factor Scoring System. Br J Surg 77:1260–4

4. Agarwal N, Pitchumoni CS (1991) Assessment of Severity In Acute Pancreatitis. Amer J Gastroenterol 86 (10):1385–91
5. Corfield AP, Cooper MJ, Williamson RCN, et al. (1985) Prediction of Severity In Acute Pancreatitis: Prospective Comparison of Three Prognostic Indices. Lancet 2:403–7
6. Larvin M, McMahon MJ (1989): Apache-II Score for Assessment and Monitoring of Acute Pancreatitis. Lancet 2:201–5
7. Kalfarentzos F, Kehagias J, Mead N, et al. (1997) Enteral Nutrition Is Superior to Parenteral Nutrition in Severe Acute Pancreatitis: Results of a Randomized Prospective Trial. Brit J Surg 84:1665–9
8. Windsor ACJ, Kanwar S, Li AGK, et al. (1998) Compared With Parenteral Nutrition, Enteral Feeding Attenuates the Acute Phase Response and Improves Disease Severity in Acute Pancreatitis. Gut 42:431–5
9. Bradley EL III (1993) A Cinically Based Classification System for Acute Pancreatitis. Arch Surg 128:586–90
10. Bradley EL III (1996) Acute pancreatitis: Clinical Classification and Terminology. Pract Gastroenterol 20 (5):8–24
11. Soergel KH (1989) Acute Pancreatitis, in Gastrointestinal Disease – Pathophysiology, Diagnosis, Management, Sleisenger MH, Fordtran JS (Eds), WB Saunders Co., Philadelphia, PA pp 1814–42
12. Saluja AK, Steer ML (1999) Pathophysiology of Pancreatitis. Role of Cytokines and Other Mediators of Inflammation. Digestion 60:(suppl 1):27–33
13. Norman JG (1999) New Approaches to Acute Pancreatitis: Role of Inflammatory Mediators. Digestion 60 (suppl 1):57–60
14. Banks PA (1996) Pancreatitis for the Endoscopist-Terminology, Prediction of Complications and Management. ASGE Postgraduate Course, Digestive Disease Week, San Francisco, CA, May 23–24
15. Bradley EL III (1999) Operative vs. Nonoperative Therapy in Necrotizing Pancreatitis. Digestion 60 (suppl 1):19–21
16. Renner IG, Savage WT III, Pantoja JL, Renner VJ (1985) Death Due to Acute Pancreatitis: A Retrospective Analysis of 405 Autopsy Cases. Dig Dis Sci 30:1005–18
17. Lumsden A, Bradley EL III (1990) Secondary Pancreatic Infection: Abscess, Infected Necrosis, and Infected Pseudocyst. Surg Gynecol Obstet 170:459–67
18. Fong Y, Marano MA, Barber A (1989) Total Parenteral Nutrition and Bowel Rest Modify the Metabolic Response to Endotoxin in Humans. Ann Surg 210:449–57
19. Povoski SP, Nussbaum MS (1995) Nutrition Support in Pancreatitis: Fertile Ground for Prospective Clinical Investigation. Nutr Clin Pract 10:43–44
20. McClave SA, Snider HL, Owens N, Sexton LK (1997) Clinical Nutrition in Pancreatitis. Dig Dis Sci 42:2035–44
21. Iszak EM, Shike M, Roulet M, Jeejeebuoy KN (1980) Pancreatitis In Association With Hypercalcemia In Patients Receiving Total Parenteral Nutrition. Gastroenterol 79:555–8
22. Leibowitz AB, O'Sullivan P, Iberti TJ (1992) Intravenous Fat Emulsions and the Pancreas: A review. Mt Sinai J Med 59:38–42
23. Corcoy R, Ma Sanchez J, Domingo P, Net A (1988) Nutrition in the Patient With Severe Acute Pancreatitis. Nutrition 4:269–275
24. Parekh D, Lawson HH, Segal I (1993) The Role of Total Enteral Nutrition in Pancreatic Disease. S Afr J Surg 31:57–61
25. Helton WS (1990) Intravenous Nnutrition in Patients With Acute Pancreatitis. In Rombeau JL (ED):Clinical nutrition: Parenteral nutrition. Philadelphia, PA, W.B. Saunders Co., pp442–61
26. Koretz RL (1993) Nutritional Support in Pancreatitis-Feeding an Organ That Has Eaten Itself. Semin Gastrointestinal Disease 4: 99–115
27. Niederau C, Niederau M, Luthen R, et al. (1990) Pancreatic Exocrine Secretion in Acute Experimental Pancreatitis. Gastroenterology 99:1120–1127

28. Levy P, Heresbach D, Pariente EA, et al. (1997) Frequency and Risk Factors of Recurrent Pain During Refeeding in Ppatients with Acute Pancreatitis: A Multivariant Multicenter Prospective Study of 116 patients. Gut 40:262–6
29. Cassim MM, Allardyce DB (1974) Pancreatic Secretion in Response to Jejunal Feeding of Elemental Diet. Ann Surg 180:228
30. Mitchell CJ, Playforth MJ, Kelleher J, McMahon MJ (1983) Functional Recovery of the Exocrine Pancreas after Acute Pancreatitis. Scand J Gastroenterol 18:5–8
31. Arendt T, Rogos R (1991) Pancreatic Exocrine Secretion in Acute Experimental Pancreatitis. Gastroent 101:276–8
32. Groos S, Hunefeld G, Luciano L (1996) Parenteral Versus Enteral Nutrition: Morphological Changes in Human Adult Intestinal Mucosa. J Submic Cytol Pathol 28:61–74
33. Lange JF, van Gool J, Tytgat GNJ (1987) The Protective Effect of a Reduction in Intestinal Flora on Mortality of Acute Haemorrhagic Pancreatitis in the Rat. Hepatogastroenterology 34:28–30
34. Russel JC, Welch JP, Clark DG (1983) Colonic Complications of Acute Pancreatitis and Pancreatic Abscess. Am J Surg 146:558–64
35. Sax HC, Warner BW, Talamini MA, et al. (1987) Early Total Parenteral Nutrition In Acute Pancreatitis: Lack of Beneficial Effects. Am J Surg 153 (1):117–124
36. McClave SA, Greene LM, Snider HL, et al. (1997) Comparison of the Safety of Early Enteral Versus Parenteral Nutrition in Mild Acute Pancreatitis. JPEN 21:14–20
37. Imondi AR, Stradley RP (1974) Utilization of Enzymatically Hydrolyzed Soybean Protein and Crystalline Amino Acid Diets by Rats With Exocrine Pancreatic Insufficiency. J Nutr 104:793–801
38. Milla PJ, Lilby A, Rassam UB, Harries JT (1983) Small Intestinal Absorption of Amino Acids and a Dipeptide in Pancreatic Insufficiency. Gut 24:818–24
39. Havala T, Shronts E, Cerra F (1989) Nutritional Support in Acute Pancreatitis. Gastroenterol Clin N Amer 18 (3)525–42
40. Kohn CL, Bronzenec S, Foster PF (1993) Nutritional Support for the Patient With Pancreaticobiliary Disease. Crit Care Nurs Clin North Am 5:37–45
41. Voitk A, Brown RA, Echave V, et al. (1973) Use of An Elemental Diet in the Treatment of Complicated Pancreatitis. Am J Surg 125:223–7
42. Bury KD, Stephens RV, Randall HT (1971) Use of Chemically Defined, Liquid Elemental Diet for Nutritional Management of Fistulas of the Alimentary Tract. Am J Surg 121:174–83
43. Cowley A, Dutta SK, Narang A, et al. (1983) Evaluation of the Efficacy of Elemental Diet Therapy in Patients With Chronic Alcoholic Pancreatitis (Abstr). Gastroenterology 84:1130
44. Nasrallah SM, Martin DM (1984) Comparative Effects of Criticare HN and Vivonex HN in the Treatment of Malnutrition Due to Pancreatic Insufficiency. Am J Clin Nutr 39:251–4
45. Lawson DW, Daggett WM, Civetta JM, et al. (1970) Surgical Treatment of Acute Necrotizing Pancreatitis. Ann Surg 172:605–15
46. Kudsk KA, Campbell SM, O'Brien T, Fuller R (1990) Postoperative Jejunal Feedings Following Complicated Pancreatitis. Nutrition in Clinical Practice 5:14–7

Nutrition Support of Critically Ill Obese Patients

L. Flancbaum, P.S. Choban, and S.B. Heymsfield

Introduction

The World Health Organization recently noted that the incidence of obesity is increasing worldwide at an alarming rate [1]. In the United States, obesity is already the most prevalent chronic disease, affecting one-third of American adults [2]. In Europe, Australia, New Zealand, the Middle East and the remaining portions of Americas, its incidence appears to be increasing and is now between 10% and 20%. The incidence of obesity is still fairly low in China, Japan, and many countries in Africa [1].

The significance of obesity as a public health problem is primarily due to the fact that it is a significant independent risk factor for mortality from all causes, with the death rate increasing as the degree of obesity increases [3–6], and its relationship with numerous comorbid conditions. Diseases associated with obesity include diabetes, hypertension, coronary artery disease, obstructive sleep apnea and the obesity hypoventilation syndrome, gastroesophageal reflux, gallstones, urinary stress incontinence, osteoarthritis, and several forms of cancer (breast, prostate, endometrial and colon).

Because of its high prevalence, and the predisposition of obese patients to many surgical diseases, it is common to encounter obese individuals in hospitals and intensive care units. In a retrospective review of general, thoracic, urologic, and gynecologic surgical patients at Ohio State University [7], it was noted that 37% of the elective adult surgical population were overweight, having a Body Mass Index (BMI) >27 kg/m² and 17% were severely overweight, with a BMI of greater than 31 kg/m². In a 1990 review of blunt trauma victims treated at a Level I trauma center, 24% of the population was overweight (BMI >27 kg/m²) and 10% of the overall population severely overweight (BMI >31 kg/m²) [8]. These findings emphasize the pervasive nature of this problem and an estimate for the incidence of obesity of 35%–40% for the hospitalized population in general is probably reasonable, if not low.

The optimal method for providing nutrition support to obese hospitalized patients remains a dilemma. There is a lack of consensus among nutrition support practitioners about the definition of obesity, the equations to be used to calculate estimated energy needs, whether ideal, actual or "adjusted" body weight should be used in these equations, and how much protein obese patients should be fed [9].

Similar problems exist concerning the nutrition support of critically ill patients, who comprise a progressively greater proportion of hospitalized patients as the population continues to age and advances are made in medical technology. Disagreement is widespread concerning the preferred method for nutritional assessment, route of administration and composition of the formula.

Defining Obesity

Obesity is characterized by an excess of adipose tissue which can produce adverse health effects. For the vast majority of patients, with the exception of growing children, pregnant women, well-conditioned athletes, or frail sedentary adults, obesity can be defined using height and weight. These parameters may be used to determine the percentage of ideal body weight (IBW) or a Body Mass Index (BMI).

Several commonly used methods exist for estimating IBW, such as the use of height/weight tables [10] and the Hamwi formula [11], with obesity beginning when the individual exceeds 120% of IBW. However, BMI is currently the preferred parameter for use in clinical practice. These methods are illustrated in Table 1. A normal BMI is generally considered to be between 19 and 25 kg/m^2. Obesity is usually defined as a BMI >27 kg/m^2, with severe obesity beginning above a BMI of 31 kg/m^2 and morbid obesity above a BMI of 35 kg/m^2 [1, 3, 12–14]. Health risk increases as BMI increases [3, 12].

Metabolic Changes in Obesity and Critical Illness

Both obesity and critical illness are associated with a variety of metabolic changes that affect nutritional status and requirements. As with non-obese patients, suspicion of malnutrition should be prompted by knowledge of the underlying clinical condition of the patient and confirmed by a careful history, physical examination and appropriate laboratory studies. Obesity and malnutrition are not mutually exclusive and obese individuals should be assessed using the same approach as non-obese patients. In addition, an involuntary recent weight loss is a concern in this population and may indicate a loss of lean body mass and subsequent malnutrition. On the other hand, patients who experience significant voluntary weight loss in a monitored balanced-deficit program are not at increased risk for nutrition related poor outcome [15].

Obese patients are often insulin resistant, which results in hyperinsulinemia and predisposes to glucose intolerance, coronary artery disease, hypertension and hyperlipidemia (which together are referred to as "syndrome x"). These complications, in turn, can lead to intolerance to large volumes of intravenous fluid or lipid infusion. Also, obese patients may suffer from obstructive sleep apnea and the obesity hypoventilation syndrome, which can be exacerbated by overfeeding, leading to difficulty weaning and prolonging the need for mechanical ventilation [12, 14].

As with obesity, critical illness is associated with insulin resistance and glucose intolerance. Critically ill patients with hepatic dysfunction may demonstrate lipid intolerance, manifested as lipemic serum, hypercholesterolemia and hyper-

Table 1. Comparison of Hamwi formula, Metropolitan relative weight (MRW) and body mass index (BMI) for two hypothetical persons

		Degree of Obesity		
	"Ideal"	Mild	Moderate	Clinically severe
% IBW Hamwi [3]	100	130	150	200
Patient A	100 lb.	130 lb.	150 lb.	200 lb.
Patient B	166 lb.	216 lb.	249 lb.	332 lb.
% IBW MRW [4]	100	130	150	200
Patient A	109 lb.	136 lb.	164 lb.	218 lb.
Patient B	150 lb.	195 lb.	225 lb.	300 lb.
BMI (kg/m^2)	24	27	31	40
Patient A	122 lb.	138 lb.	158 lb.	204 lb.
Patient B	167 lb.	188 lb.	216 lb.	278 lb.

Patient A, a 5-ft. woman, and patient B, a 5-ft, 10-in. man, both over 25 years of age. BMI, weight (kg)/[height (m)]^2. Hamwi, women: 100 lb. for first 5 ft+5 lb. for each inch thereafter; men: 106 lb. for first 5 ft+6 lb. for each inch thereafter 10. Metropolitan Relative Weight which is mid-point of medium frame range (modified from 1959 Metropolitan Life Desirable Weights).

triglyceridemia [16]. Also, patients with respiratory insufficiency who require prolonged mechanical ventilation can have trouble weaning if overfed. Critical illness leads to an increase in energy expenditure, protein turnover, and hence protein requirements. Lean body mass is mobilized and if protein requirements are not met by exogenous administration, malnutrition can develop rapidly [16].

Critically ill patients with catabolic illnesses (such as trauma, burns, sepsis), prolonged ventilator dependence, and cancer (especially if they are receiving chemotherapy or radiation therapy), are at greatest risk for the significant loss of lean body mass and malnutrition. Nutrition support should be initiated expeditiously in those obese patients with illnesses that produce significant catabolism. Starvation or "letting them live off their excess fat" is an inappropriate strategy, as it places these patients at risk for increased loss of lean body mass because metabolic stress results in "mixed fuel" utilization (carbohydrate, protein and fat), as opposed to the response seen with simple starvation [16]. Patients who were relatively healthy prior to the onset of their current illness, or those undergoing elective surgery, can usually withstand a period of 5–7 days without oral intake before nutrition support needs to be seriously considered.

Estimating Nutritional Needs in Obese and Critically Ill Patients

The major goals of nutrition support are to provide patients with sufficient amounts of energy and protein to meet their needs. Many strategies for estimating nutritional needs in obese patients have been proposed.

Some practitioners simply ignore the overweight and believe that obese patients can be fed in the same manner one would feed other patients, on a per kg basis adjusted for the perceived degree of stress. The problem with this approach is that it does not take into account the changes in body composition associated with obesity, nor the fact that lean body mass is metabolically active, whereas adipose tissue tends to be metabolically inactive. Body composition does not change in a linear fashion with increasing body weight; as weight increases there is some increase in lean body mass, but overall there is a disproportionate increase in body fat in the majority of individuals. These variables make it difficult to accurately estimate energy requirements in obese patients and have resulted in controversy regarding the best method.

Considerable debate exists regarding the most appropriate weight to be used when calculating energy needs, with practitioners using both actual and "adjusted" body weight [9]. Adjusted body weight is calculated by determining 25% of the obese patient's actual weight and adding it to the ideal body weight (IBW) [adjusted BW=(actual BW x.25)+IBW]. This is an attempt to account for the increase in lean body mass seen in obese patients. This value is then substituted into equations, such as the Harris-Benedict equation, to predict energy needs.

Predictive equations which are based on normal populations, such as the Harris-Benedict equations, have been shown to underestimate the resting energy expenditure of obese individuals when IBW is used and overestimate energy expenditure when actual body weight is used in the equations [17, 18]. This has resulted in individuals fudging these equations with adjusted body weights. Ireton-Jones developed a set of equations for predicting energy expenditure accurately in hospitalized patients, including obese patients, which correlated strongly with measured values [19]. These equations adjusted for the type of stress experienced by the patient as well as ventilatory status:

$$EEE\ (v)=1925-10\ (A)+5\ (W)+281\ (S)+292\ (T)+851\ (B), R^2=0.43$$
$$EEE\ (s)=629-11\ (A)+25\ (W)-609\ (O), R^2=0.5$$

EEE=kcal/day, v=ventilator dependent, s=spontaneosly breathing, A=age (years), W=wt (kg), S=sex (m=1, f=o) and T=trauma, B=burn, O=obesity (present=1, absent=0). Ireton-Jones subsequently looked at the use of ideal versus actual body weight and concluded that use of the actual body weight is preferable when determining energy needs [20].

In critically ill patients, the inaccuracy of predictive equations has been documented based upon measured values obtained by indirect calorimetry [18, 21]. This has led to several authors attempting to estimate energy requirements using hemodynamic measurements obtained from indwelling pulmonary artery catheters and the Fick equation, with variable results [22–33].

As the degree of obesity and the severity of concomitant illness increase, it becomes progressively more difficult to estimate energy needs by any method. In such a situation one should consider utilizing indirect calorimetry to obtain a measured energy expenditure (MEE). The metabolic cart, by directly measuring O_2 consumption and CO_2 production, allows the 24- h energy expenditure to be calculated. In hospitalized patients, it is difficult to meet the conditions needed for a true resting energy expenditure (REE) or basal metabolic rate (BMR). The routine provided to patients, such as baths, physical therapy, dressing changes, and respiratory therapy, make it unusual for patients to be resting quietly for 30–45 min of measurement after an overnight fast and restful sleep. For this reason, MEE is utilized as an estimate of the 24 h energy needs without requiring any stress factors. This value can be used as a guide for the provision of non-protein calories, allowing all of the protein administered to be utilized, in theory, for anabolism. This approach is similar to that advocated by others, providing 1.2–1.3× REE as total calories, to account for the thermogenic effect of food [34].

Calculation of protein needs is usually determined based upon achieving positive nitrogen balance. This is especially true in critically ill patients, where the catabolism due to the underlying illness can cause extensive mobilization and breakdown of lean body tissue and markedly negative nitrogen balance. If clinical conditions permit (i.e. renal and hepatic function are reasonable), protein should be provided in a dosage that will place the patient in+2 to+5 nitrogen balance as long as it is well tolerated (no development of azotemia, encephalopathy, or liver function test abnormality). Fortunately, the necessary dosage of protein can be estimated based upon a measurement of urine urea nitrogen (UUN), which is reasonably accurate and can be done in most institutions [35].

Hypocaloric Nutrition Support

Starvation or semi-starvation has been successfully used as a treatment for obesity in otherwise healthy obese individuals for some time [36]. Adaptive changes during starvation reduce energy requirements and allow fat depots to be utilized for energy while sparing muscle protein from excessive catabolism. In this setting, the administration of adequate amounts of exogenous protein (approximately 1 g/kg IBW) results in nitrogen equilibrium or positive nitrogen balance [37, 38]. Attenuation of tissue protein losses seen with hypocaloric diets can also be accomplished by the administration of exogenous recombinant growth hormone [39]. This reduction in tissue protein loss with the administration of recombinant growth hormone has been reported in normal patients following surgery and or trauma, as well [40]. However, the applicability of such an approach in obese patients is questionable.

During stress, high insulin levels impede normal adaptive mechanisms. As a result, muscle protein is actively catabolized for energy. It appears that stressed obese patients may be less able to mobilize fat for energy than stressed non-obese patients, at least early after trauma [41]. However the consistently low RQ values noted by Dickerson and in our studies suggest that fat is mobilized [42–44].

Data concerning the safety of hypocaloric nutritional regimens in acutely ill obese patients is accumulating. Three prospective studies have been performed to date. The first report by Dickerson et al. demonstrated that nitrogen balance could be achieved in mild to moderately stressed obese patients receiving total parenteral nutrition (TPN) containing approximately 51% of measured resting energy expenditure as nonprotein calories (NPC). These NPCs were predominantly dextrose as intravenous lipid was provided intermittently [42]. This study included morbidly obese surgical patients who were 208±114% (range 117%–577%) of IBW as calculated according to the formula of Devine [45]. The NPC intake averaged 881±393 kcal/day, and protein intake was 2.13±0.59 g/kg IBW. The patients were maintained on this regime for an average of 48 days. Serum albumin and total iron binding capacity improved significantly, while all subjects had complete tissue healing. In this study, weight reduction was an end-point and the weight change that occurred was from 120±60 kg to 110±33 kg.

Based on the information from Dickerson, we designed two prospective, randomized, double blind trials of hypocaloric nutrition support in obese hospitalized patients [43, 44]. Patients who were greater than 130% of IBW, as determined according to Hamwi, and who were expected to require parenteral nutrition support for greater than 10 days were eligible to be enrolled. Because the protocol required administration of a large dose of protein (1.5–2.0 g/kg IBW/day) patients with renal and/or hepatic dysfunction were excluded. In the initial study, patients in the intensive care unit and with pre-existing diabetes mellitus were excluded. Two parenteral formulas, shown in Table 2, were used.

In the initial study, energy expenditure was measured using indirect calorimetry and the formulas were administered at a rate to provide 100% of MEE as NPCs to the control subjects or 50% of MEE as NPCs to the hypocaloric group. The second study was performed in an attempt to eliminate the need for indirect calorimetry, making this approach more widely applicable. The same two "3-in-1" formulas were utilized, however dosing was based on the protein component adjusted. Treatment was initiated at a formula rate that provided 2 g protein/kg IBW/day. In both studies the length of time on the study formulae was limited to 14 days, following which the patient was transitioned to a standard formula as would have been the clinical practice at the time of the study. The main clinical end-point for assessment of efficacy was the achievement of positive nitrogen balance. Three-in-one solutions were chosen because they represented the norm at our institution and concern that provision of all of the NPCs as dextrose could promote metabolic and respiratory complications. Both studies showed that most patients (>90%) achieved positive nitrogen balance without adverse effects. In addition, there was no difference in the probability of a patient reaching positive nitrogen regardless of the formula they received.

While weight loss was one of the goals of Dickerson's population, it was not one of the objectives in either of our studies. Our primary aim was to achieve comparable nitrogen balance while demonstrating safety and avoiding the risks inherent in overfeeding. Our studies were of much shorter duration than that of Dickerson et al. (av. 9.6 vs 48 days). Though the methods used to determine the rate of

Table 2. Comparison of the hypocaloric and control TPN formulas

(g/l)	Amino acid (g/l)	Dextrose (g/l)	Lipid	Non-protein kcal: nitrogen	Total kcal: nitrogen
Hypocaloric	60	75	20	46:1	75:1
Control	60	150	40	93:1	150:1

formula administration differed in the first and second studies, the final daily amounts of protein and energy provided were virtually identical. Table 3 summarizes the daily protein and energy delivered in our two studies as well as those from the study by Dickerson et al. Included in this table are published recommendations from other authors as well, though the basis for these recommendations is less strongly supported [46, 47].

Of interest was the response to hypocaloric feeding of glucose control in the small number of diabetic patients included in our second study [44]. Nine of the 30 patients had glycosuria (5 hypocaloric, 4 control) and one mild ketonuria (hypocaloric) documented during the study. Forty percent of patients (6 hypocaloric, 6 control) received insulin at some time during the study, 11 of these 12 patients had an admission diagnosis of diabetes mellitus. The mean daily insulin requirements per day was 36.1 ± 47.1 units in the hypocaloric group compared to 61.1 ± 61.1 units in the control group, a clinically, but not statistically, significant finding.

An admission diagnosis of diabetes mellitus was present in 13 (43%) patients (43%; four type I, nine type II); seven patients in the hypocaloric group and six in the control group. There was a trend toward decreased insulin requirements among the diabetic patients in the hypocaloric group. There was no difference in the number of diabetic patients in each group receiving insulin; however, among the type II diabetic patients, the average number of study days on which insulin was required was significantly less in the hypocaloric group [3.2 ± 2.7 days hypocaloric (N=5), versus 8.0 ± 2.5 days control (N=4), $p<.05$]. The average daily serum glucose and average daily insulin requirements for the first 8 days of the study were also lower in the hypocaloric group, although these differences did not reach statistical significance because of large intragroup variability. Nevertheless, the impact of lower average serum glucose levels combined with lower average daily insulin requirements may be clinically significant. Though this may merely reflect the reduced substrate provided with the hypocaloric formula, reducing the need for exogenous insulin in the obese diabetic requiring nutrition support may well benefit both the patients and the healthcare providers, who will have reduced work.

Clinical Practice

The results of our experience with hypocaloric feedings have been very encouraging. In patients who require parenteral nutrition support and are greater than 130% of IBW or have a BMI>27 kg/m^2, we routinely utilize the hypocaloric formula at a rate which will provide 2 g protein/kg IBW/day, provided the patients have normal renal and hepatic function. For patients with functional GI tracts, we formulate a similar hypocaloric enteral regimen using a commercially available "high-stress" formula with high protein (>60 g/l) and a low calorie to nitrogen ratio (<100:1) supplemented with a modular protein supplement to achieve a similar composition. (The amount of protein added will vary depending upon the distribution of CHO, protein and fat in the formula, but should result in a ratio of 75 g CHO, 60 g protein and 20 g fat.) All patients then undergo weekly urine urea

Table 3. Summary of studies on nutrition support in obese patients (*DB* double blind, *rand.* randomized, *H* hypocaloric, *C* control, *+NB* positive nitrogen balance, *IBW* ideal body weight, *ABW* actual body weight, *EE* energy expenditure)

	Study design	N (H/C)	Protein (gm/kg/d) (H/C)	Total kcal/kg/d (H/C)	Non-protein kcal/kg/d (H/C)	End Point +NB (H/C)
Burge [43]	Prospective DB, rand.	9/7	2.0/2.2 IBW 1.2/1.3 ABW	22/42 IBW 14/25 ABW	10/33 IBW 7/20 ABW	8/6
Choban [44]	Prospective DB, rand.	16/14	2.0/2.0 IBW 1.2/1.2 ABW	22/36 IBW 13.5/22.4 ABW	14/28 IBW 17.5/8.6 ABW	13/13
Dickerson [42]	Prospective	13/0	2.1 IBW 1.2 ABW		15 IBW 6.9 ABW	8
Pasulka [46]			1.5–1.7 IBW	25 IBW		
Baxter [47]			1.5 IBW	300–500 less than EE		

nitrogen studies and calculation of nitrogen balance. The rate of administration is increased accordingly to reach positive nitrogen balance if the patient is found to be in negative nitrogen balance,

This strategy does not include patients with significant renal or hepatic dysfunction which generally mandate some restriction of protein intake in order to avoid severe azotemia (BUN >100 mg/dl) and hepatic encephalopathy. In such patients, protein is administered at a dose of 0.8–1.2 g/kg IBW/day and NPCs provided at a quantity based upon estimated or measured degree of stress. Indirect calorimetry is often useful in this population, particularly in those patients with concomitant health problems to avoid overfeeding.

Route of Delivery

Determination of the route of nutrition support is independent of the formula and also the same as in non-obese patients. If no contraindication to enteral support exists, an initial attempt at enteral feeding should always be made. This may be accomplished by use of a regular diet, oral supplements, or via gastric or jejunal feeding tubes placed transnasally or by surgery or endoscopy, as dictated by the clinical situation. Parenteral access can be somewhat difficult in obese patients. Central venous cannulation tends to be increasingly difficult because as body fat increases, the normal anatomic landmarks are obscured [48].

Summary

Critically ill obese patients often require nutrition support. A strategy of hypocaloric support provides sufficient protein and energy to achieve positive nitrogen balance and healing in these patients. The complications of overfeeding are avoided and in obese Type II diabetics, this method simplifies disease management. Long-term studies to corroborate these results continue, but overall this appears to be a useful strategy that can benefit the obese patients under our care.

References

1. Obesity: Preventing and Managing the Global Epidemic. Report of a World health Organization Consultation on Obesity. WHO, Geneva, 1998
2. Kuczmarski RJ, Flegal KM, Campbell SM, Johnson CL: Increasing prevalence of Overweight among US Adults. JAMA 1994; 272:205–211
3. National Institutes of Health Consensus Development Panel on the Health Implications of Obesity. Health implications of obesity: National Institutes of Health consensus development conference statement. Ann Int Med. 1985;103:1073–1078
4. Herbert HB, Feinleib M, McNamara PM, Castelli WP. Obesity as an independent risk factor for cardiovascular disease: a 26-year follow-up of participants in the Framingham Heart Study. Circulation. 1983; 67:968–977
5. Kannel WB, Brand N, Skinner JJ. The relation of adiposity to blood pressure and development of hypertension: the Framingham study. Ann Int Med. 1967;67:48–59
6. Pi-Sunyer FX. Medical Hazards of Obesity. Ann Int Med 1993; 119:655–660

7. Choban PS, Heckler R, Burge J, Flancbaum L: Nosocomial infections in Obese Surgical Patients. Am Surg 1995; 61:1001–1005

8. Choban PS, Maynes C., Weireter LJ: Obesity and Increased Mortality in Blunt Trauma. J Trauma 1991; 31:1253–57

9. Ireton-Jones CS, Francis C: Obesity: Nutrition Support Practice and Application to Critical Care. Nutr Clin Prac 1995;10:144–149

10. Simopoulos AP: Obesity and body weight standards. Ann Rev Pub Health 1986;7:481–92.23

11. Hamwi GJ. Changing dietary concepts. In, Diabetes Mellitus: Diagnosis and Treatment. Donowski TS (ed.) American Diabetes Association Inc: New York 1964

12. Bray GA. Pathophysiology of Obesity. Am J Cl Nutr. 1992;55:488S-494 S

13. St. Joer S, Meisler JG: Summary and Recommendations from the American Health Foundations Expert Panel on Healthy Weight. AJCN, 1996, S474–477

14. Dwyer JT. Medical Evaluation and Classification of Obesity. In, Obesity: Pathophysiology, Psychology and Treatment, GL Blackburn and BS Kanders (eds). New York:Chapman & Hall 1994:p9

15. Martin LF, Tjiauw-Ling T, Holmes DA, Horn J, and Bixler EO: Can Morbidly Obese Patients Safely Lose Weight Preoperatively? Am J Surg 1995, 169:245–253

16. Cerra FB: Hypermetabolosm, Organ Failure, and Metabolic Support. Surgery 10:1–14, 1987

17. Pavlou KN, Hoefer MA, Blackburn GL. Resting energy expenditure in moderate obesity. Ann Surg. 1986; 203:136–141

18. Daly JM, Heymsfield SB, Head CA, et al. Human energy requirements: Overestimation by widely used prediction equation. Am J Clin Nutr. 1985;42:1170–1174

19. Ireton-Jones CS: Evaluation of Energy Expenditures in Obese Patients. Nutrit Clin Prac 1989;4:127–9

20. Ireton-Jones CS, Turner WW Jr: Actual or ideal body weight: which should be used to predict energy expenditure? JADA 1991 91:193–5

21. Long CL, Schaffel N, Geiger JW, Schiller WR, Blakemore WS. Metabolic response to injury and illness: estimation of energy and protein needs from indirect calorimetry and nitrogen balance. JPEN 1979; 3:452–456

22. Liggett SB, St. John RE, LeFrak SS. Determination of resting energy expenditure utilizing the thermodilution pulmonary artery catheter. Chest 1987; 91:562–566

23. Sawyer M, Rolandelli R, Novick W, Marino PL. Measurement of resting energy expenditure (REE) in the ICU using pulmonary artery catheters. (Abstract) JPEN 1988; 12:5 S

24. Williams RR, Fuenning CR. Circulatory indirect calorimetry in the critically ill. JPEN 1991; 15:509–512

25. Smithies MN, Royston B, Makita K, Konieczko K, Nunn JF. Comparison of oxygen consumption measurements: indirect calorimetry versus the reversed Fick method. Crit Care Med 1991; 19:1401–1406

26. Cobean RA, Gentilello LM, Parker A, Jurkovich GJ, Maier RV. Nutritional assessment using a pulmonary artery catheter. J Trauma 1992; 33:452–456

27. Brandi LS, Grana M, Mazzanti T, et al. Energy expenditure and gas exchange measurements in postoperative patients: thermodilution versus indirect calorimetry. Crit Care Med 1992; 20:1273–1283

28. Kearney PA, Pofahl WE, Annis K, et al. A comparison of indirect calorimetry and the direct Fick method for calculating energy expenditure. (Abstract) JPEN (supp) 1992;16:

29. Ireton-Jones CS, Turner WW, Liepa GW, et al. Equations for estimating energy expenditure in burn patients with special reference to ventilatory status. J Burn Care Rehabil 1992; 13:330–333

30. Frankenfield DC, Omert LA, Badellino MM. et al. Correlation between measured energy expenditure and clinically obtained variables in trauma and sepsis. J Trauma 1994; 18:398–403

31. Fusco MA, Mills ME, Nelson LD. Predicting caloric requirements with emphasis on avoiding overfeeding. JPEN (Supp) 1995; 19:18 S

32. Mink S, Dechert R, Shane H, Bartlett R. Can thermal dilution be used to calculate REE in critically ill patients? JPEN (Supp) 1995; 19:22 S

33. Flancbaum L, Choban PS, Sambucco S, Burge JC: Comparison of indirect calorimetry, the Fick method, and prediction equations in estimating energy requirements in critically ill patients. Am J Clin Nut 1999; 69:461–466

34. Brandi LS, Bertolini R, Calafa M: Indirect Calorimetry in Critically Ill Patients: Clinical Applications and Practical Advice. Nutrition 1997 13:349–358

35. Burge JC, Choban PS, McKnight T, Flancbaum L: UUN plus Ammonia as an Estimate of TUN in Patients Receiving Parenteral Nutrition Support. JPEN 1993; 17:529–531

36. Bray GA. The obese patient. Philadelphia, PA, W.B. Saunders Company, 1976

37. Strang JM, McClugage HB, Evans FA. Further studies in the dietary correction of obesity. Am J Med Sci. 1930;179:687–694

38. Strang, JM, McClugage HB, Evans FA. The nitrogen balance during dietary correction of obesity. Am J Med Sci. 1931;181:336–349

39. Zeigler, TR, Young, LS, Manson, JM, Wilmore, DW. Metabolic effects of recombinant human growth hormone in patients receiving parenteral nutrition. Ann Surg. 1988;208:6–16

40. Ward, HC, Halliday, D, Sim, JW. Protein and energy metabolism with biosynthetic human growth hormone after gastrointestinal surgery. Ann Surg. 1987; 206:56–61

41. Jeevanandam M, Young DH, Schiller WR. Obesity and the metabolic response to severe multiple trauma in man. J Clin Invest. 1991;87:262–269

42. Dickerson RN, Rosato EF, Mullen JL. Net protein anabolism with hypocaloric parenteral nutrition in obese stressed patients. Am J Clin Nutr. 1986;44:747–755

43. Burge JC, Goon A, Choban PS, Flancbaum L: Efficacy of hypocaloric total parenteral nutrition in hospitalized obese patients: a prospective, double-blind randomized trial. JPEN, 1994;18:203–7

44. Choban PS, Burge J, Scales D, Flancbaum L: Hypocaloric Nutrition Support in Hospitalized Obese Patients: A Simplified Method for Clinical Application Am J Cl Nutr 1999; 69:461–466.

45. Devine BJ: Gentamicin therapy. Drug Intell Clin Pharm 1974, 8:650–6

46. Pasulka PS, Kohl D: Nutrition support of the stressed obese patient. Nutrit Clin Prac 1989; 4:130–2

47. Baxter JK, Bistrian BR: Moderate hypocaloric parenteral nutrition in the critically ill, obese patient. Nutrit Clin Prac 1989; 4:133–5

48. Flancbaum L and Choban PC: Surgical Implications of Obesity. Ann Rev Med, 1998; 49:215–234

Hyperglycemia and Blood Sugar Management: Implications for Infection

K.C. McCowen, L. Khaodhiar, and B.R. Bistrian

Introduction

The nature of the relationship between "critical illness hyperglycemia" and noso-comial infection is confounded by a dearth of randomized controlled trials examining the impact of good versus poor glycemic control on infection rates. It has long been clear that hyperglycemia may be a consequence of the systemic inflammatory response syndrome (SIRS) and thereby serve as a marker of severity of stress. However, evidence is emerging that hyperglycemia early in the postoperative period can be a significant risk factor for the subsequent development of nosocomial infection. Many patients with uncontrolled hyperglycemia in the intensive care unit (ICU) have underlying diabetes mellitus, either on the basis of insulin deficiency (type 1) or insulin resistance in combination with insulin deficiency (type 2) [1]. However, catabolic illness alone may produce sufficient insulin resistance that temporary hyperglycemia ("stress diabetes") can develop [2]. The major risk factors for insulin resistance in critical illness are:
- Diabetes mellitus
- Hyperglycemia (of any cause)
- Systemic inflammatory response syndrome
- Obesity
- Elevated free fatty acid concentrations
- Increasing age
- Exogenous glucocorticoid or catecholamine therapy

This situation is often compounded by the addition of nutrition support which, if administered inappropriately in the form of excessive carbohydrate, may result in dramatic and sustained hyperglycemia.

Glucose Homeostasis in the Critically III: Mechanisms of Insulin Resistance

Acute or subacute illness is accompanied by a marked increase in the plasma concentration of counterregulatory hormones, i.e. glucagon, epinephrine, cortisol and growth hormone that have multiple effects on glucose homeostasis (Table 1). Together these hormones can effect significant reductions in insulin sensitivity through poorly understood mechanisms likely related to alterations in the insulin signaling pathway [3]. Counterregulatory hormones also enhance lipolysis and elevate free fatty acids (FFA) which may contribute additional defects to the defective insulin action.

Hepatic insulin resistance leads to ongoing glucose production even in the face of hyperglycemia [4]. Peripheral insulin resistance decreases skeletal muscle glucose uptake and reduces glucose clearance. These two actions combine to elevate serum glucose sometimes to hyperglycemic levels. In the non-stressed individual, postprandial insulin and glucose concentrations are sufficient to inhibit hepatic gluconeogenesis and glycogenolysis and prevent additional glucose production [5]. In contrast, in critically ill persons, glucose infusion failed to suppress endogenous glucose production despite accompanying hyperinsulinemia. Using stable isotopes, it was demonstrated that hepatic glucose production was ~150% of the normal resting post-absorptive values of healthy subjects in spite of provision of total parenteral nutrition (TPN) with dextrose at rates exceeding the basal energy expenditure [6]. In diabetic patients an even greater derangement in glucose metabolism is noted with severe stress [3], since their ability to secrete insulin as a compensatory response is impaired. Coexisting obesity or hyperglycemia, if present, also increase insulin resistance. The cytokines, interleukin-1 (IL-1), tumor necrosis factor-α (TNFα), and interleukin-6 (IL-6) which underlie SIRS can alter glucose homeostasis, both indirectly by stimulating counterregulatory hormone secretion and by direct action themselves [7]. IL-1, TNFα and IL-6, individually and synergistically, increase net glucose flux through resistance to insulin actions in muscle and liver via poorly understood post-receptor mechanisms [8].

Table 1. Major effects of counterregulatory hormones on glucose homeostasis

Hormone	Perturbs	Effect
Catecholamines	Glycogenolysis	↑
	Gluconeogenesis[a]	↑
	Lipolysis[b]	↑
	Insulin release	↓
Glucagon	Glycogenolysis	↑
	Gluconeogenesis	↑
	Ketogenesis	↑
Glucocorticoids	Gluconeogenesis[a]	↑
	Catecholamine response	↑
	Insulin resistance	↑
Growth hormone	Gluconeogenesis	↑
	Lipolysis[b]	↑
	Insulin resistance	↑

[a]Gluconeogenesis is increased by substrate provision from both proteolysis (alanine) and lipolysis (glycerol).
[b]Lipolysis causes increases in both glycerol and free fatty acids, thus increasing gluconeogenesis and causing insulin resistance.

Hyperglycemia in Critically Ill Persons:
Multiple Mechanisms of Enhanced Risk of Infection

In diabetic persons, antibacterial function of polymorphonuclear leukocytes (PMNL) has been reported to be both normal [9, 10] and impaired [11–13], but the preponderance of evidence favors an adverse impact [14]. In patients with poorly controlled diabetes, abnormalities in PMNL adherence [15, 16], chemotaxis [17], phagocytosis [18], and bactericidal function [19] improve with more aggressive glycemic control. In ketoacidosis, phagocytosis and bactericidal killing by PMNLs appear to be impaired [20]. Superoxide radical production in PMNLs from both poorly controlled diabetics and from healthy non-diabetic controls that have been exposed to high concentrations of glucose ex vivo has been reported to be abnormal [21–23], suggesting that hyperglycemia itself may cause the impairment in immune function. Glycosylation of immunoglobulin can result in its inactivation [24]. Intracellular calcium concentrations in PMNL from diabetic patients have been shown to be elevated in association with reduction in ATP content and impaired phagocytosis [25]; institution of improved glycemic control in this population with use of oral hypoglycemic therapy was associated with reversal of these abnormalities. Other work has documented that therapeutic use of calcium channel blocking drugs also reverses the calcium abnormality as well as the phagocytic defect [26].

In one recent study of the effects of acute hyperglycemia in non-diabetic rodents, some of these immunologic deficits were confirmed [27]. Rats were infused with either saline or hypertonic dextrose, the latter to produce plasma glucose levels of 300 mg/dl over 3 h. Various cell lines (alveolar and peritoneal macrophages, and peripheral neutrophils) were harvested. Hyperglycemia significantly reduced the oxidative burst and phagocytic abilities of the alveolar macrophage. Peritoneal macrophages were less affected, with only a trend to reduced oxidative burst but no change in ability to phagocytose. In contrast, the respiratory burst was increased in PMNLs. The authors were unable to make clinical inferences directly, although the study does indicate that hyperglycemia per se in the absence of diabetes can alter immune function.

Insulin infusion has been demonstrated to improve PMNL function in diabetics in a study of 26 patients who underwent coronary bypass surgery [28]. Participants were randomized to receive either aggressive insulin therapy or standard care during surgery. The experimental group received continuous insulin by infusion, the controls intermittent boluses of insulin during the perioperative period. Blood was drawn for PMNL testing before surgery, 1 h after completion of bypass and on the first postoperative day. PMNL phagocytic activity was reduced in both groups, but was significantly worse in the group randomized to standard care (47% of baseline versus 75% in the aggressive insulin group, $P<0.05$). The authors made no attempt to correlate these laboratory abnormalities with clinical outcome, an important next step.

Hyperglycemia in Critically III Persons: Risk of Infection

A study from our institution [29] has demonstrated that hyperglycemia on the first postoperative day (POD#1) in diabetics undergoing major cardiac or abdominal surgery is a sensitive predictor of subsequent nosocomial infection. This observational study included 97 diabetics consecutively admitted for elective surgery, who did not have any signs of preoperative infection. Blood sugar was controlled in a routine manner by the patient's endocrinologist or surgeon. In patients with hyperglycemia (>220 mg/dl) on POD#1, the infection rate was 2.7 times that observed (31.3% vs 11.5%, $P<0.05$) in diabetics with all glucose measurements below this cutoff. The threshold value of 220 mg/dl was chosen because older studies have shown that values above this are associated with poor granulocyte function. When minor infection of the bladder was excluded, the relative risk for serious infection increased to 5.8 (24.6% vs 4.2%, $P<0.03$) when any POD#1 blood glucose level exceeded 220 mg/dl.

However, there was significant correlation between APACHE II scores and maximum POD#1 glucose values in this study, which might support the alternative explanation that the sickest patients developed both infections and hyperglycemia, as opposed to the elevated glucose being etiologic in the later infectious process. The authors addressed this issue by pointing out both that the magnitude of the correlation was low ($r=0.42$) and that the mean POD#1 glucose was not correlated with APACHE II score, making this explanation less likely. Interestingly, the study did not show the same association between POD#2 blood glucose level and rate of nosocomial infection. This might be because the period of highest risk for the development of postoperative infection is early, when the patient is maximally stressed, and therefore most immunosuppressed. Moreover, during this time the potential exposure to pathogens is most likely due to the surgical procedure, either by technical error or via bacterial translocation from the gut. It might also lead to the tentative conclusion that, since hyperglycemia did not occur on the days leading up to the diagnosis of infection, postoperative hyperglycemia was not a marker of infection that was already present.

Other recent results provide support for this proposed relationship. One study [30] found that early postoperative hyperglycemia in elderly patients undergoing cardiac surgeries was a significant predictor of early postoperative mortality on multivariate analysis. Hyperglycemia was a risk factor with univariate analysis for postoperative morbidity. Also noted was that the patients who died in the early postoperative period had a significantly higher rate of nosocomial infection than those who survived (39% in non-survivors vs 5% in survivors). Although there is no way to know from the published data whether hyperglycemia and nosocomial infection occurred in the same patients or what the temporal relationship might have been, it is reasonable to assume that the patients were not infected preoperatively given the nature of the surgery, and that most nosocomial infections would develop later in the postoperative period.

Does Treating Hyperglycemia Reduce Postoperative Infection Risk?

More direct evidence of this relationship can be found when the effects of treating hyperglycemia are examined. In a retrospective, observational study, Zarr et al. studied 8910 patients who underwent cardiac surgeries from 1987–1993 [31]. Of these, 1585 (18%) had diabetes mellitus. The rate of deep wound infection was significantly higher in diabetic patients than in non-diabetics (1.7% vs 0.4%). The mean glucose level on the first 2 postoperative days was higher in infected diabetic patients than non-infected diabetics (208±7.1 versus 190±0.8 mg/dl, $P<0.003$). Once again, hyperglycemia appears to occur much earlier in the postoperative period than nosocomial infections developed – generally after discharge. The deep infection rate increased dramatically as the POD#1 glucose increased, being 6 times higher with 250–300 mg/dl compared to 100–150 mg/dl.

In a second study from the same authors, their experience with aggressive insulin therapy to prevent hyperglycemia was reported in 1499 diabetic patients undergoing cardiac surgery between 1991 and 1997 [32]. In their protocol, continuous insulin infusion was used to maintain blood glucose <200 mg/dl in the perioperative period with hourly fingersticks initially, then 2-hourly as the patient stabilized. The infusion was continued until the patient was tolerating a full liquid diet. Implementation of this regimen resulted in a decrease in mean blood glucose level compared with controls from the same institution who received otherwise the same care. Mean glucose was lower each day with the intensive therapy: on the day of operation (199±1.4 versus 241±1.9 mg/dl), POD#1 (176±0.8 versus 206±1.2 mg/dl), POD#2 (181±1.2 versus 195±1.3 mg/dl) and POD#3 (179±1.5 versus 188±1.4 mg/dl), with $P<0.0001$ for all comparisons. Mean blood glucose levels in persons that went on to deep sternal wound infection (DSWI) were significantly increased on POD#1 and #2, compared with those remaining without infection. The rate of DSWI also decreased to 1.3% overall, a significant reduction over that seen in their historic controls. During the same time period there had been no difference in rate of DSWI in non-diabetic patients (0.4% vs 0.38%), indicating that the likely cause of the reduction in the infection rate in the diabetics was improved glycemic control.

These studies have suggested that hyperglycemia in the perioperative period increases infection risk in diabetes and that aggressive diabetic control can diminish infection rate and improve outcome. Prospective, randomized controlled trials of good versus poor glycemic control have never been performed to examine this question. A potentially analogous study was performed examining the effects of tight control versus usual care in diabetic patients ($n=620$) with acute myocardial infarction – the "DIGAMI" study [33–35]. Implementation of strict euglycemia using insulin infusions and multiple daily injections caused a prompt and sustained improvement in all-cause mortality (30% reduction at 1 year). One might consider that repair of a myocardial infarct resembles healing of a surgical wound; thus this study strengthens the theory that hyperglycemia hinders wound healing which is one important component of immune function. However, improved glucose homeostasis is likely to impact on many other components of immune function including non-specific glycation of complement or immunoglobulin in addition to those mentioned earlier.

Hyperglycemia and Infections: The Implications for Nutrition Support

Endogenous production of glucose is almost 2 mg/kg/minute (approximately 200 g/day) in normal subjects; about 60% of this is oxidized. In contrast, hepatic glucose production in critically ill persons can rise to as much as 3 mg/kg/minute with about a similar amount oxidized [36]. The provision of dextrose at high rates to such patients does not significantly enhance glucose oxidation; with the resistance to insulin-mediated glucose uptake that is universal in such patients, hyperglycemia results and de novo lipogenesis from glucose (which creates its own set of problems) is enhanced. Thus extreme care is needed when using nutrition support therapy to prevent additional disturbances in glucose homeostasis. In a retrospective study of 37 non-diabetic patients receiving TPN, 18 of 37 patients who received dextrose at rates >5 mg/kg/minute exhibited hyperglycemia, as opposed to none of 19 in whom the dextrose was infused at 4 mg/kg/min [37]. In addition, TPN dextrose infusion rate was positively correlated with blood glucose concentration, over and above other variables considered in a multiple regression analysis.

In the Veteran's Administration trial of TPN versus no additional nutrition support in preoperative patients, there was a twofold increase in risk of infectious complications in the TPN group versus controls (14.1% vs 6.4%) [38]. Since the patients in this trial were allowed eat ad libitum in addition to TPN, the total caloric intake in the TPN group was approximately 45 kcalories/kg body weight. Based on measurements in patients with similar ages and conditions, their estimated REE would be approximately 22–25 kcal/kg [39]. This presumably was the major cause for the severe hyperglycemia of >300 mg/dl that occurred in significantly more (20% vs 1%) of the TPN patients compared to the control group. Although not stated, it could be estimated that the majority of patients in the TPN group would likely have had a blood glucose >200 mg/dl which would put them at increased infectious risk. If hyperglycemia is allowed to occur, any potential benefits from nutrition support are potentially negated through an increased risk of infectious complications.

A meta-analysis of randomized trials comparing TPN with enteral nutrition concluded that the former is associated with a higher infection rate [40]. However, close analysis of the data reveals that the greatest difference between the 2 groups was that the TPN recipients were fed significantly more calories and had much higher rates of hyperglycemia. It is likely that the ease with which TPN can be administered (in comparison with tube feeding which often is poorly tolerated, necessitating reductions in feeding rates) leads to rapid advances in dextrose loads [41]; in turn, hyperglycemia results. It is clear that this approach to nutrition support is associated with an increased risk of infection in an already vulnerable population.

The practical implications are that glucose tolerance should be tested by the introduction of TPN that contains low quantities of dextrose, that all patients undergo blood sugar monitoring and that goal glucose values of <200 mg/dl be achieved through aggressive use of insulin which can most easily be delivered admixed with TPN [42], although subcutaneous sliding scale regular insulin is usually also required. No attempt should be made to advance dextrose calories unless glucose values are controlled. The principles of TPN provision for hyperglycemia avoidance are:

– Calculate total caloric goal, 25 kcal/kg dry (usual) weight. If obese, 25 kcal/kg ideal body weight.
– Provide protein at 1.5 g/kg dry (usual) weight. If obese, 2 g/kg ideal weight.
– Fat emulsion can be used to provide up to 30% of total calories if not otherwise contra-indicated.
– Begin with 150 g dextrose (maximum) on first day of TPN. Consider addition of regular insulin to TPN, approximately 50% of total home dose or previous day's requirement.
– Monitor blood glucose fingersticks 6-hourly; give additional regular insulin by algorithm, using lower doses for type 1 diabetics (~50% of type 2 doses).
– Advance dextrose to goal by 50–75 g/day if patient remains euglycemic.
– Dextrose should not be provided at >4 mg/kg/min.
– Underfeeding calories is less likely to cause complications than overfeeding and will have only limited impact on protein metabolism if protein intake optimal (1.5 g/kg/d).

Older persons are particularly at risk of hyperglycemia, as one study has shown that serum glucose in response to TPN increased as a function of patient age, while the serum insulin level was inversely related to the patient age [43].

Traditional beliefs about feeding requirements for ICU patients were based on indirect calorimetric studies that suggested resting energy expenditures (REE) of up to 200%, depending on the underlying illness. However, more recent work has demonstrated that REE is usually close to normal [39] and rarely more than what has been calculated using the Harris-Benedict equation, approximately 20–25 kcal/kg. While critically ill persons are not necessarily hypermetabolic, certainly they are hypercatabolic and thus provision of generous amounts of protein rather than calories in excess of requirement should be emphasized for nutrition support. Thus, there is an increasing literature concerning the deliberate use of hypocaloric nutrition support in the critically ill to prevent many of the metabolic complications that are associated with provision of excessive TPN.

One potential risk of underfeeding calories is a negative impact upon nitrogen balance. However in a study of 30 hospitalized obese (>130% of ideal body weight) patients randomized to hypocaloric versus traditional TPN, no deleterious effects on any measures of nutritional status occurred [44]. Those randomized to hypocaloric TPN were fed 22 kcal/kg ideal body weight (IBW), which averaged 14 kcal/kg actual weight, whereas controls received 36 kcal/kg IBW, averaging 22 kcal/kg actual weight. The only significant difference between the 2 groups was that the hypocaloric group had fewer days requiring exogenous insulin. Generous provision of protein (2 g/kg IBW in all participants) enabled attainment of equivalent nitrogen balance in the 2 groups.

In a retrospective analysis of 107 critically ill persons in a surgical ICU in Colombia, the impact of hypocaloric, hyperproteinemic TPN was assessed [45]. Glucose was provided in amounts approximating physiologic hepatic production, i.e.180 g daily, while protein was 1.5–2 g/kg IBW daily. No attempt was made to match the study participants to others from the same institution who had received more traditional nutrition support. However, despite average APACHE II scores of 11–12, hyperglycemia never occurred and no insulin therapy was required. Average blood sugars between the various subgroups described in this study ranged from 121–135 mg/dl. It is worth noting that nitrogen balance, averaging –9 g/day, is possibly less negative than what might be expected in ICU patients, suggesting again an absence of negative impact of hypocaloric support upon anabolism.

How Strong Is the Argument that Hyperglycemia Is a Warning of Intercurrent Infection?

There is no doubt that the presence of nosocomial infection in the postoperative setting is associated with elevations in counterregulatory hormones and consequent deterioration in glucose homeostasis. Many older experiments have confirmed this repeatedly. It may be difficult in certain clinical situations to distinguish such an infection from one that arises as a result of immune dysfunction consequent to hyperglycemia. The evidence presented above clearly demonstrates that when hyperglycemia occurs in the first days following surgery, subsequent rates of infection are higher. However, often this hyperglycemia is short-lived. In contrast, hyperglycemia that accompanies infection is not easily controlled without specific antibiotics or wound débridement. These considerations aside, one can hardly recommend poor glucose control as optimal therapy given the relative ease of accomplishing improvement through nurse-directed algorithms and the substantial suggestive clinical evidence that failure to achieve reasonable control has serious adverse consequences.

Conclusions

In summary, it is the timing of hyperglycemia that provides the best clue as to whether this heralds underlying infection versus a potential risk factor for future infection. If the latter, recent evidence would indicate that aggressive management with normalization of blood glucose may be an effective means to combat perioperative infection. Nevertheless, improved glycemic control is indicated as well when hyperglycemia develops as a consequence of infection, since immune function should be optimized in the treatment of infection as well as in its prophylaxis. The high risk of hyperglycemia in the setting of TPN therapy in critically ill persons should lead to extreme caution with the quantity of nutrition support provided.

References

1. McCowen KC, Smith RJ (1999) Diabetes Mellitus: Classification and Chemical Pathology. In: Sadler, Strain (eds): Encyclopedia of Nutrition, 1st edn. Academic Press, London pp 508–514
2. Mizock BA (1995) Alterations in carbohydrate metabolism during stress: a review of the literature. Am J Med 98:75–84
3. Shamoon M, Hendler R, Sherwin R (1980) Altered responsiveness to cortisol, epinephrine and glucagon in insulin-infused juvenile-onset diabetes. Diabetes 29:284–291
4. Wolfe RR (1997) Substrate utilization/insulin resistance in sepsis/trauma. Balliere's Clin Endocrinol Metab 11:645–57
5. Rizza RA, Mandarino LJ, Gerich JE (1981) Dose-response characteristics for effects of insulin on production and utilization of glucose in man. Am J Physiol 240:E630–9
6. Tappy L, Schwarz JM, Schneiter P et al. (1998) Effects of isoenergetic glucose-based or lipid-based parenteral nutrition on glucose metabolism, de novo lipogenesis, and respiratory gas exchanges in critically ill patients. Crit Care Med 26:860–7
7. Webber J (1998) Abnormalities in glucose metabolism and their relevance to nutrition support in the critically ill. Curr Opin Clin Nutr and Metab Care 1:191–194
8. Chang HR, Bistrian B (1998) The role of cytokines in the catabolic consequences of infection and injury. JPEN 22:156–166
9. Richardson R (1994) Immunity in diabetes. IV Measurement of phagocytic activity in diabetes mellitus. Am J Med Sci 204:29–35
10. Bybee J, Roberts D (1964) The phagocytic activity of polymorphonuclear leukocytes obtained from patients with diabetes mellitus. J Lab Clin Med 64:1–13
11. Walters M, Lessler M, Stevenson T (1971) Oxidative metabolism of leukocytes from nondiabetic and diabetic patients. J Lab Clin Med 78:158–166
12. Delamaire M, Maugendre D, Moreno M, Le Goff MC, Allannic H, Genetet B (1997) Impaired leucocyte functions in diabetic patients. Diabet Med 14:29–34
13. Sawant JM (1993) Biochemical changes in polymorphonuclear leucocytes in diabetic patients. J Postgrad Med 39:183–6
14. McMahon MM, Bistrian BR (1995) Host defenses and susceptibility to infection in patients with diabetes mellitus. Infect Dis Clin North Am 9:1–9
15. Bagdade J, Koot R, Bulger R (1974) Impaired leukocyte function in patients with poorly controlled diabetes. Diabetes 23:9–15
16. Bagdade J, Stewart M, Walters E (1978) Impaired granulocyte adherence: A reversible defect in host defense in patients with poorly controlled diabetes. Diabetes 27:677–681
17. Mowat A, Baum J (1971) Chemotaxis of polymorphonuclear leukocytes from patients with diabetes mellitus. N Engl J Med 284:621–627
18. Bagdade J, Neilson K, Bulger R (1972) Reversible abnormalities in phagocytic function in poorly controlled diabetic patients. Am J Med Sci 263:451–456
19. Nolan C, Beaty H, Bagdade J (1978) Impaired granulocyte bactericidal function in patients with poorly controlled diabetes. Diabetes 127:889–894
20. Saeed FA, Castle GE (1998) Neutrophil chemiluminescence during phagocytosis is inhibited by abnormally elevated levels of acetoacetate: implications for diabetic susceptibility to infections. Clin Diagn Lab Immunol 5:740–743
21. Nielson C, Hindson D (1989) Inhibition of polymorphonuclear leukocyte respiratory burst by elevated glucose concentrations in vitro. Diabetes 38:1031–1035
22. Nath N, Chari SN, Rathi AB (1984) Superoxide dismutase in diabetic polymorphonuclear leukocytes. Diabetes 33:586–9
23. Muchova J, Liptakova A, Orszaghova Z, Garaiova I, Tison P, Carsky J et al. (1999) Antioxidant systems in polymorphonuclear leucocytes of Type 2 diabetes mellitus. Diabet Med 16:74–8
24. Black CT, Hennessey PJ, Andrassy RJ (1990) Short-term hyperglycemia depresses immunity through nonenzymatic glycosylation of circulating immunoglobulin. J Trauma 30:830–832; discussion 832–3

25. Alexiewicz JM, Kumar D, Smogorzewski M, Klin M, Massry SG (1995) Polymorphonuclear leukocytes in non-insulin-dependent diabetes mellitus: abnormalities in metabolism and function. Ann Intern Med 123:919–24

26. Seyrek N, Marcinkowski W, Smogorzewski M, Demerdash TM, Massry SG (1997) Amlodipine prevents and reverses the elevation in [Ca2+]i and the impaired phagocytosis of PMNL of diabetic rats. Nephrol Dial Transplant 12:265–72

27. Kwoun M, Ling PR, Lydon E et al. (1997) Immunologic effects of acute hyperglycemia in non-diabetic rats. JPEN 21:91–95.

28. Rassias AJ, Marrin CA, Arruda J, Whalen PK, Beach M, Yeager MP (1999) Insulin infusion improves neutrophil function in diabetic cardiac surgery patients. Anesth Analg 88:1011–6

29. Pomposelli J, Baxter J, Babineau T et al. (1998) Early postoperative glucose control predicts nosocomial infection rate in diabetic patients. JPEN 22:77–81

30. Rady M, Ryan T, Starr N (1998) Perioperative determinants of morbidity and mortality in elderly patients undergoing cardiac surgery. Crit Care Med 6:225–235

31. Zarr K, Furnary A, Grunkemeier G, Bookin S, Kanhere V, Starr A (1997) Glucose control lowers the risk of wound infection in diabetics after open heart operation. Ann Thorac Surg 63:356–361

32. Furnary AP, Zerr KJ, Grunkemeier GL, Starr A (1999) Continuous intravenous insulin infusion reduces the incidence of deep sternal wound infection in diabetic patients after cardiac surgical procedures. Ann Thorac Surg 67:352–360

33. Malmberg K, Ryden L, Efendic S et al. (1995) A randomised trial of insulin-glucose infusion followed by subcutaneous insulin treatment in diabetic patients with acute myocardial infarction: effect on one year mortality. J Am Coll Cardiol 26:57–65

34. Malmberg K, Ryden L, Hamsten A, Herlitz J, Waldenstorm A, Wedel H (1996) Effects of insulin treatment on cause specific one year mortality and morbidity in diabetic patients with acute myocardial infarction. Eur Heart J 17:1337–40

35. Malmberg K for the DIGAMI study group (1997) Prospective randomised study of intensive insulin treatment on long term survival after acute myocardial infarction in patients with diabetes mellitus. BMJ 314:1512–5

36. Long CL, Kinney JM, Geiger JW (1976) Nonsuppressability of gluconeogenesis by glucose in septic patients. Metabolism 25:193–201

37. Rosmarin DK, Wardlaw GM, Mirtallo J (1996) Hyperglycemia associated with high, continuous infusion rates of total parenteral nutrition dextrose. Nutr Clin Pract 11:151–6

38. VA TPN Cooperative Study (1991) Perioperative total parenteral nutrition in surgical patients. New England Journal of Medicine 325:525–532

39. Hunter DC, Jaksic T, Lewis D, Benotti PN, Blackburn GL, Bistrian BR (1988) Resting energy expenditure in the critically ill: estimations versus measurement. Br J Surg 75:875–8

40. Moore FA, Feliciano DV, Andrassy RJ et al. (1986) Early enteral feeding, compared with parenteral, reduces postoperative septic complications. The results of a meta-analysis. Ann Surg 216:172–83

41. Adams S, Dellinger EP, Wertz MJ, Oreskovich MR, Simonowitz D, Johansen K (1986) Enteral versus parenteral nutritional support following laparotomy for trauma: a randomized prospective trial. J Trauma 26:882–91

42. Hongsermeier T, Bistrian BR (1993) Evaluation of a practical technique for determining insulin requirements in diabetic patients receiving total parenteral nutrition. JPEN 17:16–9

43. Watters JM, Kirkpatrick SM, Hopbach D et al. (1996) Aging exaggerates the blood glucose response to total parenteral nutrition. Can J Surg 39:481–485

44. Choban PS, Burge JC, Scales D et al. (1997) Hypoenergetic nutrition support in hospitalized obese patients: a simplified method for clinical application. Am J Clin Nutr 66:546–550

45. Patino JF, de Pimiento SE, Vergara A, Savino P, Rodriguez M, Escallon J (1999) Hypocaloric support in the critically ill. World J Surg 23:553–9

Nutrition Support of the Septic Patient

C.J. Galbán Rodríguez

Sepsis poses a serious clinical problem with significant economic repercussions. The incidence of sepsis observed in a recent multicenter study [1] was 2 cases for every 100 admissions or 3 cases for each 1000 patient/days with 59% occurring within the intensive care unit (ICU). Sepsis carried a mortality rate of 34% at 28 days and 45% at 5 months with septic patients averaging a hospital stay of 29 days compared to 6.6 days for the general hospital population with a mean ICU stay of 17.7 days compared to 0.8 days. In Europe [2] nosocomial infections occur in 20% of ICU patients. Because of widely accepted definitions to group and stratify septic patients [3], clinicians can now reach some conclusions on therapeutic management.

Although mechanisms that regulate it are unknown, knowledge of the altered metabolism of the septic patient [4, 5] have increased considerably, and investigators are beginning to rationalize nutrition support as metabolic support and adapt it to the characteristics of the altered metabolism [6, 7]. Outcome of the septic patient depends upon correct diagnostic and therapeutic management which includes identification, medical and surgical treatment, adequate resuscitation, and prevention of multiorgan failure [8]. Multiple organ dysfunction syndrome (MODS) is potentiated through the development of nosocomial infections possibly through a "second hit" phenomenon. Provision of correct nutrition support with specific substrates may provide benefits independent of their nutritional value by modifying the immune-inflammatory response and thus improve patient outcome. This nutrition support is commonly referred to an immunonutrition, immune-enhancing nutrition, immune-specific nutrition, pharmacologic nutrition, or nutriceutical therapy [9].

Metabolic Disorder in the Septic Patient

The metabolism of septic patients is significantly altered with changes in the quantity and quality of substrate requirements. The general characteristics are hypermetabolism, increases in Resting Energy Expenditure (REE), and oxygen consumption, reduced ketogenesis, and hypercatabolism that exceeds anabolism. Only the nervous system appears to be spared significant catabolism. The metabolic state is characterized by a persistent negative nitrogen balance which usually does not exceeds 15 g/day compared to the higher rate of trauma victims.

Carbohydrate Metabolism

The most prominent characteristic of carbohydrate metabolism is hyperglycemia [10] which is speculated to be related to insulin resistance [11, 12] due to counter-regulatory hormones and mediators of inflammation [13]; insulin resistance itself, however, does not explain this increase in glucose levels. Unrestricted gluconeogenesis from lactate, glycerol, and amino acids increases glucose production. This gluconeogenesis is associated with an increase in cellular glucose uptake but a relative decrease of glucose oxidation, resulting in occasional hyperlactacidemia which is unrelated to tissue hypoxia but caused by enzyme blockade at a cellular level [14]. Hypoglycemia is a bad prognostic sign related to splanchnic hypoperfusion or hepatic failure.

Lipid Metabolism

Sepsis induces lipolysis [15] increasing free fatty acid levels due to increased tissue lipase action induced by catecholamines. In the septic patient, increased oxidation of FFA supports tissue energy needs. Other fatty acids are contained in triglycerides carried by lipoproteins synthesized by the liver. The hypertriglyceridemia of septic patients is due to an increase in the synthesis of very low density lipoproteins (VLDL) and a decrease in triglyceride clearance due to reductions in lipoprotein lipase in adipose tissue although levels of these enzymes are maintained in muscle and heart. Energy generated from fatty acid oxidation is used by the hepatocyte for gluconeogenesis. The hyperlipidemia in septic patients has been proposed as a defense mechanism by Harris et al. [16] in an experimental model of endotoxemia. Despite increases in FFA, ketone bodies remain low, indicating that ketogenesis is not part of the metabolic response as an alternative energy source.

Protein Metabolism

Accelerated protein catabolism [15, 17] increases nitrogen loss to levels of 15 g/day (and occasionally more) in association with fatty mass loss of 0.5 kg/day. Although muscle mass is primarily affected, connective tissue and intestinal losses also are significant. This protein catabolism supports gluconeogenesis and provides amino acids for hepatic synthesis of acute-phase reactants as hepatic synthesis is reprioritized from albumin and transferrin synthesis. Despite the observation that glutamine and alanine represent two-thirds of the amino acids released by muscle during stress, glutamine depletion occurs in the amino acid pool of muscle, and under conditions of experimental endotoxemia [18], glutamine release is increased in muscle and decreased in the kidney and serves as an oxidative fuel for enterocytes and cells of the immune system. As a result of the changes in amino acid metabolism, uric acid and ammonia excretion are increased. Simultaneously, there is an increase in aromatic amino acids in the plasma with a decrease in branched-chain amino acids (BCAA) as BCAA are oxidized in skeletal muscle.

Requirements of the Septic Patient

Exogenous nutrition support does not improve the metabolic situation and over-feeding must be avoided. The judicious use of substrate administration mini-mizes metabolic complications.

Caloric Needs

The most commonly employed calculation for energy needs is the Harris-Bene-dict (HB) equation that calculates needs based on weight, height, age, and gender to determine the Basal Energy Expenditure (BEE) [19]. This calculated value is then multiplied by an activity coefficient and a stress coefficient to obtain an esti-mate of The Resting Energy Expenditure (REE). The REE is commonly used but currently is considered to overestimate energy requirements [20, 21]. Because of immobilization, mechanical ventilation, sedation, and analgesia, caloric require-ments are lower than traditional estimates. In the septic patient, particularly those with peritonitis, the Total Energy Expenditure (TEE) over the first week is approximately 25 kcal/kg/day [22] which is similar to a REE obtained by multi-plying the BEE by a factor of 1.3. In this study, the TEE was calculated by measur-ing individual components of metabolic expenditure in septic and trauma patients and results from the first week was compared against the second week. Both TEE and REE (measured by indirect calorimetry) were analyzed. During the second week of sepsis, TEE increased to 47 kcal/kg/day equal to the REE obtained by indirect calorimetry and multiplied by a factor of 1.7 or the BEE obtained through HB multiplied by a factor of 2.3.

While indirect calorimetry may currently be the best way to determine caloric needs, its use is still not general practice in ICUs [23]; however, studies using indi-rect calorimetry have provided improved knowledge on the proportion and quantity of substrates that should be used in septic patients [24].

Carbohydrates

Glucose is the primary substrate for the central nervous system, erythrocytes, the immune system, and injured tissues. Endogenous glucose production in sepsis is approximately 2.5 mg/kg/min. exogenous glucose administration of 4–8 mg/kg/min does not inhibit this gluconeogenesis. It does, however, affect the respiratory quotient. Because of these observations, glucose should not be administered faster than 4 mg/kg/min and should represent 50%–60% of total calorie require-ments or 60%–70% of nonprotein calories [24]. Caloric overfeeding produces hypertriglyceridemia, hyperglycemia with potential for hyperosmolar syndrome, osmotic diuresis with dehydration, increased CO_2 production (which can aggra-vate respiratory insufficiency and prolong ventilator dependency), hepatic steato-sis, and cholestasis. In addition, hyperglycemia can glycosylate immunoglobulins and complement factors altering the respiratory burst of neutrophils and alveolar macrophages while inhibiting adhesions, chemotaxis, phagocytosis, and antimicrobial function of neutrophils and monocytes. Glucose levels should not exceed 220 mg% [25]. This recommendation is supported by two observations. First, control of glucose levels below this level in the first 24 h postoperatively reduces infectious complications in diabetic patients [26]; second, hyperglycemia with parenteral feeding appears to be associated with an increase in perioperative infectious complications [27].

Lipids

Septic patients are capable of metabolizing exogenous fats and should be administered to avoid a central fatty acid deficiency. Data from indirect calorimetry demonstrates that fat is efficiently used when it provides between 25%–30% of the total caloric requirement and 30%–40% of nonprotein calories. Fat should not be administered in quantities greater than 1 g/kg/day. A mixed fuel source reduces the need for carbohydrate and can improve glucose control while reducing insulin needs [15]. Excessive fat administration, however, results in dysfunction of neutrophils and lymphocytes, blockades the mononuclear phagocytic system, induces hypoxemia due to ventilation-perfusion disorders and injury of the alveolocapillary membrane, induces hepatic steatosis, and increases synthesis of PGE2.

The composition of fat in nutrition support is important since it is an essential component of cellular membrane phospholipids. The proportion of polyunsaturated fatty acids (PUFA) of the omega-6 and omega-3 series is responsible for membrane fluidity, ionic channel flow, activity of membrane receptors, and the mechanisms in cellular signal response. PUFAS of the omega-6 family are precursors of arachidonic acid from which eicosanoids of the 2 series and leukotrienes of the 4 series are synthesized. These products have intense inflammatory and immunosuppressive activity. PUFAS of the omega-3 series are precursors of docosahexaenoic acid (DHA) and eicosapentaenoic acid (EPA) which are synthesized to prostaglandins and thromboxanes of the 3 series and leukotrienes of the 5 series. Both of these are less inflammatory and less immunosuppressive. Both omega-3 and omega-6 PUFAS compete for the same metabolic pathways [28].

The exact proportion of essential fatty acids has not been defined. Use of physiologic mixtures of long chain and medium chain triglycerides as well as omega-3 fatty acids are a current avenue of investigation, particularly in the nutriceutical modulation of inflammation and immune-enhancing diets.

Proteins

Proteins are the crucial element in hypermetabolic patients, particularly in sepsis. During autocannibalism of lean tissue, muscular and visceral proteins are used as energy substrates in the muscle and as substrate for hepatic gluconeogenesis (alanine and glutamine) in synthesis of acute-phase protein reactants [29]. Protein needs exceed the normal requirement of 1 g/kg/protein/day and should be administered at 1.5–2 g/kg/day or 0.24–0.32 g nitrogen/kg/day [15, 29, 30, 31]. Greater amounts of protein do not improve nitrogen balance or the synthesis of short turnover proteins but increase blood urea. The quantity of protein should constitute 15%–20% of total calories and be provided in a nonprotein calorie/nitrogen ratio of 80–110:1 [4].

Branched-Chain Amino Acids

Because branched-chain amino acids are import fuels in sepsis, there was specu-lation that use of branched-chain amino acids in stress and sepsis [32, 33] would be of value, especially in multiple organ failure. BCAA are precursors of glutamine [33] in skeletal muscle. In a study of septic patients given parenteral nutrition supplemented with 45% BCAA, some positive benefits in mortality was noted with the high branched-chain formula [34]. Additional benefits have been noted in nutritional parameters [35]. The use of branched-chain amino acids, however, in general sepsis still remains controversial.

Glutamine

Glutamine represents one-third of amino acids released by muscle during stress and is used as a fuel by rapidly proliferating cells, particularly of the immune system and enterocytes and it appears to have beneficial effects on the structure and function of the gastrointestinal tract when given parenterally. Glutamine is a substrate for nucleic acid and glutathione synthesis and is an essential element for maintenance of acid-base balance in the kidney [36]. Glutamine utilization increases plasma levels of arginine through synthesis in the kidney [37]. In a recent study [38] comparing glutamine-enriched parenteral nutrition with an isonitrogenous, isocaloric control, six month mortality was reduced in critically ill patients with a decrease in cost; unfortunately, no specific analysis of septic patients was included in this study. In a second study comparing an enteral diet enriched in glutamine with an isonitrogenous, isocaloric control diet [39], there were no benefits in mortality but a reduction in cost with the enriched enteral formula. In a multicenter study of 71 critically ill patients administered a glu-tamine-enriched diet versus a control diet [40], there were no changes in gut barrier function, length of stay in the intensive care unit, or in mortality, but there appeared to be a reduction in the number of nosocomial infections from 55% in the control diet to 25% in the glutamine-supplemented diet, suggesting an improvement in the immune response. Houdijk et al. [41] studied 72 trauma patients, 60 of whom received enteral nutrition for 5 days. In a group of 29 patient receiving a glutamine-enriched diet, there were significantly fewer infec-tious complications than in the 31 patients receiving the control diet. Both pneu-monia and bacteremia were significantly less in the control diet. These studies in critically ill patients demonstrate that glutamine appears to have beneficial clinical effects while lowering costs in surviving patients. Glutamine appears to improve defensive capacities against infection in critically ill and traumatized patients although no specific study has been performed only in a septic popula-tion.

Arginine

Arginine is considered a semiessential amino acid important in immunity and wound repair [42, 43]. Arginine increases thymic size and content of lymphocytes and increases the activity of natural killer cells while enhancing lymphocyte proliferation to mitogens and alloantigens [44, 45]. In an experimental model of trauma and hemorrhage, arginine restored macrophage function [46]. Arginine is a precursor in the synthesis of nitric oxide [47] in endothelial cells, macrophages, and neutrophils and is capable of producing hemodynamic changes and increasing tumoricidal, virucidal, and bactericidal activity. Nitric oxide provides a connection between hemodynamic and immunologic responses.

Arginine is also an important secretagogue of human growth hormone, prolactin, glucagon, and insulin which may translate into improvement in nitrogen balance and wound repair. These activities led to incorporation of arginine in specific immune-enhancing diets for use in trauma, surgical, burn, and critically ill patients.

Nucleotides

Nucleotides are essential elements for the synthesis of DNA, RNA, and ATP. Purines and pyrimidines are used in nucleotide synthesis, and in healthy persons are efficiently absorbed from the diet. Following injury, demand for nucleotides is increased to maintain synthesis capacity within immune system cells [48, 49]. Restriction of nucleotides in the diet induces immunosuppressive effects that can be reversed with the parenteral or enteral administration of these components. Parenteral solutions and the majority of enteral diets do not contain nucleotides although the human diet provides 1–2 g/day. There are no clinical studies that analyze exclusively the role of nucleotide supplementation in relationship to infection, but it has become a component in some immune-enhancing diets. The contribution of nucleotides to the overall effect of immune-enhancing diets is unknown.

Vitamins

Specific needs for vitamins in the critically ill patients are unknown and there is neither experimental evidence nor clinical studies that guide us in this regard, but there is the presumption that needs are increased in the hypermetabolic condition. The concomitant use of drugs can increase the requirements and processes, such as renal insufficiency, can reduce the needs of certain vitamins such as A and C. The recommended daily allowance should be administered, recognizing that the daily dose can be increased safely up to 50–100 times the RDA for water-soluble vitamins and for vitamin E. Safety doses of fat-soluble vitamins and vitamin B6 have been noted up to 10 times their RDA. Daily micronutrient recommendations are listed in Table 1 [30, 50].

Table 1. Day micronutrients recommendations in critical illness

Fat-soluble vitamins	
Vitamin A	10,000 UI[a]
Vitamin D	200 UI
Vitamin E	400–1000 UI
Vitamin K	1 mg
Water-soluble vitamins	
Thiamin	10 mg
Riboflavine	10 mg
Niacin	200 mg
Pantothenic acid	100 mg
Biotin	5 mg
Pyridoxine	20 mg
Folic acid	2 mg
Vitamin B12	20 µg
Vitamin C	2000 mg
Microminerals	
Copper	1.5–3 mg
Manganese	3.5–5 mg
Selenium	100 µg
Zinc	50 mg

[a]Better in β-carotene form.

Micronutrients

The needs of micronutrients in septic patients are also unknown, but just as with vitamins, it is presumed that requirements are increased in sepsis. Iron should not be provided to septic patients since it is a bacterial growth factor and it can increase oxidative damage. Zinc is required in wound healing, and levels are reduced under septic conditions because of increased urinary and gastrointestinal losses. Zinc increases DNA synthesis and mitosis in lymphocytes and its deficit diminishes the activity of natural killer cells and thus appears to be important in reducing infectious complications. Similarly, copper and selenium appear to be important in sepsis. Recommendations for utilization and needs for critically ill patients are also reflected in Table 1.

Objectives of Metabolic-Nutrition Support in Sepsis

Metabolic nutritional support of septic patients should avoid the negative effects of starvation, provide appropriate/specific nutrients necessary for hypercatabolism, improve resistance against multiple organ dysfunction syndrome, and reduce subsequent septic episodes by improving immune responses against nosocomial infections. Although very little data exists in septic patients, a conservative three-steps strategy has been proposed by Wilmore et al. [29] in critically ill patients:
- 0–3 days: fluid "administration" with electrolytes, glucose, vitamins, and minerals

- 3–7 days: administration of 50% of the nutrient requirements with amino acids/proteins and nonprotein calories
- 7–10 days: administration of 80% or greater of the nutrient requirements

In addition, nutrition support should be started early in the following patients [51]: (a) Patients with existing protein-calorie nutrition, especially if there has been insufficient intake in the previous 5 days. (b) Patients with good nutritional status who have had insufficient nutrient intake meeting at least 50% of their nutrient needs over the past 7-10 days. (c) Anticipated adequate intake delayed at least 7 days.

Route of Administration

Data suggesting benefits of enteral nutrition compared to parenteral nutrition have been discussed elsewhere but include: (a) lower cost, (b) structural and functional preservation of the GI tract, (c) maintenance of the intestinal barrier, (d) maintenance of normal physiologic mechanisms of digestion. Each of these is an important consideration in the hypermetabolic, critically patient and numerous studies [52–55] have studied outcome of critically injured patients randomized to enteral rather than parenteral feeding and generally demonstrating an advantage with enteral feeding. In healthy volunteers, enteral nutrition blunted the release of cytokines and other counter-regulatory hormones following the administration of endotoxin compared to healthy patients receiving parenteral nutrition [56]. In cases where enteral nutrition is not possible because of absolute contraindications, such as persistent vomiting, intestinal obstruction, or active gastrointestinal hemorrhage, etc., parenteral nutrition should be employed until complete enteral nutrition support can be instituted.

Immunonutrition in Sepsis

The use of enteral diets containing various combinations of omega-3 fatty acids, nucleotides, branched-chain amino acids, glutamine, and arginine have been demonstrated to be effective compared to unsupplemented diets in burn patients [57], trauma patients [58, 59], following major digestive tract surgery [60–63], and critically ill ICU patients [64, 65]. In septic ICU patients, it appears that a minimal administration of 800 ml/day of an immune-enhancing diet is necessary to demonstrate improved clinical outcome [63, 64]. A multicenter, randomized study [66] compared an immune-enhancing diet (IM) to a high protein diet (HP) in septic ICU patients with an APACHE II score of at least 10 points at entry into the study. Patients were stratified according to the APACHE II score after admission to the hospital and were homogeneous in age, gender, and APACHE II score (Table 2). Primary outcome variables included mortality and length of stay in the ICU, days on mechanical ventilation, and nosocomial infections acquired after entry into the study. Secondary variables included complications of enteral nutrition measured as the number of days in which a complication was present as presently described

[67]. There were slightly but significantly more total calories (far below rates considered overfeeding) given during the first 7 days in the group receiving the high protein diet but no significant differences in total nitrogen intake (Table 3). Mortality was significantly lower in patients receiving the immune-enhancing diets, particularly in those with the APACHE II score between 10 and 15 (Tables 4, 5). There were also significant reductions in bacteremia. Significantly fewer patients sustained two or more nosocomial infections in the group receiving the immune-enhancing diet, but there were no differences in nutritional parameters or digestive complications between the two groups. These data are consistent with the findings of Atkinson et al. [65] and Bower et al. [64] which demonstrated a significant improvement in the patients tolerating an immune-enhancing diet.

Summary

Early metabolic-nutrition support benefits septic patients once resuscitation measures have been successful and hemodynamic stability reached. By early enteral feeding, subsequent infections can be reduced in severely injured patients. By multiplying the BEE (calculated by the Harris-Benedict equation) with a factor of 1.3, clinicians can estimate the appropriate amount of a high protein enteral diet necessary for support. In cases of parenteral nutrition or when using modular diets, 1.5–1.9 g protein/kg/day or 0.24–0.32 g nitrogen/kg/day should be administered with a calorie to nitrogen ratio of 80–110:1. Immune-enhancing diets enriched in arginine and/or glutamine and/or nucleotides and/or omega-3 fatty acids appear to improve clinical outcome in patients sustaining severe trauma as well as in critically ill patients. Their use in septic patients is still under investigation but appears to improve clinical outcome if administered in effective volumes.

Table 2. Demographic information concerning the study populations

	High-protein diet	Immune-enhancing diet	P
Age	57.7±16.9	53.9±18.5	0.16
APACHE II	17.9±5.2	18.4±5.6	0.49
Males	65/87 (74.7%)	64/89 (71.9%)	0.67

Table 3. Nutritional intake

	High-protein diet	Immune-enhancing diet	P
Nutrition intake in the 4° day			
kcal/day	1805±234	1784±223	0.54
Nitrogen/day (g)	15.5±4.3	16.3±4.5	0.23
Mean nutrition intake in the first 7 days			
kcal/day	1414±471	1231±411	0.004
Nitrogen	12.3±4.1	13.3±4.4	0.13

Table 4. Clinical results of trial

	High-protein diet		Immune-enhancing diet		
	n	%	n	%	P
Mortality	28/87	32.2	17/89	19.1	0.05
Mortality (APACHE II=10–15)	8/29	27.6	1/26	3.8	0.02
Bacteremias	19/87	21.8	7/89	7.9	0.01
>1 nosocomial infection	17/87	19.5	5/89	5.6	0.01
Length of stay, days	16.6±12.9		18.2±12.6		0.41
Ventilator days	12.2±10.3		12.4±10.4		0.90

Table 5. Mortality as a function of APACHE II score and feed

APACHE II score	High-protein diet		Immune-enhancing diet		Relative Risk (95% CI)	P
	n	%	n	%		
10–15	8/29	27.6	1/26	3.8	0.10 (0.01–0.87)	0.02
16–20	10/38	26.3	7/41	17.1	0.58 (0.19–1.71)	0.32
21–25	6/11	56.5	4/12	33.3	0.42 (0.08–2.25)	0.31
25+	4/9	44.4	5/10	50.0	1.25 (0.20–7.61)	0.81

References

1. Sands KE, Bates DW, Lanken PN, et al. (1997) Epidemiology of Sepsis Syndrome in 8 Academic Medical Centers. JAMA 278: 234–240
2. Vincent JL, Bihari DJ, Suter PM, et al. for the EPIC International Advisory Committee (1995) The prevalence of nosocomial infection in the intensive care units of Europe: Results of the European prevalence of infection in intensive care (EPIC) study. JAMA 274: 639–644
3. Bone RC, Balk RA, Cerra FB, et al. (1992) American College of Chest Physicians/Society of Critical Care Medicine Consensus Conference: Definitions for Sepsis and Organ Failure and guidelines for the use of innovative therapies in Sepsis. Chest 101: 644–655 and Crit Care Med 20: 864–874
4. Garcia de Lorenzo A, Ortiz C y Grupo de Trabajo de Metabolismo y Nutricion (1997) Segunda Conferencia de Consenso organizada por la SEMIUC. Respuesta a la agresión: valoración e implicaciones terapéuticas. Med Intensiva 21: 13–28
5. Michie HR, (1996) Metabolism of Sepsis and Multiple Organ Failure. World J Surg 20: 460–464
6. Cerra FB, Siegel JH, Colman B, et al. (1980) Septic autocannabalism, a failure of exogenous nutritional support. Ann Surg 192: 570–574
7. Cerra FB (1981) Sepsis, Metabolic Failure and Total Parenteral Nutrition. Nutritional Support Services 1: 26–29
8. Wheeler AP, Bernard GR (1999) Current Concepts: Treating Patients with severe sepsis. N Engl J Med 340: 207–214
9. Zaloga GP (1994) Frontiers in Critical Care Nutrition. New Horizons 2: 121
10. Elwyn DH, Bursztein S (1993) Carbohydrate metabolism and requirements for nutritional support. Part I. Nutrition 9: 50–66

11. Lang CH (1993) Mechanism of insulin resistance in infection. In: Schlang G, Redl H (eds): Pathophysiology of Shock, Sepsis, and Organ Failure. Springer-Verlag, New York, pp 609–625
12. Lang CH (1992) Sepsis-induced resistance in mediated by alfa-adrenergic mechanism. Am J Physiol 262: E703-E711
13. Lang CH (1995) Role of Cytokines in glucose metabolism. In: Puri RK, Aggarwall BB (eds): Human Cytokines: Their Role in Health and Disease: Blackwell Scientific, New York, pp 274–284
14. Gutierrez G, Wulf ME (1996) Lactic acidosis in sepsis: a commentary. Intensive Care Med 22: 6–16
15. Wojnar MM, Hawkins WG, Lang CH (1995) Nutritional Support of the Septic Patient. Crit Care Clin 11:717–733
16. Harris HW, Grunfeld C, Feingold KR, et al. (1990) Human very low density lipoproteins and chylomicrons can protect against endotoxin-induced death in mice. J Clin Invest 86: 696–702
17. Biolo G, Toigo G, Ciocchi B, Situlin R, Iscra F, Gullo A, Guarnieri G (1997) Metabolic response to injury and sepsis: Changes in protein metabolism. Nutrition: 13 (Supp): 52S-57 S
18. Souba WW, Austgen TR (1990) Interorgan glutamine following surgery and infection. JPEN 14: 68S-70 S
19. Frankenfield DC, Omert LA, Badellino MM, et al. (1994) Correlation between measured energy expenditure and clinically obtained variables in trauma and sepsis patients. JPEN 18: 398–403
20. Cortes V, Nelson LD (1989) Errors in estimating energy expenditure in critically ill surgical patients. Arch Surg 124: 287–290
21. Daly JM, Heymsfield SB, Head CA, et al. (1985) Human energy requirements: Overestimation by widely used prediction equation. AM J Clin Nutr 42: 1170–1174
22. Uehara M, Plank LD, Hill GL (1999) Components of energy expenditure in patients with severe sepsis and major trauma: A basis for clinical care. Crit Care Med 21: 1295–1302
23. Ireton Jones CS, Jones JD, McClave SA, Spain DA (1998) Should Predictive Equations or Indirect Calorimetry Be Used to Design Nutrition Support Regimens? NCP 13: 141–145
24. Garcia de Lorenzo A, Ortiz Leiba C, Montejo Gonzalez JC, Jimenez Lendinez M (1993) Requerimientos Energeticos en el soporte nutricional. Calorimetria indirecta. In: Celaya Perez S (ed) Avances en nutricion artificial. Prensa Universitaria, Zaragoza, pp 59–76
25. Cerra FB, Rios Benitez M, Blackburn GL and Nutrition Consensus Group (1997) Applied Nutrition in ICU Patients. ACCP Consensus Statement. Chest 111: 769–778
26. Baxter JK, Babineau TJ, Apovian CM, et al. (1990) Perioperative glucose control predicts increased nosocomial infection in diabetics. Crit Care Med 18: S207 (Abst)
27. Buzby GP and The Veterans Affairs Total Parenteral Nutrition Cooperative Study Group (1991) Perioperative total parenteral nutrition in surgical patients. N Engl J Med 325: 525–532
28. Peck MD (1994) Omega -3 Polynsaturated Fatty Acids: Benfit or Harm During Sepsis?. New Horizons 2: 230–236
29. DeBiasse MA, Wilmore DW (1994) What Is Optimal Nutritional Support?. New Horizon 2: 122–130
30. Ortiz Leiba C, Jimenez Limenez FJ, Garnacho Montero J (1998) Nutrición artificial en la sepsis, In: Celaya S (ed) Tratado de Nutricion Artificial, vol 2. GRUPO Aula Medica, S.A, Madrid, pp 491–505
31. Fürst P, Sthele P (1994) Are Intravenous Amino Acid Solutions Unbalanced? New Horizon 2: 215–223
32. Bower RH, Muggin-Sullam N, Valgren S, et al. (1986) Branched chain amino acid-enriched solutions in the septic patients: A randomized, prospective trial. Ann Surg 203: 13–21
33. Ski B, Kevin V, Gill KM, et al. (1990) Branched-chain amino acids: Their metabolism and clinical utility. Crit Care Med 18: 549–571
34. Garcia de Lorenz A, Orates Lye C, Planes M, et al. (1997) Administration of different amounts of branched-chain amino acids in septic patients. Clinical and metabolic aspects. Crit Care Med 25:418–424

35. Jimenez FJ, Ortiz Leyba C, Morales Mendez S (1991) Prospective study on the efficacy of branched-chain amino acids in septic patients. JPEN 15: 252–261
36. Ziegler TR, Szeszycki EE, Estivariz CF, et al. (1996) Glutamine from basic science to clinical applications. Nutrition 12: S68-S70
37. Houdijik APJ, van Leeuven PAM, Teerlink T, et al. (1994) Glutamine-enriched enteral diet increased renal arginine production. JPEN 18: 422–426
38. Griffiths RD, Jones C, Palmer TE (1997) Six-month outcome of critically ill patients given glutamine-supplemented parenteral nutrition. Nutrition 13:295–302
39. Jones C, Palmer TE, Griffiths RD (1999) Randomized clinical outcome study of critically ill patients given glutamine-supplemented enteral nutrition. Nutrition 15: 108–115
40. Planas M, Conejero R, Bonet A and SEMIUC Metabolic Working Group (1998) Glutamine enriched enteral nutrition in critically ill patients. Intensive Care Med 24: S105 (Abst)
41. Houdijk APJ, Rijnsburger ER, Jansen J, et al. (1998) Randomized trial of glutamine-enriched enteral nutrition on infectious morbidity in patients with multiple trauma. Lancet 352: 772–776
42. Redmon HP, Daly JM (1993) Arginine. In: Klurfed DM (ed): Human nutrition. A comprehensive treatise, vol 8: Nutrition and Immunology. Plenum Press, New York, pp 157–166
43. Lieberman ED, Fahey TJ 3erd, Daly JM (1998) Immunonutrition: the role of arginine. Nutrition 1998 14: 611–617
44. Kirk S, Barbul A (1990) Role of arginine in trauma, sepsis and immunity. JPEN: 14 S226-S229
45. Barbul A (1990) Arginine and immune function. Nutrition 6: 53–58
46. Angele MK, Smail N, Ayala A, et al. (1999) L- Arginine: A Unique Amino acid for Restoring the Depressed Macrophage Functions after Trauma- Hemorrhage. J Trauma 46: 34–41
47. Moncada S, Palmer RMJ, Higgs EA (1989) Biosynthesis of nitric oxide from L-arginine. A pathway for the regulation of cell function and communication. Biochem Pharmacol 38: 1709–1715
48. Kulkarni AD, Rudolph FB, Van Buren CT (1994) The 4role of dietary sources of nucleotides in immune function: A review. J Nutr 124: 1442S-1446 S
49. Jyonouchi H (1994) Nucleotides action on humoral immune response. J Nutr 124: 138S-143 S
50. Demling RH (1995) Micronutrients in Critical Illness. Crit Care Clin 11: 651–673
51. Peck MD (1994) Sepsis. In: Zaloga GP (ed) Nutrition in Critical Care. Mosby-Year Book Inc. St Louis, pp 599–616
52. Kudsk KA, Croce MA, Fabian TC, et al. (1992) Enteral versus parenteral feeding: effects on septic morbidity following blunt and penetrating trauma. Ann Surg 215: 503.513
53. Moore EE, Jones TE, (1986) Benefits of immediate jejunostomy feeding after major abdominal trauma: a prospective randomized study. J Trauma 26: 874–881
54. Moore FA, Moore EE, Jones TN, et al. (1989) TEN versus TPN following major abdominal trauma: reduced septic morbidity. J Trauma 29: 916–923
55. Moore FA, Feliciano DV, Andrassy RJ. (1992) Early enteral feeding compared with parenteral, reduce postoperative septic complications: the results of a meta-analysis. Ann Surg 216: 172–183
56. Fong Y, Marano MA, Barber AE, et al. (1989) Total parenteral nutrition an bowel rest modify the metabolic response to endotoxin in humans. Ann Surg 210: 449–457
57. Gottschlish MM, Jenkins M, Warden GD, et al. (1990) Differential effects of three enteral dietary regimens on selected outcome variables in burn patients. JPEN 14: 225–236
58. Moore FA, Moore EE, Kudsk KA, et al. (1994) Clinical benefits of an immune-enhancing diet for early postinjury enteral feeding. J Trauma 37: 607–615
59. Kudsk KA, Minard G, Croce MA, et al. (1996) A randomized trial of isonitrogenous enteral diets after severe trauma: An immune-enhancing diet reduce septic complication. Ann Surg 224: 531–543
60. Daly JM, Leberman MD, Goldfine J, et al. (1992) Enteral nutrition with supplemental arginine, RNA, and omega-3 fatty acids in patients after operation: Immunologic, metabolic and clinical outcome. Surgery 112: 56–67

61. Daly JM, Weintraub FN, Shou J, et al. (1995) Enteral nutrition during multimodality therapy in upper gastrointestinal cancer patients. Ann Surg 221: 327–338
62. SenkalM, Mumme A, Eickhoff U, et al. (1997) Early postoperative enteral immunonutrition: Clinical outcome and cost comparison analysis in surgical patients. Crit Care Med 25: 1489–1496
63. Braga M, Gianotti L, Vignaly A, et al. (1998) Artificial nutrition after major abdominal surgery: Impact of route of administration and composition of the diet. Crit Care Med 26:24–30
64. Bower RH, Cerra FB, Bershadsky B et al. (1995) Early enteral administration of a Formula (Impact) supplemented with arginine, nucleotides, and fish oil in intensive care unit patients: Results of a multicenter, prospective, randomized, clinical trial. Crit Care Med 23: 436–449
65. Atkinson S, Seiffert E, Bihari D (1998) on the behalf of the Guy's Hospital Intensive Care Group: A prospective, randomized, double-blind, controlled clinical trial of enteral immunonutrition in critically ill. Crit Care Med 26: 1164–1172
66. Galban C, Celaya S, Marco P, et al. (1998) An immune-enhancing enteral diet reduces mortality and episodes of bacteremia in septic ICU patients. JPEN 22: S13. (Abst) and Crit Care Med (in press)
67. Montejo JC for the Nutritional and Metabolic Working Group of the Spanish Society of Intensive Care Medicine and Coronary Units (1999) Enteral nutrition-related gastrointestinal complications in critically ill patients: A multicenter study. Crit Care Med 27: 1447–1453

Nutrition Support Guidelines for Therapeutically Immunosuppressed Patients

J. Hasse and K. Robien

Introduction

Solid organ and marrow transplantation present unique nutrition challenges. The increasing prevalence and success of these transplants requires that nutrition providers be aware of the specific nutritional needs and problems associated with transplantation.

Malnutrition

Malnutrition often occurs in transplant recipients either due to effects of end-stage organ failure (as in organ transplant candidates) or the conditioning regimen prior to marrow transplantation. Malnutrition increases mortality rates in organ transplant recipients [1–4]. A study of marrow transplant patients also showed a significantly greater risk (RR=2.11) of non-relapse mortality when patients were less than 85% of ideal body weight [5].

Pretransplant nutrition assessment should be performed to identify patients at nutritional risk. Appropriate assessment parameters include anthropometric measurements; current weight and weight history; diet recall focusing on adequacy of current diet and changes in ability to eat related to previous treatments, chemotherapy, or radiation; laboratory data; medical history; and a physical examination. Compared with solid organ transplants, marrow transplant candidates tend to be in better nutritional status on presentation for transplant as they tend to be in the earlier stages of their disease, and usually do not wait as long for a donor.

Because transplantable organs are a scarce resource, transplant recipients are waiting longer for a transplant than ever before. Nutritional status often continues to decline while a patient awaits transplantation [4]. In one study, the median waiting time from 1985–1991 for a liver transplant was 13 days. From 1992–1996, the median waiting time was 115 days. Figure 1 illustrates that even though survival rates among well nourished and moderately malnourished patients improved from the first to the second study period, the posttransplant survival rate declined in the severely malnourished patients. It is theorized that this decline was influenced by increased waiting times.

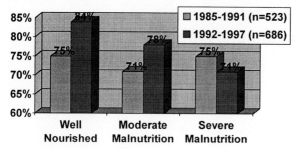

Fig. 1. Effect of pretransplant nutritional status on 3-year patient survival in liver transplant recipients at a single center

Side Effects of Immunosuppression and Conditioning Therapy

The posttransplant immunosuppression therapy and pre-marrow transplant conditioning regimen alters nutrient needs, absorption, utilization, and excretion. Tables 1 and 2 outline common nutritional side effects of these medications.

Even though organ and marrow transplant recipients are both therapeutically immunosuppressed, there are differences in the suggested supportive nutrition therapies. Therefore, specific nutrition support guidelines will be discussed separately for organ and marrow transplantation.

Solid Organ Transplantation

When providing nutrition to transplant recipients, the nutrition provider needs to consider the route of feeding (how to feed), when to initiate feedings (when to feed), the appropriate diet or nutrition support formulation (what to feed), and the amount of nutrients (how much to feed).

Route of Feeding

An oral diet is the preferred route of feeding; however, when an oral diet can be initiated will vary depending on the type of organ transplanted. For example, kidney transplant recipients begin to eat as early as postoperative day one while intestinal transplant recipients may wait more than a week to eat. Most other organ transplant recipients will begin to eat 3–5 days following surgery. Because the posttransplant state is highly catabolic, nutrition support is indicated when a patient is unable to eat adequate amounts within a few days after transplantation regardless of nutritional status.

Tube feeding (TF) is preferred over total parenteral nutrition (TPN) unless the gastrointestinal tract is not functioning (Fig. 2). Indications for TPN include ileus, severe pancreatitis, chylous ascites, immediate postoperative period following

Table 1. Immunosuppressive medications and their nutritional side effects (from [6–11])

	Antilymphocyte serum	Azathioprine	Corticosteroids	Cyclosporine	Daclizumab	Deoxyspergualin	Muromonab-CD3	Mycophenolate mofetil	Tacrolimus
Anorexia							+		
Nausea and vomiting	+	+					+		+
Diarrhea	+	+					+	+	
Sore throat, mucositis		+							
Gastrointestinal distress						+			+
Ulcers			+						
Dysgeusia		+							
Pancreatitis		+	+						
Macrocytic anemia		+							
Hyperglycemia			+	+					+
Hypertension			+	+					
Hyperlipidemia			+	+					
Hyperphagia			+						
Hyperkalemia				+					+
Hypomagnesemia			+	+					+
Sodium retention			+						
Osteoporosis			+						
Impaired wound healing			+						
Fever and chills	+				+				
No known nutrition side effect									

Table 2. Conditioning regimen related side effects impacting oral intake (from [12, 13])

Chemotherapeutic agent	Mucositis	Esophagitis	Nausea	Vomiting	Diarrhea	Anorexia	Xerostomia	Dysguesia/hypoguesia
Cyclophosphamide			Moderate-severe	+	+	+		
Busulfan	+		Mild	+		+		
Total body irradiation	+		Mild-moderate					
Melphalan			Mild-moderate	+				
Thiotepa	+		Moderate	+		+		
Ifosfamide			Mild-moderate	+				
Etoposide	+		Mild-moderate	+	+			
Carmustine		+	Moderate-severe	+		+		
Carboplatinum			Moderate-severe	+	+			
Cisplatinum	+		Severe	+	+	+[a]		+
Mitoxantrone			Mild-moderate	+				
Cytosine arabinoside	+	+	Severe	+	+	+		
Fluorouracil		+	Severe	+	+	+		+
Methotrexate	+	+	Mild-moderate	+	+	+		

[a] <1 week after transplantation.

small bowel transplantation, and possibly during infection or rejection of a small bowel graft.

Two studies compared results of providing TF or TPN to liver transplant recipients [14, 15]. In the first study [14], 63 patients fed enterally via jejunostomy tubes were compared with 21 historical control patients who received TPN. Because the study was retrospective, the type of TF formula that was infused varied. Compared with patients receiving TPN, tube-fed patients had a reduced frequency of ileus, earlier initiation of nutrition support, and achieved adequate oral intake sooner. The major metabolic complication of the TF was temporary diarrhea. Placement of jejunostomy tubes in 108 liver transplant recipients resulted in

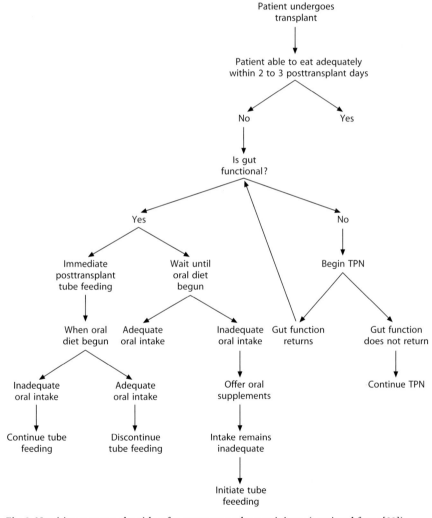

Fig. 2. Nutrition support algorithm for organ transplant recipients (reprinted from [80])

18 complications in 16 patients including mechanical obstruction of the tube, infection, small bowel obstruction, and catheter displacement [16].

Wicks et al. [15] performed a prospective study with 24 patients receiving either postoperative TF via a nasojejunal tube ($n=14$) or TPN. In this study, the number of days for patients to begin eating and to achieve adequate intake (70% of estimated needs) did not differ between the groups. Diarrhea occurred in two patients in each group and infection rates were similar between TF- (71%) and TPN-fed (70%) patients. Feeding tube access was a problem in three patients; there were no other tube-related complications. There was a delay of up to 60 h in starting TPN in three patients in the TPN group. This study also evaluated intestinal absorption and mucosal integrity. There was a decrease in absorption after transplant, but the decline was deemed clinically insignificant. Mucosal integrity/permeability also was insignificantly altered after transplant.

A final study [17] compared results of administering immediate postoperative TF ($n=14$) vs. intravenous (IV) fluid ($n=17$) in the immediate post-liver transplant period prior to the initiation of an oral diet. Nasojejunal tubes were placed during surgery in the TF group; TF infusion was initiated 12 h after surgery. A major problem with the study was placement of the tube; the surgeons forgot to place the tubes in several cases causing a higher than expected drop-out rate. No serious complications occurred when the tubes were placed. The cumulative nutrient intake over the first 12 postoperative days was significantly higher in the TF compared with the control group. The percentage of nutrient needs met during the first postoperative week was also greater in the TF vs. control group. Finally, there were fewer patients with a viral infection in the TF group and a trend for fewer patients in the TF group to have at least one documented and treated infection in the first 21 posttransplant days (TF – 21.4%; control group – 47.1%).

Some transplant centers recommend placing feeding tubes in all transplant recipients in whom there is a high rate of malnutrition or delay in the initiation of a diet. Liver, pancreas, and small bowel transplant recipients are the most likely candidates for this approach. Other centers opt to place feeding tubes only in patients in whom oral diets are contraindicated or fail to eat adequately once oral diets are initiated. Finally, some transplant centers advocate trying to predict high-risk patients and place feeding tubes during surgery. However, it is difficult to accurately predict when organ function will be delayed and affect nutrient intake.

Nasogastric and nasointestinal tubes are most frequently chosen for short-term TF therapy [15, 17]. Jejunostomy or gastrostomy tubes are beneficial for long-term therapy. Table 3 highlights suggestions for TF and TPN formulas following organ transplantation.

Posttransplant Nutrient Requirements

Following solid organ transplantation, nutrient requirements are altered. Specific nutrient recommendations are outlined in Table 4.

Researchers are evaluating the use of specific nutrients to enhance the immunosuppressive effects of anti-rejection drugs. For example, supplementing

Table 3. Selecting nutrition support formulas for acute post-organ transplant patients (adapted from [81])

Condition	Suggested tube feeding formula	Suggested parenteral nutrition formula
Immediate posttransplant-normal absorption	Polymeric, high-nitrogen formula	TPN contraindicated
Immediate posttransplant-ileus or pancreatitis (no gut function)	TF contraindicated	High-nitrogen formula
Fluid overload	Concentrated polymeric formula	Concentrated formula
Hyperglycemia	Formula with complex vs. simple carbohydrates	Start with no more than 200 g glucose; increase by 50 g daily when euglycemia achieved. Suggested initial insulin doses for diabetic patients are 0.1 U/g glucose.
Hypercarbia	Do not provide excess calories; if patients is still hypercarbic, try a high-fat formula.	Do not provide excess calories; if patients is still hypercarbic, try a high-fat formula.
Fat malabsorption	Low-fat formula or formula containing medium-chain triglycerides	Not applicable
Diarrhea or constipation	High-fiber formula (provide adequate fluid)	Provide adequate fluid
Renal failure	Concentrated formula with limited potassium, sodium, and phosphorus	Concentrated formula with limited potassium, sodium, and phosphorus
Impaired digestion or immediate post-intestinal transplant	Semi-elemental or glutamine-enhanced formula	Standard TPN may be required in the immediate post-intestinal transplant period

Table 4. Short-term posttransplant (1–3 months) nutrient recommendations for transplant recipients

Nutrient	Recommendations	Comments
Protein [18–21]	1.5–2.0 g/kg	Protein catabolic rate is increased due to surgical stress and high-dose corticosteroids. Adequate amounts of protein are required for wound healing and to prevent infection. Additional losses from surgical drains, fistulas, wounds, and dialysis should be considered.
Calories [1, 22–29]	130%–150% of calculated basal energy expenditure	The upper range of calories is recommended for underweight patients; the lower range is recommended for overweight patients. Indirect calorimetry is indicated when a patient's medical condition is complicated by co-morbidities.
Carbohydrate [30–32]	50%–70% of non-protein calories	Serum glucose levels may be increased because of medications (e.g., corticosteroids, cyclosporine, tacrolimus), metabolic stress, or infection. Treat hyperglycemia with insulin dosed on a sliding scale; add other hyperglycemic agents as needed. If hyperglycemia or diabetes mellitus is present in patient requiring TPN, limit dextrose to 200 g in initial bag. Increase dextrose by 50 g/day when euglycemia is achieved. When an oral diet is initiated, limit simple carbohydrates.
Lipid [18, 33–37]	30%–50% of non-protein calories	The higher range of lipids is recommended only when hyperglycemia is severe and not yet under control with insulin. Fat oxidation decreases following transplantation. Hyperlipidemia is common in the chronic recovery phase and can lead to vasculopathy. Fish oil (ω–3 fatty acids) may induce long-term functional transplant tolerance and may enhance immunosuppression.
Fluid [38, 39]	Solid organ transplant 1 ml/calorie; adjust based on output. Marrow transplant: 1500 ml/m^2 for patients >20 kg	Monitor output from urine, drains, wounds, diarrhea, nasogastric tube suction, fistulas, para/thoracentesis. Exocrine pancreatic secretions via urinary drainage can be as high as 2–3 l/day. Ostomy output from a small bowel transplant can be as high as 4 l/day. Restrict fluid if hyponatremia/excess water exists.
Sodium	2–4 g	Restrict if ascites or edema is severe.
Potassium	Individualize	Serum levels may increase with administration of tacrolimus, cyclosporine, or potassium-sparing diuretics; renal insufficiency; or metabolic acidosis. Serum levels may decrease with administration of potassium-wasting diuretics or amphotericin, refeeding syndrome, diarrhea, or fistulas.

Phosphorus	Individualize	Serum levels may increase with renal insufficiency.
		Serum levels may decrease with refeeding syndrome or administration of corticosteroids.
Magnesium	Individualize	Serum levels may increase with renal insufficiency.
		Serum levels may decrease with administration of cyclosporine, tacrolimus, or diuretics; refeeding syndrome; diabetic ketoacidosis; or diarrhea.
Bicarbonate	Individualize	Serum levels often decrease due to exocrine drainage of transplanted pancreas or drainage from transplanted small intestine.

heart-transplanted rats with 2% and 5% arginine improved survival rates especially when donor-specific transfusions were given [40]. Survival was also enhanced with the addition of 10% fish oil with or without donor-specific transfusions or arginine.

Fish oil also has been shown to improve renal hemodynamics in liver transplant recipients maintained on cyclosporine-based immunosuppression [41] and hasten recovery of renal function after kidney transplant rejection [42]. Fish oil also decreased serum triglycerides, platelet aggregation, and blood pressure; and improved graft survival [42–46].

Earlier studies in rat models revealed that nucleotide-free diets improved heart transplant survival [47]. Although these nutritional therapies are reported in literature; wide-spread clinical application of these practices has not occurred. It is possible that other specific nutrients, when administered, will affect (favorably or unfavorably) transplant graft function and survival.

Posttransplant Complications

There are common complications of organ transplantation that, when present, may require that nutrient composition or delivery be altered. Some of these common problems include rejection, infection, delayed wound healing, renal insufficiency, hyperglycemia, and others.

Rejection

Graft rejection is a complication unique to transplantation. There are a number of anti-rejection medications (Table 1) that are used to prevent and treat rejection. Because these medications have nutrition-related side effects, rejection treatment with additional doses of immunosuppression agents can compound nutrition problems. For example, the most common initial treatment for acute cellular rejection is to provide increased doses of corticosteroids to the patient for several days. Because corticosteroids increase the protein catabolic rate, it is important to provide at least 1.5–2.0 g protein/kg daily [18–21]. In addition, during corticosteroid therapy for rejection, protein and carbohydrate become preferential fuels for energy and hyperglycemia is likely to occur [18]. If a monoclonal antibody such as muromonab CD3 is utilized to treat rejection, common side effects of nausea, vomiting, diarrhea, and headache are likely to diminish a patient's desire to eat.

Infection

When a patient is immunosuppressed, the opportunity for infection to occur increases. Malnutrition further increases rate of infection. In a study by Harrison et al. [3], liver transplant recipients with mid-arm muscle circumference measurements less than the 25th percentile had more bacterial infections than patients whose mid-arm muscle circumference was above the 25th percentile.

Antimicrobial agents given to prevent or treat infection can cause gastrointestinal symptoms such as nausea or diarrhea and adversely affect a patient's appetite. If a patient is receiving a tube feeding infusion, antibiotics may cause or worsen diarrhea.

Wound Healing

There are several nutrition factors that affect wound healing. Patients who are malnourished or obese may experience delayed healing of their surgical wounds. The increased rate of wound complications in obese renal and liver transplant recipients is well documented [48–53]. In addition, nutrients play a major role in wound healing. For example, synthesis, hydroxylation, cross-linking, and remodeling of collagen requires adequate intake of protein, vitamins A and C, iron, copper, and manganese [54]. In addition, blood glucose needs to be maintained near normal levels to aid the healing process.

Renal Insufficiency

Renal insufficiency in the post-kidney transplant phase occurs when the transplanted kidney has not yet begun to function adequately. In addition, immunosuppressants, specifically cyclosporine and tacrolimus, are nephrotoxic. Other potential causes of renal insufficiency in transplant recipients include hypovolemia, cardiovascular failure, acute tubular necrosis, ischemia, multi-system organ failure, radiographic contrast agents, and other nephrotoxic drugs. If renal replacement therapy is initiated, nutrient requirements will change.

If renal insufficiency is accompanied by multi-organ failure, calorie requirements are most accurately determined via indirect calorimetry. Depending on the type of renal replacement therapy (hemodialysis, continuous hemofiltration or dialysis) 5–10 g of amino acids may be lost in dialysate daily; protein recommendations range from 1.1–2.5 g protein/kg/day [55]. During continuous hemofiltration, 300 g glucose can be absorbed over 24 h when glucose-rich replacement fluids are used [56]. Likewise, approximately 43%–45% of calories are absorbed from the dextrose dialysate during continuous hemodialysis [57]. This can provide over 500 calories per day and sometimes contributes to hyperglycemia. For patients with renal insufficiency, serum potassium, phosphorus, calcium, and magnesium levels should be monitored and restricted or supplemented as indicated.

Hyperglycemia

Hyperglycemia is common in the acute posttransplant phase and adversely affects infection rates and wound healing. A 50% increase in infection rates was reported in diabetic versus nondiabetic kidney transplant recipients [58]. Immunosuppressive medications contribute to hyperglycemia– corticosteroids cause insulin resistance; pancreatic islet cell function and insulin release are inhibited by cyclosporine and tacrolimus [30]. Infection and metabolic stress also contribute to hyperglycemia. Finally, a sudden increase in serum glucose concentration in a pancreas transplant recipient signals graft rejection or ischemia.

Posttransplant hyperglycemia is usually treated with regular insulin dosed on a sliding scale. When severe hyperglycemia is present, an insulin drip may be required temporarily. The carbohydrate content of nutrition support solutions should be adjusted as discussed previously. Because de novo diabetes mellitus may develop in some recipients and serum glucose levels are affected by corticosteroid doses, it is important to continue to monitor glucose levels until they are normalized.

Other Complications

Other conditions that can affect posttransplant recovery include vascular complications, postoperative bleeding, pancreatitis, edema, hypertension, and gastrointestinal complications. Any complication that requires surgery may require a period of NPO status or initiation of nutrition support. When pancreatitis is severe, TPN is indicated. Sodium restriction may help treat edema and hypertension. Finally, intestinal complications such as ileus, diarrhea, ulcers, and viral enteritis may prompt a change in nutrition route or content. For example, prolonged ileus is an indication for TPN; liquid oral nutrition supplements may be better tolerated than solid food by a patient with esophagitis; and a patient with diarrhea must consume additional fluid. It is important to be attentive to the changing medical condition of the patients. Then, nutrition support can be tailored to each patient's individual needs to achieve the overall goals of recovery and improvement in nutritional status.

Marrow Transplantation

Table 5 summarizes the medical and nutritional issues related to the marrow transplant process. Conditioning regimen related toxicities such as mucositis, esophagitis, gastritis, nausea, vomiting, and diarrhea tend to prevent the individual from meeting estimated nutritional requirements via oral intake during conditioning and the first 20–30 days posttransplant. Table 2 summarizes the effect of various cytoreductive agents on oral intake. Decreased intestinal motility due to the use of narcotics is another complicating factor.

Route of Feeding

Parenteral nutrition support is often used for sole nutrition support or to supplement oral intake during the cytoreductive and neutropenic phases because enteral feedings are generally not well tolerated and central line access has usually been established for delivery of the conditioning regimen. Weisdorf et al. [59] also found that overall survival, time to relapse, and disease-free survival were significantly improved in marrow transplant patients who received TPN during conditioning and for the first 4 weeks following marrow transplant compared with patients who received a 5% dextrose solution with vitamins, minerals, electrolytes, and trace elements.

There has been concern that the use of IV lipid emulsions may lead to an increased incidence of infections due to impairment of the normal function of the

Table 5. Typical medical and nutrition related issues during the marrow transplant process: typical allogeneic marrow transplant progression

	Cytoreduction (day –10 to day 0)[a]	Neutropenia (day 0 to day 20)	Engraftment/early recovery (days 20–100)	Long-term recovery (days 100–1 year+)
Possible medical issues:	Tumor lysis	Tumor lysis Early opportunistic infections Mucositis, esophagitis, gastritis Venooclusive disease Hyperacute GVHD[b] Conditioning related toxicities, especially blistering of feet and hands, diarrhea	Acute GVHD Opportunistic infections Idiopathic pneumonitis syndrome	Chronic GVHD Late opportunistic infections Infertility Delayed growth and development Relapse Secondary tumors Bronchiolitis obliterans Cataracts
Possible nutrition related issues:	Poor oral intake due to nausea, vomiting Fluid/electrolyte imbalances	Poor oral intake due to mucositis, nausea, vomiting Intolerance to certain foods (especially lactose, citrus, fat) Fluid/electrolyte imbalances Altered taste acuity Changes in consistency, volume of saliva	Suboptimal oral intake related to GI GVHD, altered taste acuity Transition from IV to PO medications contributing to nausea, vomiting, diarrhea Fluid/electrolyte imbalances Fluid retention	Malabsorption related to chronic GI GVHD Oral, esophageal strictures Osteopenia/osteoporosis related to chronic use of corticosteroids Pancreatic insufficiency Adrenal insufficiency related to the chronic use of corticosteroids Hyperlipidemia

Patients receiving autologous, syngeneic, or low dose TBI and PBSC infusion may be at lower risk of both medical and nutritional complications because of lower toxicity of conditioning and immunosuppressive regimens.
[a] The day of transplant is traditionally referred to as day 0.
[b] GVHD = graft-vs-host disease.

reticuloendothelial system and altered neutrophil chemotaxis. However, a study of 482 patients undergoing allogeneic or autologous marrow transplantation for hematologic malignancies failed to show an association between intravenous lipid emulsions (of 20% linoleic acid at either 6%–8% or 25%–30% of total daily energy) and an increased incidence of bacterial and fungal infections [60].

Parenteral nutrition may, however, limit oral intake, cause increases in liver function tests, and decrease gastrointestinal mucosal integrity. Charuhas et al. [61] found that providing TPN once the patient has been able to transition from the hospital to the outpatient setting (corresponding roughly to the transition between the neutropenic stage and the engraftment/early recovery phase) resulted in delayed resumption of oral intake. In their study of 258 marrow transplant patients, the patients who were randomized to receive IV hydration in place of TPN were able to meet >85% estimated caloric needs 6 days sooner than the PN group.

Parenteral feedings may contribute to hepatic abnormalities following marrow transplantation resulting in elevated serum transaminase, alkaline phosphatase, and bilirubin levels. Abnormalities related to parenteral nutrition should improve with discontinuation or cycling of the TPN solution.

The presence of nutrients in the intestinal tract is thought to maintain mucosal integrity and prevent bacterial translocation. There has been significant interest in encouraging oral intake or providing nutrition support via TF to marrow transplant patients because they have compromised gastrointestinal mucosal integrity due to conditioning regimens and are at increased risk for infections due to neutropenia. A study of 26 marrow transplant patients found increased intestinal permeability peaking at 1–2 weeks, but continuing for up to 4 weeks following marrow transplant based on mannitol and lactulose absorption studies [62].

Unfortunately, TF during the cytoreductive and neutropenic stages of the marrow transplant are generally not well tolerated due to enteritis (increased risk of ulceration at contact points with the tubing), vomiting (tube displacement and risk of aspiration), and low platelet counts (increased risk of bleeding complications during tube placement). However, TF may be beneficial for patients who are further posttransplant with a functional intestinal tract, yet suboptimal intake.

Posttransplant Nutrient Requirements

Specific nutrient recommendations for marrow transplant patients are outlined in Table 4.

Energy

Energy requirements for marrow transplant recipients during the cytoreduction and neutropenic periods average 30–35 kcal/kg [63]. During the engraftment and early recovery period, energy needs will vary significantly from patient to patient based on the individual's medical issues (including graft-versus-host disease and infections) and activity level. Indirect calorimetry may be useful in assessing an individual's actual energy requirements; however, monitoring actual intake and comparing this information with the individual's weight on a weekly (or more frequent) basis may be more practical in the clinical setting. That said, estimation of actual body weights may be difficult if patients are experiencing fluid retention as a side effect of corticosteroids.

Protein

Protein requirements are increased to as much as twice baseline following transplant to allow for tissue repair after cytoreductive therapy and to provide substrate for regenerating hematopoietic cell lines. Protein requirements may remain elevated even after the patient is engrafted, as patients will often need to rebuild lean body mass lost during earlier stages of the marrow transplant. Positive nitrogen balance is difficult to achieve in the cytoreduction and neutropenic periods despite aggressive nutrition support [64]. The use of corticosteroids for patients with graft-vs-host disease (GVHD) accelerates the rate of protein loss, with protein loss being greater in men than in women [65].

Studies have shown that the amino acid glutamine is an essential amino acid during periods of stress because it is a fuel for rapidly dividing cells and is a substrate for de novo nucleotide synthesis. Animal studies have shown decreased mucosal atrophy, more rapid mucosal recovery, and decreased incidence of bacteremia following high-dose chemotherapy in rats given glutamine-supplemented TPN [66] or diet [67]. However, the use of the glutamine in the oncology patient population has been an area of controversy due to concerns that while glutamine has been shown to be the primary fuel for enterocytes, it is also known that tumor cells are avid glutamine consumers. To test this concern, a study using a rat tumor model showed that glutamine-supplemented TPN did not increase tumor size compared to unsupplemented controls, and the glutamine-supplemented group had increased host glutamine stores [68]. It is believed that exogenous supplementation of glutamine can spare skeletal muscle breakdown and provide substrate for mucosal regeneration following chemotherapy and radiation without significantly impacting tumor burden. Glutamine may even suppress tumor growth through stimulation of the immune system [69].

Unfortunately, research into the role of glutamine supplementation in marrow transplant patients has been inconclusive. Ziegler et al. [70] reported significantly improved nitrogen balance among marrow transplant patients who received TPN supplemented with L-glutamine (0.57 g/kg body weight/day) compared with controls who received standard TPN solutions. They also found decreased incidence of infection and shortened length of stay in the glutamine-supplemented group. However, the study failed to provide objective criteria for hospital discharge, making comparisons based on length of stay difficult. They also did not compare long-term survival or relapse rate between the two groups. These findings have not been replicated when glutamine supplementation was evaluated for study populations that included both allogeneic and autologous marrow transplant patients [71, 72].

Jebb et al. [73] also failed to find a significant difference in incidence of oral mucositis or number of days of diarrhea between marrow transplant patients receiving oral glutamine supplementation vs. placebo. It is important to note that this trial of oral glutamine supplementation provided less than half the dose of glutamine provided in studies using the intravenous route. The authors felt that it would have been difficult to increase oral supplementation further due to decreased tolerance to oral intake overall.

Fluid

Fluid needs are also elevated posttransplant because of the use of nephrotoxic medications for cytoreduction, therapeutic immunosuppression, and anti-infective agents. Fluid requirements during marrow transplantation are estimated to be 1500 ml/m² [13], but may vary based on the individual's medical condition. Fluid restriction may be necessary if venoocclusive disease develops, where as increased fluid intake (>1500 cc/m²) may be needed if serum creatinine levels rise or if the patient experiences large volume stool losses. Fluid requirements should decrease as nephrotoxic medications are tapered.

Intake and output records along with daily weights are vital during the cytoreductive and neutropenic stages to monitor fluid overload or deficits. Weight gain during the early posttransplant period is most likely due to fluid retention rather than gain of body cell mass, and may indicate the presence of venoocclusive disease.

Micronutrients

Serum electrolyte status requires close monitoring throughout the transplant process. Table 1 lists electrolyte abnormalities associated with various immunosuppressive medications. Table 6 lists electrolyte abnormalities associated with selected anti-infective agents. If the patient is receiving TPN or IV hydration, it is often preferable to provide electrolyte supplementation in these solutions to avoid the GI upset common with oral supplementation, especially magnesium and potassium.

Marrow transplant patients often require several red blood cell transfusions during the transplant process, and as a result tend to be iron overloaded rather than iron deficient. Iron overload may contribute to liver disease in the posttransplant setting [75]. For this reason, iron supplementation should be avoided, including multivitamin supplements containing iron. The nutrition assessment at 1 year posttransplant should include an evaluation of transfusion requirements over the previous year to determine the appropriateness of continued iron restriction. Large doses of antioxidants, especially vitamin C, should be avoided in the setting of iron overload as antioxidants actually act as pro-oxidants in a high-iron environment.

Vitamin K deficiency is of concern in marrow transplant patients because oral intake is often minimal (especially early posttransplant) and broad spectrum and oral non-absorbable antibiotics (to prevent bacterial translocation) are commonly used. High-dose chemotherapy may impair intestinal absorption and hepatic metabolism of vitamin K [76]. Vitamin K deficiency may contribute to thrombotic events, which are relatively common posttransplant. Vitamin K is also known to play a role in the synthesis of osteocalcin, which facilitates calcium binding to

Table 6. Nutritional side effects of selected anti-infective agents (from [13, 74])

Anti-infective agent	Gastrointestinal/renal effects	Nutrient effects
Anti-fungal agents		
Amphotericin B	Anorexia, nausea, vomiting, renal insufficiency	Hypokalemia, hypomagnesemia
Fluconazole	Nausea, vomiting, increased liver function tests	Hypercholesterolemia, hypertriglyceridemia, hypokalemia
Itraconazole	Nausea, increased liver function tests	
Anti-viral Agents		
Foscarnet	Renal insufficiency	Hypokalemia, hypomagnesemia, hypophosphatemia, hypocalcemia
Ganciclovir	Nausea, vomiting, abnormal liver function tests	Hypokalemia, hypoglycemia
Ribavirin	Nausea, xerostomia, metallic taste, flatulence, increased liver function tests	
Anti-bacterial agents		
Dapsone	Nausea, vomiting, abdominal pain, anorexia, abnormal liver function tests	Hypoalbuminemia, hyperkalemia
Imipenum	Nausea, vomiting, diarrhea, heartburn, increased salivation, increased liver function tests	Hyperkalemia, hyponatremia
Isoniazid	Nausea, vomiting, anorexia, increased liver function tests	Pyridoxine (Vitamin B_6) deficiency
Metronidazole	Nausea, vomiting, epigastric distress, anorexia, metallic taste	
Trimethoprim and sulfamethoxazole	Anorexia, nausea, vomiting, glossitis, stomatitis, abdominal pain, diarrhea, increased liver function tests	Folate deficiency, hyperkalemia, possible decreased vitamin K absorption
Vancomycin	Nausea, renal insufficiency	

the hydroxyapatite matrix of bone [77]. Thus, a vitamin K deficiency might increase the risk of developing osteoporosis while receiving corticosteroids. Vitamin K should be given intravenously at a dose of 10 mg once a week or 5 mg per day [76, 78].

Posttransplant Complications

Venoocclusive Disease

Venoocclusive disease (VOD) is a syndrome of liver toxicity following cytoreduction. It is characterized by liver enlargement, fluid retention/weight gain, and hyperbilirubinemia, and typically occurs between days –3 and 20 posttransplant. The primary management objective in cases of VOD is to minimize fluid retention while maintaining adequate renal perfusion. Limiting IV sources of sodium is important, including TPN, intravenous hydration solutions, and medications. Fluid restrictions, including concentration of TPN solutions, may also become necessary to limit fluid retention. If bilirubin levels reach >10 mg/dl and persist beyond 1 week, trace minerals (manganese and copper) should be removed from the TPN solution as they are excreted via bile acids. Serum copper levels should be checked if diarrhea is present, and copper may need to be replaced if serum levels are low. Elevated serum levels of manganese have been associated with extrapyramidal symptoms [79].

Graft-vs-Host Disease

Graft-vs-host disease can occur in most organs of the body. Acute GVHD typically occurs during the first 100 days posttransplant, most commonly affecting skin, intestinal tract, and liver. First line therapy for GVDH has been corticosteroids.

The severity of GVHD of the skin will vary, but severe cases may result in increased energy expenditure and nutrient requirements comparable to those seen in patients with burn injuries. In the event of skin ulceration, attention should be paid to providing adequate energy, protein, vitamin C, and zinc for wound healing.

Symptoms of GVHD of the intestinal tract include abdominal cramping, anorexia, nausea, vomiting, and large volume, secretory diarrhea. Severe cases may result in sloughing of the mucosal membranes and thus malabsorption, increased risk of bacterial translocation, and GI bleeding.

Nutritional management of intestinal GVHD will vary with the severity of GVHD and may range from limiting dietary fat, insoluble fiber, caffeine, and lactose to discontinuing the oral diet and resuming parenteral nutrition support. Hyperglycemia is common among patients receiving high-dose corticosteroids, especially among patients receiving TPN concurrently.

Liver GVHD may result in cholestasis and consequent fat malabsorption. Anorexia is also common among patients with liver GVHD.

Infections

Patients who receive therapeutic immunosuppression are at increased risk of bacterial, viral, and fungal infections. Marrow transplant patients are at additional risk due to neutropenia following cytoreduction. The use of antibiotics can result in the reduction of the normal gastrointestinal flora, which in turn can result in vitamin K deficiency, diarrhea, and intestinal infections such as clostridium difficle or vancomycin-resistant enterococci. Many anti-infective agents will cause nausea, vomiting, and/or diarrhea, especially when taken orally. Table 6 lists nutritional side effects of selected anti-infective agents.

Reactivation of latent cytomegalovirus of donor or host origin may result in colonization in the intestinal tract. The symptoms of this complication mimic that of intestinal GVHD, making an endoscopy imperative to rule out infection prior to starting corticosteroids for presumed GVHD.

Other Complications

Other common complications following marrow transplantation include renal insufficiency and hyperglycemia as described above.

Conclusion

Patients undergoing organ and marrow transplantation are at risk for malnutrition due to disease state or therapy for the disease. Nutrient needs are altered by immunosuppressive and cytoreductive medications and the many complications associated with transplantation. Providing nutrition support is vital to the recovery and success of transplantation. Oral diet is the preferred route of nutrition, but TF or TPN is often indicated during the acute posttransplant phase when oral intake is prohibited or inadequate.

References

1. Frazier OH, Van Buren CT, Poindexter SM, Waldenberger F (1985) Nutritional management of the heart transplant recipient. Heart Transplantation 4 (4):450–452
2. Pikul J, Sharpe MD, Lowndes R, Ghent CN (1994) Degree of preoperative malnutrition is predictive of postoperative morbidity and mortality in liver transplant recipients. Transplantation 57:469–472
3. Harrison J, McKiernan J, Neuberger JM (1997) A prospective study on the effect of recipient nutritional status on outcome in liver transplantation. Transpl Int 10:369–374
4. Hasse JM, Gonwa TA, Jennings, LW, Goldstein RM, Levy MF, Husberg BS, Klintmalm GB (1998) Malnutrition affects liver transplant outcomes. Transplantation 66 (8):S53 (Abst)
5. Deeg HJ, Seidel K, Bruemmer B, Pepe MS, Appelbaum FR (1995) Impact of patient weight on non-relapse mortality after marrow transplantation. Bone Marrow Transplantation 15:461–468
6. Wahrenberger A (1995) Pharmacologic immunosuppression: cure or curse? Crit Care Nurs Q 17:27–36

7. Ohara MM (1992) Immunosuppression in solid organ transplantation: a nutrition perspective. Topics in Clinical Nutrition 7 (3):6–11
8. Manez R, Jain A, Marino IR, Thomson AW (1995) Comparative evaluation of tacrolimus (FK506) and cyclosporine A as immunosuppressive agents. Transplant Rev 9:63–76
9. Klintmalm GB (1994) FK506: an update. Clin Transplant 8:207–210
10. Gonwa TA (1996) Mycophenolate mofetil for maintenance therapy in kidney transplantation. Clin Transplant 10:128–130
11. Mueller AR, Platz KP, Blumhardt G, et al. (1995) The superior immunosuppressant according to diagnosis: FK506 or cyclosporine A. Transplant Proc 27:1117–1120
12. Charuhas PM, Aker SN (1992) Nutritional implications of antineoplastic chemotherapeutic agents. Clin Appl Nutr 2 (2):20–33
13. Lenssen P (1998) Bone marrow and stem cell transplantation. In: Matarese LE, Gottschlich MM, eds. Contemporary Nutrition Support Practice: A Clinical Guide. WB Saunders Company, Philadelphia pp 561–581
14. Mehta PL, Alaka KJ, Filo RS, Leapman SB, Milgrom ML, Pescovitz MD (1995) Nutrition support following liver transplantation: Comparison of jejunal versus parenteral routes. Clin Transplant 9:837–840.
15. Wicks C, Somasundaram S, Buarnason I, et al. (1994) Comparison of enteral feeding and total parenteral nutrition after liver transplantation. Lancet 344:837–840
16. Pescovitz MD, Mehta PL, Leapman SB, Milgrom ML, Jindal RM, Filo RS (1995) Tube jejunostomy in liver transplant recipients. Surgery 117:642–647
17. Hasse JM, Blue LS, Liepa GU, et al. (1995) Early enteral nutrition support in patients undergoing liver transplantation. JPEN 19:437–443
18. Steiger U, Lippuner K, Jensen EX, Montandon A, Jaeger Ph, Horber FF (1995) Body composition and fuel metabolism after kidney grafting. Eur J Clin Invest 25:809–816
19. Seagraves A, Moore EE, Moore, FA, Weil R (1986) Net protein catabolic rate after kidney transplantation: impact of corticosteroid immunosuppression. JPEN 10 (5):453–455
20. Hoy WE, Sargent JA, Freeman RB, Pabico RC, McKenna BA, Sterling WA (1986) The influence of glucocorticoid dose on protein catabolism after renal transplantation. Am J Med Sci 291:241–247
21. Hoy WE, Sargent JA, Hall D, et al. (1985) Protein catabolism during the postoperative course after renal transplantation. Am J Kidney Dis 5 (3):186–190
22. Poindexter SM (1992) Nutrition support in cardiac transplantation. Topics in Clinical Nutrition 7 (3):12–16
23. Evans MA, Shronts EP, Fish JA (1992) A case report: Nutrition support of a heart-lung transplant recipient. Support Line 14 (1):1–8
24. Delafosse B, Faure JL, Bouffard Y, et al. (1989) Liver transplantation – Energy expenditure, nitrogen loss, and substrate oxidation rate in the first two postoperative days. Transplant Proc 21:2453–2454
25. Plevak DJ, DiCecco SR, Wiesner RH, et al. (1994) Nutritional support for liver transplantation: Identifying caloric and protein requirements. Mayo Clin Proc 69:225–230
26. Ragsdale D (1987) Nutritional program for heart transplantation. J Heart Transplantation 6:228–233
27. Edwards MS, Doster S (1990) Renal transplant diet recommendations: results of a survey of renal dietitians in the United States. J Am Diet Assoc 90:843–846
28. Zabielski P (1992) What are the calorie and protein requirements during the acute postrenal transplant period? Support Line 14 (1)11–13
29. Kowalchuk D (1992) Nutritional management of the pancreas transplant patient. Support Line 14 (1):10–11
30. Jindal RM (1994) Posttransplant diabetes mellitus – A review. Transplantation 58 (12):1289–1298
31. Babineau TJ, Borlase BC, Blackburn GL (1991) Applied total parenteral nutrition in the critically ill. In: Rippe JM, Irwin RS, Alpert JS, Fink MP (eds) Intensive Care Medicine, 2nd ed. Little, Brown and Company, Boston, pp 1675–1691

32. McMahon M, Manji N, Driscol DF, et al. (1989) Parenteral nutrition in patients with diabetes mellitus: Theoretical and practical considerations. JPEN 13:545–553
33. Kobashigawa JA, Kasiske BL (1997) Hyperlipidemia in solid organ transplantation. Transplantation 63:331–338
34. Alexander JW (1998) Immunonutrition: The role of ω–3 fatty acids. Nutrition 14:627–633
35. Perez RV, Waymack JP, Munda R, Alexander JW (1987) The effect of donor specific transfusions and dietary fatty acids on rat cardiac allograft survival. J Surg Res 42 (4):335–340
36. Otto DA, Kahn DR, Hamm HW, Forrest DE, Wooten JT (1990) Improved survival of heterotopic cardiac allografts in rats with dietary omega-3 polyunsaturated fatty acids. Transplantation 50 (2):193–198
37. Kelley VE, Kirkman RL, Bastos M, Barrett LV, Strom TB (1989) Enhancement of immunosuppression by substitution of fish oil for olive oil as a vehicle for cyclosporine. Transplantation 48 (1):98–102
38. Bartucci MR, Loughman KA, Moir EJ (1992) Kidney-pancreas transplantation: a treatment option for ESRD and type I diabetes. American Nephrology Nursing Association Journal 19:467–474
39. Reyes J, Tzakis AG, Todo S, et al. (1993) Nutritional management of intestinal transplant recipients. Transplant Proc 25:1200–1201
40. Alexander JW, Levy A, Custer D, et al. (1998) Arginine, fish oil, and donor-specific transfusions independently improve cardiac allograft survival in rats given subtherapeutic doses of cyclosporine. JPEN 22:152–155
41. Badalamenti S, Salerno F, Lorenzano E, et al. (1995) Renal effects of dietary supplementation with fish oil in cyclosporine-treated liver transplant recipients. Hepatol 22:1695–1701
42. Homan van der Heide JJ, Bilo HJG, Donker AJM, Wilmink JM, Sluiter WJ, Tegzess AM (1992) The effects of dietary supplementation with fish oil on renal function and the course of early postoperative rejection episodes in cyclosporine-treated renal transplant recipients. Transplantation 54:257–263
43. Donker JM, van der Heide JJ, Bilo HJG, et al. (1993) Effect of dietary fish oil on renal function and rejection in cyclosporine-treated recipients of renal transplants. N Engl J Med 329 (11):769–773
44. Sweny P, Wheeler DC, Lui SF, et al. (1989) Dietary fish oil supplements preserve renal function in renal transplant recipients with chronic vascular rejection. Nephrol Dial Transplant 4 (12):1070–1075
45. Homan van der Heide JJ, Bilo HJG, Donker AJM, Wilmink JM, Sluiter WJ, Tegzess AM (1990) Dietary supplementation with fish oil modifies renal reserve filtration capacity in postoperative, cyclosporin A-treated renal transplant recipients. Transplant Int 3:171–175
46. Homan van der Heide JJ, Bilo HJG, Donker JM, Wilmink JM, Tegzess AM (1993) Effect of dietary fish oil on renal function and rejection in cyclosporine-treated recipients of renal transplants. N Engl J Med 329:769–773
47. Van Buren CT, Kulkami A, Rudolph F (1983) Synergistic effect of a nucleotide-free diet and cyclosporine on allograft survival. Transplant Proc 15 Suppl 1:2967–2968
48. Merion RM, Twork AM, Rosenberg L, et al. (1991) Obesity and renal transplantation. Surg Gynecol Obstet 172:367–376
49. Holley JL, Shapiro R, Lopatin WB, Tzakis AG, Hakala TR, Starzl TE (1990) Obesity as a risk factor following cadaveric renal transplantation. Transplantation 49 (2):387–389
50. Pirsch JD, Armbrust MJ, Knechtle SJ, D'Allesandro AM, Sollinger HW, Heisey DM, et al. (1995) Obesity as a risk factor following renal transplantation. Transplantation 59 (4):631–633
51. Keeffe EB, Gettys C, Esquivel CO (1994) Liver transplantation in patients with severe obesity. Transplantation 57:309–311
52. Testa G, Hasse JM, Jennings LW, et al. (1998) Morbid obesity is not an independent risk factor for liver transplantation. Transplantation 66 (8):S53 (abst)
53. Braunfeld MY, Chan S, Pregler J, et al. (1996) Liver transplantation in the morbidly obese. J Clin Anesth 8:585–590

54. Lown D (1998) Wound healing. In: Matarese LEM, Gottschlich MM (eds) Contemporary nutrition support practice: A clinical guide. W.B. Saunders Co., Philadelphia, pp 583–589
55. Rodriguez DJ (1997) Nutrition support in acute renal failure patients: current perspectives Support Line 19 (7):3–9
56. Monaghan R, Watters JM, Clancey SM, Moulton SB, Rabin EZ (1993) Uptake of glucose during continuous arteriovenous hemofiltration. Crit Care Med 21:1159–1163.
57. Monson P, Mehta RL (1994) Nutrition in acute renal failure: a reappraisal for the 1990s. J Renal Nutr 4:58–77
58. Eckstrand AV, Eriksson JG, Gronhagen-Riska C, et al. (1992) Insulin resistance and insulin deficiency in the pathogenesis of posttransplantation diabetes in man. Transplantation 53 (3):563–569
59. Weisdorf SA, Lysne J, Wind D, et al. (1987) Positive effect of prophylactic total parenteral nutrition on long-term outcome of bone marrow transplantation. Transplantation 43 (6):833–838
60. Lenssen P, Bruemmer B, Aker S, et al. (1994) Relationship between IV lipid dose and incidence of bacteremia and fungemia in 482 marrow transplant (MT) patients. JPEN 18:22 S (Abst)
61. Charuhas PM, Fosberg KL, Bruemmer B, et al. (1997) A double-blind randomized trial comparing outpatient parenteral nutrition with intravenous hydration: effect on resumption of oral intake after marrow transplantation. JPEN 21 (3):157–161
62. Fegan C, Poynton CH, Whittaker JA (1990) The gut mucosal barrier in bone marrow transplantation. Bone Marrow Transplantation 5:373–377
63. Stralovich A, Porter C (1991) Energy expenditure of bone marrow transplant patients. JPEN 15 (1):36 S (Abst)
64. Keller U, Kraenzlin ME, Gratwohl A, et al. (1990) Protein metabolism assessed by 1-^{13}C leucine infusions in patients undergoing bone marrow transplantation. JPEN 14 (5):480–484
65. Cheney CL, Lenssen P, Aker SN et al. (1987) Sex differences in nitrogen balance following marrow grafting for leukemia. J Am Coll Nutr 6:223–230
66. O'Dwyer ST, Scott T, Smith RJ, Wilmore W (1987) 5-Fluoruracil toxicity on small intestinal mucosa but not white blood cells is decreased by glutamine. Clin Res 35:367 (Abst)
67. Fox AD, Kripke SA, De Paula JA, Berman JM, Settle RG, Rombeau J (1988) The effect of glutamine-supplemented enteral nutrition on methotrexate-induced enterocolitis. JPEN 12:325–331
68. Austgen TR, Dudrick PS, Sitren H, Bland KI, Copeland E, Souba WW (1992) The effects of glutamine-enriched total parenteral nutrition on tumor growth and host tissues. Ann Surg 215 (2):107–13
69. Klimberg VS, McClellan JL (1996) Glutamine, cancer, and its therapy. Am J Surg 172 (5):418–424
70. Ziegler TR, Young LS, Benfell K, et al. (1992) Clinical and metabolic efficacy of glutamine-supplemented parenteral nutrition after bone marrow transplantation. Ann Intern Med 116: 821–828
71. Schloerb PR, Amare M (1993) Total parenteral nutrition with glutamine in bone marrow transplantation and other clinical applications (a randomized, double-blind study). JPEN 17:407–413
72. Schloerb PR, Skikne BS. Oral and parenteral glutamine in bone marrow transplantation: a randomized, double-blind study. JPEN 23:117–122
73. Jebb SA, Marcus R, Elia M (1995) A pilot study of oral glutamine supplementation in patients receiving bone marrow transplants. Clin Nutr 14:162–165
74. Drug Facts and Comparisons, 1999 Edition (1998) Facts and Comparisons, St. Louis, MO
75. McKay PJ, Murphy JA, Cameron S, et al. (1996) Iron overload and liver dysfunction after allogeneic or autologous bone marrow transplantation. Bone Marrow Transplantation 17: 63–66
76. Elston TN, Dudley JM, Shearer MJ, Schey SA (1995) Vitamin K prophylaxis in high dose chemotherapy. Lancet 345 (8959): 1245
77. Shearer MJ (1995) Vitamin K. Lancet 345 (8944):229–234

78. Gordon BG, Haire WD, Stephens LC, Kotulak GD, Kessinger A (1993) Protein C deficiency following hematopoietic stem cell transplantation: optimization of intravenous vitamin K dose. Bone Marrow Transplantation 12:73–76
79. Fredstrom S, Rogosheske J, Gupta P, Burns LJ (1995) Extrapyramidal symptoms in a BMT recipient with hyperintense basal ganglia and elevated manganese. Bone Marrow Transplantation 15:989–992
80. Hasse JM, Roberts S (In Press) Transplantation. In: Rombeau JL, Rolandelli RH (eds) Parenteral Nutrition, 3rd edn. Saunders, Philadelphia
81. Hasse JM (1998) Recovery after organ transplantation in adults: the role of postoperative nutrition therapy. Topics in Clinical Nutrition 13 (2):15–26

Enteral Immunonutrition in the Intensive Care Unit: A Critical Approach

G. Nitenberg, S. Antoun, and B. Raynard

The priority during the initial period of injury, trauma and sepsis in the ICU is hemodynamic and ventilatory management, without forgetting the urgent need to identify and treat the causes (particularly infections) of organ failure. As long as the situation remains unstable there is no point in starting complex nutritional support, which otherwise may even be harmful [1, 2]. However, it is important not to delay the outset of nutritional support for too long; indeed, it must be started before the onset of severe complications likely to lead to irreversible multiple organ failure. Conventional nutritional support, which can only limit the process of stressed starvation, can and should now be replaced by modern metabolic and nutritional support aimed at correcting the immune disorders associated with malnutrition and acute stress [3, 4]. However, it is difficult to demonstrate the effectiveness of nutritional support in terms of mortality and/or morbidity in these patients, in whom the exact cause of death often cannot be identified, and in whom a favorable outcome clearly results from the combined effects of optimal management options.

Over the last few years the impact of "nutritional immuno-pharmacology" has been evaluated not only in terms of biological and immunological parameters, but also in terms of clinically relevant outcomes.

Potential Factors in Nutritional Immuno-Pharmacology

In the discussion that follows, emphasis will be briefly placed on macronutrients such as lipids and amino acids, although there is abundant evidence that micronutrients such as vitamins A, E, and C, iron, zinc and selenium also affect the immune response. A detailed review of the respective value of these new immunonutrients is provided elsewhere in this book.

New Lipids

The dietary fatty acids are rapidly incorporated into cell membranes and profoundly influence cell functions and biological responses. Conventional enteral diets are relatively rich in omega-6 PUFAs (linoleic and arachidonic acids), which are responsible for immunosuppressive properties and for the generation of oxygen free radicals. Conversely, such emulsions are poor in omega-3 PUFAs which give rise to 10- to 100-fold less platelet activation and thrombogenesis compared to omega-6 PUFAs, and are therefore less prone to inducing inflammatory responses to the activation of target cells by cytokines [5, 6].

Whereas animal studies suggest that the nature of the fatty acids used in nutrition affects the post-injury response, in particular to infection, few studies are currently available on critically ill patients. Gottschlich et al. have reported that the use of a diet containing 12% of the total calories as lipids (half fish oil and half safflower oil) in burn patients reduces wound infection and shortens the hospital stay when compared with other standard enteral formulations [7]. However, other changes in nutrient composition (such as supplemental arginine) make it difficult to attribute these benefits to the lipid composition alone. In the same way, during human "sepsis syndromes", enrichment of EN in arginine, nucleic acids and fish oil improved in vitro immunity without modifying the clinical outcome, the cumulative nitrogen balance or delayed cutaneous hypersensitivity [8]. More recently, Kenler et al. compared the effects of two types of enteral nutrition, differing only by their lipid composition, on digestive tolerance and infectious complications after major gastrointestinal surgery for cancer [9]. Fifty patients were randomized to receive either Osmolite HN or an isocaloric, isonitrogenous diet containing a mixture of MCT and fish oil in the form of structured lipids (FOSL-HN). Unfortunately, only 37 patients – those having received a minimum nutritional supply of 40 ml/h – were regarded as assessable. In these 37 patients digestive complications were significantly reduced in the treated group ($P=0.05$), but the total number of postoperative infections was not significantly decreased.

Immunomodulating Amino Acids

Schematically, the objective of nitrogen supply during " modern" artificial nutrition is to allow the liver to increase its synthesis of useful proteins, such as those which take part in immune defenses, and to provide immunomodulating amino acids (AA) in pharmacological amounts [10].

Glutamine

Glutamine in inflammatory conditions, such as injury and sepsis, becomes an essential AA and the preferred fuel for rapidly dividing cells such as lymphocytes, macrophages and enterocytes. In addition, glutamine requirements increase considerably during inflammatory states, and relative glutamine deficiency may thus occur [11, 12]. Non-toxic and efficacious glutamine-enriched enteral preparations are becoming available, but the clinical efficacy of these glutamine-enriched diets is controversial, on the one hand because of the difficulty in identifying the respective effects of the individual immunonutrients (arginine, glutamine, lipids etc), and on the other hand because of the absence of a dose-effect evaluation aimed at determining the optimal proportion of glutamine. Jensen et al. obtained no convincing biological or clinical results in ICU patients, in spite of about a sixfold increase in glutamine content in the test diet (15 g/l) compared with the control isonitrogenous solution (2.6 g glutamine/l) [13]. In contrast, a Dutch group recently published a remarkable randomized study in trauma patients, using the same formula compared with a 1.8 g glutamine/l control diet, with convincing results on infectious complications [14] (see below). Finally, Jones et al. recently reported the results of a randomized study comparing a glutamine-enriched diet (by extemporaneous addition of 10 g glutamine/l) with an isonitrogenous glycine-enriched control diet in 78 ICU patients [15]. Unfortunately, 28 patients were excluded from the analysis because of early death or EN intolerance. Even in the per protocol analysis they were unable to show any difference in mortality or the length of ICU and hospital stay between the two groups. Only the cost analysis, based on questionable assumptions, showed that when patients were given glutamine there was a 30% hospital cost reduction per survivor ($P=0.036$).

Arginine

Arginine is a conditionally essential amino acid in adults and becomes essential in hypermetabolic and septic states [16]. In addition, arginine plays an essential role in the urea cycle and polyamine synthesis, and is the only precursor of nitric oxide (NO), particular at the hepatic and vascular levels [17, 18]. Addition of arginine to EN leads to T-lymphocyte stimulation in critically ill patients, and these effects are likely to translate into better clinical outcome in severely burned patients and cancer patients after GI surgery (see below). The coexistence of other EN modifications (such as fish oil supplementation) rules out any attempt to attribute the benefit to arginine itself. There is an urgent need to better define the value of enteral supplementation in arginine [19], and the optimal enrichment for critically ill patients, as certain animal data suggest that an excessive concentration could be harmful.

Ornithine α-Ketoglutarate

Ornithine α-ketoglutarate (OKG) is a nitrogen compound whose anabolic properties (stimulation of insulin and growth hormone secretion) and anti-catabolic properties (stimulation of glutamine, arginine and proline synthesis) are well adapted to ICU patients [20] (Fig. 1). Moreover, ornithine is a precursor of polyamines, which are essential for cell multiplication in the intestinal mucosa [19]. Favorable results were obtained when OKG was added to EN in traumatized and severely burned patients, in terms of both metabolic parameters and morbidity [21]. In a recent double-blind, randomized, controlled clinical trial in the burns setting, Donati et al. demonstrated a significant improvement in healing with OKG, but no effect either on the rate of infectious complications or on the length of hospital stay [22].

Nucleotides

The absence of nucleotides (purines and pyrimidines) in food leads to a selective loss of T-helper lymphocytes and a suppression of IL-2 production [23]. In clini-

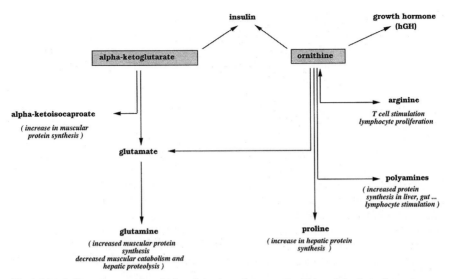

Fig. 1. Metabolic pathways of ornithine alpha-ketoglutarate. Ornithine alpha-ketoglutarate possesses anabolic properties via the stimulation of insulin and GH secretion, and anticatabolic properties via the stimulation of glutamine and arginine synthesis. These effects are theoretically adapted to hypermetabolic states. Ornithine is a precursor of polyamines that are essential for cell growth and protein synthesis

cal nutrition, adequate supplies of RNA or nucleotides seem crucial to restore intestinal function and immune status, as suggested by studies of animal models and critical-care patients.

Antioxidant Role of Certain Vitamins and Trace Elements

Some vitamins, such as vitamin C, E and beta-carotene (precursor of vitamin A) are likely to prevent or correct the cell damage caused by free radicals, which are generated during ischemia/reperfusion syndromes [24]. However, "antioxidant therapeutic" is a double-edged sword, and more information is needed before we can establish recommendations for antioxidant supplementation adapted to specific ICU settings.

EN and Nutritional Pharmacology: Do Complex Dietary Formulations Influence Patient-Related Outcomes?

Based on the assumption that modified EN might reverse the immunosuppression related to malnutrition and/or injury, the innovative concept of immuno/pharmaconutrition was used as the rationale for the development of specific solutions. Enrichment of conventional nutritive mixtures with arginine, glutamine, omega-3 fatty acids, nucleotides, antioxidants, etc., has been proposed over the last decade. Five products were thus manufactured: Modular Tube Feeding (MTF), AlitraQ (Ross Labs), Immun-Aid (McGaw Labs), Impact (Novartis Labs) and more recently Stresson (Nutricia Labs) (Table 1).

It was clearly shown that these enteral diets improve the immune response in animal models of severe burns and septic states, for example [25], but also in the clinical postoperative and ICU settings [8, 26, 27]. But the key question remained: were these immune-enhancing diets likely to improve the clinical outcome of ICU patients in terms of mortality, morbidity (especially infectious), length of stay and costs of hospitalization? Since 1995, the number of clinical trials of increasing quality addressing this question has exploded. Scepticism, governed by rigid application of "evidence-based medicine" was the rule in the middle of the 1990s [28, 29], the dawn of the 3rd millenium is seeing the pendulum swing towards almost boundless optimism [30, 31]. The available data must therefore be examined with a cool head and no prejudice. More than 20 well-designed randomized controlled studies have now been carried out, approximately half of them in various types of ICUs, with a predominance of trauma centers (Table 2). It would be too tiresome to dissect the entire dataset, so we will restrict our analysis to the most outstanding studies, and will try to propose an objective synthesis of the results.

Modular Tube Feeding

This small-scale production was started at the beginning of the 1990s by Alexander's group for the nutrition of severely burned patients. Modular tube feeding (MTF) is an original formula, but has only been validated in clinical practice by the study from Gottschlich et al. (see New Lipids above). The results are balanced, with a significant reduction in skin infections ($P<0.03$) and length of stay ($P<0.002$), and a non-significant reduction in pneumonia and mortality rates [7].

Table 1. Main characteristics of immune-enhancing diets (*MCT* medium-chain triglycerides, *LCT* long-chain triglycerides)

	Impact	Immun-Aid	AlitraQ	Stresson
Protein (cal%)	22	32	21	24
Free glutamine (g/l)	0	12.5	14.2	13
Arginine (g/l)	14.0	15.4	4.5	6.7
Nucleotides (g/l)	1.25+RNA	1.0	0	0
Lipids	Palm, Safflower and Menhaden	Canola, MCT	Safflower, MCT	Vegetable+Fish LCT/MCT=1.5
ω-3-Fatty acids (g/l)	1.68	1.1	–	30 mg
Anyioxidants	–	–	–	Vitamins A, C, E

Unfortunately, the lack of any precise definition of infections, and biased statistical treatment, considerably weaken the significance of this study, whose main merit is to have founded a far-reaching concept.

Immun-Aid

Moore et al. first claimed the clinical advantages of Immun-Aid in early EN [33]. However, their apparently strict study has some important weaknesses: (a) the nitrogen supply of the control EN was significantly lower than that of the treated group, and the control solution was an elemental diet, well known for its poor digestive tolerance and prone to compromising the integrity of the digestive barrier [50]; (b) despite the eligibility of severely stressed patients (Injury Severity Score, or ISS, of 20 on average), the total mortality rate remained very low in the two groups, preventing any conclusions from being drawn on the clinical value of the product for ICU patients; (c) no main or secondary endpoints were defined prospectively in the study protocol; (d) the positive effects of Immun-Aid on immune parameters were very limited, with a significant increase in the total, T and CD4+lymphocyte counts; (e) no difference was found in the duration of mechanical ventilation (MV) and the hospital or ICU length of stay. In fact, the only tangible result of this study is a significant reduction in the incidence of intra-abdominal abscesses and MOF in patients receiving Immun-Aid.

More convincing is the study by Kudsk et al. which compared the effects of ImmunAid and Promote (an isocaloric and isonitrogenous diet) in 33 multiple trauma patients with an ISS of 25 [37]. Patients receiving Immun-Aid had fewer septic complications (31% vs 65%; $P=0.06$), fewer intra-abdominal abscesses (6% vs 35%; $P=0.05$), reduced antibiotic consumption ($P=0.02$) and a shorter hospital stay (18.3 vs 32.6 days; $P=0.03$) (Fig. 2). Nevertheless, the incidence of abscesses in the control group, particularly in the subgroup of patients with colon injury, was surprisingly high, and this excellent study is weakened by the comparison with a historical control group having received no nutrition or TPN. As presented, the study suggests that early conventional EN has no advantages over NPT – contradicting the same group's conclusions in the same type of patients 4 years previously! [51]. It remains that this is one of the most convincing studies in favor of an immune-enhancing diet in a small subset of multiple trauma patients, who represent only approximately one-tenth of trauma center patients.

Impact

The immunostimulating effect of Impact has been evaluated in various post-insult settings, usually *after* scheduled GI surgery. Some sound studies used immunological parameters as the main endpoints [52, 53], while in others they were only secondary criteria (see below). These studies evaluated variations in a broad range of immunological parameters and/or circulating immunoglobulins.

Table 2. Prospective, randomized, clinical trials of immunonutrition in the ICU and in cancer surgery (*GI* gastrointestinal, *Std* standard enteral formula, *FOSL* fish oil structured lipid, *HN* high nitrogen, *IED* immune-enhancing diet, *LOS* length of stay, *ICU* intensive care unit)

Reference	Year	Patients	n	Diet(s)	Isocaloric Isonitrogenous	Results	Efficacy	Comments
Gottschlich [14]	1990	Burns	50	MTF vs Osmolite	– Yes	↓ Infections (P<0.07) ↓ LOS (P<0.05) in the MTF group	±	Non-commercialized diet Poor definitions of infections and LOS
Daly [42]	1992	GI surgery	77	Impact vs Osmolite HN	Yes No (ED>Std)	↓ Infections (P<0.05) ↓ LOS (P<0.05) in the Impact group	±a	*A posteriori* definition of infections and endpoints
Moore [43]	1994	Multiple trauma	98	Immun-aid vs Vivonex TEN	Yes no (ED>Std)	↓ IA abcesses (P=0.02) ↓ MOF (P=0.02) in the Immun-aid group	Yes	Elemental control diet, potentially deleterious for the digestive tract
Bower [44]	1995	ICU	326	Imapct vs Osmolite	No (IED>Std) no (IED>Std)	↑ Mortality with Impact ↓ Infections (NS) ↓ LOS (P<0.05) in the "septic" subgroup	No	Complex and questionnable *post-hoc* stratification. Marginal and partial benefit for septic patients
Daly [45]	1995	GI surgery	60	Impact vs Traumacal	Yes –	↓ Infections (NS) ↓ Wound abcesses (P<0.005) ↓ LOS (P=0.02) in the Impact group	±	high incidence of complications in the control group

	Year	Population	n	Comparison			Results		Comments
Kenler [16]	1996	GI surgery	50	FOSL-HN vs Osmolite HN	Yes	–	↓ Infections (NS) ↑ Digestive tolérance ($P=0.05$) in the FOSL-HN group	No	37/50 assesseble patients *post-hoc* stratification
Schilling [46]	1996	GI surgery	41	Impact (A) vs Std (B) and low-lipid diet (C)	No	No	↓ Infect. Compl. group A (A versus C, $P=0.15$) No difference in ICU and hospital LOS	No	Debatable statistical analysis Major differences in nutrient intakes
Kudsk [47]	1996	Multiple trauma	35	Immun-aid vs Promote	Yes	–	↓ Infections ($P=0.02$) ↓ Hospital LOS ($P=0.03$) ↓ Global cost ($P=0.10$) in Immun-aid group	Yes	Small number of patients High incidence of intra-abdominal abscesses in the control group
Mendez [48]	1996 LOS	Multiple trauma	43	Immun-aid vs Osmolite HN	Yes	–	No difference in mortality ↑ Duration MV, Hospital and ICU stay (all NS) in the test group	No	Randomization unfavorable to the test group (excess of ARDS at inclusion)
Senkal [49]	1997	GI surgery	154	Impact vs Std	–	Yes	↓ Late ($P<0.05$) and total (NS) complications in the Impact group Similar costs and LOS	±	Large and homogeneous population Weak statistical benefit

Table 2. *Continued*

	Year	Population	N	Comparison				Outcome	Comments
Heslin [40]	1997	GI surgery	195	Impact vs IV cristalloïds	–	No	No difference in minor and major complications, LOS and mortality	No	61% (Impact) and 22% (T) of energy needs Provocative study and results
Saffle [51]	1997	Burns	50	Impact vs Replete	–	Yes	No difference in mortality, LOS, duration of MV and costs ↑ Infections with Impact (NS)	No	Comparison of two ω-3-enriched IED diets More glutamine supplementation in Replete
Gianotti [52]	1997	GI surgery	260	Impact (A) vs Std vs TPN	–	Yes	% Infections: A<Std<TPN ($P=0.06$) Hospital LOS: A<Std ($P=0.01$) <TPN ($P=0.004$)	Yes	"Death knell" for postoperative TPN? "oriented" statistical analysis
Weinman [53]	1998	Multiple trauma	32	Impact vs Std	–	Yes	↓ MOF with Impact ($P<0.05$) Similar LOS, infections and mortality	±	Small number of patients, 29/32 "assessable" pts. Limited overall benefit
Braga [54]	1998	GI surgery	166	Impact vs Std vs TPN	–	Yes	↓ Infections, sepsis score and LOS (NS) in the Impact group	±	Post-hoc stratification Conflicting and inconclusive results
Atkinson [55]	1998	ICU	398/101[b]	Impact vs Std	–	Yes	Identical mortality (48% vs 44%) in ITT ↓ Duration MV, LOS, SIRS (all $P<0.05$)	Yes (?)	"Early nutrition" group defined a priori but unchanged mortality and morbidity

Reference	Year	Patients	N	Comparison			Results		Comments
Houdijk [21]	1998	Multiple trauma	72	AlitraQ vs Std identical arginine contents	–	Yes	↓ Sepsis ($P<0.02$), pneumonias bacteremias ($P<0.005$) with ($P<0.02$) and AlitraQ Similar mortality (?) and LOS in the "early nutrition" group	Yes	Strong and conclusive study Beneficial effect attributable to glutamine?
Galban [56]	1998	ICU, septic patients	176	Impact vs Std	–	Yes	↓ Mortality (19% vs 32%; $P<0.05$) ↓ Infections (7% vs 20%: $P=0.01$) in the Impact group	Yes	No difference in LOS Waiting for full publication
Gadek [57]	1998	ICU patients with or at risk of ARDS	142	ω-3- enriched diet vs Std	–	Yes	↑ PaO2/FiO2 ($P<0.05$) ↓ Duration MV and ICU LOS ($P<0.05$) In the treated group	±	Per protocol analysis (n=98) Role of lipids on lung function (?)
Jones [22]	1999	ICU patients	78	Gln-enriched EN vs Std	Yes	–	No difference in late (6 months) mortality ↓ ICU and hospital LOS (NS) ↓ ICU and hospital costs ($P=0.036$)	No	Per protocol analysis (50 "successful EN" patients) Interesting cost-efficacy evaluation

Table 2. *Continued*

Snyderman [58]	1999	Head and neck surgery	136	Impact vs Replete	– Yes	No differences in wound healing and LOS ↓ Infections in the Impact group (modified ITT-n=129; *P*=0.02) Similar LOS and wound healing problems	No (?)	Incoherent randomization (82 vs 47) 33 protocol violations 10%–50% missing data in the ITT analysis
						in the Impact group		
Braga [59]	1999	GI surgery	206	Impact vs Std	– Yes	↓ Infectious complications (ITT; *P*=0.009) ↓ Postop. LOS (per protocol; *P*=0.01) in the Impact group	Yes	Preop. home oral+postop. enteral nutrition Efficacy of IED regardless of nutritional status

aSee text.
b398 ITT, 101 "early nutrition".

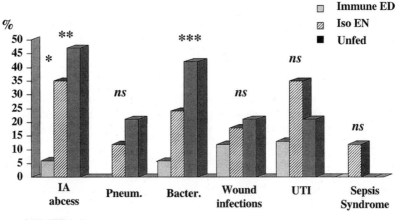

Fig. 2. Comparison of an immune-enhancing diet (Immun-Aid) with a control isoenergetic, isonitrogenous EN in severe trauma patients. Intra-abdominal abscesses and bacteremias were significantly reduced in severely injured patients receiving Immun-Aid. However, the incidence of pneumonias, wound infections and severe sepsis was not different between the two groups. This reduction in septic complications resulted in a reduced hospital stay (18.3 vs 32.6 days; P=0.03) and in decreased antibiotic usage in the IED group (P=0.02). Contemporary patients with similar severity of injury but without enteral access served as the "unfed" group. The unfed group had significantly more colon injuries than the control EN group, with a similar trend when compared with the IED group. *IED* Immune-enhancing diet; *iso* isocaloric, isonitrogenous; *Unfed* contemporary unfed trauma patients; *IA* intrabdominal; *Pneum* pneumonia; *Bacter* bacteremia; *UTI* urinary tract infections

Markers of the inflammatory reaction were sometimes added to these immunological criteria, such as plasma concentrations of TNF-α, IL-1, IL-6, gamma-interferon, and leukotrienes. The results generally favored the use of Impact over the control diets. Unfortunately, there were numerous discrepancies within and among the studies, and the positive effects were observed late, when postoperative complications are infrequent and when the patients often have left the ICU [53]. Nonetheless, there is a strong presumption in favor of Impact in the prevention of late (after the fifth potoperative day) stress-related immunosuppression, especially lymphocyte functions.

With regard to clinical efficacy, about ten randomized, double-blind placebo-controlled studies are available, including those of Daly [32, 35], the contradictory studies by Heslin [40], Senkal [39] and Braga [44] in gastrointestinal surgery for cancer, the studies by Bower [34] and Atkinson [45] in ICUs, and a stimulating abstract from Galban on septic ICU patients [46]. It is essential to discriminate between studies performed in the perioperative period and studies carried out in critically ill (ventilated and/or septic) ICU patients.

In the study by Daly, 85 patients having undergone major surgery for gastrointestinal malignancies received post-operative enteral nutrition with either Impact or Osmolite HN [32]. There was no difference between the two groups with regard to the length of hospital stay in the intention-to-treat analysis. Likewise, there was no significant reduction in individual infections (such as pneumonia) in the Impact group. But when the various infectious complications were combined with anastomotic dehiscence, the difference became statistically significant in favor of Impact. This result was confirmed by another similar study from the same group [35]. It is noteworthy, however, that the Impact group had a significantly higher nitrogen supply, and that these two studies involved only moderately stressed surgical patients: the mortality rate was only 2%, and of course was not different between the two groups.

The three studies by Heslin [40], Senkal [39] and Braga [44] are intriguing. All three evaluated the effects of Impact after major surgery in a large population of GI cancer patients, but the designs differed notably. Schematically, Senkal compared Impact with an isocaloric, isonitrogenous placebo, while Braga added a 3rd group receiving equivalent TPN and Heslin challenged the old dogma of obligatory postoperative nutrition (i.e. in line with recent European and American recommendations) by comparing Impact with simple post-operative hydration. The only convincing conclusion is that the concept of post-operative TPN is on the wane. The authors' conclusions diverged, no doubt because of the methodological biases of each study: (a) in Senkal's study only late infectious complications, after the 5th day, were reduced in the Impact group (5 vs 13; $P<0.05$), and a sound medico-economic evaluation showed a saving of approximately 22 000 euros (or dollars) per 150 patients; (b) Braga et al. found a clear clinical advantage of EN over TPN, and suggested that this advantage could be increased by the use of an "immune diet" such as Impact, especially in severely malnourished patients and patients with multiple blood transfusions ($P<0.05$), but the statistical analysis, particularly the analysis of variance, was questionable; (c) finally, Heslin found no difference between the groups in terms of the (low) mortality rate, infectious morbidity, or the length of hospital stay (on average 11 days), and stepwise logistic regression showed that the only risk factors for complication were previous malnutrition and esophageal surgery (Table 3). However, the effective calorie intake was only 61% and 22% of calculated energy needs, respectively, in the Impact and hydration groups. Overall, EN or, better, immune-enhancing EN, would appear to be effective only for particularly compliant patients, such as GI cancer patients (except patients with esophageal cancers). The possibility remains that a few days of complementary (immune?) PN might be beneficial.

The most recent studies and meta-analyses fail to answer these problems, but an innovative study by Braga et al. clearly suggests that the efficacy of immunonutrition in GI surgery is strongly dependent on the *preoperative* administration of immunonutrients. This recent and elegant study evaluated perioperative immunonutrition in cancer surgery, and could help to clarify the debate [49]. The trial was based on a double postulate: first, that it would be advisable to administer the immune-enhancing diet *before* surgery to efficiently counteract the impairment of host defense mechanisms that occurs very soon after major surgery; this is consistent with the results of Senkal's study (see above) and with a preliminary phase 2 trial by Braga et al. showing that preoperative immunonutrition resulted in upregulation of the immune system, gut microperfusion and

Table 3. Multivariate analysis for the determination of the significant predictive factors of complications in upper gastrointestinal cancer surgery (n=195; ITT intent-to-treat analysis, RR relative risk, CI confidence interval, EN enteral nutrition, NRI nutritional risk index; from [40])

Endpoint	Significant factor	P	RR	95% CI
Any complication	Early immune EN	0.10	2.1	1.1–3.9
	Esophageal surgery	0.008	4.4	1.7–11.5
	Comorbidity	0.002	2.4	1.2–4.5
	Preoperative chemotherapy	0.04	0.2	0.06–1.0
Infections/wounds complications	Early immune EN	0.66	0.8	0.4–1.6
	Esophageal surgery	0.009	3.3.8	1.3–8.2
	High NRI	0.02	–	–

oxygen metabolism [26]. The second postulate was that to ensure the adhesion of patients (and probably surgeons too!) to the protocol, preoperative nutrition should be carried out on an outpatient basis. Indeed, a recent survey in France showed that fewer than 10% of severely malnourished surgical patients effectively received the recommended preoperative nutritional support [54].

Patients were allocated to drink, for 7 consecutive days before surgery, either 1 l/d of Impact (n=102) or 1 l/d of a control isoenergetic, isonitrogenous diet (n=104); early jejunal EN with the same formulas was continued until postoperative day 7. The rate of infectious complications, based on consensual definitions, was far lower in the Impact group than in the control group, both the intention-to-treat analysis (14% vs 30%; P=0.009) and in the eligible population (11% vs 24%; P=0.02). The mean postoperative LOS was also shorter in the supplemented group than in the controls (11.1 days vs 12.9 days; P=0.01), but only in per protocol analysis and, as usual, without predefined criteria for patient discharge (Fig. 3). As expected, the total mortality rate was very low (0.6%). It is noteworthy that the daily mean postoperative energy intake was about 1000 kcal in both groups (no additional TPN was provided): as in Heslin's study, this amount is far lower than patient's needs, but clinical results were totally different, partly because a large subset of patients in Heslin's study had esophageal cancers (none in Braga's study). The need to administer immunonutrition *before* GI surgery to be effective poses economic and organisational problems. Additional post-hoc data showing that postoperative infections are significantly reduced by immunonutrition in both well-nourished and malnourished GI cancer patients argue for the administration of such immune-enhancing diets regardless of patients' nutritional status.

Bower et al. conducted a multicenter randomized, controlled, double-blind study lasting 2 years and involving 326 ICU patients (mostly young and traumatized). The patients received early EN with either Impact or an isocaloric non-isonitrogenous diet [34]. The study design was excellent, with baseline stratification into septic and non-septic patients, but the interpretation of the results is incredibly complex! If one sticks to the intention to treat analysis, *the only objective, paradoxical, result is that mortality was higher in the impact group than in the control group* (23/147 vs 10/132; P=0.05 in the χ^2 test)! The remainder of the

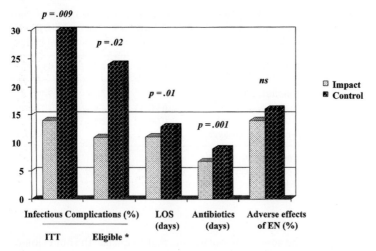

Fig. 3. Perioperative immunonutrition and reduction in postoperative infections after gastrointestinal cancer surgery. Early and late infectious complications were significantly reduced in the supplemented group, both in the ITT analysis (n=206) and in the eligible population (n=171), regardless of nutritional status. The length postoperative stay, antibiotic therapy, and the adverse effects of EN were only analyzed in the eligible population. Only one patient died in the control group. *Eligible population discarded patients with palliative surgery, anastomotic leakage (?), or who did not complete the preoperative feeding. *ITT* Intent-to-treat analysis; *LOS* length of posoperative stay; *Antibiotics* duration of curative antibiotic treatment; *EN* enteral nutrition

article is an avalanche of statistics which ends up producing "significant" results. The most astonishing feature is the distribution of the patients into four subgroups defined retrospectively according to the food really received: this approach is erroneous, as it is based on the assumption that treatment has no influence on the result. In addition, the statistical power of the trial was incompatible with such subdivision of the population. To summarize, the incidence of infections was not different between the two groups, and the shorter median length of stay in the Impact subgroup of 89 patients with sepsis (18 days vs 28 days; $P<0.05$) was no doubt explained the excess deaths!! To mediate [29, 55]

Atkinson et al. recently studied a homogeneous population in *one* medical ICU in Great Britain. Their prospective randomized, controlled study against an isocaloric, isonitrogenous enteral diet evaluated the clinical effects of Impact in 398 mechanically ventilated ICU patients [45]. A subgroup of 101 patients (50/51) having received more than 2.5 l EN in the first 72 h was identified prospectively as being on "effective early nutrition" and was evaluated separately, but the intention to treat (ITT) analysis was also performed. It is without contest the best study of this type currently available, in so far as the severity scores at admission were similar in the two arms of the subgroup thus defined. The results are interesting, but not miraculous: in the ITT analysis there was no difference between the two groups in terms of mortality (Impact 48% vs control 44%), infectious morbidity, or the ICU/hospital length of stay, either in the whole population or in any subgroup (Fig. 4). However, in the "early effective nutrition"subgroup, Impact yielded a significant reduction in the duration of mechanical ventilation (6 vs 10.5 days), the length of ICU stay (7.5 vs 12 days) and the hospital stay (15.5 vs 20 days), as well as the average duration of SIRS (3 vs 6 days) (P<0.05 for all these parameters). This work confirms that immunomodulating diets are clinically effective in ICU patients who can receive early and complete EN. However, the economic and medical questions raised by such an approach are unclear, namely, how to identify this subpopulation? Are septic patients the best candidates [34, 46]? and is it worthwhile offering this type of nutrition to all ICU patients, and then to select probable responders according to EN tolerance? The results of a strict ongoing medico-economic evaluation are eagerly awaited.

AlitraQ

No reliable clinical studies of this immunomodulating diet had been published until the work of Houdijk et al. [14]. AlitraQ is based on strong enrichment in glutamine (30.5 g per 100 g of protein) and a large percentage of arginine (8.5g%), but with no nucleotide or omega-3 lipid supply. This diet was compared with a control isocaloric, isonitrogenous enteral diet differing from AlitraQ by its glutamine content (3.5 g%) in a population of 72 polytraumatized patients defined by an ISS>20. The study design is very rigorous, with both ITT and per protocol

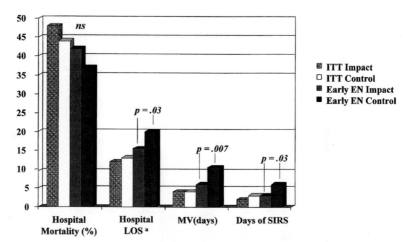

Fig. 4. Comparative effects of Impact and an isocaloric, isonitrogenous standard diet on survival in a homogeneous population of 398 ICU patients. The subgroup of 101 patients (50/51) who actually received more than 2.5 liters of EN within 72 h of ICU admission was prospectively identified as "*successful early EN*". The APACHE II score at admission was similar in these two subgroups. In the ITT analysis, hospital mortality did not differ between the two groups or between the two subgroups. MV requirements, the length of hospital stay, and the duration of the inflammatory response were significantly reduced in the supplemented early EN subgroup. *ITT* Intent-to-treat analysis; *EN* enteral nutrition; *LOS* length of stay; *SIRS* systemic inflammatory response syndrome

analyses, a precise definition of infectious complications (main endpoint) evaluated on the 15th day, and calculation of the statistical power of the study based on previous local data. The patients receiving AlitraQ had a significant reduction in the incidence of pneumonia (17% vs 43%; $P<0.02$) and bacteremia (9% vs 38%; $P<0.005$) (Fig. 5). However, the duration of mechanical ventilation and the length of hospital stay were not different, and the mortality rates (probably low) were not reported. Interestingly, the AlitraQ group had a considerable reduction in TNF p55 and p75 receptors, and in argininemia. As underlined by the authors, the results are there, but the explanations remain on standby.

Methodological Considerations: Future Directions

Thus, immune-enhancing diets significantly improve the immunosuppression induced by any kind of injury, trauma or sepsis. But are there sufficient clinical arguments to establish that they improve survival, decrease infectious complications and reduce the duration of hospitalization in major surgery and/or in critically ill patients in the ICU? The clinical results are conflicting, but nobody can deny that the majority of recent studies, and especially those with the best methodology, show one or more clinical advantages over conventional EN or PN, at least in selected patient populations. As expected, mortality is modified little if at all.

These findings have been analyzed in several articles on the effects of supplemented enteral nutrition in critically ill patients [30, 31, 56–59], yielding a much more precise estimate of therapeutic efficacy than provided by the individual studies. However, it should be stressed that the clinical trials selected for these

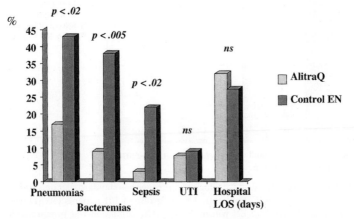

Fig. 5. Randomized trial of glutamine-supplemented EN (AlitraQ) compared with an isocaloric, isonitrogenous diet in severe trauma patients with ISS>20. Both the ITT and per protocol analyses showed that patients receiving AlitraQ had a significant reduction in the incidence of early and late infections (until day 15). However, the length of hospital stay and the duration of MV were not different between the two groups. The mortality rate (probably low) was not indicated in the study report. *UTI* Urinary tract infections; *LOS* length of stay; *EN* enteral nutrition

analyses, although similar, often differ significantly in terms of the patients' nutritional status, risk of complications, therapeutic regimens and general characteristics. Thus, they cannot reliably be aggregated and subjected to identical criteria [60].

Outstanding issues are related to research in critical care and to nutrition-centered methodological problems. They can be summarized thus:

- The era of nutritional support in the ICU is probably finished, mainly because TPN is ineffective in this setting, and potentially harmful [2]. The era of pharmacological (enteral) nutrition began 10 years ago. This switch from support to treatment first requires proof of clinical efficacy to be obtained using the same trial methodologies as for new drugs (e.g. antibiotics), although the use of physiologic parameters may be appropriate in the assessment of severity of illness and as surrogate markers of outcome.

- The debate continues as to the choice between randomized control trials (RCTs) and non-experimental outcomes research, including meta-analyses, case-control studies and quality improvement programs. It is essential to understand that the methods are complementary, because RCTs are not always applicable or generalizable, and they are also expensive and can take years to complete.

- Outcomes research is being used to guide clinical practice, but key variables such as the type of disease, the patient population, therapy, and matched control groups are difficult to handle [61].

- Because nutritional support in critical care is a component of the multidisciplinary management of complications of medical or surgical interventions, it is difficult to delineate between nutritional outcomes and the outcomes and process of care for the primary disease.

- The correct mortality and length-of-stay endpoints depend on a variety of factors related to the severity of illness, primary disease, reason for admission to the ICU (some patients who receive care in the ICU are not critically ill), the nature of nutritional treatment, as well as institutional, geographic and physician characteristics. Short-term mortality is very low in cancer surgery and is unlikely to be affected by the type of nutritional support. In contrast, it has been suggested that survival analysis techniques should be used to avoid the influence of practice patterns on the interpretation of mortality [61], and to censor the effects of death on the length of ICU or hospital stay [56]. However, event times are rarely provided for each patient in the different studies. To avoid the problem of competing mortality, another solution might be to calculate life-support-free days (e.g. the number of days without mechanical ventilation), a measure that combines mortality and morbidity.

- Despite the increasing importance given to evidence-based medicine, the conclusions of recent analyses and meta-analyses are quite contradictory, and seem to be influenced by authors' subjectiveness, particularly regarding the criteria used to select the studies analyzed. Thus, D. Heyland concludes "There is insufficient evidence to support the routine use of immune-enhanced feeding in critically ill patients" Grade A recommendation [58], while G. Zaloga claims that " using an evidence-based approach, the use of immune-enhancing enteral nutrition in critically ill patients represents a level I recommendation

[31]. Never forget that truth has variable geometry in medicine, that recommendations are not rules, and that each medical decision relies on outcomes trials but should be highly individualized. Statistics are for doctors what street lamps are for drunks: they serve more as a crutch than as a source of illumination.

- Some discrepancies among efficacy analyses of immune nutrition can be explained by the different methodological approaches of the individual studies:
  - Intention-to-treat (ITT) analyses include all randomized patients; they are less sensitive but gives the most robust estimate of the treatment effect.
  - Efficacy analyses include only patients who met the eligibility criteria and actually receive the treatment as allocated. They are more sensitive but less valid than ITT. These analyses make scientific sense, because only patients who receive enough nutrition are likely to benefit from immunonutrients. This type of analysis is very similar to the modified ITT analysis recently introduced by the FDA for the interpretation of studies on new antibiotics. However, subgroup analyses should be planned for before starting a study.
  - Compliance analysis includes only patients who receive a critical volume of study feeds. It is highly biased, and more likely to misinform the reader. These analyses must be rejected.
- In addition, sensitivity analyses of individual studies are most often found wanting. For meta-analyses, it is important to calculate how many negative studies (so difficult to publish!) are necessary to invalidate a positive observed effect. The ideal is to perform meta-analyses based on individual data, but this method is cumbersome and time-consuming.
- When all these restrictions are taken into account, it is probable that supplemented enteral nutrition for critically ill patients significantly reduces the incidence of major infectious complications and the length of hospital stay [31, 56]. However, there are important limitations.
  - In several studies immune diets were compared with control diets containing significantly less nitrogen. Although recent studies and current knowledge suggest that small differences in nitrogen intake may not be important, this weakens the practical implications of the results.
  - This reduction has only been clearly demonstrated in trauma patients, and in patients with gastrointestinal cancer in the postoperative period [56, 57]. We do not agree with the generalization of the conclusions of Heys et al. [56]. One must avoid abusive extrapolations from one population to another. The data obtained in major GI tract surgery do not necessarily apply to low-risk surgical patients, who do not require any special postoperative nutrition, except for previous malnutrition or perioperative complications [62–64].
  - The case is even more complex for ICU patients, who are sometimes intolerant of (early) enteral nutrition despite extensive use of prokinetics [65], as Atkinson et al. nicely showed. Indeed, Heys et al. show a trend towards an increased risk of death in patients receiving supplemented EN compared to standard EN (OR=1.77; 95% CI: 1.00–3.12), although the questionable study by Bower et al. [34] exerts a predominant weight on this result [56]. This raises the unsolved question of the value of mixed (immune?) enteral and

parenteral nutrition during periods of hemodynamic instability in these patients.

- The current view is that immune nutrition is more likely to benefit malnourished patients, especially after cancer surgery. However, information on preoperative nutritional status is often lacking. Furthermore, the recent data from Braga et al. suggest that postoperative infections are significantly reduced by preoperative *and* postoperative immunonutrition in both well-nourished and malnourished GI cancer patients [49].

- The timing of EN administration is another important issue. While current recommendations are to deliver nutrition for 7–10 days before surgery, in all the studies but one [49] performed in cancer surgery, all the patients were given only postoperative EN. This point is crucial and is discussed above: if the goal is to improve the impairment of host defenses that occurs early after major surgery, it would be advisable to administer the immune-enhancing diet *before* surgery [26, 39].

- Another subsidiary problem is that we cannot yet determine which pharmaco/immunonutrient (s) is (are) responsible for the improved clinical outcomes, and even less to choose between the different immune-enhancing diets: all of them seem to be so good! The concept of immune-enhancing diets is very similar to that of new cooking recipies, but we all know that good cooking requires a subtle mix of art, processing and science. To illustrate this debate, only the study by Saffle et al. compared two immune diets (Impact vs Replete), with similar omega-3 PUFA contents and different contents in glutamine and antioxidants (higher in Replete) and arginine (higher in Impact) [41]. This comparative study involving a population of 50 severely burned patients showed no difference between the two products in terms of mortality, infectious morbidity, duration of hospitalization and MV, or cost of hospitalization, but the study lacked a standard-EN arm (Fig. 6). Do these results imply that omega-3 PUFAs are the main immunomodulators, or that the enrichment of Replete in glutamine offsets the enrichment of Impact in arginine? Or, more simply, that a population of only 50 patients is unlikely to answer such questions?

- New ideas are now emerging for the evaluation of immune-enhanced EN in major surgery and critical care patients in the ICU. Clinical nutrition needs to focus on patient-centered outcomes in these settings, such as functional status, quality of life, and satisfaction with medical care. In the present and future context of scarce resources, it is essential to define more precisely the subsets of seriously ill patients who can clearly benefit for this "nutritional treatment", even if the cost of hospital care will doubtless be so high that the cost of immune EN will be negligible by comparison [59]. Cost-benefit analyses comparing total costs for all patients are urgently needed in this context.

We still have a long way to go to establish enteral immunonutrition: current research is directed (at last!) towards the evaluation of the immunomodulating effects of individual pharmaco/immunonutrients, towards the isolation and characterization of their pharmacological effects, and towards the investigation of their molecular mechanisms of action. As in other fields of intensive care medicine, and partly under pressure from pharmaceutical industry, we have probably put the cart before the horse.

Conclusion

As a whole, the results obtained with enteral immunonutrition must now be taken seriously, and we overcome the scepticism which was until recently the rule. However, economic constraints are forcing us to better define the indications of immunonutrition, and in particular the populations of stressed patients likely to benefit, before to propose immunonutrition as a standard of care. Future studies should follow the guidelines recently established for clinical trial analysis. We need well-designed PRCTs with adequate statistical power, selected ICU patient populations, clearly defined immune diets and isonitrogenous, isoenergetic control diets, and adequate outcome measures to define the indications of immunonutrition. But other types of outcome-based nutritional research, such as well-matched case-control studies and cohort studies with multivariate techniques, will be helpful. We also need to refine these new concepts of "specific" nutrition: a formula modification may be of value for polytraumatized patients but not for septic patients, and the different immune diets now available may have different optimal uses. A huge range of clinical studies are underway in the field of pharmaco/immunonutrition. These new weapons, associated with other innovative therapeutics and techniques, such as early enteral nutrition [66], will contribute effectively to the fight against infectious complications in critically ill patients.

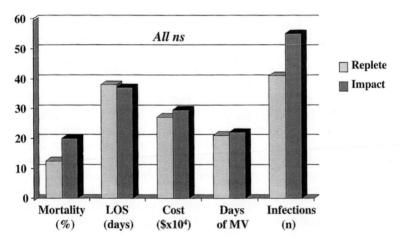

Fig. 6. Randomized trial of two different immune-enhancing diets in burn patients. The two diets had a similar omega-3 fatty acid content, and Replete was richer than Impact in glutamine (5.6 versus 0 g/l). There were no significant differences in mortality, length of stay, hospital charges per day, or duration of mechanical ventilation (*MV*) between the two feeding groups. The rate of infections was higher, but not significantly so, in the Impact group, and the mean cost of the diet was significantly higher in the Impact group. *LOS* Length of hospital stay

References

1. Koretz RL. (1995) Nutritional supplementation in the ICU. How critical is nutrition for the critically ill? Am J Respir Crit Care Med;151 (2 Pt 1):570–3
2. Heyland DK, MacDonald S, Keefe L, Drover JW. (1998) Total Parenteral Nutrition in the Critically Ill Patient. A Meta-analysis. JAMA;280:2013–9
3. Scrimshaw NS, SanGiovanni JP. (1997) Synergism of nutrition, infection, and immunity: an overview. Am J Clin Nutr;66 (2):464S-477 S
4. Alexander JW, Ogle CK, Nelson JL. (1998) Diets and infection: composition and consequences. World J Surg;22 (2):209–12
5. Pomposelli JJ, Flores EA, Blackburn GL, Zeisel SH, Bistrian BR. (1991) Diets enriched with N-3 fatty acids ameliorate lactic acidosis by improving endotoxin-induced tissue hypoperfusion in guinea pigs. Ann Surg;213 (2):166–76
6. Alexander JW. (1998) Immunonutrition: The role of omega-3 fatty acids. Nutrition;14:627–33
7. Gottschlich MM, Jenkins M, Warden GD, et al. (1990) Differential effects of three enteral dietary regimens on selected outcome variables in burn patients. JPEN;14 (3):225–36
8. Cerra FB, Lehmann S, Konstantinides N, et al. (1991) Improvement in immune function in ICU patients by enteral nutrition supplemented with arginine, RNA, and menhaden oil is independent of nitrogen balance. Nutrition;7 (3):193–9
9. Kenler AS, Swails WS, Driscoll DF, et al. (1996) Early enteral feeding in postsurgical cancer patients. Fish oil structured lipid-based polymeric formula versus a standard polymeric formula. Ann Surg;223 (3):316–33
10. Moinard C, Chauveau B, Walrand S, et al. (1999) Phagocyte functions in stressed rats: comparison of modulation by glutamine, arginine and ornithine 2-oxoglutarate. Clin Sci (Colch);97 (1):59–65
11. Hall JC, Heel K, McCauley R. (1996) Glutamine. Br J Surg;83 (3):305–12
12. Wilmore DW, Shabert JK. (1998) Role of glutamine in immunologic responses. Nutrition;14:618–26
13. Jensen GL, Miller RH, Talabiska DG, Fish J, Gianferante L. (1996) A double-blind, prospective, randomized study of glutamine-enriched compared with standard peptide-based feeding in critically ill patients. Am J Clin Nutr;64 (4):615–21
14. Houdijk AP, Rijnsburger ER, Jansen J, et al. (1998) Randomised trial of glutamine-enriched enteral nutrition on infectious morbidity in patients with multiple trauma. Lancet;352 (9130):772–6
15. Jones C, Palmer TE, Griffiths RD. (1999) Randomized clinical outcome study of critically ill patients given glutamine-supplemented enteral nutrition. Nutrition;15 (2):108–15
16. Evoy D, Lieberman M, Fahey III T, Daly J. (1998) Immunonutrition: the role of arginine. Nutrition;14:611–7
17. Geller DA, Freeswick PD, Nguyen D, et al. (1994) Differential induction of nitric oxide synthase in hepatocytes during endotoxemia and the acute-phase response. Arch Surg;129 (2):165–71
18. Rodeberg DA, Chaet MS, Bass RC, Arkovitz MS, Garcia VF. (1995) Nitric oxide: an overview. Am J Surg;170 (3):292–303
19. Cynober L. (1994) Can arginine and ornithine support gut functions? Gut;1 (Suppl.) S42-S45
20. Le Boucher J, Cynober LA. (1998) Ornithine alpha-ketoglutarate: the puzzle. Nutrition;14 (11–12):870–3
21. Coudray-Lucas C, Le Bever H, Cynober L, de Bandt J, Carsin H. (1999) Ornithine alpha-ketoglutarate improves wound healing in severe burn patients. A prospective randomized double blind trial versus isonitrogenous controls. Crit care Med; (accepted for publication)
22. Donati L, Ziegler F, Pongelli G, Signorini M. (1999) Nutritional and clinical efficacy of ornithine alpha-ketoglutarate in severe burn patients. Clin Nutr;18:307–11
23. Van Buren CT, Kulkarni AD, Rudolph FB. (1994) The role of nucleotides in adult nutrition. J Nutr:160S-164 S

24. Grimble RF. (1994) Nutritional antioxidants and the modulation of inflammation: theory and practice. New Horiz;2 (2):175–85

25. Sukumar P, Loo A, Magur E, Nandi J, Oler A, Levine RA. (1997) Dietary supplementation of nucleotides and arginine promotes healing of small bowel ulcers in experimental ulcerative ileitis. Dig Dis Sci;42 (7):1530–6

26. Braga M, Gianotti L, Cestari A, et al. (1996) Gut function and immune and inflammatory responses in patients perioperatively fed with supplemented enteral formulas. Arch Surg;131 (12):1257–64

27. van der Hulst RR, von Meyenfeldt MF, Tiebosch A, Buurman WA, Soeters PB. (1997) Glutamine and intestinal immune cells in humans. JPEN;21 (6):310–5

28. Heyland DK, Cook DJ, Guyatt GH. (1994) Does the formulation of enteral feeding products influence infectious morbidity and mortality rates in the critically ill patients, A critical review of the evidence. Crit Care Med;22:1192–1202

29. Koretz RL. (1995) The impact of immunonutrition. Gastroenterology;109 (5):1713–4

30. Beale R. (2000) Immunonutrition in the critically ill: a systematic review on clinical outcome. Crit Care Med (in press)

31. Zaloga GP. (1998) Immune-enhancing enteral diets: where's the beef? Crit Care Med;26:1143–6

32. Daly JM, Lieberman MD, Goldfine J, et al. (1992) Enteral nutrition with supplemental arginine, RNA, and omega-3 fatty acids in patients after operation: immunologic, metabolic, and clinical outcome. Surgery;112 (1):56–67

33. Moore FA, Moore EE, Kudsk KA, et al. (1994) Clinical benefits of an immune-enhancing diet for early postinjury enteral feeding. J.Trauma;37 (4):607–615

34. Bower RH, Cerra FB, Bershadsky B, et al. (1995) Early enteral administration of a formula (Impact) supplemented with arginine, nucleotides, and fish oil in intensive care unit patients: results of a multicenter, prospective, randomized, clinical trial. Crit Care Med;23 (3):436–49

35. Daly JM, Weintraub FN, Shou J, Rosato EF, Lucia M. (1995) Enteral nutrition during multimodality therapy in upper gastrointestinal cancer patients. Ann Surg;221 (4):327–38

36. Schilling J, Vranjes N, Fierz W, et al. (1996) Clinical outcome and immunology of postoperative arginine, omega-3 fatty acids, and nucleotide-enriched enteral feeding: a randomized prospective comparison with standard enteral and low calorie/low fat i.v. solutions. Nutrition;12 (6):423–9

37. Kudsk KA, Minard G, Croce MA, et al. (1996) A randomized trial of isonitrogenous enteral diets after severe trauma. An immune-enhancing diet reduces septic complications. Ann Surg;224 (4):531–40

38. Mendez C, Jurkovich GJ, Wener MH, Garcia I, Mays M, Maier RV. (1996) Effects of supplemental dietary arginine, canola oil, and trace elements on cellular immune function in critically injured patients. Shock;6 (1):7–12

39. Senkal M, Mumme A, Eickhoff U, et al. (1997) Early postoperative enteral immunonutrition: clinical outcome and cost-comparison analysis in surgical patients. Crit Care Med;25 (9):1489–96

40. Heslin MJ, Latkany L, Leung D, et al. (1997) A prospective, randomized trial of early enteral feeding after resection of upper gastrointestinal malignancy. Ann Surg;226 (4):567–77

41. Saffle JR, Wiebke G, Jennings K, Morris SE, Barton RG. (1997) Randomized trial of immune-enhancing enteral nutrition in burn patients. J Trauma;42 (5):793–800

42. Gianotti L, Braga M, Vignali A, et al. (1997) Effect of route of delivery and formulation of postoperative nutritional support in patients undergoing major operations for malignant neoplasms. Arch Surg;132 (11):1222–9

43. Weimann A, Bastian L, Bischoff WE, et al. (1998) Influence of arginine, omega-3 fatty acids and nucleotide-supplemented enteral support on systemic inflammatory response syndrome and multiple organ failure in patients after severe trauma. Nutrition;14 (2):165–72

44. Braga M, Gianotti L, Vignali A, Cestari A, Bisagni P, Di Carlo V. (1998) Artificial nutrition after major abdominal surgery: impact of route of administration and composition of the diet. Crit Care Med;26 (1):24–30

45. Atkinson S, Sieffert E, Bihari D. (1998) A prospective, randomized, double-blind, controlled clinical trial of enteral immunonutrition in the critically ill. Guy's Hospital Intensive Care Group. Crit Care Med;26 (7):1164–72

46. Galban C, Celaya S, Marco P, et al. (1998) An immune-enhancing enteral dietreduces mortality and episodes of bacteremia in septic ICU patients. JPEN;22:S13 (Abstr.)

47. Gadek J, DeMIchele S, Karlstad M, et al. (1999) Effect of enteral feeding with eicosapentaenoic acid, γ-linolenic acid, and antioxidants in patients with acute respiratory distress syndrome. Crit. Care Med. 27 (8):1409–20

48. Snyderman CH, Kachman K, Molseed L, et al. (1999) Reduced postoperative infections with an immune-enhancing nutritional supplement. Laryngoscope;109 (6):915–21

49. Braga M, Gianotti L, Radaelli G, et al. (1999) Perioperative immunonutrition in patients undergoing cancer surgery: results of a randomized double-blind phase 3 trial. Arch Surg;134 (4):428–33

50. Deitch EA. (1994) Bacterial translocation: the influence of dietary variables. Gut:S23–7

51. Kudsk KA, Croce MA, Fabian TC, et al. (1992) Enteral versus parenteral feeding. Effects on septic morbidity after blunt and penetrating abdominal trauma. Ann Surg;215 (5):503–11

52. Kemen M, Senkal M, Homann H, et al. (1995) Early postoperative enteral nutrition with arginine, omega-3 fatty acids and ribonucleic acid-supplemented diet versus placebo in cancer patients: An immunologic evaluation of Impact. Crit Care Med;23:652–659

53. Senkal M, Kemen M, Homann H, Eickhoff U, Baier J, Zumtobel V. (1995) Modulation of postoperative immune response by enteral nutrition with a diet enriched with arginine, RNA, and omega-3 fatty acids in patients with upper gastrointestinal cancer. Eur J Surg;161:115–122

54. Lanoir D, Chambrier C, Vergnon P, et al. (1998) Perioperative artificial nutrition in elective surgery: an impact study of French guidelines. Clin Nutr;17 (4):153–7

55. Atkinson S, Bihari D. (1996) Immunonutrition: we are what we eat [letter]. Gastroenterology;110 (5):1678

56. Heys SD, Walker LG, Smith I, Eremin O. (1999) Enteral nutritional supplementation with key nutrients in patients with critical illness and cancer: a meta-analysis of randomized controlled clinical trials. Ann Surg;229 (4):467–77

57. McQuiggan M, Marvin R, McKinley B, Moore F. (1999) Enteral feeding following major torso trauma: from theory to practice. New Horiz;7 (1):131–46

58. Heyland DK. (1998) Nutritional support in the critically ill patient. A critical review of the evidence. Crit Care Clinics;14:423–40

59. Barton J. (1997) Immune-enhancing enteral formulas: are they beneficial in critically ill patients? NCP;9 (4):127–139

60. Shaneyfelt TM, Mayo-Smith MF, Rothwangl J. (1999) Are guidelines following guidelines? The methodological quality of clinical practice guidelines in the peer-reviewed medical literature. Jama;281 (20):1900–5

61. Rubenfeld GD, Angus DC, Pinsky MR, Curtis JR, Connors AF, Bernard GR. (1999) Outcomes research in critical care. Results of the american thoracic society critical care assembly workshop on outcomes research. Am J Respir Crit Care Med;160 (1):358–67

62. Klein S, Kinney J, Jeejeebhoy K, et al. (1997) Nutrition support in clinical practice: review of published data and recommendations for future research directions. Summary of a conference sponsored by the National Institutes of Health, American Society for Parenteral and Enteral Nutrition, and American Society for Clinical Nutrition. Am J Clin Nutr;66 (3):683–706

63. Cerra F, Benitez M, Blackburn G, et al. (1997) Applied nutrition in ICU patients. A consensus statement of the American College of Chest Physicians. Chest;111 (3):769–78

64. Anonymous. (1995) Conférence de Consensus. Nutrition artificielle périopératoire en chirurgie programmée de l'adulte. Nutr Clin Métabol;9 (1 (Supplt)):1–148

65. Frost P, Edwatds N, Bihari D. (1997) Gastric emptying in the critically ill-the way forward? Intensive Care Med;23:243–245
66. Lipman TO. (1998) Grains or veins: is enteral nutrition really better than parenteral nutrition? A look at the evidence. JPEN;22 (3):167–82

Effects of Route and Dose of Immunonutrition Compounds

R.D. Griffiths and F. Andrews

Introduction

In the care of the critically ill patient a concept termed "immunonutrition" has developed to imply a nutritional formulation that promotes or beneficially modulates the immune system. A number of nutrients have come to be known as immunonutrients of which glutamine, arginine, ornithine-α-ketoglutarate (OKG) and ω-3 fatty acids have been the most extensively studied, but the list could also include nucleotides, trace minerals such as selenium, or even probiotic bacteria. This short review, predominantly focusing on amino acids, discusses what evidence exists on whether the route of administration of nutrients can effect their clinical action.

The article will attempt to focus on the critically ill patient who is deprived of all the advantages of maintaining an oral diet and is either dependent on enteral nutrition, if the bowel is working, or parenteral nutrition, in those few patients with gastrointestinal dysfunction. The paucity of clinical studies in genuine intensive care patients is a limiting factor to achieving this goal.

Earlier chapters have discussed the advantages or disadvantages of enteral or parenteral nutrition and also whether "immuno-nutrient" enhanced formulations collectively have been shown superior to standard formulations. Although enteral nutrition has deservedly been promoted for biological and economic reasons, and early enteral nutrition encouraged for much the same agenda as immunonutrition, it should not be forgotten that artificial nutrition is associated with significant morbidity in the very sick. Enteral and parenteral feeding are abnormal routes of nutrition, which are associated with immune dysfunction and increased infective morbidity either by nature of the route and device, or the synthetic (and possibly deficient) formulation used. One can only speculate on the morbidity consequences of a nasogastric tube alone in a ventilated ICU patient, but it is clear in colo-rectal post-operative patients its mere presence contributes significantly to atelectasis and postoperative fever [1]. Indeed early oral feeding in such patients without nasogastric tubes more rapidly advances achievement of a normal diet [2]. Perhaps the true control group to compare the efficacy of enteral immunonutrients in post-operative studies is that of patients given food by mouth who have no nasogastric tube. Obviously such an option in practice is rarely open for the intensive care patient.

Is the Enteral Route for
an Immunonutrient Always Sufficient?

In the ICU there are a variety of evolving scenarios in which gastrointestinal dysfunction can occur. Intensive care is about preventing or managing organ systems dysfunction and as far as possible aims to maintain gastrointestinal function. In recent years a culture of early and modest enteral nutrition is the norm for the majority of patients ranging from the mildly stressed post-operative patient through to the patient with severe burns, trauma or sepsis. In reality only about 5%–15% of patients have more complete gastrointestinal dysfunction and the parenteral route then becomes the only option. This shift to enteral delivery in ICU has occurred over the past 10 years such that some contest that it is the *only* route to use for nutrition in nearly all ICU patients. This approach is still held even when enteral delivery is sub-optimal. It is a generally held view that the gut is working normally when nutrient passed down a naso-gastric tube leaves the stomach. The assumption is that nutrient absorption is normal because motility is present. Despite this apparent confidence that the gut will absorb nutrients effectively intensivists nevertheless still administer nearly all their drugs parenterally citing concerns regarding disturbed absorption by the gut or clearance by first pass metabolism. Recent studies have shown that the pattern of gastrointestinal motility is disturbed in the critically ill patient due to a multitude of disease or medication related factors [3]. More importantly despite apparently successful gastric tube feeding there is a failure of conversion of a fasting to a fed pattern of gastrointestinal motility, which is considered necessary for digestion and absorption [4]. Impairment of gastrointestinal function is apparent from scrutiny of audit [5] and research studies that demonstrate either failure or inadequate delivery of nutrients with naso-gastric tube feeding. In two large studies the effect of the immunonutrient was shown in only a small proportion of patients who received an "adequate" intake, 30% [6] and 25% [7]. An alternative interpretation was that 70% and 75% of the patients were inadequately fed. This review does not intend to debate the advantages and disadvantages of NG/NJ feeding but to remind readers that IF the biological action is expected to occur sufficient dose of nutrient must be given, and if required systemically it must be absorbed and clear first pass metabolism. This is a problem if the enteral feeding policy is one of hypocaloric small volume feeds with a small dose of the immunonutrient.

It is perhaps no surprise that the majority of studies that have demonstrated clinical advantages with early enteral feeding and/or immunonutrition therapy have used jejunal feeding with tubes usually surgical placed. This is understandable considering the surgical nature of the patient population that has been studied. Normally this would ensure greater volume delivery but even some jejunal feeding studies have shown poor compliance and tolerance of feeding with limited delivery of feed. A recent, detailed, well controlled study [8] in post-operative patients fed jejunally suggests no difference in outcome between the immunonutrition fed subjects and those given IV dextrose and saline. However close inspection shows that only 35% of total goal calorie intake came from the enteral immunonutrient feed in the first 5 days, adding only about 650 kcal, 6 g N per day to that received by the control group? In a lower risk, non-malnourished population it was perhaps optimistic to expect any benefit could be demonstrated, particularly in a relatively short time frame and when many patients were soon taking oral diet.

Immunonutrients: How Much?

For glutamine, arginine and OKG there is obvious metabolic interchange (see Fig. 1) at the biochemical level. Not surprisingly in cell culture and some animal studies where the substrate supply to the cell can be assured, equivalence and lack of additive effects are seen for glutamine and arginine [9, 10]. Interestingly in the later study an upper dose limit appeared for arginine above which the effect appeared counterproductive. At the macro-cellular or organ level different immune effects are implicated for the various nutrients and the physiology of interorgan metabolism is quite different. While the other amino acids are intracellular players, glutamine is the major inter-cellular transporter and true tissue precursor for many intermediate metabolites (such as glutamate, aspartate, and glutathione) by nature of its relative abundance and effective cell transport mechanisms.

The amount of immunonutrient required will depend where the site of action is expected. Most clinical studies of enteral immunonutrients are given to patients who are non-infected following trauma or undergoing elective surgery to prevent infective complications developing. Here the presumed target is the gastrointestinal tract, liver, and the gut associated lymphoid tissue, and from this an effect on general mucosal immunity. These effects are in addition to the benefits of enteral feed alone. A direct comparison between an enteral immunonutrient, a normal enteral feed and a standard parenteral feed given to patients undergoing major upper GI surgery has recently been made [11]. All patients started TPN but two

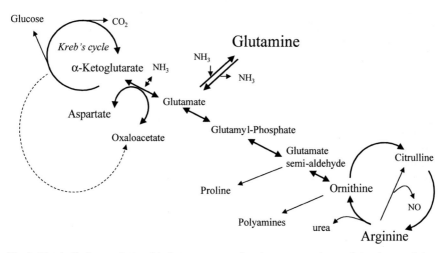

Fig. 1. Metabolic inter-relationship between some key immunonutrients, glutamine, arginine and ornithine α-ketoglutarate

groups were rapidly weaned onto one or other of the two enteral feeds. At all times calorie and nitrogen intakes were matched. The immunonutrient feed contained arginine, nucleotides and ω-3 fatty acids and this group showed a lower severity of post-operative infections, which were more marked in a malnourished sub-group compared with the TPN group. Interestingly there was little difference between the normally enteral fed patients and the TPN fed group.

To interpret any effect of the immunonutrient it is necessary to reflect whether it was not due to a fault of the other artificial feeds that were inadequate to maintain optimal immune function. Current TPN is a synthetic compromise for technical and pharmaceutical reasons resulting in a number of recognised deficiencies that are only now are being addressed [12]. In a series of small-animal studies it has been shown that conventional TPN impairs IgA mediated respiratory mucosal immunity. Immunity is maintained with a normal diet and only partly restored by giving the TPN intragastrically [13]. However the immunity against viruses [14] and pseudomonas [15] can also be restored by the addition of glutamine to the TPN even when given parenterally.

Glutamine

Glutamine has a range of other metabolic functions in addition to its marked stimulatory and modulatory action on the immune system [16]. Through animal and human studies it has been shown that following surgical stress, trauma or severe illness plasma glutamine declines. Therefore it is generally given from the position of a state of deficiency and the supplementation of feeds may merely reflect replacing a nutrient that has become essential during that catabolic state. Recent stable isotope studies in the critically ill confirm a systemic demand for glutamine with large fluxes of glutamine from skeletal muscle [17]. Despite increased glutamine synthesis normal intramuscular glutamine levels could not be maintained. Immune system activation with its requirement for increased glutamine utilisation [18] is one hypothesis to explain the observed fluxes from skeletal muscle [19]. Both animal and ex-vivo studies on lymphocytes demonstrate a striking dose response relationship at physiological plasma glutamine concentrations which is critical for T lymphocyte function [20] and can be related to the clinical immunological response and patient outcome [21].

In human volunteer studies sustained elevations in normal plasma levels of glutamine could be achieved with IV doses between 0.285 g Gln/kg/day and 0.570 g Gln/kg/day which for a 70 kg male would require between 20 and 42 g glutamine per day [22]. Physiological studies of enteral glutamine given at doses ranging from 7 and 21 g glutamine ingested as a bolus elevates plasma levels acutely proportional to the dose. This returns to normal levels after about 2–3 h with the different doses respectively [22, 23]. A non-significant rise in glutamate and ammonia was observed proportional to the glutamine dose. Significant increases occurred in the amino acids that are products of glutamine metabolism, alanine, citrulline and arginine while total branch chain amino acids fell. In normal subjects ingestion of an amino acid mixture containing glutamine (about 2 g/h) still resulted in more than 2/3rds of the ingested glutamine being extracted by the splanchnic region with only modest rises in plasma glutamine [24]. This confirms earlier work showing that only with large doses of glutamine (9 g/h) was the splanchnic extraction exceeded [25].

If enteral delivery is to achieve significant plasma changes it either requires large bolus administration, or a much larger daily dose if infused continuously. A study in 60 severe multiple-trauma patients illustrates the challenge to deliver an adequate dose to prevent infective complications. In a randomised, controlled study [26] nutrition was commenced within 48 h via a naso-duodenal tube for a minimum of 5 days. There was a significantly reduced pneumonia, bacteraemia, and severe sepsis (Fig. 2). The glutamine group of patients had faster rising (although not normal) plasma levels of glutamine, and arginine levels that were near normal by the third day. The precise amount of glutamine actually received by these patients is not given in the paper. Based on a letter published later [27] it can be estimated to have been as much as 25 g (0.35 g/kg/d) to 30 g (0.42 g/kg/d) of glutamine with an average volume of feed received after 3 days of 1800 ml. Dedication to naso-jejunal insertion so early and feed delivery so consistently is a challenge in so very ill multi-trauma ventilated ICU patients. Tube placements in such sick patients usually require endoscopic or radiological screening methods that take time and conflict with other treatment agendas.

Enteral and parenteral delivery of glutamine containing feeds have been compared directly in 20 post-surgical patients. Using continuous infusion, an elemental jejunal feed and a conventional TPN were enriched with 10 g/l glutamine to give a target of 0.3 g gln/kg BW/day. While all 10 TPN patients were successfully fed, 3 of the jejunal fed subjects had to stop because of delivery problems. Both groups showed a significant post-operative fall in plasma glutamine, with a trend towards a faster plasma glutamine recovery in the TPN fed patients. Glutamine intake by day 4 was 16 g (0.23 g/kg/d) enterally and 18.5 g (0.26 g/kg/d) in the par-

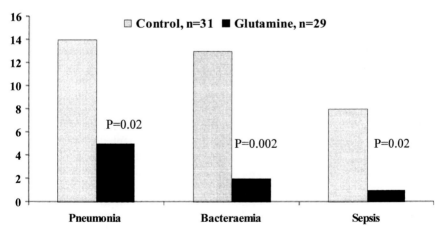

Fig. 2. Early enteral glutamine supplemental feeding in multi-trauma ICU patients within 48 h. Rapid increase in feed volume via naso-jejunal tube such that by 3rd–4th day receiving about 1800 ml feed and between 25–30 g glutamine per day. No overall survival difference but significant reductions in infectious morbidity in first 15 days. (From [26])

enteral group. On day 5 only the enteral fed patients still had significantly lower plasma glutamine levels.

Clinical morbidity or outcome studies in the intensive care patient using enteral glutamine alone are limited. Enteral feeding of low-birth weight neonates (all initially non-infected) given up to 0.31 g/kg/d glutamine improved indices of immune function and reduced morbidity due to sepsis [28]. In a mixed group of adult ICU patients, some already infected, 18 g (0.25 g/kg/d) glutamine within a feed given naso-gastrically over 20 h/day resulted in significantly reduced post-intervention hospital costs, and need for parenteral nutrition supplements. This was associated with a lower incidence of new infections in intensive care [29]. No difference in six-month mortality was observed.

The Parenteral Route for Glutamine

In the stressed or already septic patient immune activation may lead to a greater systemic demand for glutamine. The nutrient flow of glutamine is from muscle where it is synthesised and released to the tissues, and not from the gut to the tissues. It is perhaps heretical to suggest that in this situation IV glutamine might be considered a more physiological supplement as it mimics the systemic rather than portal flux.

Early clinical studies were performed on patients undergoing elective operations with a predictable degree of stress and decline of free glutamine in muscle. The depletion of glutamine could be prevented by parenteral nutrition supplemented with glutamine [30], ornithine-alpha-ketoglutarate [31], alanyl-glutamine [32], or glycyl-glutamine [33]. In the last example stopping the IV giutamine on day three led to a subsequent fall in muscle glutamine by day 10 despite resuming a normal diet. More recent studies have examined whether glutamine could replete the intracellular muscle glutamine pool and stimulate protein synthesis. Elective colon surgery patients were studied 2–3 days post-operatively with an acute infusion of 0.285 g/kg BW (about 20 g) glutamine over 5.5 h. Despite a doubling in plasma glutamine there was no increase in the low intramuscular free glutamine and no stimulation of the depressed protein synthesis rates. The clinical extreme is the critically ill patient with an intramuscular glutamine pool depleted some 70%–80% prior to commencing nutrition [34, 35] and 20 g glutamine per day for 5 days could not return this to normal. It was not possible to show a statistical elevation in plasma glutamine when infused over 24 h, perhaps not unexpected given the increased demands now documented from stable isotope studies [17]. A sustained elevation in plasma glutamine has been shown in multiple trauma patients in ICU only when given as a larger dose equivalent to 28 g (0.4 g/kg/d) of glutamine (as 40 g dipeptide Gly-Gln) [36]. Studies are awaited on the effect on the muscle glutamine pool in the critically ill patients at these higher doses. A dose however infused at three times this rate given over 2 h (7 g) in normal subjects double plasma levels and elevates muscle glutamine. Detailed stable isotope studies in normal subjects have confirmed that while enteral amino acid mixtures with glutamine increase glutamine availability to the muscle and stimulate uptake, they do this without an increase in the intramuscular glutamine because there is a simultaneous increase in glutamine release [24]. Maintaining the muscle glutamine may not be as important as maintaining the supply of glutamine.

The high rate of glutamine utilisation by immune cells results from glutaminolysis in macrophages and lymphocytes to maintain important substrate intermediaries [18]. This is necessary particularly for nucleotide synthesis for protein synthesis and division but also energy supply. Some of the substrates produced are returned to the circulation and can participate in glucose metabolism. This is no surprise as exercise physiology [37] has shown how closely glutamine is involved in glucose and glycogen metabolism [38, 39]. Recently the importance of glutamine to gluconeogenesis by the kidney [40] has added to the view that glutamine may have potential significance as a nutrient adjuvant in clinical situations with insulin resistance.

The first clinical trial of glutamine supplemented parenteral nutrition was in allogenic bone marrow transplant patients using between 35 g and 40 g (0.57 g/kg/d) [41]. Fewer glutamine recipients developed clinical infection and hospital stay was significantly shorter with cost savings. Lower doses of parenteral glutamine have been used in post-operative studies. After colorectal surgery T-cell DNA synthesis was restored with 5 days of 12 g (0.17 g/kg/d) glutamine compared with an isonitrogenous control [42]. The same group has also shown that 15 g (0.21 g/kg/d) glutamine reduces mononuclear cell interleukin-8 release in severe acute pancreatitis [43], both these studies using a dipeptide. In another post-operative study the patients randomised to TPN with 12 g (0.17 g/kg/d) of glutamine (20 g Ala-gln dipeptide) following bowel surgery showed improved nitrogen balances, shorter length of stay. Improved recovery of lymphocyte counts and improved generation of cysteinyl-leukotrienes from polymorphonuclear neutrophil granulocytes were markers of improved immune status [44]. These positive studies contrast with a large study that failed to show benefit from supplementation with 20 g (0.28 g/kg/d) of glutamine parenterally [45]. Unfortunately the design of the study may have reduced the chances to demonstrate any clinical benefit in the heterogeneous patient population that was studied. The referral pattern and patient selection recruited a lower risk group of patients such that the overall mortality was half that of a pre-study prediction. Only in a subgroup of surgical patients was the length of stay significantly reduced, but because this group included most of the deaths the observation may not be relevant. The failure to show a treatment effect may be because the patients who were more deficient of glutamine for a longer time and therefore more likely to benefit have been excluded from study.

The patients most likely to benefit are those in intensive care. Deaths are either due to the magnitude of the presenting problem or arise later as second hit episodes of sepsis, a recognised risk of a sustained ICU stay, and overtake the mortality risk of the initial illness. Correcting any deficiency of glutamine would be seen by the prevention of late deaths, with deaths due to Multiple organ failure (MOF) the most frequent. In a randomised, controlled, double-blind study 84 critically ill adult patients with APACHE II score at least greater than 10, were started on parenteral nutrition if enteral nutrition was contraindicated or unsuccessful, i.e. had gastrointestinal failure [46]. Over three-quarters of the patients had major sepsis with intra-abdominal causes the most common. Despite differences in the initial illness the patient population is more homogeneous by the nature of the multiple organ failure they develop. Although they represent only a very small proportion of ICU admissions their stay is often long and costly. Daily median glutamine intakes were 18 g (0.25 g/kg/d) rising to 21 g (0.3 g/kg/d). Survival measured at 6 months was significantly better with glutamine 57% v control 33%, $P=0.049$.

A "dose" effect was evident in that patients who needed to receive parenteral nutrition for more than 10 days had a significantly greater mortality on the control (and therefore glutamine deficient) formulation compared with those receiving a glutamine containing feed ($P=0.03$; Fig. 3). The difference in mortality, predominantly due to multiple organ failure, increased with time on parenteral feed and was only related to glutamine use and not to the age, the illness severity or total amount of other nutrition received.

The cost of any immunonutrient product alone is a weak argument for the choice of route unless the overall influence on hospital costs can be shown to be different. This is illustrated by the glutamine studies in ICU involving patients either with or without gut failure. Both studies showed reductions in the costs per survivor [29, 46]. In the parenteral study, the effect on survival was such that the increased costs per survivor were brought down to values similar to less sick patients who were fed in the enteral study (Fig. 4).

While 12–15 g/day of glutamine may be adequate for the less stressed patient it is likely that an excess of 20 g/day is the minimum glutamine requirement for the already critically ill patient. It may be that the enteral route alone would be unable to achieve this higher dosing given that the human gut extracts 50%–85% of enteral glutamine and much is converted to citrulline (for arginine synthesis) and alanine. The gut utilises glutamine from the arterial and luminal side equally well for both metabolic conversions and oxidative metabolism [47], yet arterial glutamine uptake continues during fasting suggesting arterial glutamine is more important for synthetic processes. Glucose can partly substitute as a metabolic fuel as can glutamate from luminal absorption suggesting that glutamine for oxidation is dispensable. However disturbance of glutamine utilisation either for metabolic conversion or donation of nitrogen for purines and pyrimidines lead to a graded deterioration in tissue function in the gut [48]. This may be linked to the need for de novo nucleotide synthesis (see below). The distribution of the key enzymes involved in glutamine synthesis (glutamine synthetase) and breakdown (glutaminase) have been mapped along the human gastrointestinal tract [49]. The small bowel and to some extent the large bowel have the greatest ability to utilise glutamine, but have little synthesising capacity. In contrast neither the oesophagus nor stomach have much glutaminase and therefore probably use little glutamine.

The kidney utilises the citrulline produced from glutamine metabolism in the gut, as the sole precursor for the synthesis of arginine [50]. Recent work suggests however that the kidney is not the only site for arginine production as a 75% enterectomy in the rat while reducing renal arginine production does little to effect the whole body arginine production [51]. The enzyme capability for mouse macrophages and human monocytes to utilise glutamine to produce argi-

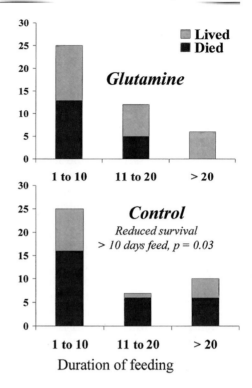

Fig. 3. Survival related to duration of parenteral nutrition support in ICU patients. Reduced survival seen in control (glutamine deficient) group with increasing duration of feeding, which was significant in those on feed for 10 days or more. (From [46])

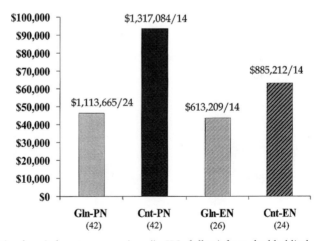

Fig. 4. Total post-intervention hospital costs per survivor (in U.S. dollars) from double-blind, randomized studies for glutamine (*Gln*) parenteral (*PN*) and enteral (*EN*) feeding in adult ICU patients. *Cnt* Control subjects received matched isonitrogenous, isoenergetics feeds. (From [29, 46])

nine has now been demonstrated [52] adding a further component confirming the importance of glutamine to the immune system. While glutamine increases arginine production, it has been shown to paradoxically reduce NO production playing an as yet poorly explored role in endothelial metabolism and vascular control [53].

Arginine

Arginine, a semi-essential amino acid, participates in the urea cycle and in the citric acid cycle, precursor for polyamine synthesis, is a nitrogen source for the nitric oxide synthesis and stimulates the secretion of anabolic hormones (GH, Insulin). Its role in immunonutrition and wound healing are well documented [54, 55]. Intravenous administration has involved doses of 15 g/d while enteral studies using arginine alone have used between 17 and 24 g/d free arginine. A possible concern is that too large a dose could induce lysine deficiency by competing for tubular reabsorption. In most of the large scale clinical studies where arginine has been used it is difficult to interpret individual dose requirements as it has been part of a combined immunonutrient feed. Close examination of the studies shows that the average amount of arginine that actually gets delivered to all the patients (when quoted) is of the order of only 10–14 g/d. In upper GI surgery 5–7 days of naso-jejunal feeding from 12 h after theatre containing 12 g/day arginine (as a combination feed) reduced the incidence of late complications and as a consequence had a significant effect on costs [56] (Fig. 5). Standard parenteral amino acid solutions deliver a similar amount of arginine, 8–11 g/d. In post-operative studies these enteral doses may be sufficient, but doses less than this, such as only 8 g arginine given in the study discussed earlier [8], may be worthless.

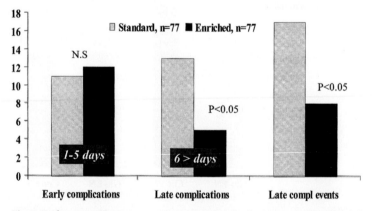

Fig. 5. Early upper GI cancer surgery post-operative immunonutrition (arginine, ω-3 FA, RNA) in 154 patients fed via jejunostomy tube 12 h following operation. Includes about 12 g arginine/day. A significant reduction in the number of late patient complications and late complication events with a 32% overall cost reduction is seen. (From [56])

In the ICU studies also mentioned earlier, where only a small sub-group of full feeders had a clinical outcome benefit, the amount received was between 16–19 g/day of arginine [6, 7]. A study, at present only in abstract form, suggests improved ICU survival and less bacteraemia in the whole group of patients fed the same immunonutrient via the naso-jejunal route [57]. No dose information is yet available, but it is likely to be higher than that received in studies using the naso-gastric route. Arginine can be readily incorporated into enteral feeds, unlike glutamine, which presents more of a challenge. The clinical studies combining arginine have generally been given to subjects before they are septic. Once septic there may be concern that intestinal absorption of arginine could be reduced [58], suggesting higher doses would be needed enterally or supplementation by the parenteral route. Whether the addition of arginine is necessary with a plentiful glutamine supply is unclear.

Ornithine α-Ketoglutarate

α-Ketoglutarate (OKG) is a salt formed from one molecule of α-ketoglutarate and two of ornithine. It is recognised as a nutritional modulator with anticatabolic activity, an immunomodulator and promotor of wound healing [59]. Its mode of action is not fully understood but the secretion of anabolic hormones (insulin and growth hormone) and the synthesis of metabolites such as glutamine, arginine, polyamines and proline may be involved. Supplementation of TPN regimens with OKG improved nitrogen balance and preserved intramuscular glutamine as equally effective as glutamine [31].

It is through enteral nutrition studies in septic, trauma, and burns patients where OKG has shown clinical benefits. The theory of its mode of action has been termed "push-pull", that is stimulation of anabolic hormones and synthesis of key metabolites. Animal studies would suggest this might be best achieved through altering the equilibrium of a number of enzyme systems through bolus loading rather than through continuous infusion. Human stable-isotope studies confirm that continuous enteral delivery of OKG cannot alter glutamine kinetics in burn patients [17]. Two recent studies in burn patients have done most to explore the problem of dose and route of delivery. Burn patients were randomly assigned a single 10 g bolus or a continuous infusion in three doses 10, 20, 30 g/d or a control. Glutamine, arginine and proline were the main metabolites with the bolus dose leading to greater production [60]. In a larger study involving some 54 burn patients the same group examined the effect of three doses 10, 20, 30 g/d by bolus or continuous infusion and compared this to matched nitrogen controls on some clinical outcomes. The bolus doses were given as 10 g either daily, twice or thrice daily as larger single doses produce diarrhoea. OKG administration significantly improved nitrogen balance and reduced 3-methylhistidine excretion that was dose related. OKG lead to a rise in glutamine that was greater with bolus administration. The greatest effects were seen with bolus administration leading to significant better wound healing and a trend to shorter hospital stay. In these very catabolic patients a bolus dose of 30 g/d may be necessary.

Nucleotides

In clinical studies nucleotides have been added to multi-component immunonutrient feeds because unlike normal diet synthetic enteral and parenteral feeds do not contain nucleotides. However most of the evidence that nucleotides have a unique and direct action is drawn from animal and in vitro studies and there is little convincing evidence in the adult that nucleotides are utilised directly from a diet adequate in protein. In principle purines and pyrimidines are synthesised either de novo or salvaged from RNA turnover. Where protein intake is adequate de novo synthesis probably provides the main source of nucleotides for protein synthesis with glutamine as the main nitrogen precursor. De novo synthesis provides most of the nucleotide flux for increased RNA and DNA synthesis in stimulated lymphocytes as suggested by the limited ability of exogenous nucleobases and nucleosides (salvage pathway) to relieve the inhibition of growth induced by limiting glutamine in the medium (de novo pathway) [61]. Although some believe that the intestinal mucosa has specific requirement for dietary nucleosides enteral tracer studies in mice suggest that most mucosal nuclear acid nucleotides come from de novo synthesis [62, 63]. It would seem therefore that dietary uptake of purines and pyrimidines are probably modest and if not absorbed are presented to the colonic microflora. While this may or may not be of benefit we lack any firm clinical evidence to suggest that nucleotides specifically either enterally or parenterally are essential dietary constituents in the critically ill.

Conclusion

It is accepted that maintaining gastrointestinal function and enteral nutrition is necessary to reduce infective morbidity. Evidence suggests these effects may be enhanced by immunonutrient formulations. It however remains unclear how much of this effect is related to improvements in nutrition for the gut and immune system directly or whether it is due to any influence that enteral nutrition or its immunonutrient may play on gastrointestinal micro-organisms. The delivery of immunonutrients via the parenteral route in circumstances where enteral nutrition is not possible has shown benefits. These modified parenteral formulations probably exert their benefits by reversing the immune dysfunction that arises from a non-functional gastrointestinal system. Along with larger doses, the systemic and portal delivery is assured. In situations where enteral administration aims to alter systemic metabolite delivery the studies that show real clinical outcomes would suggest that bolus or large dose delivery is required. Most of the small animal studies providing the scientific basis for these clinical approaches do not use continuous enteral tube feeding and many employ a dose of immunonutrient some 5–10 times greater that given in clinical studies [64].

The use of parenteral nutrition *alone* when the gut is at least partly functional is not recommended based upon current evidence. However ruling out parenteral nutrition to *supplement* enteral nutrition based upon poor or inadequate evidence gathered outside intensive care can be questioned. Preliminary evidence in genuine intensive care patients suggests that parenteral nutrition added to compliment a limited, but on-going enteral nutrition does not carry any increased risks, and may even improve long-term outcome [65]. In the very sick and already severely stressed or septic patient adequate immunonutrition may not be assured if systemic demand exceeds the functional gastrointestinal absorption possible. Continued research is needed to explore the optimal route for immunonutrient delivery in the different circumstance that occur in the critically ill and relate this to inter-organ nutrition in the critically ill.

References

1. Petrelli NJ, Stulc JP, Rodriguez-Bigas M, Blumenson L. (1993) Nasogastric decompression following elective colorectal surgery. Am Surg 59: 632–635
2. Sands DR, Wexner SD. (1999) Nasogastric tubes and dietary advancement after laparoscopic and open colorectal surgery. Nutrition 15: 347–350
3. Dive A. (1999) Enteral Nutrition in the critically ill: Is the gut working properly? Nutrition 15: 404–405
4. Bosscha K, Nieuwenhuijs VB, Vos A, Samson M, Roelofs JMM, Akkermans LMA. (1998) Gastrointestinal motility and gastric tube feeding in mechanically ventilated patients. Crit Care Medicine. 26: 1510–1517
5. Adam S, Batson S. (1997) A study of problems associated with the delivery of enteral feed in critically ill patients in five ICU's in the UK. Intensive Care Medicine. 23:261–266
6. Bower RH, Cerra FB, Bershadsky B, Licari JJ, Hoyt DB, Jensen GL, Van Buren CT, Rothkopf MM, Daly JM, Adelsberg BR. (1995) Early enteral administration of a formula (Impact) supplemented with arginine, nucleotides, and fish oil in intensive care unit patients: results of a multicenter, prospective, randomized, clinical trial. Crit Care Med 23: 436–49
7. Atkinson S, Sieffert E, Bihari D. (1998) A prospective, randomized, double-blind, controlled clinical trial of enteral immunonutrition in the critically ill. Critical Care Medicine. 26: 1164–1172
8. Heslin MJ, Latkany L, Leung D, Brooks AD, Hochwald SN, Pisters PWT, Shike M, Brennan MF. (1997) A prospective, randomized trial of early enteral feeding after resection of upper gastrointestinal malignancy. Annals of Surgery, 226: 567–580
9. Gennari R, Alexander JW. (1997) Arginine, glutamine, and dehydroepiandrosterone reverse the immunosuppressive affect of prednisolone during gut-derived sepsis. Crit Care Med. 25: 1207–1214
10. Alexander JW, Valente JF, Greenberg NA, Custer DA, Ogle CK, Gibson S, Babcock G. (1999) Dietary amino acids as new and novel agents to enhance allograft survival. Nutrition 15: 130–134
11. Braga M, Gianotti L, Vignali A, Cestari A, Bisagni P, Di Carlo V. (1998) Artificial nutrition after major surgery: impact of route of administration and composition of the diet. Crit Care Med. 26:24–30
12. Furst P, Stehle P. (1994) Are Intravenous amino acid solutions unbalanced. New Horizons. 2: 215–223
13. Wu Y, Kudsk KA, DeWitt C, Tolley EA, Li J. (1999) Route and type of nutrition influence IgA-mediating intestinal cytokines. Annals of Surgery 229:662–668
14. Li J, King BK, Janu PG, Renegar KB, Kudsk KA. (1998) Glycyl-L-Glutamine-Enriched total parenteral nutrition maintains small intestine gut-associated lymphoid tissue and upper respiratory tract immunity. JPEN, 22: 31–36
15. DeWitt RC, Wu Y, Renegar KB, Kudsk KA. (1999) Glutamine-enriched total parenteral nutrition preserves respiratory immunity and improves survival to a psuedomonas pneumonia. J Surg Res. 84: 13–18
16. Griffiths RD. (1999) Glutamine: establishing clinical indications. Current Opinion in Clinical Nutrition and Metabolic Care. 2: 177–182

17. Mittendorfer B, Gore DC, Herndon DN, Wolfe RR. (1999) Accelerated glutamine synthesis in critically ill patients cannot maintain normal intracellular free glutamine concentrations. JPEN (in press)
18. Newsholme P, Curi R, Pithon Curi TC, Murphy CJ, Garcia C, Pires de Melo M. (1999) Glutamine metabolism by lymphocytes, macrophages, and neutrophils: Its importance in health and disease. J Nutr Biochem 10: 316–324
19. Newsholme EA, Calder PC. (1997) The proposed role of glutamine in some cells of the immune system and speculative consequences for the whole animal. Nutrition 13:728–730
20. Yaqoob P, Calder PC (1997) Glutamine requirements of proliferating T Lymphocytes. Nutrition 13: 646–651
21. Wilmore DW, Shabert JK. (1998) Role of glutamine in immunologic responses. Nutrition 14: 618–626
22. Ziegler TR, Benfell K, Smith RJ, Young LS, Brown E, Ferrari-Baliviera E, Lowe DK, Wilmore DW. (1990) Safety and metabolic effects of L-Glutamine administration in humans. Journal parenteral and enteral nutrition. 14: 137S-146 S
23. Castell LM, Newsholme EA. (1997) The effects of oral glutamine supplementation on athletes after prolonged, exhaustive exercise. Nutrition. 13: 738–742
24. Mittendorfer B, Volpi E, Wolfe RR. (1999) Whole-Body and skeletal muscle glutamine metabolism in healthy man. Am J Physiol (in press)
25. Hankard RG, Darmaun D, Sager BK, d'Amore D, Reed Parsons W, Haymond M. (1995) Response of glutamine metabolism to exogenous glutamine in humans. Am J Physiol. 269: E663-E670
26. Houdijk APJ, Rijnsburger ER, Jansen J, Wesdorp RIC, Weis JK, McCamish MA, Teerlink T, Meuwissen SG, Haarman HJ, Thijs LG, van Leeuwen PA. (1998) Randomised trial of glutamine-enriched enteral nutrition on infectious morbidity in patients with multiple trauma. Lancet 352: 772–776
27. Houdijk APJ, van Leeuwen PAM, Haarman HJThM. (1998) Glutamine-enriched enteral nutrition in patients with multiple trauma. Lancet, 352:1553 (letter)
28. Neu J, Roig JC, Meetze WH, Veerman M, Carter C, Millsaps M, Bowling D, Dallas MJ, Sleasman J, Knight T, Auestad N. (1997) Enteral glutamine supplementation for the very low birth weight infants decreeases morbidity. J Pediatr 131:691–699
29. Jones C, Palmer TEA, Griffiths RD. (1999) Randomized clinical outcome study of critically ill patients given glutamine-supplemented enteral nutrition. Nutrition 15:108–115
30. Hammarqvist F, Wernerman J, Ali R, von der Decken A, Vinnars E. (1989) Addition of glutamine to total parenteral nutrition after elective abdominal surgery spares free glutamine in muscle, counteracts the fall in muscle protein synthesis, and improves nitrogen balance. Ann Surg. 209: 455–461
31. Wernerman J, Hammarqvist F, Ali MR, Vinnars E. (1989) Glutamine and ornithine-alpha-ketoglutarate but not branched-chain amino acids reduce the loss of muscle glutamine after surgical trauma. Metabolism 38 (8 suppl 1):63–6
32. Stehle P, Zander J, Mertes N, Albers S, Puchstein C, Lawin P, Furst P. (1989) Effect of parenteral glutamine peptide supplements on muscle glutamine loss and nitrogen balance after major surgery. Lancet 1 (8632):231–3
33. Petersson B, Waller S-O Vinnars E, Wernerman J. (1994) Long-term effect of glycyl-glutamine after elective surgery on free amino acids in muscle. J of Parenteral and Enteral Nutrition 18: 320–325
34. Roth E, Funovics J, Muhlbacher F et al. (1982) Metabolic disorders in severe abdominal sepsis: glutamine deficiency in skeletal muscle. Clin Nutr. 1: 25–41
35. Palmer TEA, Griffiths RD, Jones C. (1996) Effect of parenteral l-glutamine on muscle in the very severely ill. Nutrition. 12 (5): 316–320
36. Weingartmann G, Fridrich P, Mauritz W, Götzinger P, Mittlböck M, Germann P, Karner J, Roth E. (1996) Safety and efficacy of increasing dosages of glycyl-glutamine for total parenteral nutrition in polytrauma patients. Wien Klin Wochenschr. 108/21:683–688

37. Wagenmakers AJ. (1998) Muscle amino acid metabolism at rest and during exercise: role in human physiology and metabolism. Exerc. Sport Sci Rev. 26: 287–314

38. Varnier M, Leese GP, Thompson J, Rennie MJ. (1995) Stimulatory effect of glutamine on glycogen accumulation in human skeletal muscle. Am J Physiol. 269 (Endocrinol. metable 32): E309-E315

39. Nurjhan N, Bucci A, Perriello G, Stumvoll M, Daily G, Bier DM, Toft I, Jenssen TG, Gerich JE. (1995) Glutamine: a major gluconeogenic prescursor and vehicle for interorgan carbon transport in man. J Clin Invest 95:272–277

40. Stumvoll M, Meyer C, Perriello G, Kreider M, Welle S, Gerich J. (1998) Human kidney and liver gluconeogenesis: evidence for organ substrate selectivity. Am J Physiol. 274: E817-E826

41. Ziegler TR, Young LS, Benfell K, Scheltinga M, Hortos K, Bye R, Morrow FD, Jacobs DO, Smith RJ, Antin JH, Wilmore DW. (1992) Clinical and metabolic efficacy of glutamine-supplemented parenteral nutrition after bone marrow transplantation. Annals of Internal Medicine 116: 821–828

42. O'Riordain MG, Fearon KCH, Ross JA, Rogers P, Falconer JS, Bartolo DCC, Garden OJ, Carter DC. (1994) Glutamine-supplemented total parenteral nutrition enhances T-lymphocyte response in surgical patients undergoing colorectal resection. Annals of Surgery. 220: 212–221

43. De Beaux AC, O'Riordan MG, Ross JA, Jodozi L, Carter DC, Fearon KCH. (1998) Glutamine-supplemented total parenteral nutrition reduces blood mononuclear cell interleukin-8 release in severe acute pancreatitis. Nutrition, 14:261–265

44. Morlion BJ, Stehle P, Wachter P, Siedhoff HP, Koller M, Konig W, Fürst P, Puchstein C. (1998) Total parenteral nutrition with glutamine dipeptide after major abdominal surgery – a randomized, double-blind, controlled study. Annals of Surgery, 227: 302–308

45. Powell-Tuck J, Jamieson CP, Bettany GEA, Obeid O, Fawcett HV, Archer C, Murphy DL. (1999) A double blind, randomised, controlled trial of glutamine supplementation in parenteral nutrition. Gut, 45:82–88

46. Griffiths RD, Jones C, Palmer TEA. (1997) Six-month outcome of critically ill patients given glutamine supplemented parenteral nutrition. Nutrition 13:295–302

47. Plauth M, Schneider BH, Raible A, Hartmann F. (1999) Effects of vascular or luminal administration and and of simultaneous glucose availability on glutamine utilization by isolated rat small intestine. Int J Colorectal Dis. 14 (2):95–100

48. Plauth M, Riable A, Vieillard-baron D, Bauder-Gross D, Hartmann F. (1999) Is glutamine essential for the maintenance of intestinal function? A study in the isolated perfusd rat small intestine. Int J Colorectal Dis, 14 (2):86–94

49. James LA, Lunn PG, Middleton S, Elia M. (1998) Distribution of glutaminase and glutamine synthetase activities in the human gastrointestinal tract. Clinical Science 94:313–319

50. Houdjik APJ, Van Leeuwen PAM, Teerlink T, Flinkerbusch EL, Boermeester MA, Sauerwein HP, Wesdorp RI. (1994) Glutamine-enriched enteral diet increases renal arginine synthesis. Journal of Parenteral and Enteral Nutrition 18: 422–426

51. Dejong CHC, Welters CFM, Deutz NEP, Heineman E, Soeters PB. (1998) Renal arginine metabolism in fasted rats with subacute short bowel syndrome. Clinical Science 95:409–418

52. Murphy C, Newsholme P. (1998) Importance of glutamine metabolism in murine macrophages and human monocytes to L-arginine biosynthesis and rates of nitrite or urea production. Clinical Science 95:397–407

53. Roth E. (1998) L-arginine-nitric oxide metabolism. Glutamine: a new player in this metabolic game. Editorial. Clinical Nutrition. 17:1–2

54. Evoy D, Lieberman MD, Fahey TJ, Daly JM. (1998) Immunonutrition: the role of arginine. Nutrition 14: 611–617

55. Ziegler TR, Leader LM, Jonas CR, Griffith DP. (1997) Adjunctive therapies in Nutritional Support. Nutrition 13: 64S-72 S

56. Senkal M, Mumme A, Eickhoff U, Geier B, Spath G, Wulfert D, Joosten U, Frei A, Kemen M. (1997) Early postoperative immunonutrition: clinical outcome and cost-comparison analysis in surgical patients. Crit Care Med. 25: 1489–1496

57. Galban C, Montejo JC, Mesejo A, Marco P, Celaya S, Sanchez-Segura JM, Farre M, Bryg DJ. (1998) An immune-enhancing enteral diet reduces mortality and episodes of bacteraemia in septic ICU patients. Intensive Care Medicine. 24: S123 (abstract)

58. Gardiner KR, Gardiner RE, Barbul A. (1995) Reduced intestinal absorption of arginine during sepsis. Crit Care Med. 23 (70): 1227–32

59. Cynober L. (1991) Ornithine α-ketoglutarate in nutritional support. Nutrition 7: 313–322

60. Le Bricon T, Coudray-Lucas C, Lioret N, Lim SK, Plassart F, Schlegel L, De Bandt J-P, Saizy R, Giboudeau J, Cynober Luc. (1997) Ornithine α-ketoglutarate metabolismafter enteral administration in burn patients: bolus compared with continuous infusion. Am J Clin Nutr. 65: 512–518

61. Szondy Z, Newsholme EA. (1990) The effect of various concetrations of nucleobases, nucleosides or gluatmine on the incorporation of [3H]thymidine inot DNA in rat mesenteric-lymph-node lymphocytes stimulated by phytohaemagglutinin. Biochemical Journal. 270:437–440

62. Berthold HK, Crain PF, Gouni I, Reeds PJ, Klein PD. (1995) Dietary pyrimidines but not dietary purines make a significant contribution to nucleic acid synthesis. Proc Natl Acad Sci USA. 92:10123–10127

63. Boza JJ, Jahoor F, Reeds PJ. (1996) Ribonucleic acid nucleotidesin maternal and fetal tissue derive almost exclusively from synthesis de novo in pregnant mice. J Nutr. 126:1749–1758

64. Moinard C, Chauveau B, Walrand S, Felgines C, Chassagne J, Caldefie F, Cynober LA, Vason M-P. (1999) Phagocyte functions in stressed rats: comparison of modulation by glutamine, arginine and ornithine 2-oxoglutarate. Clinical Science 97:59–65

65. Bauer P, Charpentier C, Bouchet C, Raffy F, Gaconnet N, Larcan A. (1998) Short parenteral nutrition coupled with early enteral nutrition in the critically ill. Intensive Care Medicine, 24: S123 (abstract)

Stress-Related Catabolism: Countermeasures

C. Pichard, L. Genton, and P. Jolliet

Introduction

Critically ill patients undergo prolonged severe metabolic stress and immobilization leading to major muscle wasting, as reflected by a negative nitrogen balance [1–3]. In addition to muscle mass catabolism, major muscle dysfunctions such as prolonged relaxation rate, decreased maximal force, and increased fatigability are observed [4]. These alterations are characteristic of protein calorie malnutrition, which is related to immune dysfunction and increased risk of infection, in turn responsible for the initiation of a vicious circle ultimately promoting further catabolism. Protein calorie malnutrition is correlated with increased prevalence of morbidity, prolonged duration of mechanical ventilation, as well as increased length of stay and duration of rehabilitation [5,6]. Optimization of enteral or parenteral nutrition has been shown to improve outcome in these patients [7]. Nevertheless, patients with prolonged metabolic stress and muscle disuse continue to undergo body protein catabolism and muscle wasting [5,8]. This observation has led to research on the combined effects of anabolic agents and nutritional support to reduce the negative effects related to stress and immobilization [2] (Fig. 1).

Strategies to Promote Anabolism

Promoting anabolism or limiting catabolism requires modulation of the metabolic pathways altered by stress in order to modify the protein kinetics occurring in muscle tissues and, to a lesser extent, in the major organs.

Four major classes of anabolic compounds can potentially be used in ICU patients to limit their stress-related catabolism: recombinant human growth hormone (rhGH), insulin-like growth factor-1 (rhIGF-1), testosterone derivatives or insulin, rhGH being the molecule with the strongest anabolic effect. These compounds will be reviewed in detail below.

In addition, other drugs acting along catecholamine-atypical β-2 axis (β$_2$-adrenoceptor agonists) can favorably influence protein metabolism. It was found that clenbuterol and cimaterol induce a protein-sparing effect and improve protein restoration in several animal models of muscle wasting such as malnutrition, muscular dystrophy and endotoxemia [9]. Other molecules such as BRL 47672 or 46104 delay the onset of cachexia in tumour-bearing mice, and torbafylline accel-

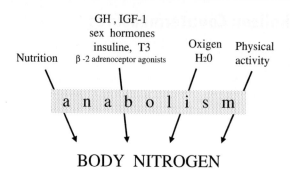

GH , IGF-1
sex hormones
insuline, T3
Nutrition   β -2 adrenoceptor agonists

Oxigen   Physical
H₂0   activity

a n a b o l i s m

BODY NITROGEN

Fig. 1. Factors of protein synthesis and catabolism. Apart from macronutrients (lipids and carbohydrate) that alter protein metabolism, endogenous and exogenous factors contribute to the regulation of body nitrogen homeostasis

erates the recovery of muscle structural and functional properties following immobilization-induced muscle atrophy. Moreover, TNF and other cytokine antisera have recently been presented as new agent s potentially capable of an anticatabolic action. These products may contribute to control stress-related catabolism in the future, but clinical data are yet very insufficient to support any sound clinical use. Research in this area is promising, since the diversity of effects of β-2-adrenoceptor agonists among different tissues provides an interesting potential for the design of more specific and efficacious agonists targeted at muscle tissue.

From a theoretical point of view, mechanical anticatabolic therapies actions should also be discussed. Indeed, when contractile tissue is considered, muscle tone is also a very important factor influencing protein synthesis and degradation. This is clearly demonstrated by simple disuse atrophy observed during prolonged bedrest (a daily loss of about 0.3 kg, representing about 2% of body protein), microgravity or muscle atrophy following nerve section or, at the opposite, muscle hypertrophy secondary to regular physical exercise or electrical stimulation [10]. Unfortunately, practical application of such physical muscle activation are almost impossible in ICU patients.

Growth Hormone

The level of natural pituitary secretion of growth hormone (hGH) depends on sleep pattern, age, stress, exercise and nutritional status. hGH has powerful anabolic effects on most body cells, either through direct action or in response to liver insuline-like growth factor-1 (IGF-I) secretion secondary to plasma hGH. In addition, hGH stimulates lipolysis with increased plasma levels of free fatty acids, inhibits glycolysis while stimulating glycogenesis, reduces nitrogen, phosphorus and potassium urinary losses. hGH (Fig. 2). hGH secretion is massively increased during a few days after any metabolic stress, but to a lesser extent for elderly patients or those with malnutrition.

Recombinant hGH (rhGH) administration in patients with prolonged stress has therefore been tested with the goal of decreasing muscle catabolism by shifting glycolysis and proteolysis to lipolysis, while promoting synthesis of protein.

This concept is further supported by the fact that severely ill patients developed reduced levels of plasma hGH, IGF-I and altered concentrations of IGF-I binding proteins which significantly impair their nitrogen economy. Many clinical trials in ICU patients have shown favorable effects on nitrogen, potassium and phosphorus retention as well as on functions such as healing processes after surgery or burns, and immunity [11–18] (Figs. 3, 4). Some discrepancies between reported results suggest that the substrate-mobilizing effects of rhGH might be dissociated from its positive nitrogen-sparing effect, which in turn raise a clinically relevant question about the potential use of rhGH therapy in critically ill patients: does rhGH improve functional and clinical outcome? Is rhGH a cost-effective therapy?

Does rhGH Improves Functional and Clinical Outcome?

Protein sparing has long been regarded as a surrogate marker for improved outcome, but a critical review of the evidence indicates that this relation is difficult to establish, especially in case of short hospital stay. Thus, more specific endpoints to evaluate outcome are needed to assess the efficacy of a specific rhGH treatment [19]. A major benefit would be to improve respiratory muscle performance and thereby shorten weaning from the ventilator and reduce the risk of ventilator-associated morbidity. Another benefit would be improvement in nonrespiratory muscle function leading to a more rapid recovery of physical mobility, and a shorter rehabilitation period and hospital stay. In ICU patients, an early study in burned children on rhGH treatment demonstrated a reduction of the duration needed between serial skingrafts and of the length of stay in the hospital [16]. In 1995, Knox et al. reported increased survival after major thermal injury in adults on rhGH [20]. More recently, the efficacy of rhGH in patients dependent on mechanical ventilation who were being weaned from the respirator was examined in a prospective unblinded trial [21]. Fifty-three patients suffering from a high incidence of co-morbid conditions and infectious

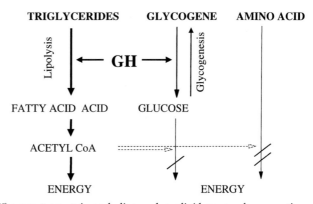

Fig. 2. Growth hormone (*GH*) promotes protein anabolism, reduces lipid reserves by promoting lipolysis, limits the use of glucose and favors nitrogen body economy. (From [25])

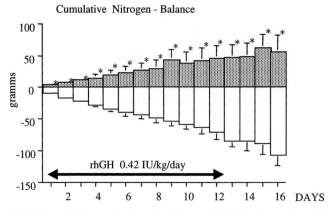

Fig. 3. Cumulative crude nitrogen balances in ICU patients of mechanical ventilation treated with 0.42 IU (0.14 mg) rhGH/kg body weight/day (*filled bar*) or with normal saline (*open bar*) during 12 days. The nitrogen-sparing effect of rhGH is carried over after ending its administration. Values expressed as mean±SEM, *$P<0.02$ (C. Pichard, unpublished data)

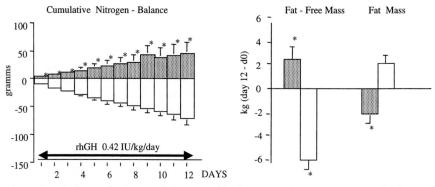

Fig. 4. Cumulative crude nitrogen balances and body composition measurements (bioelectrical impedance analysis) in ICU patients of mechanical ventilation treated with 0.42 IU (.14 mg) rhGH/kg body weight/day (*filled bar*) or with normal saline (*open bar*) during 12 days. Protection of fat-free mass with decreased fat mass is observed in rhGH-treated patients. The opposite situation is observed in control subjects. Values expressed as mean±SEM, *$P<0.02$. (Adapted from [11])

complications received standard ICU support. Those who failed to succeed the standard ventilator weaning protocol were treated with rhGH for about 38 days in an attempt to increase respiratory muscle strength and facilitate weaning from mechanical ventilation. Eighty-one percent of the previously unweanable patients were eventually weaned from mechanical ventilation with an overall survival of 76%. Mortality as predicted by the APACHE II score was significantly less than actual mortality (actual 24% versus predicted 42%, $P\leq0.05$). These results were interpreted as clinical evidence supporting the safety and efficacy of rhGH in promoting respiratory independence in a selected group of surgical ICU patients.

rhGH in Bone Marrow Transplantation

Bone marrow transplantation (BMT) is being utilized with increasing frequency in the treatment of patients with malignancy, genetic diseases and solid organ transplantation [22]. The high dose cytotoxic chemotherapy, often accompanied by total body irradiation, results in severe catabolism, disruption of the gastrointestinal mucosa and marked immunosuppression. The quantity of 0.3 IU or 0.1 mg rhGH every other day for a total of 10 injections was administered to mice after syngeneic BMT [23]. Mice on rhGH exhibited significant increases in total hematopoietic progenitor cell content in both bone marrow and spleen. Analysis of peripheral blood indicated that administration of rhGH resulted in significant increases in the rate of white and red blood cells and platelet recovery. Thus, rhGH administration after syngeneic BMT promoted multilineage hematopoietic reconstitution and may be of clinical use for accelerating hematopoiesis after autologous BMT.

rhGH in Respiratory Insufficiency

Maximal inspiratory pressure has been reported to increase in stable chronic respiratory insufficiency, whereas no increase of maximal inspiratory pressure and exercise capacity was found in patients during a controlled rehabilitation program after prolonged mechanical ventilation [24, 25]. Beneficial effects related to two subsequent 3-week courses of 0.42 IU or 0.14 mg rhGH/d were observed in a severely malnourished woman before lung transplantation [26]. Weight gain of 14.7% and 12.8% fat-free mass, as measured by 50-kHz bioelectrical impedance analysis, during treatment during a 3.5-month period was documented. Nitrogen excretion decreased from 23.7 g/day before treatment to 8.0 g/day during rhGH administration. Improvement of pulmonary function was also noted, and allowed discharge of the patient from the hospital after the second course of rhGH. She underwent successful lung transplantation 2 months later and reached 48.8 kg of body weight 6 months later. On this basis, rhGH treatment is a possible strategy that could be used with malnourished patients who are awaiting lung transplantation, to improve their nutritional status and respiratory muscle function to prevent recurring respiratory infection and postoperative complications favored by malnutrition and possibly to decrease the length of hospital stay.

In a randomized controlled trial in 20 patients requiring prolonged mechanical ventilation on the effects of rhGH on peripheral and respiratory muscle function [11], 0.42 IU or 0.14 mg rhGH/kg body weight/day for 12 days resulted in a positive nitrogen balance and an increase in lean body mass, but no improvement in peripheral muscle function assessed by electrical stimulation, and no reduction in ventilatory support duration was documented. This discrepancy is surprising, because muscle mass and function are interdependant in animal models of malnutrition and refeeding [4]. This difference may be explained, however, by various factors such as the ratio between anabolic and catabolic hormone profiles, i.e. some patients with a very high level of catabolic hormones could present a resistance to rhGH. This resistance to rhGH in stressed patients has been correlated with a decrease in the synthesis of IGF-1 secondary to circulating rhGH, plasma availability of IGF-I binding proteins, or to an abnormal response of peripheral cells to the GH signal [27]. This suggests that only a subgroup of patients may benefit from rhGH administration after early determination of their anabolic/catabolic profile using costly hormonal assays. To bypass this problem, an attempt was made to predict the level of metabolic stress by a clinical score easily and rapidly performed by any trained ICU physician [28]. The score integrates routinely assessed clinical parameters (body temperature; physical agitation; heart rate; arterial blood pressure; presence of an active infection; respiratory rate; exogenous catecholamines administration). These parameters were compared to anabolic (insulin, IGF-1, GH) and catabolic (cortisol, glucagon) hormones and nitrogen balance for each of the patients within 8 h after admission to the ICU. Comparison showed that clinical stress assessment by ICU physicians correlates with metabolic measurements. These findings require further validation, but it seems at least possible to select a subgroup of patients most likely to benefit from rhGH administration.

rhGH and Intestinal Absorption

Efficient nutrient absorption remains a key issue for ICU patients since enteral nutrition is nowadays proposed as the priority route for nutritional support despite the fact that stress and acute disease alter gut fonction. The factors that predict a successful outcome in patients who receive pharmacologic agents to promote bowel absorption after massive intestinal resection have recently been examined by Wilmore et al. [29]. Forty-five adults with an average of jejunal-ileal length of 23 cm and an average duration of home total parenteral nutrition (TPN) of 4.3 years were treated with rhGH, glutamine, and a standardized diet for 4 weeks and observed for an average of 1.8 years. After 4 weeks of therapy, 58% were free of TPN support! At follow-up, the percentage of patients who were not receiving TPN had fallen to 40%. It was concluded that approximately half of a group of patients thought to have an absorptive surface area insufficient to acheive independence from TPN support, could sustain themselves on enteral feeding after an intestinal rehabilitation program. ICU patients with major small bowel alterations (such as in case of extensive surgical resection, radio – or chemo-therapy related damages, etc.) could also benefit form such an approach.

On the other hand, some key issues about stimulating the gut by rhGH remain opened after the study published by Eizaguirre et al. [30]. In an animal model of short-bowel syndrome on TPN, 0.3 IU or 1 mg rhGH/d massively triggered the adaptive process (30% and 35% increase of thickness jejunal wall and cell proliferation index, respectively) in the remaining intestine [30]. However, translocation of gut lumen bacteria to the general circulation, defined as the presence of organisms in systemic blood, was detected in 0% of control animals and 44% of rhGH -treated rats ($P<0.05$). The authors concluded that rhGH improves gut mucosal structure in rats with short-bowel syndrome, but seems to increase mucosal permeability to intestinal bacteria [30]. The signification of this observation in humans remains debatable since the existence of bacterial translocation from the human intestine is still controversial, but this finding certainly deserves further exploration in view of the potential hazard it could represent.

Does rhGH Have Significant Adverse Effects?

Significantly increased mortality associated with rhGH treatment in 532 critically ill patients on mechanical ventilation has just been reported [31]. A total of 247 Finnish patients and 285 patients from other European countries (International study) were included in a prospective, multicenter, double-blind, randomized, placebo-controlled trial. Admission criteria included age over 18 years, elective abdominal or cardiac surgery or acute respiratory failure or polytrauma and anticipated ICU stay for at least 10 days. Patients received a daily dose of either rhGH according to their body weight ($\leq$60 kg: 6 mg or 18 IU; $\geq$60 kg: 8 mg or 24 IU) or placebo until discharge from ICU but for a maximum of 21 days. The mean APACHE score of the patients at admission was about 14±6 and 15±6 (Finnish versus International study, respectively). The range of daily energy intake was about 22±9 kcal/kg body weight in all patients and the daily nitrogen intake about 0.2±0.0 versus 0.1±0.1 g/kg weight day (Finnish vs. international study, respectively). In the Finnish study, the mortality rate was 39 versus 20% (treated versus control groups). The respective rates in the International study were 44 versus 18%. The relative risk of death for patients receiving rhGH was 1.9 (95% confidence interval, 1.3–2.9) in the Finnish study and 2.4 (95% confidence interval, 1.6–3.5) in the International study. This substantial difference remained similar if the patients were stratified according to their diagnosis at inclusion. Deaths occurred in both groups up to the 30th day after ICU admission. Among the survivors, the length of ICU and hospital stay, the duration of mechanical ventilation were prolonged in the rhGH -treated patients. No significant differences were found in terms of handgrip strength, fatigue score or exercise tolerance between groups. The authors provide no explanation for the mechanisms responsible for such a considerable increase in mortality. One may hypothesize that rhGH prevents mobilization of muscle glutamine, which reduces its availability for rapidly dividing immune cells such as leukocytes and enterocytes. This may have reduced both the efficacy of the gut as a barrier against microbial invasion, as suggested in an animal model [30] and the bactericidal capacity of immune cells.

The increase in mortality may also be explained by the theoretical potential of rhGH to stimulate the protein synthesis, including protein-based pro-inflammatory factors. This concept was not verified by Chrysopoulo et al. [32] who examined whether or not rhGH attenuates the elevated tumor necrosis factor alpha (TNF-alpha) levels that correlate with increased multiorgan failure and mortality in burned adults and children. Twenty children with burns ($\geq$40% of the total body surface area) were randomly divided into 2 groups to receive placebo or rhGH (0.6 IU or 0.2 mg/kg/d). No difference between groups were found for plasma TNF-alpha levels at admission and then 21 and 42 days after injury. In addition, 21 and 42 days after rhGH administration, plasma TNF-alpha levels were significantly decreased compared to those observed at baseline ($P \leq 0.05$), while no significant change was observed in the patients receiving placebo. The conclusion is that rhGH significantly lowers plasma TNF-alpha levels after severe burn injury which suggest that rhGH might have a beneficial effect on the acute-phase response.

Takala et al.'s study raises many unanswered questions such as: – What is the basis for administering a constant dose of rhGH not proportional to body weight when most studies on rhGH supplementation used body weight or lean body mass proportional doses?; – What was the impact of low nitrogen intake (mean and range are 9 ± 3 g/day) in a subgroup of patients at a time of strong protein synthesis stimulation?; – Were the patients consistently fed enterally or parenterally, and how soon were they fed after admission?; – What was the effect on immune function and cytokines production of the lipid profile (ratio of Omega 3/6 fatty acids) of the nutritional intakes?; What doses and types of micronutrients potentially capable of modulating the immune response were administered?; – What was the respective contribution of the many pathologies and treatments to the mortality rate and of rhGH therapy considering an enrollment of unstable patients with a spontaneous mortality rate of about 20%?; – Were patients with such a high mortality rate suitable for studying the effects of rhGH? This study clearly shows the risks of large scale multicentric trial initiated at a time when the physiologic mechanisms of action of a molecule remain poorly understood. Other authors report safe outcome related to rhGH utilization in ICU patients. The safety and efficacy of rhGH in the treatment of severely burned children was specifically assessed by Ramirez et al. [33]. During the last decade, this group has used rhGH (0.6 IU or 0.2 mg/kg/day s.q.) to successfully treat 130 children with more than 40% total body surface area burns to enhance wound healing and decrease protein loss. In addition, the records of 263 children who were burned were reviewed. Patients receiving either rhGH at 0.6 IU or 0.2 mg/kg/day subcutaneously as part of a randomized clinical trial ($n=48$) or therapeutically ($n=82$) were compared with randomized placebo- administered controls ($n=54$), contiguous matched controls ($n=48$), and matched patients admitted after August 1997, after which no patients were treated with rhGH ($n=31$). Morbidity and mortality, which might be altered by rhGH therapy, were considered with specific attention to organ function or failure, infection, hemodynamics, and calcium, phosphorous, and albumin balance. A 2% mortality was observed in both rhGH and saline placebo groups in the controlled studies, with no differences in septic complications, organ dysfunction, or heart rate pressure product identified. In addition, no difference in mortality could be shown for those given rhGH therapeutically versus their controls. No patient deaths were attributed to rhGH in autopsies reviewed by observers blinded to treatment. Hyperglycemic episodes and exogenous insulin requirements were higher among rhGH recipients, whereas exogenous albumin requirements and the development of hypocalcemia were reduced. In conclusion, these data strongly suggest that rhGH treatment is safe in severely burned children.

In summary, we firmly believe that rhGH remains an attractive agent to counteract stress-related catabolism in ICU patients. This is substantiated by our clinical experience in over 50 catabolic patients treated with 0.42 IU or 0.14 mg rhGH/kg/body weight during the last 6 years as well as by the report of hundreds of patients treated by rhGH without reported noticeable adverse effects. Based on these facts, we continue to use rhGH in some selected *non-septic* ICU patients to optimize their metabolic response to stress. Cauton is warranted however, and ICU clinicians should pay careful attention to patient selection, and should probably avoid rhGH administration to septic patients until more insight is gained into the possible deleterious effects of this agent in this specific population. Furthermore, optimal nutritional support should be considered a high priority issue if anabolic stimulation is planned.

Insulin-like Growth Factor-1

Recombinant insulin-like growth factor-1 (rhIGF-I) is a short-duration acting compound, mostly secreted in response to circulating level of endogenous hGH, which reduces protein breakdown, increases protein synthesis, and causes abrupt and severe hypoglycemia.

Critical illness and trauma modify this regulation and ICU patients are prone to have low IGF-1 levels in spite of elevated hGH values [34]. In addition, some degree of resistance to rhGH due to high stress has been documented, although administration of rhGH in these patients results in significant rise of IGF-1 plasma levels but to a lesser extend than in healthy subjects, without noticeable positive effect on nitrogen retention [35, 36]. In severely burned patients, the experimental administration of rhIGF-I has a clear anabolic effect without causing hypoglycemia, but this action is progressively blunted and is not sustainable for therapeutic purpose [34]. The effects of rhIGF-I on the catabolic and immune response induced by thermal injury were studied in burned rats fed parenterally [37]. An increase in protein synthesis greater than the increase in breakdown resulted in improved nitrogen retention in the rhIGF-I group. There was no effect on the mRNA in the structural proteins of the skeletal muscle and liver. However, the gene expression of albumin and the structural proteins of the diaphragm increased significantly in the rats receiving rhIGF-I. The proliferation of the gut mucosa and the fractional protein synthesis rate of the small intestine increased, and the endotoxin content of the liver and spleen were smaller in the burned rats that received rhIGF-I. Delayed type hypersensitivity increased significantly ($P<0.01$) in the rhIGF-I group. In conclusion, rhIGF-I improved whole-body protein metabolism, as well as albumin and respiratory muscle protein synthesis in the burned rats. It significantly promoted the proliferation of the intestinal mucosa, and reduced the intestinal translocation of endotoxin. Cellular immunity was also enhanced. After superficial intestinal injury, the mucosal integrity is reestablished by rapid migration of epithelial cells from the adjacent area in a process called restitution. Chen et al.'s study [38] was aimed at assessing the role of IGF-1 in mucosal epithelial restitution using an in vitro epithelial wound model. Wounds were established in confluent monolayers of the intestinal cell line,

IEC-6. Migration was quantitated in the presence or absence of rhIGF-I as the number of cells migrating across the wound edge. Proliferation was assessed by thymidine incorporation. rhIGF-I-enhanced epithelial cell migration, the first step involved in gastrointestinal wound healing, by 2- to 2.5-fold after 12- and 24-h treatment, respectively. Cell proliferation was significantly stimulated by rhIGF-I as well. In addition, expression of transforming growth factor-beta (TGF-beta) mRNA was significantly enhanced in the wounded monolayers treated with rhIGF-I. IGF-1 receptor mRNA was found to be detectable throughout the gastrointestinal mucosa and in the intestinal epithelial cells. In conclusion, these findings suggest that rhIGF-I plays an important role in the reconstitution of intestinal epithelial integrity after mucosal injury.

Studies with rhIGF-I alone or combined with rhGH in animal models and in ICU patients suggest that the anabolic potency of rhIGF-I is smaller than that observed with rhGH, possibly because of a secondary decrease of IGF-1 plasma binding protein-3 (IGFBP-3) associated with high levels of IGFBP-1. These observations suggest the existence of a counter-regulatory mechanism to the anabolic action of rhIGF-1 [39, 40]. Furthermore, adverse effects related to the use of rhIGF-I, such as acute hypoglycemia, edema, low arterial blood pressure and increased intracranial pressure have been described and have weakened interest in the clinical administration of rhIGF-1 [41] at the present time. The binding of IGF-1 with its plasma transporter, IGF-1 binding protein type 3 complex (IGF-1/IGFBP-3) was found to circumvent this problem and was tested in both burned adults and children [42]. Twenty- nine severely burned patients were randomly assigned to receive either IGF-BP3 complex (dosis escalating from 0.5–4.0 mg/kg/d) or saline on the 5th. day after burn to determine net balance of protein across the leg, muscle protein fractional synthetic rates, and glucose metabolism. The infusion of 1.0 mg/kg/day rhIGF-I/IGFBP-3 increased serum IGF-1, which did not further increase with 2.0 and 4.0 mg/kg/day. rhIGF-I/IGFBP-3 complex at 1–4 mg/kg/day improved net protein balance and increased muscle protein fractional synthetic rates. This study highlights the existence of a threshold action for the rhIGF-I/IGFBP-3 complex, as previously documented for rhGH administration, and also shows that this complex does not alter glucose uptake or promote hypoglycemia. Further exploration is now necessary to determine its effect on overall protein balance and clinical outcome.

Insulin

Insulin strongly reduces cellular proteolysis and increases amino-acid intracellular transport and protein synthesis. The resistance of muscle tissue to glucose during critical illness may be seen as a survival strategy to prevent the uptake of glucose in non-vital tissues and to favor its use for repairing damaged tissues. This mechanism becomes un-adapted with the emergence of prolonged catabolic state as seen in ICU setting, since without insulin the gluconeogenic precursors are provided through continued muscle catabolism, which results in patient debilitation. The anabolic effects of extremely high doses of insulin and carbohydrate to ICU patients with various levels of stress have been repeatedly reported

[43, 44] and shown to improve formation of the wound matrix in severely burned patients [45]. Nowadays, it is generally admitted that insulin administration in ICU patients is limited to the control of glycemia. Future research into the clinical use of very high dose of insulin to stimulate anabolism should focus on its effects on patient outcome and on the consequences of hyperglycemia on immune status [46].

Anabolic Steroids

Testosterone and derivatives promote anabolism, and increase lean body mass and muscle force in healthy subjects under physical training [47, 48]. Steroid hormones pass through the cell membrane of the target tissue, bind to the specific receptor and enter the nucleus to attach to the nuclear chromatin and stimulate specific messenger RNA by transcription. Then ribosomal DNA transforms into de novo proteins that represent the hormone's specific action. Anabolic steroids mainly act on muscle, bone and hematopoietic cells. Aging, chronic diseases such as HIV-infection and chronic obstructive pulmonary disease, have been correlated to hypopituitarism and secondary hypogonadism with low circulating levels of testosterone. In elderly men with hypogonadism, bi-weekly administration of testosterone has been shown to normalize its plasma levels and increase both muscle protein synthesis and strength [49]. In 217 COPD patients, Schols et al. demonstrated in a prospective controlled studio that 50 mg/2 weeks (for 8 weeks) of Nandrolone decanoate, a potent testosterone derivative, significantly improved body weight, fat-free mass, albumine, prealbumin and transferin plasma levels, as well as maximal inspiratory mouth pressure [50]. The hypothalamo-pituitary-gonadal axis responds to stress by reducing both the luteinizing hormone and the synthesis of testosterone.

In ICU patients, 50 males and 50 females were included in a prospective controlled study and classified according to their initial stress level (score APACHE) at admission in the ICU (high=group A; very high=group B) [51]. Plasma levels of dehydroepiandrosterone sulfate and testosterone were below normal values of sex- and age- matched healthy subjects. In men only, both hormones plasma concentrations were inversely correlated to the stress levels and significantly different between groups A and B. Mens' survival rate (32 versus 13) was higher (P<0.001) when plasma testosterone was higher (12.3 versus 3.5 nmol/l). No such difference was present in women. In burned patients, not only are testosterone plasma levels low initially, but they remain below normal for several months after discharge [52]. This observation has triggered the use of testosterone and derivatives to ICU patients [53]. However, unlike high levels of insulin and hGH, testosterone does not stimulate amino acid uptake by muscle, but promotes optimal utilization of intracellular amino acids. Since metabolic stress is related to high protein breakdown and readily available intracellular amino acids, the hypothesis that testosterone should promote protein synthesis during critical illness is sound. The use of testosterone and derivatives in severely ill patients is sometimes viewed with skepticism because of their potential adverse effects on liver function, at a time of liver aggression due to concomitant problems such as infection, low blood pressure, etc. Nevertheless, it should be noted that therapeutic correction of normal plasma testosterone was not related to liver abnormalities in hypogonadic men [49]. Preliminary data on testosterone administration in burn patients have shown comparative anabolic efficacy between testosterone and insulin, without adverse effects on liver function [54].

Twenty polytrauma patients on nutritional support were randomized in a placebo controlled double blind study to receive either nandrolone decanoate (50 and 25 mg, on the 3rd and 6th posttrauma days, respectively) or placebo [55]. Treated patients had increased amino acids plasma levels, improved nitrogen balance, and improved urinary output of 3-methyl-histidine (a marker of muscle protein breakdown). Clinical outcome is not reported.

Hansell et al. randomly and blindly assigned 60 patients on intravenous amino acid infusion after elective surgery for colorectal cancer, to receive either stanozolol (once 50 mg, intramuscular) or placebo on the day before surgery [56]. Nitrogen balance measured during the 4 postoperative days was improved in the treated (–7 g) vs. controlled groups (–14 g). Subsequently, no additional protein-sparing effect of stonazolol was found when patients received similar amount of amino acids and proper energy (carbohydrate and fat) load.

Oxandrolone (10 mg orally twice day) or placebo was randomly administered in 13 patients during the first 3 weeks of the recovery phase after burn injury (30%–50% of total body surface area) in association with a high protein and calorie diet. Patients also underwent a physical activity training programme. Both groups of patients had similar food intake but those on oxandrolone gained more body weight (+7 kg vs.+3.8 kg).

In summary, no published study has correlated the administration of testosterone or derivatives with improved muscle function (respiratory or peripheral) or outcome in ICU patients. Therefore their routine use cannot be presently recommended.

Stimulation of Anabolism: When and How?

Anabolic strategy may aim at different objectives: – a preventive action before elective treatment leading to probable prolonged intensive care, – a limitation of catabolism during the acute phases of illness, – an initiation or a stimulation of anabolism during the very early phase of recovery after acute illness.

Barry's study [18] typically illustrates the preventive action mediated by the effects of perioperative rhGH on nutritional markers, skeletal muscle function, and psychological well-being in patients undergoing infrarenal, abdominal aortic aneurysm repair. Thirty-three patients undergoing elective infrarenal abdominal aortic aneurysmrepair were randomized to one of three groups: 12 control patients (placebo for 6 days before and after surgery); 10 patients treated by 0.3 IU or 0.1 mg rhGH/kg/d for 6 days before and after surgery; and 11 patients on placebo for 6 days before and rhGH 0.3 IU or 0.1 mg/kg/d for 6 days after surgery. Patients were assessed on days –7 and –1 before surgery and days 7, 14, and 60 after surgery. rhGH resulted in increased insulin-like growth factor 1 levels, the increase being significantly more marked in the group given rhGH preoperatively. Preoperative and postoperative rhGH administration reduced the postoperative decrease in both serum transferrin and grip strength at day 7 by 30% and 70%, respectively. Postoperative respiratory function and arterial oxygenation also were improved, with significant differences in arterial oxygenation between rhGH-treated and untreated groups. No difference in mood was seen between groups after surgery, nor was there any difference between subjective assessment of fatigue scores between groups. This study suggests that rhGH administered preoperatively has beneficial effects on skeletal muscle and respiratory function and may be more useful than postoperative rhGH administration alone.

The prospective, randomized, controlled study by Burdet et al. addresses the issue of a strategy aimed at accelerating the recovery phase after a prolonged catabolism related to stress due to acute decompensation in 16 COPD patients on mechanical ventilation [24]. The effects of rhGH administration on the nutritional status, resting metabolism, muscle strength, exercise tolerance, dyspnea, and subjective well-being of underweight patients with stable COPD were assessed before and during the rehabilitation programme. Sixteen elderly malnourished COPD patients attending a pulmonary rehabilitation program were randomly treated daily with either 0.15 IU or 0.05 mg/kg rhGH or placebo for 3 weeks in a double-blind fashion. Measurements were made at the beginning (DO) and at the end (D21) of treatment and 2 months later (D81). Body weight was similar in the two groups during the study, but lean body mass was significantly higher in the rhGH group at D21 ($P<0.01$) and D81 ($P<0.05$). The increase in lean body mass was 2.3±1.6 kg in the rhGH group and 1.1±0.9 kg in the control group at D21 and 1.9±1.6 kg in the rhGH group and 0.7±2.1 kg in the control group at D81. At D21, the resting energy expenditure was increased in the rhGH group (107.8% of DO, $P<0.001$ compared with the control group). At D21 and D81, the changes in maximal respiratory pressures, handgrip strength, maximal exercise capacity, and subjective well-being were similar in the two groups. At D21, the 6 min walking distance decreased in the rhGH group (−13±31%) and increased in the control group (+10±14%; $P<0.01$). The authors concluded that the daily administration of 0.15 IU or 0.05 mg/kg rhGH during 3 weeks increases lean body mass but did not improve muscle strength or exercise tolerance in underweight patients with COPD.

Conclusion

Limitation of catabolism during the initial phase of stress resolution and promotion of anabolism as soon as the catabolic phase is over are among the major nutritional therapeutic goals in ICU patients with severe and prolonged illness. Nowadays, insulin and testosterone derivates offer too limited clinical advantages to be recommended for routine use. rhGH treatment potentiates the anticatabolic effect of nutritional support, but a better understanding of potential adverse effects of rhGH treatment is urgently required as well as the demonstration of its impact in shortening ICU stay. Identification of patients who could benefit from rhGH, as well as dose and timing of administration all still require to be clarified. Meanwhile, the use of rhGH should be strictly reserved to clinicians with extensive experience in its utilization. Combination with other therapeutic agents (e.g. rhIGF-I, rhIGF-I-I/BP3 complex, beta 3-receptor agonists) are very attractive but are still under investigation.

References

1. Jolliet P, Pichard C (1997) Growth hormone therapy in intensive care patients: from bio-chemistry to muscle function. Nutrition 13: 815–817
2. Jolliet P, Pichard C, Chevrolet JC (1998) Nutritional support in the ventilator-dependent patient. European Respiratory Monography 8: 84–113
3. Kinney JM, Duke JH, Long CL, Gump FE (1970) Tissue fuel and weight loss after injury. J Clin Pathol 4: 65–72
4. Pichard C, Jeejeebhoy KN (1988) Muscle dysfunction in malnourished patients. Q J Med 260: 1021–1045
5. Cerra FB, Benitez MR, Blackburn GL, et al. (1997) Applied nutrition in ICU patients. A consensus statement of the American College of Chest Physicians. Chest 111: 769–778
6. Giner M, Laviano A, Meguid MM, Gleason JR (1996) In 1995 a correlation between malnutrition and poor outcome in critically ill patients still exists. Nutrition 12: 23–29
7. Jolliet P, Pichard C, Biolo G, et al. (1999) Enteral nutrition in intensive care patients: a practical approach. A position paper. Clin Nutr 18: 47–56
8. Berger MM, Chioléro RL, Pannatier A, Cayeux MC, Tappy L (1997) A 10-year survey of nutritional support in a surgical ICU: 1986–1995. Nutrition 13: 870–877
9. Dulloo AG, Girardier L (1992) Influence of dietary composition on energy expenditure during recovery of body weight in the rat: implications for catch-up growth and obesity relapse. Metabolism 41: 1336–1342
10. Gibson JNA, Smith K, Rennie MJ (1988) Prevention of disuse muscle atrophy by means of electrical stimulation: maintenance of protein synthesis. Lancet i: 767–769
11. Pichard C, Kyle U, Chevrolet JC, et al. (1996) Lack of effects of recombinant growth hormone on muscle function in patients requiring prolonged mechanical ventilation: a prospective randomized controlled study. Crit Care Med 24: 403–413
12. Jiang Z, He G, Zhang S, et al. (1989) Low dose growth hormone and hypocaloric nutrition attenuate the protein-catabolic response after major operation. Ann Surg 210: 513–524
13. Voerman BJ, Strak van Schijndel RJM, Groeneveld ABJ, et al. (1995) Effects of human growth hormone in critically ill nonseptic patients: results from a prospective, randomized, place-bo-controlled trial. Crit Care Med 23: 665–673
14. Roth E, Valentini L, Semsroth M, et al. (1995) Resistance of nitrogen metabolism to growth hormone treatment in the early phase after injury of patients with multiple injuries. J Trauma 38: 136–141
15. Ziegler TR, Young LS, Ferrari-Baliviera E, Demling RH, Wilmore DW (1990) Use of human growth hormone combined with nutritional support in a critical care unit. J Parent Enteral Nutr 14: 574–581
16. Herndon DN, Barrow RE, Kunkel KR (1990) Effects of recombinant human growth hormone on donor-site healing in severely burned children. Ann Surg 212: 424–429
17. Douglas RG, Humberstone DA, Haystead A, Shaw JHF (1990) Metabolic effects of recombinant human growth hormone: isotopic studies in the postabsorptive state and during total parenteral nutrition. Brit J Surg 77: 785–790
18. Barry MC, Mealy K, O'Neil S, et al. (1998) Nutritional, respiratory, and psychological effects of recombinant growth hormone in patients undergoing abdominal aortic aneurysm repair. J Parent Enteral Nutr 23: 128–135
19. Wilmore DW (1999) Postoperative protein sparing. World J Surg 23: 545–552
20. Knox J, Demling R, Wilmore D, Sarraf P, Santos A (1995) Increased survival after major thermal injury: the effect of growth hormone therapy in adults. J Trauma 39: 526–530

21. Knox J, Wilmore D, Demling R, Sarraf P, Santos AA (1996) Use of growth hormone for post-operative respiratory failure. Am J Surg 171: 576–580
22. Wilmore DW (1999) Deterrents to the successful clinical use of growth factors that enhance protein anabolism. Curr Opinion Clin Nutr 2: 15–21
23. Tian ZG, Woody MA, Sun R, et al. (1998) Recombinant human growth hormone promotes hematopoietic reconstitution after syngeneic bone marrow transplantation in mice. Stem Cells 16: 193–9
24. Burdet L, De Muralt B, Schutz Y, Pichard C, Fitting JW (1997) Administration of growth hormone to underweight patients with chronic obstructive pulmonary disease patients: a prospective randomized controlled study. Am J Resp Crit Care Med 156: 1800–1806
25. Pichard C, Jolliet P, Chevrolet JC, Romand JA, Slosman D (1996) Recombinant human growth hormone in chronic and acute respiratory insufficiency. Horm Res 46: 222–229
26. Pichard C, Kyle UG, Jolliet P, et al. (1999) Treatment of cachexia with recombinant growth hormone in a pre-lung transplantation patient: a case report. Crit Care Med 27: 1639–1642
27. Timmins AC, Cotteril AM, Hughes SCC, et al. (1996) Critical illness is associated with low circulating concentrations of insulin-like growth factors-I and -II, alterations in insulin-like growth factor binding proteins, and induction of an insulin-like growth factor binding protein 3 protease. Crit Care Med 24: 1460–1466
28. Eggimann P, Pichard C, Kyle U, et al. (1995) Validation of stress state of ICU patients by clinical assessment. Intens Care Med 21: S62
29. Wilmore DW, Lacey JM, Soultanakis RP, Bosch RL, Byrne TA (1997) Factors predicting a successful outcome after pharmacologic bowel compensation. Ann Surg 226: 288–293
30. Eizaguirre I, Aldazabal P, Barrena MJ, et al. (1997) Effect of growth hormone on bacterial translocation in experimental short-bowel syndrome. Ped Surg Intern 15: 160–163
31. Takala J, Ruokonen E, Webster NR, et al. (1999) Increased mortality associated with growth hormone treatment in critically ill adults. New Engl J Med 341: 785–792
32. Chrysopoulo MT, Jeschke MG, Ramirez RJ, Barrow RE, Herndon DN (1990) Growth hormone attenuates tumor necrosis factor alpha in burned children. Arch Surg 134: 283–286
33. Ramirez RJ, Wolf SE, Barrow RE, Herndon DN (1998) Growth hormone treatment in pediatric burns: a safe therapeutic approach. Ann Surg 4: 439–448
34. Gibson FAM, Hinds CJ (1997) Growth hormone and insulin-like growth factors in critical illness. Intens Care Med 23: 369–378
35. Dahn MS, Lange MP, Jacobs LA (1998) Systemic and splanchnic metabolic response to exogenous human growth hormone. Surgery 123: 528–538
36. Gianotti L, Broglio F, Aimaretti G, et al. (1998) Low IGF-1 levels are often uncoupled with elevated GH levels in catabolic conditions. J Endocrinol Invest 21: 115–121
37. Tashiro T, Sugiura T, Morishima Y, et al. (1999) Effect of IGF-1 on protein metabolism in burned rats. J Parent Enteral Nutr 23: S93–97
38. Chen K, Nezu R, Sando K, et al. (1999) Insulin-like growth factor-1 modulation of intestinal epithelial cell restitution. J Parent Enteral Nutr 23: S89–S92
39. Goeters C, Mertes N, Tacke J, et al. (1995) Repeated administration of recombinant human insulin-like growth factor-I in patients after gastric surgery. Effect on metabolic and hormonal patterns. Ann Surg 222: 646–653
40. Cioffi WG, Gore DC, Rue III LW, et al. (1994) Insulin-like growth factor-1 lowers protein oxidation in patients with thermal injury. Ann Surg 220: 310–319
41. Bondy CA, Underwood LE, Clemmons DR, et al. (1994) Clinical uses of insulin-like growth factor-1. Ann Int Med 120: 593–601
42. Herndon DN, Ramzy PI, DebRoy MA, et al. (1999) Muscle protein catabolism after severe burn: effect of age and IGF-1/IGFBP3 treatment. Ann Surg 229: 713–720
43. Hinton P, Allison SP (1971) Insulin and glucose to reduce catabolic response to burns. Lancet 1: 767–769
44. Biolo G, Declan Fleming RY, Wolfe RR (1995) Physiologic hyperinsulinemia stimulates protein synthesis and enhances transport of selected amino acids in human skeletal muscle. J Clin Invest 95: 811–819

45. Pierre EJ, Barrow RE, Hawkins HK, et al. (1998) Effects of insulin on wound healin. J Trauma 44: 342–345
46. Kwoun MO, Ling PR, Lydon E, et al. (1997) Immunologic effects of acute hyperglycemia in nondiabetic rats. J Parent Enteral Nutr 21: 91–95
47. Bhasin S, Storer TW, Berman N, et al. (1996) The effects of supraphysiologic doses of testosterone on muscle size and strength in normal men. New Engl J Med 335: 1–7
48. Elashoff JD, Jacknow AD, Shain SG, Braunstein GD (1991) Effects of anabolic-androgenic steroids on muscular strength. Ann Int Med 115: 387–393
49. Urban RJ, Bodenburg YH, Gilkison C, et al. (1995) Testosterone administration to elderly men increased skeletal muscle strength and protein synthesis. Am J Physiol 269: E820–826
50. Schols AMWJ, Soeters PB, Mostert R, Pluymers RJ, Wouters EFM (1995) Physiological effects of nutritional support and anabolic steroids in COPD patients. A placebo controlled randomized trial. Am J Resp Crit Care Med 152: 1268–1274
51. Luppa P, Munker R, Nagel D, Weber M, Engelhardt D (1991) Serum androgens in intensive-care patients: correlations with clinical findings. Clin Endocrinol 34: 305–310
52. Woolf PD (1992) Hormonal responses to trauma. Crit Care Med 20: 216–226
53. Chang DW, DeSanti L, Demling RH (1998) Anticatabolic and anabolic strategies in critical illness: a review of current treatment modalities. Shock 10: 155–160
54. Ferrando AA (1999) Anabolic hormones in critically ill patients. Curr Opinion Clin Nutr 2: 171–175
55. Hausmann DF, Nutz V, Romelsheim K, Caspari R, Mosebach KO (1990) Anabolic steroids in polytrauma patients. Influence on renal nitrogen and amino acid losses: a double blind study. J Parent Enteral Nutr 14: 111–114
56. Hansell DT (1989) The effects of an anabolic steroid and peripherally administered intravenous nutrition in the early postoperative period. J Parent Enteral Nutr 13: 349–358

New Nitrogen-Containing Substrates in Artificial Nutrition

P. Fürst, K.S. Kuhn, and P. Stehle

> I am convinced that it is the right way to explain the phenomena of nutrition... as one investigates what substances are destroyed under different circumstances... and how much of the different materials (substrates) must be fed to maintain the body in condition.
>
> Lusk, *Science of Nutrition*, 1926

Introduction

As both common and specific mechanisms for alterations in substrate metabolism are being discovered, there arise unique opportunities to intervene in the disease process. Undoubtedly, the efficacy of providing substrate to the injured, immunocompromised and/or malnourished host has caused a renaissance in the clinical application of dietary intervention in the treatment and prevention of disease [1–3].

In the past the major nutritional efforts were directed to introduce therapeutic measures by which nitrogen load could be improved in the presence of illness, malnutrition or organ dysfunction rather than to provide specific nutrients for individual organs or tissues [4]. In contrast, current research considers individual substrates as tissue- or organ-specific single nutrients as an alternative and probably better approach. Certain diseases accompanied by deficiencies, antagonism or imbalances in a particular compartment or in various organ tissues might selectively require one or more nutrients which are appropriate for use to support the attenuated organ and/or tissue [2]. Pharmacological nutrition is a novel approach serving as a promising future tool in clinical nutrition. Using this new nutritional measure it might be feasible to adequately nourish critically ill patients, newborn and pre-term infants and patients with hepatic or renal failure. It might be a valuable therapy to improve immunity, to reduce frequency of inflammation, to regulate cellular hydration and to improve gut barrier function [5]. Indeed, delivery of a balanced diet including an adequate amount of protein or suitable amino acid preparation with required substrates might greatly facilitate an anabolic response to a life-threatening disease [6, 7]. This approach, however, is not feasible in clinical practice since limited solubility and instability prevent inclusion of glutamine, tyrosine and cysteine into the presently available amino acid preparations [3].

Recent knowledge concerning the efficient utilization of di- and tripeptides opens up the possibility of substituting available amino acid preparations with glutamine, cystine and tyrosine containing stable and highly soluble short-chain peptides. These synthetic substances are definitely to be classified as true new substrates. Their use shows great promise as an avenue for the provision of amino acids that may be otherwise difficult to deliver. Taurine is postulated as an indispensable substance during many catabolic conditions and uremia. Its intracellular transport and utilization might be considerably improved by the use of synthetic taurine conjugates which are also to be considered as true new substrates.

At the time being, the implication of these new substrates has been restricted to parenteral use. Consequently, this review is devoted to the description of the basic notion of new substrates. Their potential implications in the experimental and clinical setting will be recapitulated in the light of known nutritional deficiencies and disorders. Finally, the prospective importance of new substrates in the developing field of clinical nutrition will be considered and new strategies proposed.

Synthetic Short-Chain Peptides: Properties

Owing to their high solubility in water and sufficient stability during sterilization procedures (Table 1), synthetic dipeptides containing glutamine, tyrosine or cystine at the C-terminal position fulfil all chemical/physical criteria approved by the authorities for constituents of parenteral solutions. Indeed, synthetic dipeptides might be considered as brand new candidates for parenteral nutrition. Basic studies with various synthetic glutamine-, tyrosine- and cystine-containing short-chain peptides provide convincing evidence that these new substrates are rapidly cleared from plasma after parenteral administration without being accumulated in tissues and with inconsequential losses in urine. Considerable hydrolase activ-

Table 1. Chemical/physical characteristics of selected free amino acids and synthetic short chain peptides

	Solubility (g/l H_2O at 20°C)	Stability
Cystine	0.1	Yes
Cysteine-HCl	252.0	No
Bis-L-alanyl-L-cystine	>500.0	Yes[a]
Bis-glycyl-L-cystine	541.0	Yes[a]
Tyrosine	0.4	Yes
L-Alanyl-L-tyrosine	14.0	Yes
Glycyl-L-tyrosine	30.0	Yes
Glutamine	36.0	No
L-Alanyl-L-glutamine	568.0	Yes
Glycyl-L-glutamine	154.0	Yes

[a]Sterile filtration.

ity in extra-/intracellular tissue compartments [8–14] ensures a quantitative peptide hydrolysis, the liberated amino acids being available for protein synthesis and/or generation of energy.

Industrial production of dipeptides at a reasonable price is an essential prerequisite for implications of future dipeptide containing solutions in clinical practice. Recently we have been engaged in studies dealing with the development of novel synthesis procedures using native and/or immobilized plant proteases as biocatalysts [15, 16]. Compared with classical synthesis methods, this biotechnological approach offers advantages, like (stereo-)selectivity of the reaction, minimal protection of functional groups and simplified purification procedures. These advantages enable increased capacity and reduced production costs.

Dipeptides: Experimental Studies

Glutamine-Containing Dipeptides

L-Alanyl-L-glutamine (ala-gln) and glycyl-L-glutamine (gly-gln) are available products. They are stable during heat sterilization and storage and are highly soluble (ala-gln: 568 g/l, gly-gln: 154 g/l). Infusion of these dipeptides is well tolerated and not accompanied by any side effects.

Following a bolus injection or under conditions of continuous total parenteral nutrition (TPN) these peptides provide glutamine for the maintenance of the intra- and/or extracellular glutamine pool [11, 17–19]. Parenteral dipeptide nutrition promotes growth and nitrogen retention [17, 20, 21]. Intravenous provision of glutamine dipeptides reduces muscle loss of glutamine during stress [22]. In this respect it is interesting that infusion of this dipeptide in fasting mongrel dogs is associated with a shift of net glutamine equilibrium to glutamine utilization in the liver. Thus, parenteral administration of ala-gln after fasting is not used preferentially by skeletal muscle or by gut tissues, but rather is used predominantly by the liver [23]. Addition of glutamine dipeptides as a stable glutamine source or free glutamine to a standard TPN solution preserves or even enhances mucosal cellularity and function and reverses atrophy-associated gut dysfunction in parenterally fed rats without or with systemic septic complications [17, 24–29].

Monosaccharide transport, water absorption, and mucosal morphology are preserved with ala-gln enriched TPN following an experimental two-step small bowel transplantation procedure. It is concluded that glutamine is essential for physiological absorptive and barrier function of the intestinal graft [26, 30].

Direct intraluminal infusion of glutamine into the graft (segmental small bowel autotransplantation) improves mucosal structure and absorption of D-xylose (Li et al. personal communication). In this context it is notable that glutamine apparently induces heat shock protein (HSP) 70 and its RNA transcription in epithelial cells. This would mean that glutamine protects intestinal mucosa during critical illness against exogenous (chemotherapy, radiation) or endogenous (oxygen free radicals, endotoxinemia) insults [31]. Parenteral glutamine dipeptide supplementation reversed TPN induced gut asociated lymphoid tissue (GALT) atrophy and attenuated the TPN associated reduction of intestinal IgA.

Interestingly, parenteral glutamine improved IgA mediated protection in the upper respiratory tract [32, 33]. In a rat model of protracted peritonitis, protein synthesis in liver and skeletal muscle were improved, the morphology of the gastrointestinal tract protected and survival improved with supplemental ala-gln which may may thus be beneficial in sepsis [29].

A recent report emphasized that supplemental glutamine preserved hepatic and intestinal stores of glutathione [34]. The biochemical explanation for this finding rests in the fact that the highly charged glutamic acid molecule, one of the direct precursors of glutathione, is poorly transported across the cell membrane whereas glutamine is readily taken up by the cell. Glutamine is then deaminated and thus can serve as glutamic acid precursor [35] (Fig. 1). The effects of glutamine dipeptide supplementation are summarized in Table 2.

Tyrosine-Containing Dipeptides

A great deal of information about the mechanisms of dipeptide utilization is largely the result of carefully conducted studies performed by Adibi and colleagues with glycine di- and tripeptides, including glycyl-L-tyrosine (gly-tyr) [36, 37]. In a highly relevant publication, Daabees and Steglink reported the synthesis of 10 tyrosine-containing peptides [38]. All synthetic peptides were more soluble than free tyrosine. In a subsequent paper from the same group, utilization of L-alanyl-L-^{14}C tyrosine (^{14}C ala-tyr) in adult rats was examined [38]. When the peptide was infused as part of an intravenous nutrition solution, plasma and tissue pools were rapidly labelled. In contrast to the results obtained with Adibi's glycyl-peptides, Daabees and Steglink found high enrichment in the muscle pool when infusing the ala-tyr peptide. Little radioactivity was lost in the urine. Recent experiments indicate that a substantial rate of infusion of the peptide (2 mmol/kg/day) was not associated with an increase of urinary tyrosine excretion.

Intravenous administration of glycyl dipeptides was associated with an increase in the constituent free amino acids in most tissues except in muscle [36, 39]. Long term TPN studies in a rat model indicate that supplemental tyrosine dipeptide (gly-tyr) maintains intra- and extracellular tyrosine pools and supports growth and nitrogen balance [40]. Gly-tyr was not detectable in plasma and tissues; urinary excretion was inconsequential suggesting a virtually quantitative utilization of the infused dipeptide.

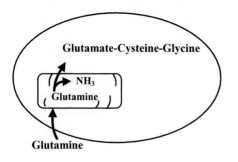

Fig. 1. The role of glutamine in glutathione synthesis. (Modified from [35])

Table 2. The effects of glutamine dipeptide supplemented parenteral nutrition: animal studies

	Observation	References
Intra-/extracellular glutamine pools	Maintained	17, 11, 18, 96, 19
Growth and nitrogen retention	Supported	17, 20, 21
Muscle loss during stress	Reduced	22
Mucosal cellularity and function	Preserved/enhanced	17, 24, 25, 26, 97, 27, 28, 29
Monosaccharide transport, water absorption, mucosal morphology after small bowel transplantation	Preserved	26, 30
Hepatic, plasma and intestinal stores of GSH	Preserved	34
TPN induced GALT atrophy and decreased respiratory tract immunity	Reversed	32, 33
Outcome in protracted peritonitis	Improved	29

The authors also investigated the utilization of N-acetyl-tyrosine. It is obvious that N-acetyl-tyrosine is well utilized in rats in contrast to humans (c.f. N-acetylated amino acids). This difference between animals and humans is probably due to the fact that animals, but not humans, possess high acylase activity in liver, mucosa and kidney.

Administration of parenteral gly-tyr during phenylalanine deficiency provides free tyrosine, thereby facilitating normal growth, promoting nitrogen metabolism and maintaining intra- and extracellular tyrosine pools [41].

An alternative tyrosine source, namely L-γ-glutamyl-L-tyrosine (γ-glu-tyr), was proposed by Hilton and colleagues. Experimental studies with this dipeptide following intravenous bolus injection demonstrate prompt hydrolysis by γ-glutamyl transpeptidase (gGT) [42]. Supplementation of TPN with γ-glu-tyr restores decreased tyrosine concentrations in plasma and improves the supply of tyrosine to the brain [43, 44].

Cystine-Containing Peptides

Intravenous provision of cystine containing peptides (bis-glycyl-cystine, bis-alanyl-cystine) results in taurine and glutathione formation. Intravenous cystine peptides are efficiently hydrolyzed and subsequently provide cystine/cysteine to maintain the extracellular pool (Fig. 2). This might be of essential importance in situations with impaired transsulphuration pathway activity [45].

Dipeptides: Healthy Volunteers

Human studies in healthy volunteers demonstrated that ala-gln [46], gly-tyr [46] and ala-tyr [47] are readily hydrolysed after their bolus injection; the elimination half-lives ranging between 3.3 and 3.8 min (Table 3). Continuous infusion of a

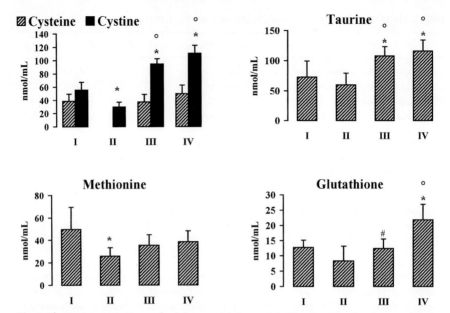

Fig. 2. Plasma concentrations of sulphur-containing metabolites (cysteine/cystine, methionine, glutathione, and taurine) in parenterally fed rats. *Group I* conventional TPN; *group II* methionine-deficient TPN; *group III* (Gly-Cys)₂ (359 mg/kg BW per day) supplemented TPN; *group IV* (Ala-Cys)₂ (385 mg/kg BW per day) supplemented TPN. * significant vs group I, ° significant vs group II, # significant vs group IV (see [45])

commercial amino acid solution supplemented with ala-gln and gly-tyr was not accompanied by any side effects and no complaints were reported [48]. Infusion of the peptide-supplemented solution resulted in a prompt increase in alanine, glutamine, glycine, and tyrosine concentrations. During the entire infusion period, only trace amounts of the dipeptides could be measured in plasma, the values being just at the detection limit. Since none of the dipeptides were detected in the 6-h urine, the results suggested that quantitative hydrolysis of the infused peptides, and subsequent utilization of the constituent free amino acids, had occurred. Adibi and colleagues have demonstrated similar results with gly-gln in postabsorptive and starved humans [49, 50].

Dipeptides: Clinical Studies

Glutamine-Containing Dipeptides

The first clinical study with a synthetic glutamine dipeptide was performed in 1986 in patients undergoing elective resection of the colon or rectum. Infusion of ala-gln supplemented TPN over 5 days resulted in a 60% improvement of the nitrogen balance compared with controls receiving isonitrogenous and isoener-

Table 3. Kinetic values (±SD) for l-alanyl-l-glutamine (Ala-Gln), glycyl-l-tyrosine (Gly-Tyr) and l-alanyl-l-tyrosine (Ala-Tyr) (r^2 coefficients of determination, K^{el} elimination rate constants, $t_{1/2}$ elimination half-lives, V distribution volumes; V' coefficients of distribution, Cl plasma clearance)

	Ala-Gln (n=10)[a]	Gly-Tyr (n=11)[a]	Ala-Tyr (n=7)[b]
r^2	0.975±0.024	0.975±0.028	–
K^{el} (min^{-1})	0.185±0.024	0.203±0.019	–
$t_{1/2}$ (min)	3.80±0.50	3.44±0.32	3.30±0.56
V (l)	10.52±2.431	3.08±2.34	5.30±0.79
V' (l/kg)	0.140±0.028	0.176±0.032	–
Cl (l/min)	1.92±0.36	2.65±0.48	3.17±0.53

[a]Data adopted from [46, 48].
[b]Data adopted from [47].

getic TPN without peptide [51, 52]. The improved net nitrogen balance was associated with maintenance of the intracellular glutamine pool whereas in patients receiving the control solution glutamine levels were markedly decreased compared to preoperative values (Fig. 3). The peptide was not detectable in plasma and muscle, and the plasma concentrations of the constituent amino acids did not differ between the treatment groups. The infusion of the solution was free of any side effects, and postoperative recovery was normal for each patient. In good agreement with these results, intravenous supply of ala-gln following cholecystectomy preserved the intracellular glutamine pool (91% of preoperative value) and the characteristic postoperative decline in muscle ribosomes was abolished [53].

Petersson and colleagues studied the long-term effect of postoperative TPN supplemented with gly-gln on protein synthesis in skeletal muscle [54]. In the glutamine group, the decrease in protein synthesis (assessed by ribosome profiles) was less pronounced compared with controls. Beneficial effects of short-term infusion of ala-gln on muscle protein synthesis assessed by [^{13}C]leucine incorporation were reported by Barua and colleagues in post-surgical patients receiving glutamine free parenteral nutrition [55]. In patients undergoing major abdominal operations we were able to confirm the beneficial effects of glutamine dipeptide supplemented TPN on nitrogen economy, lymphocyte recovery, maintenance of plasma glutamine concentration and shortened hospital stay [56].

There are numerous data emphasizing the immunostimulatory role of supplemental glutamine dipeptides [56–59]. A novel finding is the striking influence of supplemental glutamine dipeptide on cysteinyl-leukotriene (Cys-LT) metabolism. Cys-LTs are potent lipid mediators. It has been emphasized that diminished release of this mediators is accompanied with an attenuated endogenous host defense [60]. After operation the low Cys-LT concentration in isolated polymorphonuclear leukocytes was completely restored with supplemental dipeptide while remaining low with conventional TPN [56]. Keeping with these observations it is of interest that in a current study critically ill (sepsis, SIRS, sepsis syn-

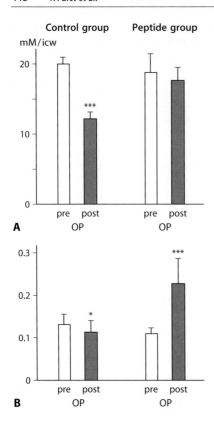

Fig. 3. Intracellular muscle glutamine (**A**) and tyrosine (**B**) concentrations (means±SEM, $n=6$) in control patients and in patients receiving Ala-Gln (280 mg/kg BW per day) and Gly-Tyr (50 mg/kg BW per day) supplemented TPN (peptide group). *ICW* intracellular water; *P<0.05; ***P<0.001 (see [52])

drome) non-surviving patients revealed low LTC_4 generation while in surviving patients LTC_4 generation was normalized during convalescence (Fig. 4).

In these patients LTC_4 correlated to sepsis severity score whereas in non-surviving patients the high sepsis severity score showed no correlation with LTC_4 generation [61]. Reduced LTC_4 generation in critically ill might be due to the anergic state caused by the underlying illness and/or lack of available fatty acid precursor at the site of the membrane. The likely explanation, however, is a decrease in antioxidant capacity during critical illness. It is to remember that intracellular stores of both glutathione and glutamine are depleted in these situations. Thus, the major question may be raised whether the combined deficiencies are intrinsically related to LTC_4-synthesizing capacity of the sick cell. We propose thus that the capacity of cysteinyl-leukotriene generation might be a biomarker for survival in the critically ill [61] and the system related to LTC_4 and glutathione might be normalized with supplemental glutamine [56].

In the presence of ala-gln or gly-gln, release of pro-inflammatory cytokines (IL-8, TNF-α) by polymorphonuclear leukocytes (PMN) was decreased while the ability to express the anti-inflammatory IL-10 was enhanced [58, 62, 63] suggesting that glutamine selectively influences the generation of lipid mediators and certain cytokines.

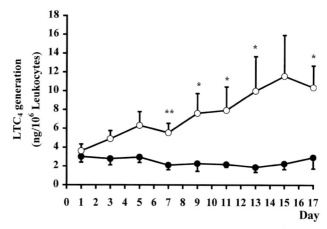

Fig. 4. Course of LTC$_4$ generation in surviving (*open circles*) and non-surviving (*black circles*) patients during a 2-week observation period. Mean, SEM. *$P<0.05$, **$P<0.01$. (Modified from [61])

Increased counts of circulating total lymphocytes and enhanced T-cell lymphocyte synthesis are consistently found in stressed patients following provision of glutamine or glutamine dipeptide-containing nutrition [56, 57, 59, 64].

As in animal experiments it could be demonstrated that glutamine dipeptide-containing TPN may avoid trauma related intestinal atrophy, associated with glutamine-free TPN. In patients with inflammatory bowel disease and neoplastic disease, intestinal permeability could be maintained and villus height preserved with gly-gln supplementation [65]. In another study, ala-gln supplemented TPN maintained absorptive capacity (assessed by D-xylose absorption test) in the proximal portion of the small intestine in critically ill patients, compared with patients receiving conventional glutamine free TPN [66, 67].

In patients with metastatic colorectal cancer receiving chemotherapy, parenteral gly-gln supplementation (0.4 g/kg b.w.) reduced mucositis and ulcerations of the gastric and colorectal mucosa. Glutamine dipeptide supplementation was also associated with a higher villous height/crypt depth ratio than in the unsupplemented group [68]. Following bone marrow transplantion high amount of parenteral gly-gln (50 g corresponding to 38 g glutamine) reduced the measure of small intestinal permeability and less episodes of fever were observed in comparison with controls.

As the large intestine harbours far more bacteria than duodenum, jejunum or ileum, the maintenance of an intact colonic barrier may be crucial. The postulate that glutamine or glutamine dipeptides exert beneficial effects on the mucosa is strongly supported by the results of a current study in which biopsies from normal human ileum, proximal colon and rectosigmoid were incubated with glutamine, ala-gln and saline. Glutamine and ala-gln equally stimulated crypt cell proliferation, the trophic effect was mainly confined to the basal crypt compartments [69]. The link between depletion, glutamine and diminished gut function was recently reviewed [70].

A current European multi-center study with ala-gln provides convincing evidence that the clinical use of glutamine dipeptide spares nitrogen and shortens length of hospital stay as compared with the controls [71, 72]. Importantly, glutamate concentrations remain unchanged compared to the pre-operative levels whether supplemented or not. Table 4 summarizes the effects of glutamine dipeptide therapy in various clinical trials.

Implications for Glutamine Dipeptide Therapy

Obviously glutamine is to be considered as a "conditionally indispensable" amino acid during stress. It is of great importance to define guidelines for routine clinical dipeptide nutrition with respect to- which patients?- which biochemical indications?- how much?- when to start and which route of administration?

Available data indicate that glutamine is an important amino acid in a number of clinical settings. The following are patient categories suggested as benefitting from glutamine dipeptide therapy:

- Severe catabolic illness
  - Burn/trauma/major operation
  - Acute/chronic infection
  - Bone marrow transplantation
  - Other critical illness
- Intestinal dysfunction
  - Inflammatory bowel disease
  - Infectious enteritis
  - Intestinal immaturity or necrotizing enterocolitis
  - Short bowel syndrome
  - Mucosal damage following chemotherapy, radiation or critical illness
- Immunodeficiency syndromes
  - Immune system dysfunction associated with critical illness or bone marrow transplantation
  - AIDS (?)
- Patients with advanced malignant disease
  - Glutamine depleted patients suffering from cancer cachexia

In general, poor nutritional status as assessed by body weight, BMI, anthropometric measures, low plasma albumin as well as severe losses of nitrogen and functional tissues are useful indications for glutamine dipeptide therapy. Poor immune status is always a strong signal for a glutamine deprivation. Decreased body cell mass in combination with decreased intracellular and increased extracellular water (easily measured by modern bioimpedance spectroscopy) is a clear hint for glutamine dipeptide administration. Please note that plasma free glutamine concentrations are not always reflecting body glutamine status. A normal plasma glutamine level might be associated with severe intracellular glutamine depletion.

Administration of glutamine by the intravenous route is the most reliable method to achieve a prolonged constant elevation of the body free glutamine

Table 4. The effects of glutamine dipeptide supplemented parenteral nutrition – Clinical trials

	Observation	References
Muscular glutamine concentration	Maintained	52, 53
	Not influenced	98, 99
Nitrogen balance	Improved	52, 99, 56, 67, 72
Protein synthesis	Increased	53, 54, 55
Trauma related intestinal atrophy	Avoided	65
Chemotherapy induced mucositis	Reduced	68
Weight gain in non-selected hematological patients	Improved	100
Length of hospital stay	Reduced	56, 67, 72
Release of pro-inflammatory cytokines (IL6, IL8, TNF α)	Reduced	63, 62
Expression of anti-inflammatory cytokines (IL 10)	Enhanced	58
Lymphocyte proliferation	Enhanced	63
Hepatic dysfunction during BMT	Improved	101
Immunity	Improved	56, 59, 62

pool. Glutamine dipeptides should be provided immediately following the catabolic insult in order to initially support the attenuated tissues with glutamine. Tube feeding trials to date have shown that hypocaloric glutamine-supplemented enteral diets will not provide the necessary amount of glutamine that can escape the splanchnic bed and elevate blood and muscle concentrations [73–77]. Enteral supplements with glutamine do carry risks since the formulations become a vigorous culture medium for micro-organisms if strict care is not taken [77, 78].

It is generally accepted that a 60–70 kg patient after major injury, uncomplicated elective operations, with gastrointestinal malfunctions or cachexy should be provided 18–30 g glutamine dipeptides (12–20 g glutamine). A severely injured patient with multiple injury, burns, sepsis, SIRS, serious immune deficiency as well as following BMT may require higher doses of glutamine dipeptide [52, 74, 77–79].

Indeed, lack of glutamine from conventional TPN and its subsequent supplementation should be considered as a replacement of a deficiency rather than a supplementation. It might thus be conceivable that the beneficial effects observed with glutamine dipeptide nutrition is simply a correction of disadvantages produced by an inadequacy of conventional amino acid solutions [3, 77, 80]. The availability of stable glutamine dipeptide containing preparations now facilitate glutamine nutrition in routine clinical setting.

Other Synthetic Short-Chain Peptides

Tyrosine containing synthetic dipeptides are commercially available and enable adequate tyrosine nutrition in clinical practice. Gly-tyr/ala-tyr supplementation may be of value in acute renal failure [81]. New, specialized amino acid solutions for patients with acute renal failure have been prepared to compensate for the specific amino acid abnormalities. One solution, containing both essential and non-essential amino acids, includes tyrosine (as dipeptide), serine and a reduced amount of phenylalanine. It has been shown to correct the plasma amino acid pattern and the phenylalanine/tyrosine ratio [81].

As already mentioned, the first study with dipeptides was performed in patients undergoing abdominal surgery [52]. These patients received gly-tyr in addition to ala-gln. Importantly, muscle free tyrosine concentrations declined in the controls without gly-tyr supplementation, while provision of the dipeptide highly enhanced the intracellular value (Fig. 3).

Acute and chronic hepatic dysfunction does not affect elimination and hydrolysis of the dipeptides gly-tyr and ala-tyr and the constituent amino acids are released immediately. Both dipeptides may serve as parenteral tyrosine source in liver disease. Moreover, by its rapid hydrolysis, the use of ala-tyr, for the first time, enables a simple rapid nonisotope evaluation of tyrosine kinetics for assessment of liver function [82].

Powerful arguments have been advanced in favor of clinical application of cysteine [83, 84]. Many potential clinical applications (proteins, peptides, amino acids – basics) are outlined by Stehle et al. (this volume). Clinical studies using the proposed strategies are not yet available, probably due to lack of suitable preparations. As emphasized the use of N-acetyl-cysteine is not appropriate in humans because of the lack of tissue acylases except in the kidney (c.f. N-acetylated amino acids). Cysteine containing dipeptides are highly soluble (Table 1). They are easily available, their half-lifes being less than 3 min [79]. After the introduction of glutamine and tyrosine containing dipeptides in routine clinical setting, the clinical use of cyst(e)ine containing dipeptides should be taken as an aim, not only to ensure the provision of an important nutrient but also an important antioxidant and intracellular regulator.

N-Acetylated Amino Acids

Early studies in experimental rats undergoing long-term TPN clearly have shown that highly soluble and stable N-acetylated amino acids, acetylcysteine, acetyltyrosine and acetylglutamine, are rapidly taken up and are subsequently hydrolyzed by acylases after their parenteral administration [40, 85, 86]. In a subsequent study in dogs, Abumrad et al. observed only poor utilization of parenterally supplied acetylglutamine associated with a large urinary excretion (38% of the amount infused) [18]. Among the organs studied, only kidney cleared acetylglutamine to a measurable extent. This was confirmed in healthy humans because continuous infusion of acetylglutamine [87], acetyltyrosine or acetylcysteine [88] resulted in an accumulation of the respective solute in plasma whereas plasma levels of the respective free amino acids were only slightly increased (Fig. 5). The urinary excretion rate of the acetylated amino acids approached 40%–50% of the amount given. After bolus injection of acetyltyrosine, Druml and coworkers observed little if any hydrolysis of the acetylated amino acid [47]. Pharmacokinetic evaluation after intravenous supply of acetyl-cysteine in humans exhibited an elimination half-life of 2.3 h, a value which is indeed ca. 40-fold higher than those observed for cystine-containing peptides [89].

It can be concluded that N-acetylated amino acids are poorly utilized in humans due to restricted acylase capacities.

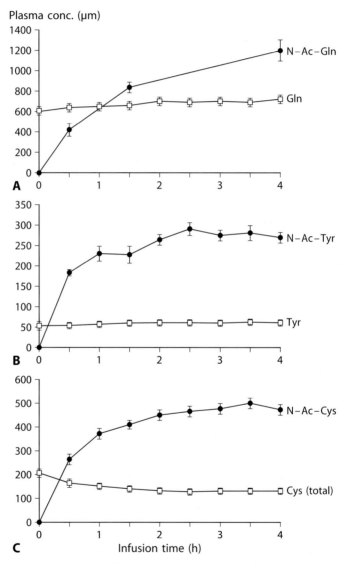

Fig. 5 A–C. Human plasma concentrations of acetylglutamine (*AcGln*), acetyltyrosine (*AcTyr*) and acetylcysteine (*AcCys*) before and during intravenous infusion of AcGln, AcTyr and AcCys, respectively. (Modified from [87, 88])

Short-Chain Protein Hydrolysates

Purified short-chain protein hydrolysates (>67% di- and tripeptides, <10% free amino acids) have been discussed as a low osmolality alternative to free amino acid solutions and synthetic dipeptides for peripheral parenteral nutrition [90, 91]. In an enzymatically prepared short-chain casein hydrolysate, less than 10% of those amino acids which are themselves relatively insoluble or unstable (tyrosine, cystine, glutamine, tryptophan) were found to exist in free form [92].

During intravenous infusion of a short-chain ovalbumin hydrolysate in healthy human subjects, excess peptide excretion during the infusion period accounted for only 6% of total nitrogen excretion, suggesting that a large proportion of the hydrolysate was metabolized [93]. Marked differences between infused and excreted peptide profiles indicated that utilization of peptides from the hydrolysate was sequence specific.

Taurine

The multitudenous chemical properties of taurine (proteins, peptides, amino acids – basics) are outlined by Stehle et al. (this volume). Indeed, the question should be raised whether taurine supplementation might be beneficial in chronic renal failure, during episodes of catabolic stress and in other conditions in which taurine may beneficially influence morbidity and/or outcome. Free crystalline taurine is available for inclusion in intravenous or enteral preparations. However, we hypothesize that the extremely high intra-/extracellular transmembrane gradient (250:1) might limit its cellular uptake. Clinical trials to supplement patients suffering from severe chronic uremia with parenteral free taurine failed to be efficient, its administration being associated with nausea, dizziness, profound accumulation of taurine in body fluids and considerable urinary losses [Bergström, personal communication, 1999]. These observations underline our hypothesis proposing limited transport of taurine accross cell membranes.

Binding of taurine to a suitable amino acid carrier yielding novel synthetic taurine conjugates has been proposed. The existence of considerable membrane-bound as well as intracellular hydrolase activity suggests that amino acid-taurine conjugates might be used as efficient sources of taurine in clinical nutrition. We investigated vascular and intestinal utilization of three taurine conjugates, L-alanyl-taurine (ala-tau), L-tyrosyl-taurine (tyr-tau) and L-phenylalanyl-taurine (phe-tau) in a perfusion model employing isolated rat small intestine [94, 95]. During single pass perfusion the conjugates were well extracted from vascular and luminal perfusates. The constituents of the conjugates were liberated suggesting intracellular hydrolysis or vascular/luminal cleavage. In contrast to previous experiments with synthetic dipeptides [46] the elimination of conjugates and appearance of free taurine in the vascular perfusate was not equimolar. This suggests intracellular transport (cellular uptake); the rate of uptake being higher for the aromatic conjugates than for ala-tau.

It is to conclude that intravenous supplementation with suitable taurine conjugates might be considered as a novel therapeutical tool during episodes of taurine depletion. Indeed, taurine might possess biological properties to act as a potent molecule in the regulation of inflammatory and immunological processes as well as serve as a powerful antioxidant. It is certainly worthwhile to consider taurine as a future important member in the growing family of pharmacological nutrients.

Conclusion

The main focus of this compilation concerns the evaluation of the clinical use of nitrogen containing new substrates exerting a selective action on the immune system, in the maintenance of gut mucosal integrity, and in reducing morbidity and mortality. From the experimental and clinical studies to date the strongest candidates would appear to be glutamine and tyrosine containing dipeptides. Cysteine and taurine are highly interesting substrates with several new functional properties. The growing body of evidence seen in experimental studies should be critically evaluated in future clinical investigations using highly soluble cysteine containing dipeptides and taurine conjugates.

Clinical studies reveal overwhelming evidence that the currently applied concept of dipeptide nutrition is beneficial in providing patients with conditionally indispensable amino acids which are otherwise difficult to deliver. Indeed, omission of glutamine, cysteine and tyrosine from conventional clinical nutrition and their subsequent supplementation should be considered as eliminating a deficiency rather than supplementing current concentrations. It might thus be conceivable that the beneficial effects observed with dipeptide nutrition are simply a correction of disadvantages produced by an inadequacy of conventional clinical nutrition.

This compilation may well illustrate how far we have advanced in our knowledge of the importance of new substrates in modern artificial nutrition. An attempt was also made to highlight directions that hold promise for advancing conditionally essential amino acids in future patient care. There is little question that efforts made to modify the response to disease by nutritional means will be rewarded with improved patient outcome. Surprising and exciting medical progress of yesterday today belongs to the daily medical exercise.

References

1. Fürst P and Stehle P (1994) Are intravenous amino acid solutions unbalanced? New Horizons 2:215–223
2. Fürst P (1994) New parenteral substrates in clinical nutrition. Part I. Introduction. New substrates in protein nutrition. Eur J Clin Nutr 48:607–616
3. Fürst P (1998) Old and new substrates in clinical nutrition. J Nutr 128:789–796
4. O'Dwyer ST, Smith R J, Kripke S A, Settle R G and Rombeau J L (1990) New fuels for the gut. In: Rombeau J L and Caldwell M D (eds) Clinical nutrition: enteral and tube feeding. Sounders Co., Philadelphia. pp. 540–555
5. Lin E, Goncalves JA and Lowry SF (1998) Efficacy of nutritional pharmacology in surgical patients. Curr Opin Clin Nutr Met Care 1:41–50

6. Wilmore DW (1989) The practice of clinical nutrition: how to prepare for the future. JPEN 13:337–343
7. Wilmore DW (1991) Catabolic Illness. Strategies for enhancing recovery. N Engl J Med 325:695–702
8. Adibi SA (1987) Experimental basis for use of peptides as substrates for parenteral nutrition: a review. Metabolism 36:1001–1011
9. Stehle P and Fürst P (1990) In vitro hydrolysis of glutamine-, tyrosine- and cystine-containing short chain peptides. Clin Nutr 9:37–38
10. Plauth M, Kremer I, Raible A, Stehle P, Fürst P and Hartmann F (1991) Dipeptide metabolism in the isolated perfused rat small intestine. Clin Nutr 10 (spec. suppl.):25–32
11. Lochs H, Williams PE, Morse EL, Abumrad NN and Adibi SA (1988) Metabolism of dipeptides and their constituent amino acids by liver, gut, kidney, and muscle. Am J Physiol 254:E588-E594
12. Hundal HS and Rennie MJ (1988) Skeletal muscle tissue contains extracellular aminopeptidase activity against Ala-Gln but no peptide transporter. Europ.J.Clin.Invest. 18:163-A34 (Abstract)
13. Ahmed A, Herzog B, Stehle P, Fürst P and Rennie MJ (1991) Skeletal muscle clearance of L-alanyl-L-glutamine: in vitro peptidase activity of rat sarcolemmal vesicles. Clin.Nutr. 10 (spec.suppl. 2):10–10 (Abstract)
14. Herzog B, Frey B, Stehle P and Fürst P (1991) In vitro peptidase activity of different cell fractions of rat mucosa: kinetic studies using glutamine-containing dipeptides. Clin.Nutr. 10 (spec.suppl. 2):32–32 (Abstract)
15. Stehle P, Bahsitta H-P, Monter B and Fürst P (1990) Papain-catalyzed synthesis of dipeptides. A novel approach using free amino acids as nucleophiles. Enzyme Microb Technol 12:56–60
16. Monter B, Herzog B, Stehle P and Fürst P (1991) Kinetically controlled synthesis of dipeptides using ficin as biocatalyst. Biotechnol Appl Biochem 14:183–191
17. Jiang Z-M, Wang L-J, Qi Y, Liu T-H, Qiu M-R, Yang N-F and Wilmore DW (1993) Comparison of parenteral nutrition supplemented with L-glutamine or glutamine dipeptides. JPEN 17:134–141
18. Abumrad NN, Morse EL, Lochs H, Williams PE and Adibi SA (1989) Possible sources of glutamine for parenteral nutrition: impact on glutamine metabolism. Am J Physiol 257:E228-E234
19. Stehle P, Ratz I and Fürst P (1991) Whole-body autoradiography in the rat after intravenous bolus injection of L-alanyl-L-[U-^{14}C]glutamine. Ann Nutr Metab 35:213–220
20. Karner J, Roth E, Ollenschläger G, Fürst P and Simmel A (1989) Glutamine-containing dipeptides as infusion substrates in the septic state. Surgery 106:893–900
21. Babst R, Hörig H, Stehle P, Brand O, Filgueira L, Marti W, Fischer M, Oberholzer M, Gudat F, Fürst P and Heberer M (1993) Glutamine peptide-supplemented long-term total parenteral nutrition: effects on intracellular and extracellular amino acid patterns, nitrogen economy, and tissue morphology in growing rats. JPEN 17:566–574
22. Roth E, Karner J, Ollenschläger G, Simmel A, Fürst P and Funovics J (1988) Alanylglutamine reduces muscle loss of alanine and glutamine in postoperative anaesthetized dogs. Clin Sci 75:641–648
23. Borel MJ, Williams PE, Jabbour K and Flakoll PJ (1996) Chronic hypocaloric parenteral nutrition containing glutamine promotes hepatic rather than skeletal muscle or gut uptake of glutamine after fasting. JPEN 20:25–30
24. Tamada H, Nezu R, Imamura I, Matsuo Y, Takagi Y, Kamata S and Okada A (1992) The dipeptide alanyl-glutamine prevents intestinal mucosal atrophy in parenterally fed rats. JPEN 16:110–116
25. Tamada H, Nezu R, Matsuo Y, Imamura I, Takagi Y and Okada A (1993) Alanyl glutamine-enriched total parenteral nutrition restores intestinal adaptation after either proximal or distal massive resection in rats. JPEN 17:236–242

26. Schröder J, Wardelmann E, Winkler W, Fändrich F, Schweizer E and Schroeder P (1995) Glutamine dipeptide-supplemented parenteral nutrition reverses gut atrophy, disaccharidase enzyme activity, and absorption in rats. JPEN 19:502–506

27. Bai M-J, Jiang Z-M, Liu Y-W, Wang W-T, Li D-M and Wilmore DW (1996) Effects of Alanyl-Glutamine on Gut Barrier Function. Nutrition 12:793–796

28. Liu YW, Bai MX, Ma YX and Jiang ZM (1997) Effects of alanyl-glutamine on intestinal adaptation and bacterial translocation in rats after 60% intestinal resection. Clin Nutr 16:75–78

29. Naka S, Saito H, Hashiguchi Y, Lin M-T, Furukawa S, Inaba T, Fukushima R, Wada N and Muto T (1996) Alanyl-Glutamine-Supplemented Total Parenteral Nutrition Improves Survival and Protein Metabolism in Rat Protracted Peritonitis Model. JPEN 20:417–423

30. Li YS, Li JS, Jiang JW, Liu FN, Li N, Qin WS and Zhu H (1999) Glycyl-glutamine-enriched long-term total parenteral nutrition attenuates bacterial translocation following small bowel transplantation in the pig. J Surg Res 82:106–111

31. Wischmeyer PE, Musch MW, Madonna MB, Thisted R and Chang EB (1997) Glutamine protects intestinal epithelial cells: Role of inducible HSP70. Am J Physiol 272:G879-G884

32. Li J, Kudsk KA, Janu P and Renegar KB (1997) Effect of glutamine-enriched total parenteral nutrition on small intestinal gut-associated lymphoid tissue and upper respiratory tract immunity. Surgery 121:542–549

33. Li J, King BK, Janu PG, Renegar KB and Kudsk KA (1998) Glycyl-L-glutamine-enriched total parenteral nutrition maintains small intestine gut-associated lymphoid tissue and upper respiratory tract immunity. JPEN J Parenter Enteral Nutr 22:31–36

34. Yu JC, Jiang ZM, Li DM, Yang NF and Bai MX (1996) Alanyl-glutamine preserves hepatic glutathione stores after 5-FU treatment. Clin Nutr 15:261–265

35. Hong RW, Rounds JD, Helton WS, Robinson MK and Wilmore DW (1992) Glutamine preserves liver glutathione after lethal hepatic injury. Ann Surg 215:114–119

36. Adibi SA, Krzysik BA and Drash AL (1977) Metabolism of intravenously administered dipeptides in rats: effects on amino acid pools, glucose concentration and insulin and glucagon secretion. Clin Sci Mol Med 52:193–204

37. Adibi SA and Johns BA (1983) Utilization of intravenously infused tripeptides in baboons: effect on plasma concentration and urinary excretion of amino acids. Metabolism 32: 103–105

38. Daabees TT and Steginck LD (1977) Soluble tyrosine peptides during total parenteral nutrition: studies of alanyl-tyrosine (Ala-Tyr). Federation Proc 36:1164

39. Adibi SA and Morse EL (1982) Enrichment of glycine pool in plasma and tissues by glycine, di-, tri-, and tetraglycine. Am J Physiol 243:E413-E417

40. Neuhäuser M, Wandira JA, Göttmann U, Bässler KH and Langer K (1985) Utilization of N-acetyl-L-tyrosine and glycyl-L-tyrosine during long-term parenteral nutrition in the growing rat. Am J Clin Nutr 42:585–596

41. Stehle P, Weber S and Fürst P (1996) Parenteral glycyl-L-tyrosine maintains tyrosine pools and supports growth and nitrogen balance in phenylalanine-deficient rats. J Nutr 126:663–667

42. Hilton MA, Hilton FK, Montgomery W, Hocker J and Adamkin DH (1991) Use of the stable peptide, gamma-L-glutamyl-L-tyrosine, as an intravenous source of tyrosine in mice. Metabolism 40:634–638

43. Radmacher PG, Hilton MA, Hilton FK, Duncan CA and Adamkin DH (1993) Use of the soluble peptide τ-L-glutamyl-L-tyrosine to provide tyrosine in total parenteral nutrition in rats. JPEN 17:337–344

44. Berger DC, Hilton MA, Hilton FK, Duncan SD, Radmacher PG and Greene SM (1996) Intravenous gamma-glutamyl-tyrosine elevates brain tyrosine but not catecholamine concentrations in normal rats. Metabolism 45:126–132

45. Fürst P, Pogan K, Hummel M, Herzog B and Stehle P (1997) Design of parenteral synthetic dipeptides for clinical nutrition: in vitro and in vivo utilization. Ann Nutr Metab 41:10–21

46. Albers S, Wernerman J, Stehle P, Vinnars E and Fürst P (1988) Availability of amino acids supplied intravenously in healthy man as synthetic dipeptides: kinetic evaluation of L-alanyl-L-glutamine and glycyl-L-tyrosine. Clin Sci 75:463–468

47. Druml W, Lochs H, Roth E, Hübl W, Balcke P and Lenz K (1991) Utilization of tyrosine dipeptides and acetyltyrosine in normal and uremic humans. Am J Physiol 260:E280-E285

48. Albers S, Wernerman J, Stehle P, Vinnars E and Fürst P (1989) Availability of amino acids supplied by constant intravenous infusion of synthetic dipeptides in healthy man. Clin Sci 76:643–648

49. Lochs H, Hübl W, Gasic S, Roth E, Morse EL and Adibi SA (1992) Glycylglutamine: Metabolism and effects on organ balances of amino acids in postabsorptive and starved subjects. Am J Physiol Endocrinol Metab 262:E155-E160

50. Lochs H, Roth E, Gasic S, Hübl W, Morse EL and Adibi SA (1990) Splanchnic, renal, and muscle clearance of alanylglutamine in man and organ fluxes of alanine and glutamine when infused in free and peptide forms. Metabolism 39:833–836

51. Fürst P, Albers S, Stehle P, Pollack L, Mertes N and Puchstein C (1988) Parenteral use of L-alanyl-L-glutamine (Ala-Gln) and glycyl-L-tyrosine (Gly-Tyr) in postoperative patients. Clin.Nutr 7:S41-S41 (Abstract)

52. Stehle P, Zander J, Mertes N, Albers S, Puchstein Ch, Lawin P and Fürst P (1989) Effect of parenteral glutamine peptide supplements on muscle glutamine loss and nitrogen balance after major surgery. Lancet i:231–233

53. Hammarqvist F, Wernerman J, Von der Decken A and Vinnars E (1990) Alanyl-glutamine counteracts the depletion of free glutamine and the postoperative decline in protein synthesis in skeletal muscle. Ann Surg 212:637–644

54. Petersson B, Waller S-O, Von der Decken A, Vinnars E and Wernerman J (1991) The long-term effect of postoperative TPN supplemented with glycyl-glutamine on protein synthesis in skeletal muscle. Clin.Nutr. 10 (spec.suppl. 2):10–10 (Abstract)

55. Barua JM, Wilson E, Downie S, Weryk B, Cuschieri A and Rennie MJ (1992) The effect of alanyl-glutamine peptide supplementation on muscle protein synthesis in post-surgical patients receiving glutamine-free amino acids intravenously. Proc Nutr Soc 51:104 A

56. Morlion BJ, Stehle P, Wachtler P, Siedhoff HP, Koller M, Konig W, Furst P and Puchstein C (1998) Total parenteral nutrition with glutamine dipeptide after major abdominal surgery – a randomized, double-blind, controlled study. Ann Surg 227:302–308

57. Calder PC (1994) Glutamine and the immune system. Clin Nutr 13:2–8

58. Morlion BJ, Köller M, Wachtler P, Wrenger K, Fürst P, Puchstein C and König W (1997) Influence of L-alanyl-L-glutamine (ala-gln) dipeptide on the synthesis of leukotrienes and cytokines in vitro. 4th International Congress on The Immune Consequences of Trauma, Shock and Sepsis 269–272

59. O'Riordain MG, Fearon KC, Ross JA, Rogers P, Falconer JS, Bartolo DC, Garden OJ and Carter DC (1994) Glutamine-supplemented total parenteral nutrition enhances T-lymphocyte response in surgical patients undergoing colorectal resection. Ann Surg 220:212–221

60. Köller M, König W, Brom J, Raulf M, Gross-Weege W, Erbs G and Müller FE (1988) Generation of leukotrienes from human polymorphonuclear granulocytes of severely burned patients. J Trauma 28:733–740

61. Morlion B J, Torwesten E, Kuhn K S, Lessire H, Puchstein C and Fürst P (2000) Cysteinyl-leucotriene generation as a biomarker for survival in the critically ill. Crit Care Med (in press)

62. Jacobi CA, Ordeman J, Zuckermann H, Döcke W, Volk HD and Müller JM (1998) The influence of Alanyl-Glutamine in postoperative total parenteral nutrition on immune functions and morbidity: Preliminary results of a prospective randomized trial. Langenbecks Arch Chir 1998:605–611

63. de Beaux AC, O'Riordain MG, Ross JA, Jodozi L, Carter DC and Fearon KC (1998) Glutamine supplemented total parenteral nutrition reduces blood mononuclear cell interleukin-8 release in severe acute pankreatitis. Nutrition 14:261–265

64. Ziegler TR, Bye RL, Persinger RL, Young LS, Antin JH and Wilmore DW (1998) Effects of glutamine supplementation on circulating lymphocytes after bone marrow transplantation: a pilot study. Am J Med Sci 315:4–10
65. Van der Hulst RRWJ, Van Kreel BK, Von Meyenfeldt MF, Brummer R-JM, Arends J-W, Deutz NEP and Soeters PB (1993) Glutamine and the preservation of gut integrity. Lancet 341:1363–1365
66. Tremel H, Kienle B, Weilemann LS, Stehle P and Fürst P (1994) Glutamine dipeptide supplemented parenteral nutrition maintains intestinal function in critically ill. Gastroenterol 107:1595–1601
67. Jiang Z M, Cao J D, Zhu X G, Cao W X, Yu J C, Ma E L, Wang X R and Liu Y W (1999) The impact of glutamine dipeptide on nitrogen balance, intestinal permeability and clinical outcome of post operative patients. JPEN (in press)
68. Decker-Baumann C, Frohmüller S, v.Herbay A, Dueck M and Schlag PM (1999) Reduction of chemotherapy-induced side-effects by parenteral glutamine supplementation in patients with metatstatic colorectal cancer. Eur J Cancer 35:202–207
69. Scheppach W, Loges C, Bartram P, Christl SU, Richter F, Dusel G, Stehle P, Fürst P and Kasper H (1994) Effect of free glutamine and alanyl-glutamine dipeptide on mucosal proliferation of the human ileum and colon. Gastroenterol 107:429–434
70. Soeters PB (1996) Glutamine: The link between depletion and diminished gut function. J Am Coll Nutr 15:195–196
71. Schulzki C, Goeters C, Stehle P, Benzing S, Herzog B, Mertes N and Fürst P (1999) Supplemental Alanyl-glutamine dipeptide improves nitrogen balance and reduces length of hospitalization in patients after severe operative injury. JPEN 23:S4-S4 (Abstract)
72. Fürst P (1999) Effects of supplemental parenteral L-Aanyl-L-glutamine (ALA-GLN) following elective operation A European Multicenter Study. Clin Nutr (in press)
73. Long CL, Nelson KM, DiRienzo DB, Weis JK, Stahl RD, Broussard TD, Theus WL, Clark JA, Pinson TW, Geiger JW, Laws HL, Blakemore WS and Carraway RP (1995) Glutamine supplemented enteral nutrition: Impact on whole body protein kinetics and glucose metabolism in critically ill patients. JPEN 19:470–476
74. Wilmore DW, Schloerb PR and Ziegler TR (1999) Glutamine in the support of patients following bone marrow transplantation. Curr Opin Clin Nutr Met Care 2:323–328
75. Jensen GL, Miller RH, Talabiska DG, Fish J and Gianferante L (1996) A double-blind, prospective, randomized study of glutamine- enriched compared with standard peptide-based feeding in critically ill patients. Am J Clin Nutr 64:615–621
76. Moore FA (1994) Issues in nutritional management of critically ill patients. Nutr Clin Prac 9:125–125
77. Griffiths RD (1999) Glutamine: establishing clinical indications. Curr Opin Clin Nutr Met Care 2:177–182
78. Wilmore DW and Shabert JK (1998) Role of glutamine in immunologic responses. Nutrition 14:618–626
79. Fürst P and Stehle P (1995) Parenteral nutrition substrates. In: Payne-James J, Grimble G and Silk D (eds) Artificial nutrition support in clinical practice. Edward Arnold, London. pp. 301–322
80. Fürst P, Pogan K and Stehle P (1997) Glutamine dipeptides in clinical nutrition. Nutrition 13:731–737
81. Druml W (1994) Nutritional considerations in the treatment of acute renal failure in septic patients. Nephrology, Dialysis and Transplantation 9:S219-S223
82. Druml W, Hübl W, Roth E and Lochs H (1995) Utilization of tyrosine-containing dipeptides and N-acetyl-tyrosine in hepatic failure. Hepatology 21:923–928
83. Fürst P (1996) The role of antioxidants in nutritional support. Proc Nutr Soc 55:945–961
84. Grimble RF (1994) Nutritional antioxidants and the modulation of inflammation: theory and practice. New Horiz 2:175–185

85. Neuhäuser M, Grötz KA, Wandira JA, Bässler KH and Langer K (1986) Utilization of methionine and N-acetyl-L-cysteine during long-term parenteral nutrition in the growing rat. Metabolism 35:869–873

86. Neuhäuser-Berthold M, Wirth S, Hellmann U and Bässler KH (1988) Utilisation of N-acetyl-L-glutamine during long-term parenteral nutrition in growing rats: significance of glutamine for weight and nitrogen balance. Clin Nutr 7:145–150

87. Magnusson I, Kihlberg R, Alvestrand A, Wernerman J, Ekman L and Wahren J (1989) Utilization of intravenously administered N-acetyl-L-glutamine in humans. Metabolism 38 (suppl 1):82–88

88. Magnusson I, Ekman L, Wangdahl M and Wahren J (1989) N-acetyl-L-tyrosine and N-acetyl-L-cysteine as tyrosine and cysteine precursors during intravenous infusion in humans. Metabolism 38:957–961

89. Stehle P, Albers S, Pollack L and Fürst P (1988) In vivo utilization of cystine-containing synthetic short chain peptides after intravenous bolus injection in the rat. J Nutr 118:1470–1474

90. Grimble GK and Silk DA (1989) Peptides in human nutrition. Nutr Res Rev 2:87–108

91. Grimble GK, Aimer PC, Morris P, Raimundo A, Weryk B and Silk DBA (1992) Plasma amino acids and peptiduria during intravenous infusion of a short-chain ovalbumin hydrolysate, or its equivalent amino acid (AA) mixture, in man. Proc Nutr Soc 51:103 A

92. Grimble GK, Rees RG, Keohane PP, Cartwright T, Desreumaux M and Silk DBA (1987) Effect of peptide chain length on absorption of egg protein hydrolysates in the normal human jejunum. Gastroenterol 92:135–142

93. Grimble GK, Raimundo A, Rees RG, Hunjan MK and Silk DA (1988) Parenteral utilisation of a purified short-chain enzymic hydrolysate of ovalbumin in man. JPEN 12 (Suppl.):15 S

94. Fürst P, Hummel M, Pogan K and Stehle P (1997) Potential use of dipeptides in clinical nutrition. In: Tessari P, Pittoni G, Tiengo A and Soeters P B (eds) Amino acid/protein metabolism in health and disease. Smith-Gordon, London. pp. 237–252

95. Plauth M, Kremer I, Raible A, Stehle P, Fürst P and Hartmann F (1992) Nitrogen absorption from isonitrogenous solutions of L-leucyl-L-leucine and L-leucine: a study in the isolated perfused rat small intestine. Clin Sci 82:283–290

96. Stehle P, Ratz I and Fürst P (1989) In vivo utilization of intravenously supplied L-alanyl-L-glutamine in various tissues of the rat. Nutrition 5:411–415

97. Scheppach W, Dusel G, Kuhn T, Loges C, Karch H, Bartram HP, Richter F, Christl SU and Kasper H (1996) Effect of L-glutamine and n-butyrate on the restitution of rat colonic mucosa after acid induced injury. Gut 38:878–885

98. Karner J, Roth E, Stehle P, Albers S and Fürst P (1989) Influence of glutamine-containing dipeptides on muscle amino acid metabolism. In: Hartig W, Dietze G, Weiner R and Fürst P (eds) Nutrition in Clinical Practice. Karger, Basel. pp. 56–70

99. Fürst P, Albers S and Stehle P (1990) Glutamine-containing dipeptides in parenteral nutrition. JPEN 14:118S-124 S

100. van Zaanen HCT, van der Lelie J, Timmer JG, Fürst P and Sauerwein HP (1994) Parenteral glutamine supplementation does not ameliorate chemotherapy-induced toxicity. Cancer 74:2879–2884

101. Brown SA, Goringe A, Fegan C, Davies SV, Giddings J, Whittaker JA, Burnett AK and Poynton CH (1998) Parenteral glutamine protects hepatic function during bone marrow transplantation. Bone Marrow Transplant 22:281–284

Merging Evidence-Based Medicine and Nutrition Support Practice for Critically Ill Patients: The (Mis)interpretation of Randomized Trials and Meta-Analyses

D.K. Heyland and R. Koretz

Introduction

In recent years, the principles and practices of "evidence-based medicine" have received increasing attention and scrutiny in critical care medicine [1–3]. Evidence-based medicine is defined as the explicit consideration of the best available evidence from scientific research in clinical decision-making. It is acknowledged that scientific knowledge is only one of many determinants to a clinical decision. Said differently, the results of randomized clinical trials (RCTs) (or meta-analyses) do *not* make clinical decisions, they inform decision makers. Evidence-based medicine provides both a paradigm and a set of principles to help establish the validity of scientific observations.

A basic tenet of evidence-based medicine is that good methods of clinical observation lead to correct conclusions (i.e., observations that are relatively free of systematic error and that cannot be easily discounted as arising from chance alone are likely to be correct). The critical appraisal exercise, applying key criteria to establish the strength of validity (and therefore, the clinical inference) of an individual study, is a hallmark of evidence-based medicine practice. Critically appraising original scientific research should not lead to a dichotomous categorization of good or bad. Rather, it is probably more helpful to judge where a particular study lies on a continuum of validity (see Fig. 1). From studies where there is minimal bias or a low chance of error, one can make strong inferences. Conversely, from studies with substantial bias or a high chance of error, one can only make weak inferences or no inferences at all.

Critical appraisal of the evidence allows us to put forward clinical recommendations based on rules of evidence [4]. Strong clinical recommendations can be made (i.e. Grade A recommendations) when supported by rigorous randomized trials or meta-analyses in critically ill patients with a low chance of error (Level I evidence). Moderately strong recommendation (Grade B) can be made from randomized trials or meta-analyses in critically ill patients with a high risk of error (Level II evidence). Weaker recommendations (Grade C) are based on less rigorous studies or randomized trials in different patient populations or randomized trials focusing on surrogate outcomes. Finally, no clinical recommendations can be made from evidence that comes from non-randomized studies in non-critically ill patients, animal studies or studies based on biological rationale. This relationship between levels of evidence and grades of recommendations is outlined in Table 1.

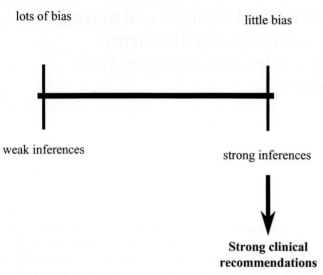

Fig. 1. Making inferences from scientific research

Table 1. Levels of evidence and grades of recommendations (modified from [39])

Level of evidence	Grade of recommendation
1: Randomized trial or meta-analysis with low risk of error	A: Supported by level 1 evidence
II: Randomized trial or meta-analysis with high risk of error	B: Supported by at least one level II study
III: Non-randomized trial or randomized trial of patients other that population of interest or randomized trial of measuring surrogate outcomes	C: No support from level I or II studies
IV: Non-randomized trial in patients other than population of interest or animal studies or biological rationale	No recommendation

Given the degree of malnutrition amongst seriously ill hospitalized patients and its association with increased morbidity, prolonged hospital stay, and increased costs to the health care system [5, 6], nutritional support has become a standard of care for seriously ill hospitalized patients. Increasingly, randomized trials and meta-analyses are used to determine the efficacy of nutritional interventions. However, not all randomized trials (or meta-analyses) are created equally. The purpose of this paper is to illustrate the application of evidence-based medicine principles and practices to the current nutrition support literature related to the care of critically ill patients. The intent is not to be critical in the pejorative sense; rather, by illuminating current misunderstandings related to the interpretation of RCT's and meta-analyses, we hope to increase the level of scientific rigor of clinical recommendations related to nutrition support.

Randomized Clinical Trials

Methodological Quality

Studies in which treatment is allocated in any other method than randomization tend to show larger (and frequently "false-positive") treatment effects than do randomized trials [7]. A randomized trial is the only experimental design in which a deliberate attempt is made to alter only one variable; any change in outcome can then be attributed to that single intervention. Non-randomized controls differ from the experimental patients in at least two variables, (a) the receipt or non-receipt of the intervention in question and (b) the reason why the intervention was or was not provided. Hence, randomized trials have become the gold standard for determining efficacy.

However, as previously noted, not all RCT's are conducted equally. Recent publications in the *Journal of American Medical Association* have outlined key criteria that need to be considered when evaluating the strength of individual trials [8, 9]. To assess the validity of randomized trials, one needs to consider the extent to which studies reported that their randomization schema was concealed, whether or not blinding occurred, the extent to which consecutive, eligible patients were enrolled in the trial, whether groups were equal at baseline, if cointerventions were adequately described, whether objective definitions of clinically important outcomes were employed and whether all patients were properly accounted for in the analysis. Obviously, one can make stronger clinical inferences from randomized trials that use more rigorous methods (see Fig. 2).

The methodological quality of randomized trials highly correlates with the estimate of treatment effect [10]. For example, in a meta-analysis of TPN in critically ill patients [11], the quality each individual study was critically appraised using a standardized scoring system. Trials with the higher methods score demonstrated a trend towards an increase in mortality associated with TPN (RR=1.17, 95% confidence intervals, 0.88–1.56) while there was a trend towards a lower mortality rate in studies with a lower methods score (RR=0.76, 95% confidence intervals, 0.49–1.19). The difference between these two subgroups was short of conventional levels of significance (P=0.12). Similarly, with respect to complication rates, studies with a higher methods score demonstrated no treatment effect (RR=1.13, 95% confidence intervals, 0.86–1.50) while those with a lower methods score showed a significant reduction (RR=0.54, 95% confidence intervals, 0.33–0.87). The difference in complication rates between these sub-

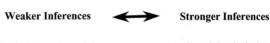

Weaker Inferences		Stronger Inferences
• Randomization not concealed		• Concealed randomization
• No blinding		• Blinded
• Groups not comparable at baseline		• Comparable at baseline
• Co-interventions		• Treated equally
• Incomplete follow-up		• Complete follow-up
• Randomized patients eliminated from analysis		• Intention-to-treat analysis

Fig. 2. Making inferences from randomized trials

groups was significant ($P=0.02$). If the results of the more rigorous trials are considered the best estimate of treatment effect, then TPN is consistent with no beneficial effect and it may do more harm than good in seriously ill patients!

The meta-analysis of TPN in critically ill patients highlights some of the other deficiencies in the methodological quality of RCT's cited earlier. For example, failure to conceal the randomization process (so the investigator has no foreknowledge to which group the patient would be allocated) can lead to an overestimation of treatment effect in RCTs [12]. Of the 26 trials in the meta-analysis, only 3 (11.5%) studies reported on methods of randomization in sufficient detail to allow a reader to discern if that process was concealed (sealed envelopes). In only two studies (7.6%) were clinicians clearly blinded to treatment allocation, while 17 studies (65%) analyzed all patients who were randomized (an intention-to-treat analysis).

Given the inherent difficulties in blinding caregivers and patients when nutritional interventions are evaluated, it is not surprising that most of these studies are not blinded. Notwithstanding these difficulties, to minimize bias, investigators must make additional efforts to standardize patient care and/or use third-party (blinded) adjudicators to determine study outcomes. For example, in a recent randomized, unblinded, multicenter trial of trauma patients, the efficacy of an "immune-enhancing" formula was compared with a standard enteral product [13]. Study feeds were started within 24 h of admission to the ICU. On average, patients receiving the "immune-enhancing" feed were on the ventilator for 1.9±0.4 days versus 5.3±2.9 days for patients receiving the control feed. It is not likely, based on scientific rationale, that a nutrition intervention initiated on the first day in ICU would result in patients coming off the ventilator 1 day later. Perhaps the baseline characteristics of these patients were somehow systematically different or they were managed differently compared to control patients. Unfortunately, the manuscript does not provide any details on other cointerventions, especially how patients were weaned from mechanical ventilators. The likelihood of such a bias weakens (if not invalidates) any inferences that can be made from this study.

Data from trials can be analyzed in several ways. An intention-to-treat analysis requires that all patients originally randomized in the trial be accounted for in the group to which they were randomized (even if they did not receive the intervention). In an efficacy analysis, the investigator states a priori that certain groups of patients will be omitted from the analysis based on scientific rationale. For example, patients who were not "truly eligible" or patients who never received the intervention might be excluded. A third type, a "compliance" analysis, is one in which the patients can only be identified after the fact because they completed all or a prespecified portion of the treatment protocol.

Increasingly, studies of enteral nutrition are basing clinical recommendations on the results of one or more "compliance" analyses [14–16]. For example, Atkinson and colleagues recently reported a large, multicenter trial that compared an immune-enhancing formula to a standard formula in critically ill patients [16]. A total of 398 patients were entered into the study. On an intention-to-treat basis, 48% of the patients who received the immune-enhancing formula died compared to 44% in the control group (NS). There was no significant difference in length of stay. A priori, the investigators had planned on analyzing the data only in those who received a specified amount of whichever diet they were given. When the investigators restricted the data analysis to patients who received more than 2.5 l enteral nutrition within the first 72 h (about 25% of the randomized patients), they found a significant reduction in duration of mechanical ventilation and length of ICU stay in patients receiving the immune-enhancing formula. However, patients receiving immunonutrition also tended to have an increased mortality and to die earlier (which may explain why length of stay was reduced!). The authors concluded, "those patients in whom it was possible to achieve early enteral nutrition... had a significant reduction in the morbidity of their critical illness." An editorial accompanying the paper [17] stated, "the analysis of subgroups who received critical amounts of formula is valid. Intention-to-treat analysis is less valid since it would also fail to demonstrate the beneficial effects of drugs in patients who fail to receive adequate amounts."

This editorial opinion contradicts current teaching in clinical epidemiology [8]. An intention-to-treat analysis is generally considered to be the most *valid* estimate of treatment effect although it may be less *sensitive* in detecting the effect. The goal of randomization is to equally distribute known and unknown prognostic variables between study groups so that observed differences can be attributed to the study intervention and not differences in patient populations. When randomized patients are dropped or excluded from the analysis, the distribution of these prognostic variables may be disturbed and the study results biased. Compared to the intention-to-treat analysis, an efficacy analysis would be more sensitive to detecting a treatment effect (because some patients who were not eligible or who did not receive the intervention were eliminated) but it is more likely to be biassed. The burden rests with the investigators to convince the scientific community that an efficacy analysis has not been biassed. Analyses classified by variables measured *after baseline* (such as compliance or tolerance) are more likely to mislead rather than inform as interactions between the treatment and its compliance may result in the systematic elimination of certain patients from one arm of the trial [18, 19]. For example, if one of the treatment arms has an adverse effect that cause intolerable symptoms in the sickest subgroup, and those patients disappear from the analysis, the ones remaining in that group, on average, will be less sick than the entire population in the other group. Hence, an apparent better effect in this group (demonstrated by the compliance analysis) may only represent a selection bias and not a true benefit of therapy. In general, study subjects should not be withdrawn from the analysis for compliance reasons [20].

Returning to our clinical example [16], the investigators stated, a priori, that only patients who tolerated more than 2.5 l within 72 h would be included in the analysis (just because the investigators state a priori their decision rule does not eliminate the risk of bias). If only 25% of randomized patients are compliant with this amount, it raises questions as to the utility of the intervention. Furthermore, patients purported to benefit cannot be identified a priori. Therefore, if this benefit is to be gained, all of the patients would have to be treated. However, we already know that, when all of them were treated, no advantage ensued. Therefore, there must be some subgroup in whom the treatment was disadvantageous. Whatever gain is achieved in one subgroup would be lost in another. The good would be negated by harm.

Use of Intermediate or Surrogate Endpoints

Since our objective is to improve the health outcomes of our patients, we should be primarily concerned with studies that evaluate the impact of health interventions on clinically important outcomes (outcomes that patients experience and are important to them).

Often, surrogate or intermediate endpoints are used in clinical trials of nutrition interventions. In non-nutrition support studies, several therapeutic interventions have been shown to have a significant impact on the surrogate outcome whereas later trials demonstrate that these interventions actually increase mortality rates (e.g., suppressing extraventricular premature beats [21], maximizing oxygen delivery in critically ill patients [22]). These surrogate endpoints do not always correlate with clinically important health outcomes [23]. In fact, it would appear that improving body weight or nitrogen balance with nutritional interventions does not correlate with improvements in clinical outcomes [24]. One can make stronger inferences from studies evaluating clinically important outcomes whereas studies evaluating surrogate endpoints primarily serve to generate future hypotheses.

Systematic Reviews and Meta-Analyses

The traditional narrative review article is one in which an "expert" in a field presents the information which he or she believes to be important. Obviously, the data which are presented or excluded are subject to the biases of that reviewer. The systematic review process is different. The process requires that the review article be created by, and thus subjected to, the same scientific rigor that is employed in original research. The steps in performing a systematic review are the same as those in designing a research project. The "investigator" (i.e., the reviewer) poses a specific question. He or she then devises a strategy (methods) whereby all of the pertinent information is identified, collected and analyzed. The process is then carried out (results) and the findings are interpreted (discussion). Systematic reviews are less likely to be biased than narrative reviews. Recommendations found in narrative reviews published in journals and textbooks often differ from recommendations found in systematic reviews. For example it has been shown that narrative reviews may lag behind by more than a decade in endorsing a treatment of proven effectiveness or they may continue to advocate therapy long after it is considered harmful or useless [25].

Meta-analyses are a subset of systematic reviews. Meta-analyses employ similar methods in finding and appraising data but include a statistical analysis that summarizes the results numerically as the best estimate of treatment efficacy. In so doing, it compensates for individual studies of small numbers of patients in which power concerns are present. All of the studies are mathematically combined; the studies are weighted according to their variance (studies with the greatest variance having the least weight). It is this last step, reducing variable data to one number, that has generated considerable controversy.

In a recent study published in the New England Journal of Medicine, LeLorier and colleagues compared the results of large randomized, controlled trials and the results of meta-analysis published on the same topic [26]. They found that agreement between meta-analyses and the large clinical trial was only fair (kappa=0.35) and concluded that "if there had been no subsequent randomized, controlled trial, the meta-analysis would have led to the adoption of an ineffective treatment in 32% of cases and to the rejection of useful treatment in 33% of cases." In an accompanying editorial, the writer concluded, "I still prefer conventional narrative reviews of the literature" [27].

While it may be true that the conclusions of some meta-analyses do disagree with large RCT's, it is premature to dismiss them as quickly as might be implicated from these findings and opinions. Several counter-arguments should be considered. The measures of disagreement utilized by LeLorier et al. tend to overestimate the degree of statistical discrepancy. In addition, they based their agreement statistics on the presence or absence of a statistically significant p-value and ignored the fact that the point estimates were similar (although the confidence intervals may be different). Moreover, the authors' methods may have been flawed in that they chose to compare meta-analyses and RCTs from select, high-profile journals which may only publish such RCTs because their results differ from previous meta-analyses. Finally, the authors seemed to be selective (biased) in their choice of comparators [28]. Other published papers that compare the results of large RCTs and meta-analyses suggest that there is concordance in the direction of the conclusions in 80%–90% of cases [29, 30].

Because meta-analyses have come under such scrutiny [31] and because they are being used more in evaluating the efficacy of nutritional interventions, it is important to point out the limitations of comparing RCTs to meta-analysis. The controversy focuses around distilling many RCTs into an overall point estimate. The controversy is not about whether the methods employed in a systematic review (comprehensive search, critical appraisal, etc.) are invalid or more misleading than narrative reviews and the editorial comments above are really not relevant. A rigorous, qualitative systematic review would still be less biased than a narrative review. The issue is the believability of the numeric results of the meta-analysis.

This whole argument assumes that RCTs are the gold standard and both meta-analyses and RCT's measure the same thing. This is not necessarily the case. Potential biases exist in both randomized trials and meta-analyses. One cannot assume that either is more valid than the other. Discrepancies might be expected between the results of large RCTs and meta-analyses because they often differ in their patient populations, treatment protocols, duration of follow-up, cointerventions, etc. It is by careful exploration of these differences that we gain further insights into why our treatments are or are not effective in different situations.

In principle, randomized trials are only generalizable to the patients included in the study and, depending on the eligibility criteria, this can be quite limited. By adding additional studies with varying patient populations, the meta-analysis has greater generalizability. The bottom line is that both randomized trials and meta-analyses are useful tools, if properly used, in discerning the truth about the effectiveness of medical interventions.

Just as not all randomized trials are created equally, meta-analyses vary in their methodological rigor (and therefore in the strength of inferences that can be generated from their results). To assess the validity of systematic reviews (or meta-analyses if a quantitative summary is provided), one needs to consider whether a comprehensive search strategy was employed to find all relevant articles, whether the validity of the original articles was appraised, whether study selection, validity assessments and data abstraction were done in a reproducible fashion and whether the results were similar from study to study (statistical homogeneity) [32]. Obviously, we can make stronger inferences from meta-analyses that employ more rigorous methods (Fig. 3).

When interpreting a meta-analysis, one must give consideration to clinical and statistical heterogeneity (major differences in the individual studies included in a meta-analysis). Clinical heterogeneity refers a clinical judgement as to the appropriateness of combining different kinds of studies. If trials are too heterogeneous, it does not make sense to combine them (the old adage of mixing apples and oranges). For example, it is reasonable to add together studies that evaluated the use of nutrition support in patients receiving cancer chemotherapy with studies in patients on mechanical ventilators? Statistical heterogeneity is a mathematical manipulation that is usually done by a computer. It produces a number that reflects the probability that the treatment effects across various studies are similar. However, the test is not very sensitive and substantial heterogeneity can be overlooked.

When heterogeneity is present, it weakens any inferences that can be made from the aggregated results and makes the results of the pre-specified subgroups more compelling. The possible sources of variation include the role of chance, or differences across studies in population, intervention, outcome and methods. For example, consider the meta-analysis comparing TPN to no TPN in critical illness [11]. An exploration of the statistical heterogeneity present in the TPN meta-analysis revealed that the treatment effect associated with TPN is systematically different in surgical patients compared to critically ill patients. TPN may be of benefit in surgical populations but most likely does more harm than good in critically ill ones [11].

Recent published meta-analyses of nutrition support in critical illness highlight the challenges in making inferences from meta-analyses [11, 33, 34]. Due to the vagaries of the reporting methods of primary studies, the TPN meta-analysis [11] was not able to assess the effect of different dosing strategies across studies. Perhaps studies that overfed patients or did not control serum glucose levels were responsible for the apparent increase in morbidity and mortality associated with TPN [35, 36].

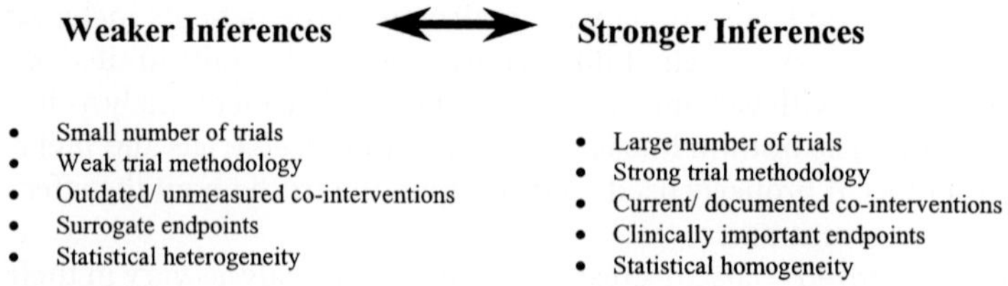

Weaker Inferences ⟵⟶ **Stronger Inferences**

- Small number of trials
- Weak trial methodology
- Outdated/ unmeasured co-interventions
- Surrogate endpoints
- Statistical heterogeneity

- Large number of trials
- Strong trial methodology
- Current/ documented co-interventions
- Clinically important endpoints
- Statistical homogeneity

Fig. 3. Making inferences from a meta-analysis of randomized trials

The use of unpublished studies in meta-analyses remains controversial [37]. If included, most agree that the unpublished studies should undergo the same rigorous critical appraisal as published studies. A meta-analysis of RCTs comparing enteral nutrition to TPN included eight studies, but six of them were unpublished [34]. There was no validity assessment of the individual studies in this work. Without knowing the quality of the primary studies, it is impossible to judge the quality of the meta-analysis.

A recent meta-analysis [33] of immunonutrition included 11 studies of cancer and critically ill patients. To date, there have been more than 30 RCTs of immunonutrition (unpublished data: Daren Heyland). Lack of a comprehensive search strategy and explicit selection criteria make it unclear why certain studies were not included in this meta-analysis [16, 38] and weaken any inferences from this paper. In addition, while purporting to do an intention-to-treat analysis, the authors of the meta-analysis actually utilized the results of the efficacy analysis from the individual studies (for example, in Bower's study [14], 326 patients were randomized but only 247 were included in the meta-analysis). More importantly, the authors seemed to ignore the substantive trend towards increased mortality associated with immunonutrition (odds ratio of 1.77 (95% confidence intervals 1.00–3.12). Just short of conventional levels of significance, this finding is clinically important and may explain why length of stay is reduced in patients who receive immunonutrition. Finally, one wonders about the sensibility of combining studies of well surgical patients (note that in some studies of surgical patients there were no deaths!) or other relatively well populations with studies of critically ill ones (with an average baseline death rate around 20%) [17, 33] especially given the aforementioned results of the TPN meta-analysis [11]. There is no evidence that the effect of nutritional intervention in obese patients, patients with HIV disease or patients with fractured hips will be consistent in critically ill ones.

Conclusions

Merging evidence-based medicine with nutrition support literature related to the care of critically ill patients presents numerous challenges to the interpretation and integration of results of clinical trials and meta-analyses. The methodological quality of RCTs and meta-analyses clearly affects the results and interpretation of the findings. Fortunately, randomized trials published within the last decade seem to be more rigorously designed [11]. Future studies of nutritional support in critically ill patients need to have adequate sample sizes to detect important differences in clinically important outcomes. Methods of randomization should be noted. Where possible, blinding of patients and caregivers should be done. If this is not possible, standardizing and documenting cointerventions and using blinded third-party adjudicators may help reduce the bias. Using rules of evidence will make transparent the strength of inference underlying clinical recommendations regarding the use of nutritional support in critically ill patients.

References

1. Cook DJ, Sibbald WJ, Vincent J-L, Cerra FB, for the Evidence Based Medicine in Critical Care Group (1996) Evidence based critical care medicine: What is it and what can it do for us? Crit Care Med 24:334–337
2. Shoemaker WC, Belzberg H (1997) Maximizing oxygen delivery in high-risk surgical patients. (letter) Crit Care Med 25:714–6
3. Khaodhiar L, Bistrian BR (1999). TPN in the critically ill patient: A meta-analysis. (letter) JAMA 282:1424–1425
4. Sackett DL (1989) Rules of evidence and clinical recommendations on the use of antithrombotic agents. Chest 95 (2):2S-4 S
5. Warnold I, Lundholm K (1984) Clinical significance of preoperative nutritional status in 215 non-cancer patients. Ann Surg 199:299–305
6. Dempsey DT, Mullen JL, Buzby GP (1988) The link between nutritional status and clinical outcome: Can nutritional intervention modify it? Am J Clin Nutr 47:351–356
7. Sacks HS, Chalmers TC, Smith H Jr (1983) Randomized versus historical assignment in controlled trials. N Engl J Med 309:1353–1361
8. Guyatt GH, Sackett DL, Cook DJ, for the Evidence-Based Medicine Working Group (1993) Users' guides to the medical literature. II. How to use an article about therapy or prevention. A. Are the results of the study valid? JAMA 270:2598–2601
9. Guyatt GH, Sackett DL, Cook DJ, for the Evidence-Based Medicine Working Group (1994) Users' guides to the medical literature. II. How to use an article about therapy or prevention. B. What were the results and will they help me in caring for my patients? JAMA 271:59–63
10. Schulz KF, Chalmers I, Hayes RJ, Altman DG (1995) Empirical evidence of bias: Dimensions of methodological quality associated with estimates of treatment effects in controlled trials. JAMA 273:408–412
11. Heyland DK, MacDonald S, Keefe L, Drover JW (1998) Total parenteral nutrition in the critically ill patient: A meta-analysis. JAMA 280:2013–2019
12. Chalmers TC, Celano P, Sacks HS, Smith H (1988) Bias in treatment assignment in controlled clinical trials. N Engl J Med 309:1358–61
13. Moore FA, Moore EE, Kudsk KA, et.al. (1994) Clinical benefits of an immune-enhancing diet for early postinjury enteral feeding. J Trauma 37:607–615
14. Bower RH, Cerra FB, Bershadsky B, Licari JJ, Hoyt DR, Jensen GO, Van Buren CT, Rothkopf MP, Daly JO, Adelsberg BR (1995) Early enteral administration of a formula (Impact) supplemented with arginine, nucleotides, and fish oil in intensive care unit patients: Results of a multicenter, prospective, randomized, clinical trial. Crit Care Med 23:436–449
15. Kenler AS, Swail WS, Driscoll DF, et al. (1996) Early enteral feeding in postsurgical cancer patients: Fish oil structured lipid-based polymeric formula versus a standard polymeric formula. Surgery 223:316–333
16. Atkinson S, Sieffert E, Bihari D (1998) A prospective, randomized, double-blind, controlled clinical trial of enteral immunonutrition in the critically ill. Crit Care Med 26:1164–1172
17. Zaloga GP (1998) Immune-enhancing enteral diets: Where is the beef? Crit Care Med 26:1143–1145
18. Oxman AD, Guyatt GH (1992) Apples, oranges and fish: A consumer's guide to subgroup analyses. Ann Intern Med 116:78–84
19. Yusuf S, Wittes J, Probstfiel J, Tyroler HA (1991) Analysis and interpretation of treatment effects in subgroups of patients in randomized clinical trials. JAMA 266 (1): 93–98
20. Friedman LM, Furberg CD, DeMets DL. Fundamentals of clinical trials. 2nd edition.PSG Publishing Co., Littleton, Massachusetts, 1985, pp. 241–249.
21. Pratt CM, Moye LA (1990) The cardiac arrhythmia suppression trial: background, interim results and implications. Am J Cardiol 65:20B-29B
22. Heyland DK, Cook D, King D, Kernerman P, Bruin-Buisson C (1996) Maximizing Oxygen Delivery in Critically ill Patients: A Methodologic Appraisal of the Evidence. Crit Care Med 24:517–524

23. Fleming TR, DeMets DL (1996) Surrogate end points in clinical trials: Are we being misled? Ann Intern Med 125:605–613
24. Koretz RL (1994) Is nutritional support worthwhile? In Heatley RV, Green JH, Losowsky MS, (eds): Consensus in Clinical Nutrition. Cambridge University Press;Cambridge, England, 158–191
25. Antman EM, Lau J, Kupelnick B, Mosteller F, Chalmers TC (1992) A comparison of results of meta-analyses of randomized controlled trials and recommendations of clinical experts. Treatments for myocardial infarction. JAMA 298:240–8
26. LeLorier J, Gregoire G, Benhaddad A, Lapierre J, Derderian F (1997) Discrepancies between meta-analyses and subsequent large randomized controlled trials. N Engl J Med 337:536–42
27. Bailar JC (1997) The promise and problems of meta-analysis. New Engl J Med 337:559–60
28. Naylor D (1997) Meta-analysis and the meta-epidemiology of clinical research. Br Med J 315:617–619
29. Cappelleri JC, Ioannidis JPA, Schmid CH, de Ferranti SD, Aubert M, Chalmers T, Lau J (1996) Large trials vs. meta-analysis of smaller trials: How do they compare? JAMA 276:1332–1338
30. Villar J, Carroli G, Belizian JM (1995) Predictive ability of meta-analyses of randomized controlled trials. Lancet 345:772–76
31. Editor (1997) Meta-analysis under scrutiny. Lancet 350:675
32. Oxman AD, Cook DJ, Guyatt GH, for the Evidence-Based Medicine Working Group (1994). Users' guides to the medical literature. VI. How to use an overview. JAMA 272:1367–1371
33. Heys SD, Walker LG, Smith I, Eremin O (1999) Enteral nutritional supplementation with key nutrients in patients with critical illness and cancer: A meta-analysis of randomized controlled clinical trials. Ann Surg 229:467–477
34. Moore FA, Feliciano DV, Andrassy RJ, McArdle AH, McL. Booth F, Morgenstein-Wagner TB, et al. (1992) Early enteral feeding, compared with parenteral, reduces septic complications-The results of a Meta-analysis. Ann Surg 216 (2);172–183
35. Schloerb PR, Henning JF (1998) Patterns and problems of adult total parenteral nutrition use in US academic medical centers. Arch Surg 133:7–12
36. Pomposelli JJ, Baxter JK, Babineau TJ, et al. (1998) Early postoperative glucose control predicts nosocomial infection rate in diabetic patients. JPEN 22:77–81
37. Meade MO, Richardson WS (1997) Selecting and appraising studies for a systematic review. Ann Intern Med 127:531–537
38. Brown RO, Hunt H, Mowatt-Larssen CA, Wojtysiak SL, Henningfield MF, Kudsk KA (1994) Comparison of specialized and standard enteral formulas in trauma patients. Pharmacotherapy 14:314–320
39. Heyland DK, Cook DJ, Guyatt G (1993) Enteral nutrition in the critically ill patient: a review. Intensive Care Med 19:435–442

Subject Index

DATE DUE

Demco, Inc. 38-293

Printing: Mercedes-Druck, Berlin
Binding: Buchbinderei Lüderitz & Bauer, Berlin